FIRST AID

Q&A FOR THE USMLE STEP 1

Second Edition

SENIOR EDITORS

Tao Le, MD, MHS
Assistant Clinical Professor
Chief, Section of Allergy and Clinical Immunology
Department of Medicine
University of Louisville

Seth K. Bechis, MS
University of California, San Francisco
Class of 2010

EDITORS

Karen A. Adler, MD
Resident
Department of Psychiatry
Massachusetts General Hospital

Jacob S. Appelbaum
Yale School of Medicine
Class of 2012

Carina H.G. Baird, MD
Resident
Department of Pediatrics
University of California, San Francisco

Xuemei Cai
Harvard Medical School
Class of 2009

Phillip J. Gray, Jr.
Johns Hopkins University School of Medicine
Class of 2009

Christopher R. Kinsella, Jr.
Drexel University College of Medicine
Class of 2009

Gabriel J. Martinez-Diaz
Stanford University School of Medicine
Class 2010

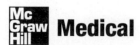
Medical

New York / Chicago / San Francisco / Lisbon / London / Madrid / Mexico City
Milan / New Delhi / San Juan / Seoul / Singapore / Sydney / Toronto

The **McGraw·Hill** Companies

First Aid™ Q&A for the USMLE Step 1, Second Edition

1 2 3 4 5 6 7 8 9 0   QPD/QPD   12 11 10 9

ISBN 978-0-07-159794-4
MHID 0-07-159794-8
ISSN 1932-5207

NOTICE

Medicine is an ever-changing science. As new research and clinical experience broaden our knowledge, changes in treatment and drug therapy are required. The authors and the publisher of this work have checked with sources believed to be reliable in their efforts to provide information that is complete and generally in accord with the standards accepted at the time of publication. However, in view of the possibility of human error or changes in medical sciences, neither the authors nor the publisher nor any other party who has been involved in the preparation or publication of this work warrants that the information contained herein is in every respect accurate or complete, and they disclaim all responsibility for any errors or omissions or for the results obtained from use of the information contained in this work. Readers are encouraged to confirm the information contained herein with other sources. For example and in particular, readers are advised to check the product information sheet included in the package of each drug they plan to administer to be certain that the information contained in this work is accurate and that changes have not been made in the recommended dose or in the contraindications for administration. This recommendation is of particular importance in connection with new or infrequently used drugs.

This book was set in Electra LH by Rainbow Graphics.
The editor was Catherine A. Johnson.
The production supervisor was Phil Galea.
Project management was provided by Rainbow Graphics.
Quebecor Dubuque was printer and binder.

This book is printed on acid-free paper.

To the contributors to this and future editions, who took time to share their knowledge, insight, and humor for the benefit of students, residents, and clinicians.

and

To our families, friends, and loved ones, who supported us in the task of assembling this guide.

CONTENTS

SECTION I GENERAL PRINCIPLES 1

SECTION II ORGAN SYSTEMS 143

AUTHORS

REBECCA AHRENS

Tri-Institutional MD/PhD Program
Weill Medical College of Cornell University

SARA ALCORN

Harvard Medical School
Class of 2010

VIJAY BABU, MD

Intern
Department of Internal Medicine
The Reading Hospital
Reading, Pa.

PAULA BORGES, MS

Stanford University Medical School
Class of 2009

RACHEL BORTNICK, MPhil

Medical Scientist Training Program, Year V
Harvard Medical School

STEVEN CHEN

Johns Hopkins University School of Medicine
Class of 2010

JOHN CHILDRESS III

University of Michigan Medical School
Class of 2010

RAGHU CHIVUKULA

Medical Scientist Training Program, Year IV
Johns Hopkins University School of Medicine

JUSTIN BRENT COHEN

Yale School of Medicine
Class of 2009

ANA COSTA, MD

Resident
Department of Anesthesiology
Weill Medical College of Cornell University

ANDRES E. CRUZ-INIGO

Weill Medical College of Cornell University

MARTIN H. DOMINGUEZ

MD/PhD Program
Yale School of Medicine

ALLEN OMID EGHRARI

Johns Hopkins University School of Medicine
Class of 2009

SHARIFEH (SHERI) FARASAT

Johns Hopkins University School of Medicine
Class of 2009

JAMES A. FEINSTEIN, MD

Resident
Department of Pediatrics
Seattle Children's Hospital and Regional Medical Center

SHENNEN FLOY

Harvard Medical School
Class of 2009

ARIELLA FRIEDMAN

Weill Medical College of Cornell University
Class of 2008

ROBERT J. GIANOTTI, MD

Resident
Department of Internal Medicine
New York University

PHILIP HALL

Yale School of Medicine
Class of 2010

DANIEL M. HALPERIN

Weill Medical College of Cornell University
Class of 2009

COLLEEN M. HARRISON

Harvard Medical School
Class of 2009

CHLOE HILL

Weill Medical College of Cornell University
Class of 2010

SELENA LIAO

Harvard Medical School
Class of 2009

KEN LIN

Medical Scientist Training Program, Year V
Harvard Medical School
Class of 2010

SUSAN MATHAI

Yale School of Medicine
Class of 2009

HEATHER MCGEE, MPhil

Medical Scientist Training Program, Year IV
Yale School of Medicine

LEAH MCNALLY

Yale School of Medicine
Class of 2009

EMILY PFEIL

Johns Hopkins University School of Medicine
Class of 2009

MICHELLE RIOS, MD

Resident
Department of Internal Medicine
University of California, Los Angeles Medical Center

MAYA ROBERTS

Yale School of Medicine and Harvard School of Public Health
Class of 2009

MARIANELI RODRIGUEZ

Medical Scientist Training Program
Johns Hopkins University School of Medicine

SEPIDEH SABER

Stanford University School of Medicine
Class of 2010

BENJAMIN SMITH

Harvard Medical School
Class of 2010

SARA STERN-NEZER

Stanford University School of Medicine and
  University of California, Berkeley School of Public Health

TOMEKA L. SUBER

Medical Scientist Training Program
Johns Hopkins University School of Medicine

CARLOS A. TORRE

University of Puerto Rico, Medical Science Campus
Class of 2009

JONATHAN TZU

Johns Hopkins University School of Medicine
Class of 2009

BRANT W. ULLERY, MD

Resident
Department of General Surgery
Hospital of the University of Pennsylvania

KELLY VRANAS, MD

Resident
Department of Internal Medicine
Hospital of the University of Pennsylvania

FREDERICK WANG

Yale School of Medicine
Class of 2010

MARC WEIN

Medical Scientist Training Program, Year VI
Harvard Medical School

RASIKA WICKRAMASINGHE, PhD

Medical Scientist Training Program, Year VI
Johns Hopkins University School of Medicine

ASSOCIATE AUTHORS

JAN BROWN II

St. George's University School of Medicine
Class of 2010

PAUL D. DI CAPUA

Yale School of Medicine
Class of 2009

LARS GRIMM

Yale School of Medicine
Class of 2009

NICOLE M. HSU

Second Lieutenant, United States Air Force Medical Service Corps
F. Edward Hébert School of Medicine
Uniformed Services University of the Health Sciences
Class of 2009

BENJAMIN SILVERBERG, MS

University of Connecticut School of Medicine
Class of 2009

HARRAS ZAID

University of California, San Francisco School of Medicine
Class of 2010

FACULTY REVIEWERS

R. SHARON CHINTHRAJAH, MD

Chief Resident
Department of Internal Medicine
California Pacific Medical Center
San Francisco, Calif.

RACHEL CHONG, MD, PhD

Endocrinologist
Lakeridge Health Corporation
Ontario, Canada

RONALD D. COHN, MD

Assistant Professor, Pediatrics and Neurology
McKusick-Nathans Institute of Genetic Medicine
Director, Medical Genetics Residency Program
Director, Johns Hopkins University Center for Hypotonia
Johns Hopkins University School of Medicine

ALEXIS DANG, MD

Resident
Department of Orthopedic Surgery
University of California, San Francisco

GWENDOLYN J. GODFREY, DO, MPH

Resident
Department of Pathology and Laboratory Medicine
University of Louisville School of Medicine

KURT E. JOHNSON, PhD

Professor of Anatomy and Regenerative Biology
The George Washington University School of Medicine

WILLIAM KONIGSBERG, MD

Professor
Department of Molecular Biophysics and Biochemistry
Yale University School of Medicine

NABIL KOTBI, MD

Assistant Professor of Psychiatry
Weill Medical College of Cornell University
New York-Presbyterian Hospital

NAHLA A. MAHGOUB, MD

Instructor
Department of Psychiatry
Weill Medical College of Cornell University

JOHN R. McARDLE, MD

Assistant Professor of Medicine
Section of Pulmonary & Critical Care Medicine
Yale School of Medicine

ANDREW MILLER, DO

Fellow
Division of Rheumatology & Immunology
Department of Medicine
Vanderbilt University Medical Center

TRACEY A. MILLIGAN, MD, MS

Associate Neurologist
Brigham and Women's Hospital
Instructor in Neurology
Harvard Medical School

MICHAEL J. PARKER, MD

Assistant Professor of Medicine
Division of Pulmonary and Critical Care Medicine
Beth Israel Deaconess Medical Center
Senior Interactive Media Architect
Center for Educational Technology
Harvard Medical School

MICHAEL S. RAFII, MD, PhD

Assistant Professor
Department of Neurosciences
University of California, San Diego School of Medicine

GEORGE A. SAGI, MD

New York-Presbyterian Hospital

LAWRENCE SIEGEL, MD, MPH

Instructor
Division of International Medicine & Infectious Diseases
Department of Medicine
Weill Medical College of Cornell University

RICHARD S. STEIN, MD

Professor
Department of Medicine
Vanderbilt University School of Medicine

JANIS M. STOLL, MD

Resident
Departments of Internal Medicine and Pediatrics
The University of Chicago Hospitals

ANTHONY STURZU, MD

Fellow
Division of Cardiology
Massachusetts General Hospital
Harvard Medical School

EDWARD TANNER, MD

Chief Resident
Department of Gynecology and Obstetrics
Johns Hopkins University School of Medicine

MUTHUKUMAR THANGAMANI, MD

Resident
Division of Nephrology
Department of Medicine
Weill Medical College of Cornell University

EUNICE S. WANG, MD

Assistant Professor
Leukemia Service, Department of Medicine
State University of New York at Stony Brook School of Medicine
Roswell Park Cancer Institute
Buffalo, N.Y.

SCOTT WEISENBERG

Weill Medical College of Cornell University

MICHAEL WEST, MD, PhD

Departments of Endocrinology and Metabolism
Department of Medicine
Johns Hopkins University School of Medicine

With the second edition of *First Aid Q&A for the USMLE Step 1*, we continue our commitment to providing students with the most useful and up-to-date preparation guides for the USMLE Step 1. This new edition represents an outstanding effort by a talented group of authors and includes the following:

- Almost 1000 high-yield USMLE-style questions based on the top-rated *USMLERx Qmax Step 1 Test Bank* (www.usmlerx.com).
- Concise yet complete explanations to correct and incorrect answers
- Questions organized by general principles and organ systems
- Seven full-length test blocks simulate the actual exam experience
- High-yield images, diagrams, and tables complement the questions and answers
- Organized as a perfect complement to *First Aid for the USMLE Step 1*

We invite you to share your thoughts and ideas to help us improve *First Aid Q&A for the USMLE Step 1*. See How to Contribute, p. xvii.

Louisville   Tao Le
San Francisco   Seth K. Bechis

ACKNOWLEDGMENTS

This has been a collaborative project from the start. We gratefully acknowledge the thoughtful comments and advice of the medical students, international medical graduates, and faculty who have supported the authors in the continuing development of *First Aid Q&A for the USMLE Step 1.*

Additional thanks to the following for reviewing manuscript: Rachel Glaser, MD; Niccolò Della Penna, MD; and Nathan Stitzel, MD.

For support and encouragement throughout the project, we are grateful to Thao Pham, Louise Petersen, Selina Franklin, Jonathan Kirsch, and Vikas Bhushan. Thanks to our publisher, McGraw-Hill, for the valuable assistance of their staff. For enthusiasm, support, and commitment to this challenging project, thanks to our editor, Catherine Johnson. For outstanding editorial work, we thank Steve Freedkin, Isabel Nogueira, Mike Shelton, and Emma D. Underdown. A special thanks to Rainbow Graphics for remarkable production work.

For contributions, correction, and surveys we thank Utkarsh Acharya, Achal Achrol, Mohamad Alsabbagh, Mahyar Badrei, Judith Bellamy, Fernando Bolaños, Mohit Chaudhary, Alice Ching, Elizabeth Chisholm, Jenny Chua-Tuan, Horacio Contreras, Navid Eghbalieh, Felix Geissler, George Ghobrial, Aaron Goldsmith, Ruben Gonzalez, Leo Han, Scott Herd, Alex Hunter, Atul Jain, Katherine Kline, Michael R. Krainock, Ella Leung, Kelvin Li, Milay Luis, Elizabeth Lynn, Adrienne Ma, Eiyu Matsumoto, Francois Merle, Andrew Nakamoto, Jessica Newbury, Jacqueline Ng, Stephanie Nguyen, Ismari Ortiz, Puneet Panda, Gia Patel, Charles Pearlman, Laura Petrillo, Jason L. Pirga, Jessica Rabbitt, Joseph Richards, Oliver Rothschild, Abhit Singh, Stephen Squires, Hugo Torres y Torres, Jennifer Turley, Ben Watters, Ben Weinberg, Jed Wolpaw, Vincent Yang, and Jun Yin.

Louisville	Tao Le
San Francisco	Seth K. Bechis

HOW TO CONTRIBUTE

This edition of *First Aid Q&A for the USMLE Step 1* incorporates hundreds of contributions and changes suggested by faculty and student reviewers. We invite you to participate in this process. We also offer paid internships in medical education and publishing ranging from three months to one year (see next page for details). Please send us your suggestions for

- Corrections or enhancements to existing questions and explanations
- New high-yield questions
- Low-yield questions to remove

For each entry incorporated into the next edition, you will receive a $10 gift certificate, as well as personal acknowledgment in the next edition. Diagrams, tables, partial entries, updates, corrections, and study hints are also appreciated, and significant contributions will be compensated at the discretion of the authors.

The preferred way to submit entries, suggestions, or corrections is via our blog:

www.firstaidteam.com

Otherwise, please send entries, neatly written or typed or on disk (Microsoft Word), to:

First Aid Q&A for the USMLE Step 1, Second Edition
914 North Dixie Avenue, Suite 100
Elizabethtown, KY 42701

All entries become property of the authors and are subject to editing and reviewing. Please verify all data and spellings carefully. In the event that similar or duplicate entries are received, only the first entry received will be used. Include a reference to a standard textbook to facilitate verification of the fact. Please follow the style, punctuation, and format of this edition if possible.

INTERNSHIP OPPORTUNITIES

The First Aid Team is pleased to offer part-time and full-time paid internships in medical education and publishing to motivated medical students and physicians. Internships may range from three months (e.g., a summer) up to a full year. Participants will have an opportunity to author, edit, and earn academic credit on a wide variety of projects, including the popular *First Aid* and *USMLERx* series. Writing/editing experience, familiarity with Microsoft Word, and Internet access are desired. For more information, e-mail a résumé or a short description of your experience along with a cover letter to **firstaidteam@yahoo.com**.

General Principles

SECTION 1

General Principles

CHAPTER 1

Behavioral Science

QUESTIONS

1. A group of researchers conducted a large double-blind, randomized trial comparing the efficacy of a new antibiotic with penicillin in treating streptococcal pneumonia. The results showed that 95% of the patients taking the new antibiotic cleared their pneumonia, while 90% of those taking penicillin cleared their pneumonia. A large sample size was chosen in order to generate a statistical power of 80% with a P value of .21. Which of the following represents the probability that there is a difference between the two treatment groups despite the study's failure to show this difference?

(A) 0.05
(B) 0.20
(C) 0.21
(D) 0.80
(E) 0.90
(F) 0.95

2. A 16-year-old boy is brought to the pediatrician by his mother because of excessive daytime sleepiness. She states that over the past 6 months she has received numerous phone calls from the boy's school informing her that her son sleeps throughout all of his afternoon classes and is often difficult to arouse at the end of class. The patient reports that occasionally when he wakes up in the morning he cannot move for extended periods. He says that sometimes when he laughs at jokes or becomes nervous before a test, he feels as if he cannot move his legs. He admits that he has even fallen to the floor because of leg weakness while laughing. Which of the following is the best choice for treating this patient?

(A) Chloral hydrate
(B) Hydroxyzine
(C) Modafinil
(D) Prochlorperazine maleate
(E) Zolpidem

3. A 52-year-old woman is being treated by a male psychiatrist for depression stemming from her recent divorce. Recently, the patient has been coming to her appointments dressed up and wearing expensive perfumes. She has also started to flirt with the doctor. The patient's demeanor and appearance had initially reminded the psychiatrist of his aunt. He is uncomfortable with the patient's new behavior patterns and tells her so. She becomes very angry and storms out of the office, canceling all remaining appointments on her way out. Which of the following behaviors is an example of negative transference?

(A) The doctor seeing the patient as his aunt
(B) The doctor telling the patient he is uncomfortable
(C) The patient being angry with the doctor
(D) The patient dressing up for appointments
(E) The patient flirting with the doctor

4. A 24-year-old woman presents to her primary care physician because of depression and insomnia for the past 6 months. The patient states that she feels bad about herself almost all of the time. A review of the patient's history shows that she has had frequent physician visits with complaints of stomachaches, headaches, and fatigue for the past 2 years. Which of the following characteristics would support a diagnosis of major depressive disorder rather than dysthymic disorder in this patient?

(A) Changes in appetite
(B) Changes in sleep patterns
(C) Depressed mood
(D) Fatigue/lack of energy
(E) Remittance and recurrence
(F) Two-year duration of symptoms

5. An infant presents to the pediatrician for a routine check-up. His mother reports that he plays peek-a-boo at home, waves bye-bye, and will say "dada." He cannot yet drink from a cup. He seemed somewhat apprehensive when the physician entered the room. He can lift his head when lying on his stomach, sit unassisted, and

stand with help. He has a positive Babinski's reflex. If this infant has met all his developmental milestones appropriately, how old is he?

(A) 4–5 months
(B) 7–11 months
(C) 12–15 months
(D) 18 months
(E) 24 months

6. A 20-year-old man became very agitated at a party, and as a result was brought to the emergency department, where he is belligerent and uncooperative. A physical examination reveals fever, tachycardia, horizontal nystagmus, and hyperacusis. Which of the following substances may cause the behavioral changes and physical findings exhibited by this patient?

(A) Alcohol
(B) Amphetamines
(C) Cocaine
(D) Lysergic acid diethylamide
(E) Nicotine
(F) Phencyclidine

7. The image below is a common representation used in studying the characteristics of a test's results. Using the letters in the figure, which of the following accurately describes the prevalence of the disease?

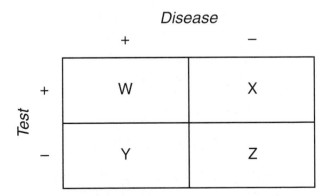

Reproduced, with permission, from USMLERx.com.

(A) W / (W + X + Y + Z)
(B) (W + X) / (W + X + Y + Z)
(C) W / (X + Y + Z)
(D) W / (X + Z)
(E) (W + Y) / (W + X + Y + Z)

8. A third-year medical resident is driving home after being on call and witnesses a car accident. He sees one person leave the car and collapse at the side of the road. He pulls over to help. The person appears to be a female in her 30s with a large laceration across her forehead. She is barely conscious. Which of the following is required and/or implied under the Good Samaritan Law?

(A) Compensation for actions
(B) Continued care until emergency services are contacted
(C) Freedom from legal action
(D) Implied consent of patient in situations in which patient cannot give voluntary consent
(E) Use of standard procedure

9. A battery of tests is used to evaluate a 13-year-old child's readiness to skip from seventh to ninth grade. Both her mother, who has requested the grade change, and many of her teachers express the belief that she functions on the intellectual level of most adults. As part of the battery, she is given an IQ test. Which of the following is an appropriate IQ test to use?

(A) Iowa Test of Educational Development
(B) Vineland Social Maturity Scale
(C) Wechsler Adult Intelligence Scale-Revised
(D) Wechsler Intelligence Scale for Children-Revised
(E) Wide-Range Achievement Test

10. A 43-year-old woman comes to her physician's office extremely nervous because she just tested positive for HIV according to a newly designed serum test. Of the 1,000 patients tested, 200 patients had HIV; the test came back positive for 180 of them, while the remaining 20 tested negative. Eight hundred of the patients did not have HIV; however, the test was positive for 40 of them. The remaining 760 patients tested negative for HIV. Given this patient's positive test, which of the following is the probability that she does have HIV?

(A) 20%
(B) 24%
(C) 82%
(D) 90%
(E) 97%

11. A 56-year-old man presents to his family doctor for a regular check-up visit. His past medical history is significant for long-standing hypertension and coronary artery disease. He had a myocardial infarction and percutaneous angioplasty 1 year ago. The patient initially reports no complaints, but as his physician is heading toward the door, the patient states with some embarrassment that he has had problems achieving erections since he was released from the hospital last year. He says that he has morning erections. His current medications include simvastatin and lisinopril. Which of the following is a likely cause for this man's acquired erectile dysfunction?

(A) Decreased interest in sexual activity
(B) Fear of another myocardial infarction
(C) Increasing age of the patient
(D) Medication side effects
(E) Physical inability after the heart attack

12. A 17-year-old girl presents to her primary care physician with a complaint of missed menses. Tests reveal she is pregnant. She returns to the office 2 weeks later asking for recommendations on obtaining an abortion. She explains that she works, lives with her husband, and is not ready for a child. She decides that she does not want to notify anyone, and says she has chosen not to talk with her parents for many months. Her doctor understands that he must abide by her wishes because she is emancipated. Which of the following makes this patient emancipated?

(A) Age 17 years is considered an adult
(B) Full-time work
(C) High school diploma
(D) Living separately from her parents
(E) Marriage

13. A group of oncologists is interested in determining whether a relationship exists between alcohol use and pancreatic cancer. The researchers enroll 1,000 patients, and subjects are placed into different groups depending on their level of alcohol consumption. The subjects are followed for 10 years; the data show no statistical difference in the number of pancreatic cancers between the groups. The above research is an example of which of the following kind of study?

(A) Case-control study
(B) Clinical treatment trial
(C) Cross-sectional study
(D) Prospective cohort study
(E) Retrospective cohort study

14. An 11-year-old girl is brought to the pediatrician with complaints of back pain. On physical examination, a right thoracic scoliotic curve is noted. An x-ray film indicates that the curve is 25 degrees. Girls with scoliosis need to be especially carefully watched during peak height velocity, during which the curvature can dramatically worsen. Given that peak height velocity occurs during a particular Tanner stage, what other physical attributes would one expect to occur in the girl at the same time?

(A) Elevation of the breast papilla only and no pubic hair
(B) Enlargement of the breast and areola with a single contour and darker, coarse curled pubic hair
(C) Mature breast adult quantity and pattern of pubic hair that extends to the thighs
(D) Projection of the areola and papilla with separate contours and adult-type pubic hair limited to the genital area
(E) Small breast buds with elevation of breast

and papilla and sparse, straight, downy hair on the labial base

15. A 10-year-old Hispanic boy is admitted for bone marrow transplantation as treatment for acute lymphocytic leukemia. The doctor wants to enroll the patient in a clinical trial for a new pain medication, but upon arriving to discuss the study, she finds that both of the patient's parents speak only Spanish. The consent form is in English, and the physician has a limited knowledge of Spanish. What is the physician's best option for obtaining consent from this patient?

   (A) Exclude non-English-speaking patients from the study
   (B) Explain the study to the whole family in Spanish, to the best of the physician's ability
   (C) Have the parents sign the English form after discussing the study via an interpreter
   (D) Have the patient translate the form for his parents
   (E) Wait to obtain a translated consent form and discuss the study via an interpreter

16. A new antihypertensive medication is being investigated in a clinical trial. Investigators have noted a decrease in blood pressure in the group treated with the drug compared to the placebo group. While examining the study's participants, investigators notice that the experimental group has a lower mean age. What is this an example of?

   (A) Confounding error
   (B) Random error
   (C) Recall bias
   (D) Selection bias
   (E) Systematic error

17. A 45-year-old patient with borderline personality disorder on a psychiatry ward is told by a staff psychiatrist to spend 2 hours in a quiet room after violently disrupting a meeting. The next morning the psychiatrist interviews her. She complains bitterly about how the nursing staff is so mean to her even though she is always nice to them. She says she has no idea why they locked her in the quiet room yester-

day. This patient is using which of the following defense mechanisms?

   (A) Dissociation
   (B) Isolation
   (C) Projection
   (D) Splitting
   (E) Suppression

18. A new serum test was recently developed to detect antibodies to a certain virus in order to diagnose the infection. One thousand patients received the test, and while 100 people had the infection, only 80 of them tested positive. Of the 900 people who did not have the infection, 800 tested negative and 100 tested positive. Which of the following percentages indicates the specificity of this new test?

   (A) 10%
   (B) 44%
   (C) 80%
   (D) 89%
   (E) 98%

19. A retrospective cohort study is examining birth complications in women with diabetes. The study determines that babies are more likely to be born large for gestational age (LGA) if the mother has diabetes. The relative risk for the study is calculated to be 4. Which of the following accurately describes this relative risk?

   (A) The incidence rate of diabetes among mothers with LGA babies is 4 times that of non-LGA mothers
   (B) The incidence rate of LGA among women with diabetes is 4 times that of women without diabetes
   (C) The incidence rate of LGA among women without diabetes is 4 times that of women with diabetes
   (D) The odds of diabetes among mothers with LGA babies is 4 times that of non-LGA mothers
   (E) The odds of LGA among women with diabetes is 4 times that of women without diabetes

20. A 45-year-old man presents to a marriage counselor at his wife's prompting. He has been mar-

ried for 10 years and believes that his wife has been unfaithful for the entire marriage, despite her protests to the contrary. He says that everyone is always betraying him, and he has a litany of slights, insults, and injuries that have been perpetrated against him. He is very defensive with the counselor and reads an attack in almost every statement. This patient most likely has which of the following personality disorders?

(A) Antisocial
(B) Avoidant
(C) Obsessive-compulsive
(D) Paranoid
(E) Schizoid
(F) Schizotypal

ANSWERS

1. **The correct answer is B.** This question is asking for the b or type II error. The P value in the trial is .21, which is greater than .05 (p < .05 is commonly accepted as statistically significant), and therefore we cannot reject the null hypothesis. Because we do not reject the null hypothesis, there is a possibility for a type II error. A type II error occurs when we state that no difference exists when in fact one does exist. b is the probability of making a type II error; in other words, the probability that we fail to reject the null hypothesis when in fact it is false. b is related to power, calculated as 1 - b, or 1 - 0.2 = 0.80.

   Answer A is incorrect. The *P* value represents the probability of making a type I error. If *P* < .05, there is less than a 5% chance that the null hypothesis was incorrectly rejected.

   Answer C is incorrect. The figure 0.21 simply represents the *P* value, which is greater than .05. We therefore fail to reject the null hypothesis (no difference between treatment groups).

   Answer D is incorrect. The figure 0.80 represents the power of the study. Power = 1 - β. The power increases when the sample size does.

   Answer E is incorrect. The figure 0.90 represents the percentage of patients taking penicillin who were able to clear the pneumonia.

   Answer F is incorrect. The figure 0.95 represents the percentage of patients taking the new antibiotic who were able to clear the pneumonia.

2. **The correct answer is C.** This patient exhibits some of the classic symptoms of narcolepsy, including cataplexy and sleep paralysis. Cataplexy is defined as brief episodes of bilateral weakness, without alteration in consciousness that is often brought on by strong emotions such as laughing or fear. Sleep paralysis is an episode of partial or total paralysis that occurs at the beginning or end of a sleep cycle. Patients are often aware that they are awake, but may suffer from frightening hallucinations known as hypnagogic when they occur at the start of sleep or hypnopompic when they occur at the end. Modafinil is a psychostimulant with proven effectiveness for treating excessive daytime sleepiness. Patients suffering from cataplexy and sleep paralysis may also benefit from the initiation of tricyclic antidepressants or selective serotonin reuptake inhibitors.

   Answer A is incorrect. Chloral hydrate is a nonbenzodiazepine hypnotic that is used for sedation and insomnia. This patient does not need help sleeping.

   Answer B is incorrect. Hydroxyzine is a nonselective antihistamine that is used in the treatment of anxiety, pruritus, nausea/vomiting, sedation, and insomnia.

   Answer D is incorrect. Prochlorperazine maleate is a typical antipsychotic used in the treatment of nausea, vomiting, anxiety, and psychosis.

   Answer E is incorrect. Zolpidem is a nonbenzodiazepine hypnotic that is used in the treatment of insomnia.

3. **The correct answer is C.** Transference occurs when a patient projects feelings from his or her personal life onto a doctor; countertransference takes place when the doctor projects feelings onto the patient. These feelings can be either positive or negative. The patient's anger at the doctor when her sexual advances are rebuffed is an example of negative transference.

   Answer A is incorrect. The doctor being reminded of his aunt by this patient is an example of countertransference.

   Answer B is incorrect. The doctor telling the patient that he is uncomfortable is not an example of countertransference or transference.

   Answer D is incorrect. The patient dressing up for appointments is positive transference.

Answer E is incorrect. The patient flirting with the doctor is positive transference. In its most extreme form, positive transference can take the form of sexual desire.

4. **The correct answer is E.** Mood disorders are extremely common in primary care offices. Distinguishing between dysthymia and a major depressive episode has clinical implications for this patient. This patient displays somatic symptoms in addition to a depressed mood. Dysthymic disorder requires the presence of two of six symptoms for at least 2 years, including change in appetite, change in sleep patterns, decreased energy, decreased self-esteem, decreased concentration, and increased hopelessness. Major depressive disorder is diagnosed in patients when they have five of nine symptoms for at least 2 weeks, including Sleep changes, loss of Interest (anhedonia), Guilt, Energy loss, Concentration changes, Appetite changes, Psychomotor abnormalities, and Suicidal thoughts (**SIG E CAPS**). Thus, major depression is more severe, presenting with the onset of a greater number of symptoms; more importantly, however, this constellation of symptoms is episodic in major depression, whereas dysthymia does not remit and recur.

Answer A is incorrect. Changes in appetite and/or weight are characteristics shared by major depression and dysthymia. Patients can exhibit an increased or decreased appetite or weight.

Answer B is incorrect. Changes in sleep patterns are also characteristics shared by major depression and dysthymia. Patients can have insomnia or hypersomnia.

Answer C is incorrect. Depressed mood is another characteristic shared by the two disorders. The depressed mood tends to last longer in patients with dysthymia, although there can be variation in their moods. Diagnostic criteria for dysthymia require that the depressed mood be present for more days than not.

Answer D is incorrect. Fatigue/lack of energy is a characteristic shared by the two disorders.

Answer F is incorrect. A 2-year duration could support either diagnosis, but is essential for the diagnosis of dysthymic disorder.

5. **The correct answer is B.** This baby is displaying motor, social, verbal, and cognitive skills appropriate for a 7- to 11-month-old baby. A 7- to 11-month-old baby should be able to sit alone, crawl, and stand with aid. He is displaying age-appropriate social skills such as playing peek-a-boo and displaying stranger anxiety. He is displaying age-appropriate verbal and cognitive skills such as saying "dada" even in a nonsensical manner. Babinski reflex ordinarily disappears by 12 months of age.

Answer A is incorrect. A 4- to 5-month-old baby can sit with support. In terms of motor development he can follow objects to midline, put his feet in his mouth, and laugh aloud.

Answer C is incorrect. A 12- to 15-month-old baby can use a pincer grasp and demonstrates stranger anxiety. He can turn to someone speaking to him and can gesture to objects of interest and use different sounds to convey meaning.

Answer D is incorrect. An 18-month-old child can climb stairs alone and demonstrates hand preference. He can stack three cubes, kick a ball, and use two-word sentences and demonstrates at least a 250-word vocabulary.

Answer E is incorrect. A 24-month-old child has high activity level, can walk backward, and turn doorknobs. They are often selfish and imitative. They can stack 6 cubes and stand on tiptoes.

6. **The correct answer is F.** This patient has taken phencyclidine, or PCP. Patients with PCP intoxication show signs of belligerence, impulsiveness, fever, psychomotor agitation, vertical and horizontal nystagmus, tachycardia, ataxia, homicidality, psychosis, and delirium. On withdrawal, patients may demonstrate a recurrence of intoxication when the PCP, which was trapped in an ionized form in the acidic gastric lumen, is reabsorbed in the alkaline duodenum. PCP users will have normal or small

pupils. Death can result from a variety of causes, including respiratory depression and violent behavior.

Answer A is incorrect. Patients presenting with acute alcohol intoxication will show symptoms of disinhibition, emotional lability, slurred speech, ataxia, coma, and blackouts. On withdrawal, they will demonstrate a tremor, tachycardia, hypertension, malaise, nausea, seizures, delirium tremens, tremulousness, agitation, and hallucinations.

Answer B is incorrect. Patients presenting with amphetamine intoxication will display psychomotor agitation, impaired judgment, pupillary dilation, hypertension, tachycardia, euphoria, prolonged wakefulness and attention, cardiac arrhythmias, delusions, hallucinations, and fever. On withdrawal, they will show a post-use "crash" that includes depression, lethargy, headache, stomach cramps, hunger, and hypersomnolence.

Answer C is incorrect. Patients presenting with acute cocaine intoxication will show symptoms of euphoria, psychomotor agitation, impaired judgment, tachycardia, pupillary dilation, hypertension, hallucinations, paranoid ideations, angina, and sudden cardiac death. On withdrawal, they will show a post-use "crash" that includes severe depression, hypersomnolence, fatigue, malaise, and severe psychological craving.

Answer D is incorrect. Patients presenting with acute lysergic acid diethylamide intoxication will display marked anxiety or depression, delusions, visual hallucinations, flashbacks, and pupillary dilation.

Answer E is incorrect. Patients presenting with acute nicotine intoxication will show symptoms of restlessness, insomnia, anxiety, and arrhythmias. On withdrawal, they will have symptoms of irritability, headache, anxiety, weight gain, craving, and tachycardia.

7. **The correct answer is E.** The prevalence is the number of individuals with a disease in a given population at a given time. Prevalence is estimated by test results but is not a measure of a test's validity. In the chart shown, the prevalence can also be determined by calculating the number of true-positive plus false-negative results divided by the total number of patients.

Answer A is incorrect. This represents true-positive results divided by the total number of patients. This would be the percent of true-positive results of all tested, but it is not used very often.

Answer B is incorrect. This term represents the incidence of positive test results.

Answer C is incorrect. This represents true-positive results divided by the total number of patients tested less those with true-positive results, and would not be a meaningful calculation.

Answer D is incorrect. This represents the number of true-positive results over the total number of patients without disease. This would not be a meaningful calculation.

8. **The correct answer is E.** The Good Samaritan Law is meant to protect people (including off-duty medical professionals) who help others in emergency situations such as this. The law differs in each state, but the general concepts are the same: care providers must use standard procedures. Note that the law does not protect volunteers from gross negligence. Volunteers should limit their actions to their field of training.

Answer A is incorrect. The Good Samaritan Law stipulates that the care provider cannot request or receive any compensation for his or her actions.

Answer B is incorrect. The provider should call for help as soon as possible. The law requires that once a provider assumes the role, he or she must stay with the victim until further help arrives, someone of equal or greater capability takes over, or it becomes unsafe to continue to give aid, not simply until help is called.

Answer C is incorrect. The Good Samaritan Law does not protect the volunteer from legal action. The patient is free to pursue legal recourse if the care provided is negligent and results in injury.

Answer D is incorrect. As with any other medical intervention, the patient has the right to refuse care from the provider.

9. **The correct answer is D.** Many different intelligence quotient scales have been devised. One of the first was the Stanford-Binet. The Wechsler Intelligence Scale for Children-Revised is used to evaluate children between the ages of 6 and 16½ years. The girl should be administered a test corresponding to her age group.

Answer A is incorrect. The Iowa Test of Educational Development is an achievement test, not an intelligence test. It is used to evaluate older children through the end of high school.

Answer B is incorrect. The Vineland Social Maturity Scale is a test used to evaluate adaptive behavior. It is typically used to evaluate children with mental retardation, but its use has been expanded to include children with other learning disabilities.

Answer C is incorrect. The Wechsler Adult Intelligence Scale-Revised is used to evaluate those patients who are older than 16½ years.

Answer E is incorrect. The Wide-Range Achievement Test is another achievement test. Unlike the Iowa tests, which are given in a group setting to almost every child in the United States, the Wide-Range Achievement Test is used for individual testing.

10. **The correct answer is C.** The probability of having a condition, given a positive test, represents the positive predictive value. This is calculated by TP / (TP + FP), where TP means true-positive and FP means false-positive. Therefore, the positive predictive value is 180 / (180 + 40), or 82%. As the prevalence of the disease increases in a population, so does the positive predictive value.

Answer A is incorrect. The figure 20% is the prevalence of the disease among tested patients (200 / 1,000).

Answer B is incorrect. The figure 24% is the number of positive tests divided by the total number of patients.

Answer D is incorrect. The figure 90% is the sensitivity of the new HIV test. It is given by TP / (TP + FN), where TP means true-positive and FN means false-negative, or those with the disease who test negative.

Answer E is incorrect. The figure 97% is the negative predictive value, or the probability of not having a condition given a negative test. It is calculated by TN / (TN + FN), where TN means true-negative and FN means false-negative.

11. **The correct answer is B.** There is a temporal association between this man's myocardial infarction and his subsequent erectile dysfunction (ED). The presence of morning erections indicates that the cause of this patient's ED is psychological rather than physical. The patient should be reassured that if he can tolerate climbing two flights of stairs, he can tolerate sexual activity.

Answer A is incorrect. It is unlikely that a patient would complain of ED if he had a decreased interest in sexual activity. A problem with decreased interest is more likely to be brought up by a partner or spouse.

Answer C is incorrect. Sexual desire/interest does not decrease with age. Men can have a longer refractory period and can take longer to achieve an erection as they age.

Answer D is incorrect. This patient's medications are low on the sexual side effect scale. While antihypertensives in general can cause impotence, angiotensin-converting enzyme inhibitors are the least likely to do so. Statins are not known to cause sexual problems.

Answer E is incorrect. If patients can climb two flights of stairs without becoming short of breath or experiencing chest pain, limits on sexual activity are unnecessary.

12. **The correct answer is E.** Emancipation is a legal definition through which minors become independent of their parents and are free to

make medical decisions for themselves. A minor, which is a legal condition defined by age, can generally acquire emancipation through court order or marriage. These situations usually suggest that the minor will be financially independent of his or her parents. This patient is married and is therefore emancipated.

Answer A is incorrect. While this patient has many adult responsibilities, 18 years is the legal age of consent and adulthood.

Answer B is incorrect. Full-time work suggests that the patient is financially independent, but taken alone it is not proof of emancipation.

Answer C is incorrect. A high school diploma does not provide emancipation. Even though a minor becomes the primary decision maker after high school graduation, he or she is not necessarily financially independent of the parents.

Answer D is incorrect. A teenager may state he or she has separated from the parents, but unless the courts have approved a legal separation, merely saying she is "separated" from her parents is not enough; legally the parents are still financially responsible for the child until he or she turns 18.

13. **The correct answer is D.** This vignette illustrates a prospective cohort study. This is an observational study in which a specific population is identified that is free of the illness at the beginning of the study and monitored for the development of disease over time. Samples are chosen based on the presence or absence of risk factors (alcohol in this case), and the incidence rate of a certain disease is compared between exposed and unexposed members.

Answer A is incorrect. Case-control studies are also observational studies, but the sample is chosen based on the presence (case) or absence (control) of a disease (pancreatic cancer). Information is then gathered regarding prior exposures of cases and controls to certain risk factors.

Answer B is incorrect. Clinical treatment trials are examples of cohort studies; however, they are interventional as opposed to observational.

Study participants with a specific illness are given a treatment, while others with the same illness are given a different therapy or a placebo. Information is collected regarding the efficacy of treatment compared with other therapies or placebo.

Answer C is incorrect. This vignette does not exemplify a cross-sectional study. These studies involve the collection of information on a disease and risk factors in a population at a single point in time.

Answer E is incorrect. This vignette is an example of a prospective cohort study, in which the start time for gathering information about the sample is the present day and data collection extends into the future. In contrast, a retrospective cohort study is one in which the relevant data are obtained from historical records (eg., medical charts), as are some or all of the outcomes being measured.

14. **The correct answer is B.** Tanner stage 3 is the stage when most girls experience peak height velocity. Peak height velocity occurs approximately 1 year after the initiation of breast development.

Answer A is incorrect. This description corresponds to Tanner stage 1.

Answer C is incorrect. This description corresponds to Tanner stage 5.

Answer D is incorrect. This description corresponds to Tanner stage 4.

Answer E is incorrect. This description corresponds to Tanner stage 2.

15. **The correct answer is E.** Obtaining informed consent from the patient means that the patient understands the risks, benefits, and alternatives to the study and pertinent matters are given to them by their doctor regarding their plan of care. For patients who do not speak English, the consent is translated into their language and discussed with them through an interpreter. This allows the patient (or in this case, his parents) freedom to read and process the consent and to discuss it later. While this option may not be possible for every language

or reasonable for every study, it is appropriate in this nonemergent situation.

Answer A is incorrect. In a random sample study, patients speaking another language cannot be excluded because of language barriers. It is important that available language services are used to include patients of all backgrounds. In addition, clinical trials should include a broad demographic of patients.

Answer B is incorrect. With limited knowledge of Spanish, the doctor will unlikely be able to address all the important issues delineated in the consent form.

Answer C is incorrect. In a nonemergent setting, the best approach would allow patients and the patient's family to view a translated copy of the consent and consider all their options in an unbiased manner. However, the use of an interpreter would be invaluable during emergency setting.

Answer D is incorrect. The patient is not responsible for the task of translating a consent form to his/her family. This places undue pressure on the patient and allows for misinterpretation of the information.

16. **The correct answer is A.** A confounding error is committed when a variable other than the one being studied is influencing the results. In this study, the treatment group's lower blood pressure may be secondary to their younger mean age rather than to the antihypertensive medication. A sampling bias could be involved, although it would refer to a systematic error in which the participants chosen for the study where not representative of the population from which they are drawn. This would pose a problem when attempting to generalize the study's results to other situations.

Answer B is incorrect. Random error results in decreased precision of results.

Answer C is incorrect. Recall bias is a systematic error due to the differences in accuracy or completeness in the memory of study subjects.

Answer D is incorrect. Selection bias is a systematic error resulting in differences between those who are selected for a study or for study subgroups.

Answer E is incorrect. Systematic errors result in decreased accuracy of results.

17. **The correct answer is D.** Splitting is a belief that people are either all good or all bad. Although the doctor had to approve the time in the quiet room, the patient blames only the nurses. She is also displaying a tendency toward acting out through tantrums. Splitting and acting out are two examples of immature defense mechanisms.

Answer A is incorrect. Dissociation is a temporary, drastic change in personality, memory, consciousness, or motor behavior that is used to avoid emotional stress. This is an immature defense mechanism.

Answer B is incorrect. Isolation is a separation of feelings from ideas and events. This is an immature defense mechanism.

Answer C is incorrect. Projection is when an unacceptable internal impulse is attributed to an external source. This is an immature defense mechanism.

Answer E is incorrect. Suppression is a voluntary withholding of an idea or feeling from conscious awareness. This is a mature defense mechanism.

18. **The correct answer is D.** The specificity of the test is 89%. It is calculated by dividing the true-negatives by the sum of the true-negatives and false-positives. In the above case, the specificity is 800 / (800 + 100). The specificity measures how well a test identifies people who are truly well. High specificity is most important when it means that a healthy patient might undergo unnecessary and harmful treatment because of testing positive.

Answer A is incorrect. The figure 10% simply represents the prevalence of the disease in this select population (100 / 1000).

Answer B is incorrect. The figure 44% is the positive predictive value of the test. It is calculated by dividing true-positives by the sum of true-positives and false-positives (80 / [80 + 100]). The positive predictive value is the probability that someone with a positive test actually does have the infection.

Answer C is incorrect. The figure 80% is the sensitivity of the test. It is calculated by dividing true-positives by the sum of true-positives and false-negatives (80 / [80 + 20]). It measures how well a test identifies truly ill people.

Answer E is incorrect. The figure 98% is the negative predictive value of the test. It is calculated by dividing true-negatives by the sum of true-negatives and false-negatives (800 / [800 + 20]). The negative predictive value is the probability that a person with a negative test actually does not have the disease.

19. **The correct answer is B.** A retrospective cohort study includes a group of subjects who had some condition or received some treatment that is followed over time and compared to another group (a control group) made up of subjects who did not have this condition or receive the treatment. Retrospective cohort studies are based on the presence or absence of risk factors. In this study, the risk factor is the presence of diabetes in the mothers and the outcome would be LGA babies. The incidence rate of LGA births in women with diabetes is 4 times that in women without diabetes. Relative risk is used in cohort studies. Relative risk is defined as the incidence rate of some outcome in those exposed to a risk factor divided by the incidence rate of those not exposed. This definition gives the factor at which the incidence rate of LGA among women with diabetes is larger than the incidence rate of LGA among women without diabetes.

Answer A is incorrect. This choice describes the correct type of risk analysis but describes the relationship in reverse.

Answer C is incorrect. This choice reverses the findings of the study, which shows that the incidence of LGA is four times more in women with diabetes.

Answer D is incorrect. This choice incorrectly uses odds rather than incidence rates and also

describes the relationship of the findings of the study in reverse.

Answer E is incorrect. This choice describes an odds ratio for a case-control study. A case-control study evaluates the presence of risk factors in people with and without a disease. Although this is the opposite of a cohort study, the results are still reported in terms of disease presence with respect to risk factors; that is, the presence or absence of disease is categorized in the group with risk factors and compared to the group without risk factors. The difference, however, is that odds are used rather than incidence. The incidence rate is a percentage (eg., 50 out of 100). Odds are calculated by dividing those with disease by those without (50 to 50, or 1 to 1).

20. **The correct answer is D.** Cluster A personality disorders include paranoid, schizoid, and schizotypal, and patients with these disorders are often characterized as eccentric and/or weird. They employ abnormal cognition (suspiciousness), abnormal self-expression (odd speech), and abnormal relation to others (seclusiveness). There is a genetic association with schizophrenia. Patients with paranoid personality disorder are not psychotic, but they are distrustful and suspicious and use projection as their main defense mechanism.

Answer A is incorrect. Cluster B personality disorders include antisocial, borderline, histrionic, and narcissistic. Patients with cluster B personality disorders are classically dramatic and unstable. Patients with antisocial personality disorder show a disregard for and violation of the rights of others, including a proclivity for criminal behavior. This is the only personality disorder with an age limit: patients must be ≥18 years old; minors with similar behavior are considered to have conduct disorder. This is the only conduct disorder in which males outnumber females.

Answer B is incorrect. Cluster C personality disorders include avoidant, obsessive compulsive, and dependent, and these disorders are characterized by anxiety. Patients with avoidant personality disorder are sensitive to rejection, socially inhibited, and timid with overwhelming feelings of inadequacy.

Answer C is incorrect. Patients with obsessive-compulsive personality disorder have a preoccupation with order and perfectionism.

Answer E is incorrect. Patients with schizoid personality disorder exhibit voluntary social withdrawal (unlike avoidant patients) and have limited emotional expressions. They are some-what similar to schizotypal patients, but lack the additional strange beliefs and thoughts.

Answer F is incorrect. Patients with schizotypal disorder are odd with peculiar notions, ideas of reference, and magical thinking. They tend to have difficulty with interpersonal relationships and are unlikely to be in a marriage for 10 years.

CHAPTER 2

Biochemistry

1. A 6-year-old boy presents to his pediatrician with skin lesions all over his body. For several years he has been very sensitive to sunlight. Neither the boy's parents nor his siblings have the same skin lesions or sun sensitivity. Biopsies of several of the boy's lesions reveal squamous cell carcinoma. Which mutation would one expect to see in this patient's DNA?

(A) Methylation of the gene
(B) Missense mutation in the gene
(C) Nonsense mutation in the middle of the gene
(D) Point mutation within the enhancer region
(E) Point mutation within the operator region
(F) Point mutation within the promoter region
(G) Thymidine dimers

2. A metabolic process is pictured in the image below. Which intermediate in this process inhibits the rate-limiting enzyme of glycolysis and activates the rate-limiting enzyme of fatty acid synthesis?

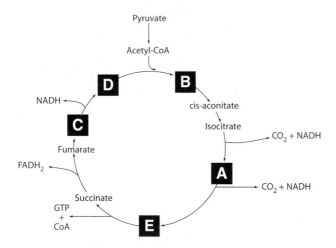

Reproduced, with permission, from USMLERx.com.

(A) A
(B) B
(C) C
(D) D
(E) E

3. A 32-year-old develops polyuria. Her nephrologist monitors her closely on a water deprivation test, and she continues to have increased urine output. A diagnosis of diabetes insipidus is made. The nephrologist orders an antidiuretic hormone level and determines that it is inappropriately elevated. Which of the following is the site of pathology in this patient?

(A) Adenohypophysis
(B) D_1
(C) Pituitary function
(D) V_1
(E) V_2

4. A 35-year-old man presents to the physician with arthritic pain in both knees along with back pain. He states that the pain has been present for months. In an effort to obtain relief, he has taken only aspirin, but this has been of little benefit. The patient is afebrile, and his slightly swollen knee joints are neither hot nor tender to palpation; however, the pain does restrict his motion. The cartilage of his ears appears slightly darker than normal. No tophi are present. A urine specimen is taken for analysis of uric acid content and turns black in the laboratory while standing. A defect in which of the following is the most likely underlying cause of the patient's condition?

(A) Galactokinase
(B) Homogentisic acid oxidase
(C) α-Ketoacid dehydrogenase
(D) Orotate phosphoribosyl transferase
(E) Phenylalanine hydroxylase

5. A patient who is a carrier of sickle cell trait presents to the clinic. The single base-pair mutation for sickle cell anemia destroys the MstII restriction enzyme recognition site represented by an asterisk in the image. The restriction enzyme-binding sites are shown as arrows on the map. DNA from this patient is treated with MstII and run on an electrophoresis gel. The DNA is then hybridized with a labeled probe that binds to the normal gene in the position

shown on the map. In the Southern blot shown in the image, which lane represents the patient?

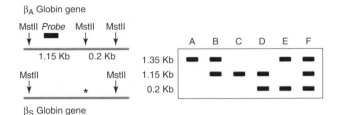

Reproduced, with permission, from USMLERx.com.

(A) A
(B) B
(C) C
(D) D
(E) E
(F) F

6. Phosphatidylcholine is a major component of red blood cell membranes, myelin, surfactant, and cholesterol. Phosphatidylcholine is synthesized through phosphorylation of choline obtained from the diet or with reused choline derived from phospholipid turnover. De novo synthesis requires an addition of three methyl groups, transferred from an amino acid. Without the turnover component, deficiency in which essential amino acid would make dietary choline essential for phosphatidylcholine synthesis?

(A) Asparagine
(B) Histidine
(C) Methionine
(D) Threonine
(E) Valine

7. A DNA fragment is added to four different tubes along with DNA polymerase, a radiolabeled primer, and the adenine, thymine, cytosine, and guanine deoxynucleotides. Each tube also contains one of the four bases as dideoxynucleotides. The four tubes are then run on electrophoresis gel and visualized by autoradiography. Which of the following laboratory techniques does this describe?

(A) Allele-specific oligonucleotide probe
(B) Enzyme-linked immunosorbent assay
(C) Northern blot
(D) Polymerase chain reaction
(E) Sequencing
(F) Southern blot
(G) Western blot

8. A DNA segment is treated with restriction enzymes, pipetted into a well of polyacrylamide gel, and subjected to an electric field. Next, the gel is stained with ethidium bromide and visualized under ultraviolet lights. What laboratory technique does this describe?

(A) Enzyme-linked immunosorbent assay
(B) Gel electrophoresis
(C) Northern blot
(D) Polymerase chain reaction
(E) Sequencing
(F) Southern blot
(G) Western blot

9. Increases in intracellular calcium can be especially detrimental to the cell. Therefore, calcium homeostasis is very tightly regulated not only across the cell membrane but also through the additional work of sequestration in endoplasmic reticulum and mitochondria. In which of the following ways does increased intracellular calcium concentration cause the most cell damage?

(A) Enzyme activation
(B) Free radical generation
(C) Increased membrane permeability
(D) Inhibition of glycolysis
(E) Inhibition of oxidative phosphorylation

10. A scientist working in a research laboratory has been examining different agonists of serotonin receptor 1B (5-HT$_{1B}$), a G-protein-coupled receptor. Compound A has a much higher affinity for 5-HT$_{1B}$ than compound B. Both compounds have a higher affinity for the receptor than serotonin. Which of the following describes the relationship between compound A and compound B when considering the guanine-nucleotide exchange activity of 5-HT$_{1B}$?

(A) K$_m$ for the exchange reaction with compound A is higher than that with compound B

(B) K$_m$ for the exchange reaction with compound A is lower than that with compound B

(C) K$_m$ values with compounds A and B are the same

(D) The maximum reaction rate with compound A is greater than that with compound B

(E) The maximum reaction rate with compound B is greater than that with compound A

11. An 18-year-old woman presents to the emergency department with acute onset of severe abdominal pain. She says she had a similar attack 1 year earlier after taking some barbiturates. At that time she underwent an exploratory laparotomy, which revealed nothing. The patient no longer takes barbiturates but recently started an extremely low-carbohydrate and low-calorie diet. She has a temperature of 37°C (98.6°F), a respiratory rate of 16/min, and a blood pressure of 128/83 mm Hg. Her WBC count is normal. Laboratory studies reveal a sodium level of 127 mEq/L, and urinalysis shows increased porphobilinogen levels. The physician tells the patient that she has a genetic condition involving her RBCs. What congenital disorder did the physician most likely tell the patient she has?

(A) Acute intermittent porphyria
(B) Fanconi's anemia
(C) Hereditary spherocytosis
(D) Porphyria cutanea tarda
(E) Sickle cell disease

12. A 48-year-old woman presents to a new physician because of the recent onset of fatigue, arthralgias, discomfort in her right upper quadrant, and polyuria. On physical examination, her skin seems somewhat browner than would be expected. Laboratory tests are remarkable for an elevated glucose level, indications of hemolysis, and increased transferrin saturation. Cardiac testing shows moderate restrictive cardiomyopathy. She mentions that she regularly requires blood transfusions. Which of the following is the cause of this patient's condition?

(A) Absence of the hemoglobin α chain
(B) Mutation of the hemoglobin β chain
(C) Mutation resulting in increased absorption of dietary iron
(D) Mutations in the gene encoding ankyrin
(E) Mutations resulting in copper accumulation

13. A 52-year-old man with a 12-year history of poorly controlled diabetes mellitus presents to his physician complaining of changes in his vision. Physical examination reveals opacities on the lens of the eye similar to those seen in the image. Which enzyme most likely contributed to this complication?

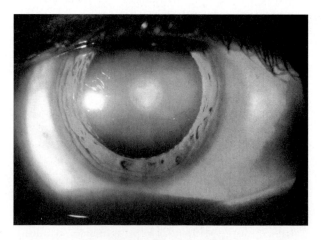

Reproduced, with permission, from Wikipedia.

(A) Adenosine deaminase
(B) Aldose reductase
(C) Galactose-1-phosphate uridyltransferase
(D) Hexokinase

(E) 3-Hydroxy-3-methylglutaryl coenzyme A reductase
(F) Insulin-like growth factor

14. Glucose is transported into human cells by two different families of membrane-associated carrier proteins: the glucose transporter facilitators (GLUT) and the sodium-coupled glucose transporters (SGLT). If a patient has a defect in the non-sodium-coupled glucose transporters, which cell line is still able to acquire glucose?

(A) Adipocytes
(B) Enterocytes
(C) Erythrocytes
(D) Hepatocytes
(E) Myocytes
(F) Pancreatic beta cells

15. A 31-year-old white woman is trying to get pregnant. She has a niece who suffers from a genetic disease characterized by recurrent respiratory infections and pancreatic failure. She would like to assess her chances of having a child with this disease. Which of the following laboratory techniques could be used to determine if this woman and/or her husband is a carrier of the mutant gene?

(A) Enzyme-linked immunosorbent assay
(B) Gel electrophoresis
(C) Northern blot
(D) Polymerase chain reaction and sequencing
(E) Western blot

16. A 32-year-old woman presents to her physician for the third time in 6 months. She has been feeling very tired and depressed, and has come to talk about starting antidepressants. She also complains of a 4.5-kg (10-lb) weight gain over the past 3 months. During her physical examination the physician notices that she is wearing a sweater and a coat, despite the room being at a warm temperature. Problems with the thyroid are suspected, and a biopsy is performed (see image). This woman may have a human leukocyte antigen subtype that also increases her risk of which disease?

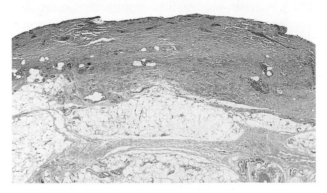

Reproduced, with permission, from PEIR Digital Library (http://peir.net).

(A) Multiple sclerosis
(B) Pernicious anemia
(C) Psoriasis
(D) Steroid-responsive nephrotic syndrome

17. A 65-year-old woman develops a urinary tract infection. Urine cultures are positive for *Enterococcus faecium*. Treatment with vancomycin is attempted but is unsuccessful. Which of the following molecular changes is responsible for this patient's vancomycin resistance?

(A) D-ala D-ala to D-ala D-lac
(B) D-ala D-ala to D-ala D-leu
(C) D-ala D-lac to D-ala D-ala
(D) D-ala D-leu to D-ala D-ala
(E) D-leu D-ala to D-ala D-ala

18. A 2-year-old boy presents to the pediatrician with fever, facial tenderness, and a green, foul-smelling nasal discharge. The patient is diagnosed with sinusitis, and the physician notes that he has a history of recurrent episodes of sinusitis. X-ray of the chest is ordered because of the fever; it reveals some dilated bronchi and shows the heart situated on the right side of his body. A congenital disorder is diagnosed. Which other finding would this patient be most likely to have?

(A) Defective chloride transport
(B) Elevated blood sugar
(C) Infertility
(D) Reactive airway disease
(E) Tetralogy of Fallot

19. A 9-month-old boy is brought to the emergency department after his mother is unable to rouse him. His past medical history is significant for the onset of seizures at the age of 4 months and for a delay in reaching developmental milestones. On examination, the patient is found to have poor muscle tone and an enlarged liver. Laboratory studies show a blood urea nitrogen level of 3.2 mg/dL, a creatinine level of 0.4 mg/dL, and a serum ammonia level of 300 mg/dL. A plasma amino acid analysis fails to detect citrulline, while his urinary orotic acid level is increased. This patient suffers from a deficiency of which of the following enzymes?

(A) Argininosuccinate lyase
(B) Carbamoyl phosphate synthetase II
(C) Glutamate dehydrogenase
(D) Ornithine transcarbamoylase

20. A 42-year-old woman presents to her physician with generalized itching. Physical examination reveals scleral icterus. Laboratory tests show:

Total bilirubin: 2.7 mg/dL
Conjugated bilirubin: 2.4 mg/dL
Alkaline phosphatase: 253 U/L
Aspartate aminotransferase: 36 U/L
Alanine aminotransferase: 40 U/L

What is the most likely mechanism underlying this patient's jaundice?

(A) Absence of UDP-glucuronyl transferase
(B) Decreased levels of UDP-glucuronyl transferase
(C) Extravascular destruction of the patient's RBCs
(D) Intrahepatic or extrahepatic biliary obstruction
(E) Intravascular destruction of the patient's RBCs

21. A 29-year-old woman with a long-standing history of asthma and eczema presents with watery, itchy eyes and a stuffy nose of 3 days' duration. The woman states that her symptoms are similar to those she experiences during the spring. Her heart rate is 82/min, blood pressure is 117/80 mm Hg, respiratory rate is 14/min, and oxygen saturation is 96%. This patient's symptoms are due to the activation of which of the following receptors?

(A) α_1
(B) β_1
(C) β_2
(D) Histamine$_1$
(E) Histamine$_2$

22. An 8-month-old boy is brought to the pediatrician by his parents because he has recently lost the ability to crawl or hold his toys. On examination the patient is tachypneic and breathing with considerable effort; the liver is palpable five fingerwidths below the right costal margin. X-ray of the chest reveals cardiomegaly. He has a difficult time sitting upright and cannot squeeze the physician's fingers or the ring of his pacifier with any noticeable force. Despite a number of interventions, the child's symptoms continue to worsen until his death 2 weeks later. On autopsy, it is likely that this patient's cells will contain an accumulation of which of the following substances?

(A) Glucose
(B) Glycogen
(C) Oxaloacetate
(D) Pyruvate
(E) Urea

23. After consumption of a carbohydrate-rich meal, the liver continues to convert glucose to glucose-6-phosphate. The liver's ability to continue this processing of high levels of glucose is important in minimizing increases in blood glucose after eating. What is the best explanation for the liver's ability to continue this conversion after eating a carbohydrate-rich meal?

(A) The hepatocyte cell membrane's permeability for glucose-6-phosphate
(B) The high maximum reaction rate of glucokinase
(C) The inhibition of glucokinase by high glucose-6-phosphate
(D) The lack of glucokinase level regulation by insulin
(E) The low Michaelis-Menten constant of glucokinase

24. A 30-year-old man is diagnosed with type I familial dyslipidemia. He has had recent laboratory studies showing elevated triglycerides and normal cholesterol levels. Which of the following explains the pathophysiology of this disease?

(A) Apolipoprotein E deficiency
(B) LDL cholesterol receptor deficiency
(C) Lipoprotein lipase deficiency
(D) VLDL cholesterol clearance deficiency
(E) VLDL cholesterol overproduction

25. A 36-year-old woman returned from a trip to Japan 2 days ago. Yesterday she started experiencing left calf pain. The woman is afebrile with a heart rate of 82/min, a blood pressure of 129/86 mm Hg, and a respiratory rate of 14/min. On examination, the patient's calf pain is found to intensify on dorsiflexion of the left foot. Suspecting a deep venous thrombosis (DVT), the physician performs a venous ultrasound, which confirms the diagnosis. Which of the following factors is most responsible in the formation of the DVT?

(A) Leukotriene C_4
(B) Prostaglandin I_2
(C) Renin
(D) Thromboxane A_2
(E) Vascular endothelial growth factor

26. A 53-year-old man comes to his physician because he noticed blood in his urine and has been having some low back pain. Physical examination reveals palpable flank masses felt bilaterally as well as mild hypertension. CT of the abdomen is shown in the image. Which of the following conditions is also associated with this disorder?

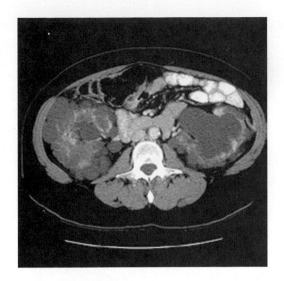

Reproduced, with permission, from PEIR Digital Library (http://peir.net).

(A) Astrocytomas
(B) Berry aneurysm
(C) Ectopic lens
(D) Optic nerve degeneration
(E) Squamous cell carcinoma

27. The bacterial ribosome and its involvement in protein synthesis pathways hold great importance to the function of various antibiotics that antagonize various steps in the process. Which of the following is true of the 50S ribosomal subunit in bacterial protein synthesis?

(A) Proteins in the 50S subunit are responsible for the creation of a peptide bond
(B) Streptomycin binds to the 50S subunit, disrupting the translocation step
(C) The 23S rRNA molecule within the 50S subunit is responsible for the creation of a peptide bond
(D) The 50S subunit holds the binding site for both the aminoacyl-tRNA (A site) and the elongating peptide chain (P site)
(E) The 50S subunit is a part of the initiation complex

28. A researcher investigating mechanisms of intracellular signaling develops a mouse model using recombinant DNA technology to generate a gene knockout. The F2 progeny exhibit dwarfism, hypogonadism, and hypothyroidism with low levels of follicle-stimulating hormone, luteinizing hormone, and thyroid-stimulating hormone but normal levels of ACTH. In addition, the female progeny exhibit impaired milk secretion. Which of the following is the second-messenger molecule for the intracellular signaling system that is most likely impaired in this mouse model?

    (A) cAMP
    (B) cGMP
    (C) Inositol trisphosphate
    (D) Steroid nuclear hormone receptor
    (E) Tyrosine kinase

29. Hemoglobin consists of 2 α subunits and 2 β subunits. Each α unit is bound to a β unit by strong hydrophobic bonds. The β units and α units are each bound to one another by weaker polar bonds that are somewhat mobile. This change in quaternary structure changes the affinity for oxygen that hemoglobin exhibits as it shifts between its taut (T) form and relaxed form. At a given partial pressure of oxygen, which of the following will increase the amount of T hemoglobin?

    (A) Binding of carbon dioxide to hemoglobin
    (B) Decreasing the amount of 2,3-bisphospho-glycerate in RBCs
    (C) Increasing the number of oxygen molecules bound to a hemoglobin from one to three
    (D) Increasing the pH by moving from peripheral tissue to lung
    (E) The presence of excess carbon monoxide from carbon monoxide poisoning

30. A group of scientists have recently discovered a new drug for treating hypercholesterolemia. In vitro studies with a hepatocyte cell line have revealed that the drug increases the number of LDL cholesterol receptors by acting in a manner similar to steroids. What is the mechanism by which this drug is acting on hepatocytes?

    (A) Allosteric regulation
    (B) Cell surface receptor antagonism
    (C) G-protein-cell receptor-mediated phosphorylation
    (D) Hormone-receptor complex formation
    (E) Proteolytic modification

31. A 30-year-old patient comes to the physician to explore the possibility of an endocrine disorder. Physical examination reveals a solitary thyroid nodule. Laboratory studies show an increased serum calcitonin level and a pentagastrin-induced rise in the secretion of calcitonin. A biopsy confirms the presence of a carcinoma. The patient is scheduled for a total thyroidectomy. Which of the following is a potential complication of this treatment?

    (A) Acromegaly
    (B) Cretinism
    (C) Hypertension
    (D) Hypoparathyroidism
    (E) Renal osteodystrophy

32. Heme synthesis occurs in the bone marrow and liver. Deficiency of δ-aminolevulinic acid hydrase would lead to the accumulation of which of the following?

    (A) δ-Aminolevulinic acid
    (B) Coproporphyrinogen
    (C) Glycine
    (D) Porphobilinogen
    (E) Succinyl-CoA

33. A group of scientists is investigating the anti neoplastic properties of a new drug. In an in vitro experiment, cancer cells exposed to the drug are found to be uniformly arrested in metaphase. The mechanism of action of this new drug is similar to the action of which of the following drugs?

    (A) Bleomycin
    (B) Cyclophosphamide
    (C) 5-Fluorouracil
    (D) Methotrexate
    (E) Paclitaxel

34. A woman gives birth to a full term baby. Upon delivery, the baby is small and has a musty

odor. Upon questioning the woman says that she did not smoke or drink alcohol during the pregnancy, and she only drinks diet soda and water. Which of the following amino acids is most likely to be deficient in the newborn?

(A) Alanine
(B) Cysteine
(C) Glutamine
(D) Phenylalanine
(E) Proline
(F) Serine
(G) Tyrosine

35. A 78-year-old man with asthma presents to his primary care physician for an annual check-up. The physician performs a physical examination and orders routine blood work, which reveals a macrocytic anemia. Subsequent laboratory tests show an elevated serum methylmalonic acid level. A peripheral blood smear is shown in the image. If this patient's vitamin deficiency is not corrected, what neurological symptoms is he most likely to experience?

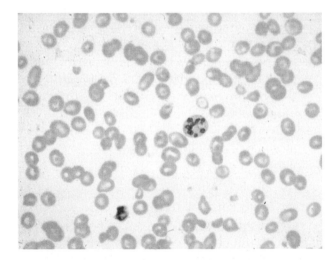

Reproduced, with permission, from PEIR Digital Library (http://peir.net).

(A) Confusion and confabulation
(B) Deficiency in this vitamin does not cause neurological symptoms
(C) Dysarthria and diplopia
(D) Paresthesias and ataxia
(E) Syncope and lethargy

36. A group of scientists is interested in studying how vesicles synthesized in the cell bodies of neurons are transported down the axon to the terminal boutons. Which of the following make up the cellular structures involved in axonal transport of vesicles?

(A) Desmin
(B) Keratin
(C) Titin
(D) Tubulin
(E) Vimentin

37. A term child is delivered by spontaneous vaginal delivery without complications. Upon physical examination the child has bilateral hip dislocations, restricted movement in shoulder and elbow joints, and coarse facial features. Laboratory studies show that the activities of β-hexosaminidase, iduronate sulfatase, and arylsulfatase A are deficient in cultured fibroblasts, but are 20 times normal in serum. This disease is associated with which of the following abnormal cellular components?

(A) Apolipoprotein B-48
(B) Collagen
(C) Mannose-6-phosphate
(D) Rough endoplasmic reticulum
(E) Sphingomyelinase

38. Patients who are said to be albino appear white-pink, have white hair, and have nonpigmented irises. In many cases these individuals may have melanocytes, but lack melanin in their skin. Which of the following is the most likely cause of congenital albinism?

(A) Acetaldehyde dehydrogenase deficiency
(B) Congenital abnormality in amino acid absorption
(C) Decreased consumption of phenylalanine
(D) Tryptophan hydroxylase deficiency
(E) Tyrosinase deficiency

39. Obstructive liver disease is usually characterized by which of the following qualities?

Choice	Type of Hyperbilirubinemia	Urine Bilirubin	Urine Urobilinogen
A	Conjugated	↑	Normal
B	Conjugated	↑	↓
C	Unconjugated	↑	↓
D	Unconjugated	↓	↑
E	Unconjugated	↓	↓

(A) A
(B) B
(C) C
(D) D
(E) E

40. The muscles that control the diameter of the pupil are triggered by a cascade of molecular events within a muscle cell. What is the function of the enzyme activated by the calcium-calmodulin complex?

(A) Binding to troponin
(B) Dephosphorylation of actin
(C) Dephosphorylation of myosin
(D) Phosphorylation of actin
(E) Phosphorylation of myosin

41. A 56-year-old man who is an alcoholic presents to the emergency department with severe epigastric pain radiating to his back. The pain was preceded by nausea and vomiting. His past medical history is notable for gallstones. Laboratory testing reveals a lipase level of 800 U/L (normal 10–140 U/L), a serum amylase level of 1020 U/L (normal 25–115 U/L), and a WBC count of 13,200/mm^3. Which of the following pathophysiologic mechanisms is most likely responsible for this patient's presentation?

(A) Exhaustion of enzyme reserve
(B) Hyperactive renin-angiotensin system

(C) Inappropriate enzyme activation
(D) Inappropriate enzyme deactivation
(E) pH alteration of the surrounding milieu

42. A 3-year-old girl who was born at home in a rural area is brought to the local clinic because of seizures. She is pale skinned, shows marked mental retardation, and has a musty body odor. The doctor diagnoses her with a defect in tetrahydrobiopterin metabolism. Which of the following is a correct therapeutic measure for this child?

(A) Branched-chain amino acid-free diet
(B) Fructose-free diet
(C) Ketogenic diet
(D) Low-phenylalanine diet
(E) Low-tyrosine diet

43. A 3-month-old infant is rushed to the emergency department in respiratory distress. Her mother notes that she is "always sick." She has had multiple hospitalizations over the past months, including one for a severe bout of pneumonia with *Pneumocystis jiroveci* (formerly *carinii*) and another for respiratory syncytial virus. On admission, she is noted to be below the 5th percentile for weight and length and appears pale and lethargic. Her vital signs include a pulse of 150/min, respirations of 20/min, and a temperature of 38.9° C (102° F). Her mouth is coated with whitish bumps that scrape off easily. This patient is most likely to have a deficiency of which of the following enzymes?

(A) Adenosine deaminase
(B) Aldolase B
(C) Arylsulfatase A
(D) B-cell tyrosine kinase
(E) HGPRTase

44. A mass is felt in the groin of an infant girl during a physical examination. Surgical resection shows that it is a testicle. The baby is diagnosed with testicular feminization syndrome. In this syndrome, androgens are produced but cells fail to respond to the steroid hormones because they lack appropriate intracellular receptors. After binding intracellular receptors, steroids regulate the rate of which of the following?

(A) Initiation of protein synthesis
(B) mRNA degradation
(C) mRNA processing
(D) Protein translation
(E) Transcription of genes

45. A 27-year-old man develops a deep venous thrombosis in his left lower leg after a 4-hour car ride. His 59-year-old father had a thrombosis in a mesenteric vein last year, and his 52-year-old mother has had repeated superficial venous thromboses. Which of the following disorders does this patent most likely have?

(A) Factor V Leiden thrombophilia
(B) Familial hypercholesterolemia
(C) Fanconi's anemia
(D) von Hippel-Lindau disease
(E) von Willebrand's deficiency

46. A pediatrician examines two babies with two separate deficiencies in fructose metabolism. The first child has a deficiency of fructokinase, and the second has a deficiency of aldolase B. Although the physician states with confidence that the first child has a benign prognosis, he is concerned about the second child. What best explains the clinical severity of aldolase B deficiency?

(A) Increased ATP
(B) Increased circulating free phosphate
(C) Increased circulating fructose
(D) Sequestration of phosphate
(E) Upregulated fructokinase

47. A patient presents to the emergency department with nausea, headache, and dizziness. On physical examination his lips and fingernail have a bluish tint. Arterial blood gas sampling reveals arterial partial oxygen pressure of 100 mm Hg and an arterial partial carbon dioxide pressure of 40 mm Hg. The nurse who drew blood for the gas analysis notes that the patient's blood looked oddly brown in the collecting tube. Which of the following is the most appropriate treatment for this condition?

(A) Hyperbaric oxygen
(B) Methylene blue
(C) N-Acetylcysteine

(D) Protamine
(E) Thiosulfate

48. A neonate born 4 hours ago is having difficulty breathing. The baby was born at 28 weeks' gestation. He is tachypneic and is flaring and grunting. The baby's heart rate is 120/min, blood pressure is 100/60 mm Hg, and respiratory rate is 55/min. What is this baby's lung lacking?

(A) Angiotensin-converting enzyme
(B) Collagen
(C) Dipalmitoyl phosphatidylcholine
(D) Elastase
(E) Functional cilia
(F) Myelin

49. A 69-year-old woman diagnosed with rheumatoid arthritis is being given antimetabolite therapy with methotrexate. Her physician explains to her that she can expect the greatest toxicity of the drug to cells with the shortest G_1 phase. Which cell has the shortest G_1 phase?

(A) Hepatocyte
(B) Intestinal mucosal cell
(C) Neuron
(D) Oocyte in the adult female
(E) RBC

50. A group of investigators is studying a segment of the human genome that evidences an interindividual variation in the number of nucleotides. They isolate a DNA segment of interest by running it on electrophoresis gel. They remove the portion of gel with the DNA and subsequently expose it to a labeled DNA probe. Which of the following laboratory techniques does this describe?

(A) Enzyme-linked immunosorbent assay
(B) Northern blot
(C) Polymerase chain reaction
(D) Sequencing
(E) Southern blot
(F) Southwestern blot
(G) Western blot

ANSWERS

1. **The correct answer is G.** This patient has xeroderma pigmentosa, an autosomal recessive disease characterized by a defect in excision repair. This disease results in an inability to repair thymidine dimers that can form in the presence of ultraviolet light. This can lead to the development of skin cancer and photosensitivity.

Answer A is incorrect. Methylation of a particular gene does not cause xeroderma pigmentosum.

Answer B is incorrect. A missense mutation does not cause xeroderma pigmentosum.

Answer C is incorrect. A nonsense mutation does not cause xeroderma pigmentosum.

Answer D is incorrect. A mutation in the enhancer region of a gene does not cause xeroderma pigmentosum.

Answer E is incorrect. A mutation in the operator region of a gene does not cause xeroderma pigmentosum.

Answer F is incorrect. A mutation in the promoter region of a gene does not cause xeroderma pigmentosum.

2. **The correct answer is B.** Citrate, formed from oxaloacetate and acetyl CoA by the enzyme citrate synthase, inhibits phosphofructokinase and allosterically activates acetyl CoA carboxylase. Citrate synthase regenerates a molecule of CoA and is an important regulator of the tricarboxylic acid cycle. It is inhibited by adenosine triphosphate.

Answer A is incorrect. α-Ketoglutarate is not an important regulator of the tricarboxylic acid cycle, but it is an important intermediate in protein metabolism.

Answer C is incorrect. Malate is not an important regulator of the tricarboxylic acid cycle, but it is important in the malate shuttle.

Answer D is incorrect. Oxaloacetate is not an important regulator of the tricarboxylic acid cycle, but it is important in glyconeogenesis.

Answer E is incorrect. Succinyl-CoA downregulates its own synthesis by inhibiting the enzyme responsible for dehydrogenation of α-ketoglutarate.

3. **The correct answer is A.** The adenohypophysis is not related to the pathology of diabetes insipidus.

Answer B is incorrect. D_1 receptors are not involved in nephrogenic diabetes insipidus.

Answer C is incorrect. This is nephrogenic, not central, diabetes insipidus.

Answer D is incorrect. The V_1 receptor is involved in vascular smooth muscle contraction.

Answer E is incorrect. This scenario describes nephrogenic diabetes insipidus, which is pathology at the antidiuretic hormone receptor in the kidney. This receptor is the V_2 receptor.

4. **The correct answer is B.** The patient has alkaptonuria, a condition corresponding to the one described in the stem. A deficiency of the enzyme homogentisic acid oxidase leads to deposition of homogentisic acid in the joints and cartilage, giving them a dark color (ochronosis) and resulting in degenerative changes. Classically, the urine of these patients turns black on contact with air or when the urine is made alkaline. The associated defect is on chromosome 3.

Answer A is incorrect. A deficiency in galactokinase causes galactosemia and galactosuria, but is otherwise a fairly benign condition and would not present with any of the symptoms seen in this patient. Other symptoms would be cataracts in affected children, owing to the accumulation of galactitol, a by-product of galactose metabolism when galactokinase is not present.

Answer C is incorrect. A deficiency in α-ketoacid dehydrogenase causes maple syrup urine disease, a metabolic disorder of autosomal recessive inheritance that affects the metabolism of branched-chain amino acids (leucine, isoleucine, and valine) and causes the urine of affected patients to smell like maple syrup. The urine does not, however, turn black upon standing. The disease is not classically associated with arthritis in middle-aged individuals.

Answer D is incorrect. Orotate phosphoribosyltransferase is an enzyme involved in pyrimidine synthesis. Deficiencies in this enzyme or in orotidine 5′-monophosphate decarboxylase (an enzyme involved in the same pathway and located on the same chromosome) cause a very rare disorder called hereditary orotic aciduria. Symptoms include poor growth, megaloblastic anemia, and orate crystals in urine. Treatment involves cystidine or uridine to bypass this step in pyrimidine synthesis and also to negatively downregulate orotic acid production.

Answer E is incorrect. A congenital deficiency of phenylalanine hydroxylase causes phenylketonuria. This enzyme converts phenylalanine to tyrosine, and a deficit of this enzyme leads to a deficiency of tyrosine and a build-up of phenylketones in the urine. It is associated with mental retardation and with the presence of phenylketones in the urine (which do not classically turn black upon standing).

5. **The correct answer is B.** Lane B represents the Southern blot of a heterozygous carrier of sickle cell anemia. The β-A-globin gene results in a 1.15-kb fragment of DNA cut by the MstII restriction enzyme. The β-S-globin gene results in a 1.35-kb band because the single base-pair mutation responsible for sickle cell anemia eliminates an MstII restriction site.

Answer A is incorrect. The band in lane A is from a sickle cell anemia patient with two copies of the β-S-globin gene. This gene results in a 1.35-kb band because the single base-pair mutation responsible for sickle cell anemia eliminates an MstII restriction site.

Answer C is incorrect. The band in lane C is from an unaffected patient with two copies of the β-A-globin gene. The gene results in a 1.15-kb fragment of DNA cut by the MstII restriction enzyme.

Answer D is incorrect. The bands in lane D could not result from any patient. The labeled DNA probe does not bind to the 0.2-kb DNA fragment and therefore would not be visualized on the Southern blot.

Answer E is incorrect. The bands in lane E could not result from any patient. The labeled DNA probe does not bind to the 0.2-kb DNA fragment and therefore would not be visualized on the Southern blot.

Answer F is incorrect. The bands in lane F could not result from any patient. The labeled DNA probe does not bind to the 0.2-kb DNA fragment and therefore would not be visualized on the Southern blot.

6. **The correct answer is C.** The key to answering this question correctly is an understanding that phosphatidylcholine is formed by donation of methyl groups. Methionine is the only amino acid listed that can donate methyl groups. Its activated form, S-adenosyl-L-methionine, is a very common methyl group donor.

Answer A is incorrect. Asparagine is an essential amino acid with a negative charge. It can serve as a hydrogen ion recipient.

Answer B is incorrect. Histidine is an essential amino acid with a positive charge. It can serve as a hydrogen ion donor.

Answer D is incorrect. Threonine is an essential amino acid with an uncharged polar side chain. It contains a hydroxy group that can serve as a hydrogen ion donor or recipient.

Answer E is incorrect. Valine is an essential amino acid with a hydrocarbon side chain; however, it is not a methyl group donor.

7. **The correct answer is E.** This question describes sequencing. Sequencing is a laboratory technique that utilizes dideoxynucleotides to randomly terminate growing strands of DNA. Gel electrophoresis is used to separate the varying lengths of DNA. The DNA sequence can then be read based on the position of the bands on the gel.

Answer A is incorrect. Allele-specific oligonucleotide probes are short, labeled DNA sequences complementary to an allele of interest. These probes can be used to detect the presence of disease-causing mutations.

Answer B is incorrect. Enzyme-linked immunosorbent assay (ELISA) is an immunologic technique used to determine whether a particular antibody is present in a patient's blood. Labeled antibodies are used to detect whether the serum contains antibodies against a specific antigen precoated on an ELISA plate.

Answer C is incorrect. In a Northern blot procedure, RNA is separated by electrophoresis, denatured, and transferred to a filter. RNA is hybridized to a labeled radioactive DNA probe. The radioactive hybridized RNA/DNA strand is radioactive and visualized when the filter is exposed to film.

Answer D is incorrect. Polymerase chain reaction (PCR) is a laboratory technique used to produce many copies of a segment of DNA. In the procedure, DNA is mixed with two specific primers, deoxynucleotides and a heat-stable polymerase. The solution is heated to denature the DNA and then cooled to allow synthesis. Twenty cycles of heating and cooling amplify the DNA more than a million times. Dideoxynucleotides are not used in PCR techniques.

Answer F is incorrect. In a Southern blot procedure, DNA is separated with electrophoresis, denatured, transferred to a filter, and hybridized with a labeled DNA probe. Regions on the filter that base-pair with the labeled DNA probes can be identified when the filter is exposed to film that is sensitive to the radiolabeled probe.

Answer G is incorrect. In a Western blot procedure, protein is separated by electrophoresis and labeled antibodies are used as a probe. This technique can be used to detect the existence of an antibody to a particular protein.

8. **The correct answer is B.** This question describes gel electrophoresis. Gel electrophoresis uses an electric field to separate molecules based on their sizes. The negatively charged DNA migrates in the electric field toward the positive end. Smaller fragments move more rapidly through the gel. Bands of DNA can be visualized by staining the gel with dyes such as ethidium bromide.

Answer A is incorrect. ELISA is an immunologic technique used in laboratories to determine whether a particular antibody is present in a patient's blood. Labeled antibodies are used to detect whether the serum contains antibodies against a specific antigen precoated on an ELISA plate. This is not the technique described above.

Answer C is incorrect. Northern blots are similar to Southern blots except that in Northern blotting, mRNA is separated by electrophoresis instead of DNA. This is not the technique described above.

Answer D is incorrect. PCR is a laboratory technique used to produce many copies of a segment of DNA. In this procedure, DNA is mixed with two specific primers, deoxynucleotides and a heat-stable polymerase. The solution is heated to denature the DNA and is then cooled to allow synthesis. Twenty cycles of heating and cooling amplify the DNA more than a million times. This is not the procedure described above.

Answer E is incorrect. Sequencing is a laboratory technique that utilizes dideoxynucleotides to randomly terminate growing strands of DNA. Gel electrophoresis is used to separate the varying lengths of DNA. The DNA sequence can then be read based on the position of the bands on the gel. This is not the technique described above.

Answer F is incorrect. In a Southern blot procedure, DNA is separated with electrophoresis, denatured, transferred to a filter, and hybridized with a labeled DNA probe. Regions on the filter that base-pair with the labeled DNA probes can be identified when the filter is exposed to film that is sensitive to the radiolabeled probe. This is not the technique described above.

Answer G is incorrect. In a Western blot procedure, protein is separated by electrophoresis and labeled antibodies are used as a probe. This technique can be used to detect the existence of an antibody to a particular protein.

9. **The correct answer is A.** Calcium is maintained in high concentrations outside the cell and within discrete compartments within the cell (ie., mitochondria). Free intracellular calcium can activate several enzymes whose cumulative effect is to induce significant cell injury. A few important enzyme classes include ATPases, which decrease ATP supply; phospholipases, which decrease membrane stability; endonucleases, which induce DNA damage; and several proteases.

Answer B is incorrect. Free radical generation is a common mechanism of cell injury, but calcium excess does not induce free radical generation.

Answer C is incorrect. Activation of proteases and phospholipases induces the breakdown of necessary components of cell membranes.

Answer D is incorrect. ATP depletion, resulting from the activation of ATPases, can contribute to the inhibition of glycolysis

Answer E is incorrect. Inhibition of oxidative phosphorylation is an effect of ATP depletion caused by enzyme activation. Although this may contribute to cell damage, it is not the best answer.

10. **The correct answer is B.** G-protein-coupled receptors exist in an equilibrium between their active and inactive states that depends on whether ligand is present and the affinity of ligand for the receptor. When active, these receptors catalyze guanine-nucleotide exchange (GTP for GDP) of their associated G-proteins. The Michaelis-Menten constant (K_m) for any enzyme-catalyzed reaction is inversely proportional to the affinity of the enzyme for its substrate. Therefore, the K_m with compound A will be lower than that with compound B because compound A has a higher affinity for the receptor than compound B. The maximum rate of reaction (V_{max}) will be reached at a lower concentration of A than it would for B, although the V_{max} is unchanged.

Answer A is incorrect. The K_m of compound A will be lower than that of compound B.

Answer C is incorrect. Given that compounds A and B have different affinities for the receptor, their Michaelis-Menten constant values cannot be the same.

Answer D is incorrect. V_{max} is directly proportional to the enzyme concentration, and is unaffected by the concentration of substrates or competitive inhibitors.

Answer E is incorrect. V_{max} is directly proportional to the enzyme concentration, and is unaffected by the concentration of substrates or competitive inhibitors.

11. **The correct answer is A.** Acute intermittent porphyria (AIP) is a blood disorder caused by a deficiency of uroporphyrinogen I synthetase. δ-Aminolevulinic acid and porphobilinogen are found in the urine. Patients often present with hyponatremia and recurrent episodes of abdominal pain and can even develop neuropsychiatric problems. Barbiturates (among other drugs) and starvation diets can precipitate attacks. Patients with AIP do not have the cutaneous photosensitivity seen in other porphyrias.

Answer B is incorrect. Fanconi's anemia is an autosomal recessive disorder in which DNA repair is defective. This results in aplastic anemia and defective DNA. Patients are at increased risk of malignancy. Abdominal pain and hyponatremia are not hallmarks of this illness.

Answer C is incorrect. Hereditary spherocytosis is an autosomal dominant disorder of the erythrocyte structural protein spectrin. The defective membrane causes erythrocytes to be culled in the spleen. While some patients may develop an anemia, abdominal pain, hyponatremia, and porphobilinogen in the urine are not observed.

Answer D is incorrect. Porphyria cutanea tarda describes a group of disorders characterized by a deficiency in the enzyme uroporphyrinogen decarboxylase. Common symptoms are cutaneous fragility of the hands and forearms after sun exposure, hypertrichosis, and scleroderma-like plaques. Reddish urine is indicative of renal excretion of increased levels of uroporphyrin. Porphyria cutanea tarda is not associated with neurological symptoms, however.

Answer E is incorrect. Sickle cell disease is an autosomal recessive disease characterized by a point mutation in the β-globin chain. While painful episodes (crises) are frequent in sickle cell disease, it is not classically associated with hyponatremia or barbiturates. Additionally, urine porphobilinogen levels are normal in sickle cell disease.

12. **The correct answer is B.** This woman suffers from β-thalassemia major. Clinically, β-thalassemia major manifests as severe hemolysis and ineffective erythropoiesis. These individuals are transfusion-dependent and frequently develop iron overload. The consequences of iron overload due to transfusion dependency or secondary hemochromatosis are described in the question stem. These manifestations are due to iron deposition in various tissues, including the pancreas, heart, and skin.

Answer A is incorrect. Absence of α chains describes the most severe form of α-thalassemia. In this form, no functional α chains are made, and the fetus is unable to make any functional hemoglobin aside from the γ_4 tetramer, also called Hb Barts. Hb Barts' high oxygen affinity results in poor oxygen delivery to peripheral tissues and ultimately congestive heart failure, anasarca, and intrauterine fetal death.

Answer C is incorrect. This answer describes hereditary hemochromatosis, a condition caused by iron overload due to an intrinsic defect in the body's ability to control the absorption of iron. Iron overload in hemochromatosis is not due to transfusions, and the laboratory picture is

not characterized by hemolysis. Otherwise, the clinical manifestations are the same for both genetic and secondary hemochromatosis.

Answer D is incorrect. Hereditary spherocytosis is caused by mutations in either the ankyrin or the spectrin gene, both of which contribute to the erythrocyte cytoskeleton. Hereditary spherocytosisis caused by erythrocytes with abnormal membranes passing through the spleen; the reticuloendothelial cells remove pieces of the membrane causing spherocyte formation. This condition is characterized by extravascular hemolysis. Clinical manifestations include gallstones, anemia, jaundice, and splenomegaly.

Answer E is incorrect. Failure of copper to enter the circulation in the form of ceruloplasmin, resulting in copper accumulation in the liver, brain, and cornea, is also known as Wilson's disease. Clinically, Wilson's disease is characterized by parkinsonian symptoms, Kayser-Fleischer rings, asterixis, and dementia. Laboratory studies demonstrate low ceruloplasmin. Heart failure, diabetes, and skin changes, as well as the hematologic manifestations of β-thalassemia, are not associated with Wilson's disease.

13. **The correct answer is B.** Aldose reductase catalyzes the breakdown of glucose into sorbitol. Sorbitol is then metabolized to fructose, a process that is relatively slow. In patients with hyperglycemia, as would be present in this patient with poorly controlled diabetes, sorbitol accumulation with the cells of the lens leads to a rise in intracellular osmolality, causing water movement into the cells. This results in cellular swelling and osmotic damage. It also leads to a decrease in intracellular myoinositol, interfering with cellular metabolism. Swelling of lens fiber cells can lead to rupture and cataract formation (as seen in the image). Inhibition of aldose reductase could decrease sorbitol accumulation in the lens and thus prevent cataract formation. No drug is currently approved to inhibit aldose reductase, but aldose reductase inhibitors such as epalrestat and ranirestat are currently being tested.

Answer A is incorrect. Adenosine deaminase inhibition would result in problems in the purine salvage pathway. Disrupting this pathway would result in excess ATP and dATP via feedback inhibition of ribonucleotide reductase. This excess ATP prevents DNA synthesis and thus affects lymphocyte development. Congenital deficiency of this enzyme results in severe combined immunodeficiency. Inhibition of this enzyme would not prevent the development of cataracts.

Answer C is incorrect. Galactose-1-phosphate (G-1-P) uridyltransferase is important in the breakdown of galactose; it catalyzes the formation of glucose-1-phosphate from G-1-P. Hereditary deficiency of this enzyme leads to hepatosplenomegaly, mental retardation, jaundice, and cataract formation. Inhibition of this enzyme in an adult would certainly not prevent the development of cataracts.

Answer D is incorrect. Hexokinase is the enzyme that catalyzes the first step in the catabolism of glucose, converting glucose to glucose-6-phosphate. It is stimulated by insulin. Inhibition of hexokinase would not prevent the development of cataracts in this patient. Congenital hexokinase deficiency is a rare autosomal recessive condition that results in severe hemolysis. Inhibition of hexokinase would likely have a similar, albeit less severe, result.

Answer E is incorrect. 3-Hydroxy-3-methylglutaryl coenzyme A (HMG-CoA) reductase catalyzes the conversion of HMG-CoA into mevalonate and eventually into cholesterol. Inhibition of this enzyme is commonly affected by statin drugs to reduce cholesterol levels, but it would not help prevent the development of cataracts.

Answer F is incorrect. Insulin-like growth factor (IGF) is a product synthesized in the liver that mediates many of the physiologic effects of growth hormone. Its name refers to a high degree of structural similarity to insulin, and it is even capable of binding to the insulin receptor directly, although with lower affinity than insulin. Its effects include increased protein synthe-sis, and IGF levels are especially high during puberty. Inhibition of IGF would not help prevent the development of cataracts.

14. **The correct answer is B.** This patient would likely have a defect of glucose transporter 1, which transports glucose across the blood-brain barrier. A family of glucose transporters (GLUT 1-5) is responsible for cellular uptake in many cell types. However, enterocytes and nephrons acquire glucose through cotransport with sodium ion.

Answer A is incorrect. Adipocytes primarily use GLUT4 for glucose transport. GLUT4 is the transporter most affected by insulin.

Answer C is incorrect. Erythrocytes largely contain GLUT1.

Answer D is incorrect. Hepatocytes primarily contain GLUT2, the same transporter found in pancreatic beta cells. This transporter is especially important for equilibrating calcium inside and outside of the cell.

Answer E is incorrect. Myocytes also use GLUT4 for glucose transport.

Answer F is incorrect. Pancreatic beta cells contain GLUT2 transporters. This transporter is especially important for equilibrating calcium inside and outside of the cell.

15. **The correct answer is D.** PCR and sequencing can be used to determine if this woman and/or her husband is a carrier of the cystic fibrosis gene, the most common single-gene mutation in white people. This mutation commonly presents with dysfunction of the lungs, pancreas, and other organs due to buildup of thick mucus. PCR is used to amplify the region of interest, and sequencing is used to see if the cystic fibrosis mutation is present.

Answer A is incorrect. ELISA is an immunologic technique used in laboratories to determine whether a particular antibody is present in a patient's blood. This test cannot be used to determine whether the woman and her husband are carriers for the cystic fibrosis gene.

Answer B is incorrect. Gel electrophoresis uses an electric field to separate molecules based on their sizes. Gel electrophoresis cannot be used alone to determine whether the woman and her husband are carriers for the cystic fibrosis gene.

Answer C is incorrect. Northern blots test RNA levels. It cannot be used to determine whether the woman and her husband are carriers for the cystic fibrosis gene.

Answer E is incorrect. A Western blot is a test for the presence or absence of a protein. This test cannot be used to determine whether the woman and her husband are carriers for the cystic fibrosis gene.

16. **The correct answer is B.** This woman has symptoms of Hashimoto's thyroiditis, an autoimmune disorder resulting in hypothyroidism (also known as myxedema), although there may be a transient hyperthyroidism at the very onset of disease when follicular rupture occurs. It is a type IV hypersensitivity associated with autoantibodies to thyroglobulin, thyroid peroxidase, and the thyroid-stimulating hormone receptor itself. The most common presenting symptoms of Hashimoto's thyroiditis are those seen in this patient, as well as constipation and dry skin. Histologic characteristics include massive infiltrates of lymphocytes with germinal cell formation. Hashimoto's thyroiditis is associated with the DR5 human leukocyte antigen subtype, as is pernicious anemia, a disease that leads to vitamin B_{12} deficiency caused by atrophic gastritis and destruction of parietal cells.

Answer A is incorrect. Multiple sclerosis is associated with the DR2 human leukocyte antigen subtype. It is not associated with Hashimoto's thyroiditis.

Answer C is incorrect. Psoriasis is associated with the B27 human leukocyte antigen subtype. It is not associated with Hashimoto's thyroiditis.

Answer D is incorrect. Steroid-responsive nephrotic syndrome is associated with the DR7 human leukocyte antigen subtype. It is not associated with Hashimoto's thyroiditis.

17. **The correct answer is A.** Vancomycin is an antibiotic that is effective only in fighting gram-positive cocci. It binds tightly to a cell wall precursor that contains the amino acid sequence D-ala D-ala and prevents cell wall synthesis. Resistance to vancomycin is transferred via plasmids and encodes enzymes that convert D-ala D-ala to D-ala D-lac, preventing vancomycin from binding. This type of resistance is much more common with *Enterococcus faecium* than with *Enterococcus faecalis*.

Answer B is incorrect. D-ala D-leu is not seen in the bacterial wall precursor.

Answer C is incorrect. Wild-type *Enterococcus* species have a cell wall precursor containing D-ala D-ala, which is the binding site for vancomycin. After acquiring resistance, D-ala D-lac is substituted for D-ala D-ala, rendering the bacterium resistant.

Answer D is incorrect. D-ala D-leu is not seen in the bacterial wall precursor.

Answer E is incorrect. D-leu D-ala is not seen in the bacterial wall precursor.

18. **The correct answer is C.** Kartagener's syndrome, or immotile cilia, is caused by a defect in dynein that prevents effective movement of cilia. The full syndrome is characterized by sinusitis, bronchiectasis, situs inversus, and male infertility. Cilia play an important role in moving mucus along the airway and clearing debris; the absence of this function contributes to the pulmonary findings of the syndrome. Cilia are also very important for leukocyte movement and phagocytosis. Infertility is present in most patients due to immotile cilia.

Answer A is incorrect. Defective chloride transport is the cause of cystic fibrosis. Cystic fibrosis frequently causes bronchiectasis, but it is not associated with situs inversus.

Answer B is incorrect. Patients with diabetes are predisposed to developing chronic fungal sinusitis. However, the bronchiectasis and situs inversus are not consistent with diabetes.

Answer D is incorrect. Mucus plugging in reactive airway disease can cause atelectasis at the lung bases. An x-ray film of the chest of a patient with reactive airway disease would likely reveal hyperinflated lungs with areas of atelectasis, not bronchiectasis.

Answer E is incorrect. Tetralogy of Fallot is a congenital heart defect, but it not associated with infections or cardiac inversion. Patients with this condition develop early cyanosis because of the malformed right-to-left shunt. The four components of the teratology are (1) ventricular septal defect, (2) overriding aorta, (3) infundibular pulmonary stenosis, and (4) right ventricular hypertrophy.

19. **The correct answer is D.** This child is suffering from an inherited form of hyperammonemia as a result of a defect in ornithine transcarbamoylase. This enzyme is a component of the urea cycle that is responsible for combining carbamoyl phosphate and ornithine to make citrulline. As a result, the patient has an excess of ammonia in circulation, which leads to mental retardation, seizures, and ultimately death. Some patients with ornithine transcarbamoylase deficiency also exhibit a very low blood urea nitrogen level, but this is not enough to make a conclusive diagnosis.

Answer A is incorrect. A defect in argininosuccinate lyase would result in elevated citrulline levels.

Answer B is incorrect. Carbamoyl phosphate synthetase I is a component of the urea cycle, and combines carbon dioxide and ammonia to form carbamoyl phosphate. Carbamoyl phosphate synthetase II, however, is an enzyme in the pyrimidine synthesis pathway and would not result in hyperammonemia if deficient.

Answer C is incorrect. Glutamate dehydrogenase is the enzyme responsible for the conversion of glutamate to α-ketoglutarate in the liver. A defect in this enzyme would result in low levels of ammonia.

20. **The correct answer is D.** This patient has obstructive jaundice, causing her pruritus and scleral icterus. In this situation conjugated bilirubin cannot be excreted, and its levels are therefore elevated in the serum. The unconjugated bilirubin level, however, is not elevated. Alkaline phosphatase is usually elevated in cases of obstructive jaundice.

Answer A is incorrect. This is seen in Crigler-Najjar syndrome type I, which leads to kernicterus and is diagnosed during childhood. Extremely high levels of unconjugated bilirubin would be expected in this case.

Answer B is incorrect. This is seen in Gilbert's syndrome, which does not have any clinical consequence. This syndrome is more common in men, the jaundice is typically associated with stress or exercise, and alkaline phosphatase levels are normal.

Answer C is incorrect. Extravascular hemolysis (eg., hereditary spherocytosis) would lead to increased levels of unconjugated bilirubin. Hemoglobinuria would not be observed in these patients.

Answer E is incorrect. Intravascular hemolysis (eg., due to mechanical injury to RBCs, defective cardiac valves, toxic injury to RBCs) would lead to an increase in unconjugated bilirubin, which is not the case in this patient. Also, levels of alkaline phosphatase would not be elevated in a patient with increased RBC destruction. Hemoglobinuria would be expected in these patients.

21. **The correct answer is D.** The patient's symptoms are consistent with those of seasonal allergies. The patient has experienced asthma, eczema, and allergies and most likely suffers from atopy. Seasonal allergies are a result of histamine1-receptor activation, which results in pruritus, bronchoconstriction, and increased nasal and bronchial mucus production. Seasonal allergy symptoms can be treated with antihistamines such as loratadine, which are histamine1-antagonists.

Answer A is incorrect. Activation of α_1-receptors results in vasoconstriction and increased blood pressure. α_1-Receptors are primarily found in blood vessel walls and are not associated with allergies.

Answer B is incorrect. Activation of β_1-receptors leads to inotropy and chronotropy. β_1-Receptors are typically located in the heart, and stimulation of the receptors results in increased contractility (inotropy) and heart rate (chronotropy).

Answer C is incorrect. Activation of β_2-receptors leads to vasodilation and bronchodilation. β_2-Receptors are primarily located in blood vessel walls and in the respiratory tract. Drugs that agonize β_2-receptors are used in the treatment of asthma.

Answer E is incorrect. Activation of histamine$_2$-receptors leads to increased gastric acid production. Histamine$_2$-receptors are located in the stomach, and drugs that antagonize histamine$_2$-receptors are used to treat gastroesophageal reflux disease and peptic ulcer disease.

22. **The correct answer is B.** This patient has Pompe's disease, a glycogen storage disorder. Pompe's disease is an autosomal recessive disease that is characterized by a deficiency or defect in lysosomal α-1,4-glucosidase. This enzyme is necessary for the dissolution of the polymer linkages in glycogen. In its absence, glycogen accumulates to toxic levels in both the cytoplasm and lysosomes.

    Answer A is incorrect. Glucose is stored as glycogen in the cells and is also present in blood. However, hyperglycemia is not responsible for the symptoms observed in this patient.

    Answer C is incorrect. Oxaloacetate is the first intermediate in the Krebs cycle. It is regenerated with each turn of the cycle but is not present in excessive amounts in the cell.

    Answer D is incorrect. Pyruvate is a component of the cellular respiration pathway and an intermediate in gluconeogenesis. It is not stored in cells in any significant quantity.

    Answer E is incorrect. Disorders of the urea cycle leading to nitrogen accumulation in the body can result in progressive lethargy and coma but generally do not cause the myopathy observed in this patient.

23. **The correct answer is B.** Glucokinase is found in liver and pancreatic β cells. It catalyzes the initial step of glycolysis, phosphorylation of glucose to glucose-6-phosphate, which is catalyzed by hexokinase in other tissues. Both enzymes are found in the liver. Glucokinase has a higher Michaelis-Menten constant (K_m) and a higher maximum reaction rate (V_{max}) than hexokinase; therefore, glucokinase has lower affinity for glucose and a higher capacity to make glucose into glucose-6-phosphate. At low glucose levels, hexokinase, with its higher affinity for glucose, processes glucose to glucose-6-phosphate. At higher glucose levels, hexokinase is overwhelmed (operating at its low V_{max}) and sufficient substrate is available for glucokinase to process the excess glucose even with its low affinity. Glucokinase thus helps to handle large increases in glucose from the gut.

    Answer A is incorrect. The hepatocyte cell membrane is permeable to glucose, which is trapped in the cell after phosphorylation.

    Answer C is incorrect. Glucokinase is not inhibited by glucose-6-phosphate. Instead, glucokinase action is decreased with decreased insulin and carbohydrate levels.

    Answer D is incorrect. Insulin-and glucose-rich diets increase glucokinase levels.

    Answer E is incorrect. Glucokinase has a relatively high Michaelis-Menten constant.

24. **The correct answer is C.** Type I dyslipidemia is caused by a deficiency of lipoprotein lipase. This enzyme exists in capillary walls of adipose and muscle tissue and cleaves triglycerides into free fatty acids and glycerol. The enzyme is activated by apolipoprotein C-II, which is found on VLDL cholesterol and chylomicrons. Type I dyslipidemia is characterized by an accumulation of triglyceride-rich lipoproteins in the plasma. It can also occur with an alteration in apolipoprotein C-II.

    Answer A is incorrect. VLDL cholesterol remnants are removed from the circulation by apolipoprotein E receptors. Thus, apolipoprotein E deficiency results in a decreased efficiency of that clearance and elevated VLDL cholesterol, triglyceride, and cholesterol levels. Dysbetali-poproteinemia often only manifests with additional factors that cause hyperlipidemia such as diabetes. Xanthomas are often present.

Answer B is incorrect. LDL cholesterol receptor dysfunction is characteristic of familial hyperbetalipoproteinemia, also known as type II hyperlipidemia. In these cases, plasma LDL cholesterol levels rise, which causes an increase in plasma cholesterol; triglyceride levels remain normal.

Answer D is incorrect. Mixed hypertriglyceridemia (type V) is a dyslipidemia characterized by extremely high triglyceride levels and visibly foamy plasma. Unlike type I, type V is characterized by elevated VLDL cholesterol levels and is thought to be related to a VLDL cholesterol clearance problem.

Answer E is incorrect. VLDL cholesterol overproduction is another characteristic of type V dyslipidemias, as well as type IIb combined hyperlipidemia.

25. **The correct answer is D.** This patient's long airplane flight placed her at an increased risk of developing DVT. In addition, the patient has a positive Homans' sign (calf pain on dorsiflexion), which is seen in some patients with a DVT. Virchow's triad refers to three factors that predispose a patient to developing a venous thrombosis: (1) local trauma to the vessel wall, (2) stasis, and (3) hypercoagulability. Thromboxane A_2 stimulates platelet aggregation and vasoconstriction and will be elevated at the site of a clot.

Answer A is incorrect. Leukotrienes (LT) C_4, LTD_4, and LTE_4 are bronchoconstrictors that are believed to contribute to symptoms of asthma. 5-Lipoxygenase is the enzyme that converts arachidonic acid to 5-hydroperoxy-eicosatetraenoic acid, which is then used to produce leukotrienes.

Answer B is incorrect. Prostaglandin I_2 (PGI_2) is synthesized by vascular endothelium and smooth muscle. Its effects include inhibition of platelet aggregation, relaxation of smooth muscle, reduction of systemic and pulmonary vascular resistance by direct vasodilation, and natriuresis in kidney. Thus, PGI_2 is not abundant locally at the site of a deep venous thrombosis because it does not promote platelet aggregation.

Answer C is incorrect. Renin is a circulating enzyme released mainly by the kidneys in response to low blood volume or low body NaCl content. Renin activates the renin-angiotensin system by cleaving angiotensinogen in the liver to produce angiotensin I. Angiotensin I is then further converted into angiotensin II in specialized lung, ultimately leading to constriction of blood vessels, an increase in ADH and aldosterone production, and stimulation of the hypothalamus to activate the thirst reflex, leading in turn to increased blood pressure.

Answer E is incorrect. Vascular endothelial growth factor (VEGF) is a substance made by cells that stimulates new blood vessel formation. The binding of VEGF turns on the receptors, which then generate signals inside the cell, ultimately leading to the growth of new blood vessels. Although this growth factor may be elevated at the site of the clot, it is not as abundant as thromboxane A_2.

26. **The correct answer is B.** This patient has adult polycystic kidney disease, an autosomal dominant condition characterized by massive bilateral cysts in the kidneys (as shown in the image). Cysts can also sometimes be found in the liver. The renal cysts eventually lead to end-stage renal disease. In addition to the cysts, patients are more prone to mitral valve prolapse as well as berry aneurysms, which can rupture and lead to strokes.

Answer A is incorrect. Astrocytomas are seen in patients with tuberous sclerosis, an autosomal dominant disorder affecting the tuberin and hamartin proteins, which regulate cellular growth and differentiation.

Answer C is incorrect. Ectopic lens is seen in Marfan's syndrome, an autosomal dominant connective tissue disorder associated with slender body habitus and aortic dissection.

Answer D is incorrect. Optic nerve degeneration can be seen in Leber's hereditary optic neuropathy, a condition in which patients develop a rapid loss of central vision.

Answer E is incorrect. Squamous cell carcinoma is seen in increased incidence in patients with xeroderma pigmentosum, an autosomal recessive disease caused by a deficiency in DNA repair of thymine dimers.

27. **The correct answer is C.** The 50S ribosomal subunit is the larger of the two ribosomal macromolecules. Its main function in translation is the creation of a new peptide bond between the incoming aminoacyl-tRNA and the growing peptide chain. Essential for this purpose is the 23S rRNA molecule, which holds the peptidyl transferase enzyme activity. Linezolid is an antibiotic that is active against gram-positive bacteria including enterococci and staphylococci. The linezolid mechanism of action is inhibition of protein synthesis by binding to the 23S rRNA and interacting with the initiation complex. Linezolid resistance has been reported in staphylococci and enterococci. Since bacteria carry several copies of the 23S rRNA gene, the number of rRNA genes mutated seems to be a significant determinant of resistance.

Answer A is incorrect. The 50S subunit is responsible for the creation of the peptide bond, but the molecule that accomplishes this activity is the 23S rRNA strand, not proteins. If all proteins are removed, the peptidyl transferase activity remains intact.

Answer B is incorrect. Streptomycin is an aminoglycoside antibiotic that binds to the 30S subunit and disrupts formation of the initiation complex. Aminoglycosides are bactericidal and used to treat gram-negative rod infections. Major adverse effects include nephrotoxicity and ototoxicity, especially when combined with cephalosporins and loop diuretics, respectively.

Answer D is incorrect. The A site of the ribosome is the binding site for the incoming aminoacyl-tRNA complexes, whereas the P site refers to the binding site for the elongating peptide chain (which is still bound to the aminoacyl-

tRNA of the 30' amino acid). While the 50S subunit has moieties that interact with each site, the 30S subunit contains the major binding sites for each.

Answer E is incorrect. The initiation complex is the term used to describe the complex of macromolecules necessary for the onset of translation. The complex is composed of the 30S subunit, an aminoacyl-tRNA bound to N-formylmethionine, and initiation factors. The 50S subunit is not part of the initiation complex.

28. **The correct answer is C.** The knockout mouse model described exhibits a phenotype consistent with impaired function of all of the hypothalamic hormones with the exception of corticotropin-releasing hormone (CRH). The hypothalamus produces a number of important hormones, including trophic hormone-releasing hormone, that act on the anterior pituitary; these include thyrotropin-releasing hormone and gonadotropin-releasing hormone as well as hormones to be stored and released in the posterior pituitary, such as ADH and oxytocin. All of the hypothalamic hormones exert their actions on target cells via a phospholipase C (PLC) intracellular signaling cascade with inositol trisphosphate (IP_3) as the second messenger, with the exception of CRH, which acts via adenylate cyclase-cAMP. Thus, the PLC-IP_3 signaling system is the most likely target of the gene knockout described in the vignette. Important nonhypothalamic hormones that also act via this signaling system include angiotensin II and α1-adrenergic agonists.

Answer A is incorrect. cAMP is the second-messenger molecule for the signaling systems that mediate the mechanisms of corticotropin-releasing hormone, luteinizing hormone, follicle-stimulating hormone, thyroid-stimulating hormone, human chorionic gonadotropin, ADH (V2 receptor), parathyroid hormone, calcitonin, glucagon, and α_2-, β_1, and β_2-adrenergic agonists.

Answer B is incorrect. cGMP is the second-messenger molecule for the signaling systems that mediate the mechanisms of atrial natriuretic peptide, endothelium-derived relaxing factor, and nitrous oxide.

Answer D is incorrect. Steroid nuclear hormone receptors are the second-messenger molecules that mediate the mechanisms of aldosterone, glucocorticoids, testosterone, estrogen, progesterone, thyroid hormones, and 1,25-dihydroxycholecalciferol (vitamin D). Steroid nuclear hormone receptors diffuse into the nucleus of the cell and act directly on DNA.

Answer E is incorrect. Tyrosine kinases are the second-messenger molecules that mediate the mechanisms of insulin, insulin-like growth factor-1, prolactin, and growth hormone. Their primary mechanism of action is phosphorylation.

29. **The correct answer is A.** Hemoglobin carries oxygen better when it is in the relaxed (R) form, in which it has a higher affinity for oxygen. As a result, the oxygen dissociation curve shifts to the left and decreased unloading of oxygen results. Conversely, tightening hemoglobin decreases its affinity for oxygen. Hemoglobin in the T form is stabilized by all the processes that result in increased oxygen unloading. Binding of CO_2 stabilizes the T form, which decreases oxygen affinity.

Answer B is incorrect. 2,3-Bisphosphoglycerate (2,3-BPG) binds to a pocket formed by the two β subunits. It can only bind when they are close together, such as in the T form. Its binding holds the hemoglobin in this fashion and prevents oxygen binding and promotes unloading. It is essential to add inosine to stored blood for transfusions to prevent the loss of 2,3-BPG, which would make transfused blood an oxygen "trap" in peripheral tissues.

Answer C is incorrect. Binding of oxygen molecules is the major cause of the shift of hemoglobin from its T structure to the R form. The oxygen molecule disrupts the weak polar bonds and "opens up" the molecule for more oxygen to bind.

Answer D is incorrect. The Bohr effect comes from an increase in protons, which subsequently stabilize the T form of hemoglobin preferentially. In addition, an increase in protons means

an increase in CO_2 because of the bicarbonate buffer present in blood. Remember, though, that increasing the pH means a decrease in protons.

Answer E is incorrect. CO stabilizes the R form of hemoglobin so that the dissociation curve shifts dramatically to the left.

30. **The correct answer is D.** Like steroid hormones, this drug is binding to a cytosolic receptor to form a hormone-receptor complex. The complex is then transported to the nucleus, where it acts on DNA to increase the transcription of LDL cholesterol receptor mRNA, which can be translated to LDL receptors.

Answer A is incorrect. Allosteric regulation involves the binding of a drug to a protein and either increasing or decreasing the activity of that protein.

Answer B is incorrect. Antagonism of a cell surface receptor would not result in increased transcription of LDL cholesterol receptors.

Answer C is incorrect. Many drugs bind to G-protein-coupled receptors (GPCRs) located at the cell surface. This binding would then set in motion a secondary messenger system that could result in increased transcription of LDL cholesterol receptors. However, steroids and the drug described above do not work by a GPCR-mediated mechanism.

Answer E is incorrect. Proteolytic modification involves the cleavage of a zymogen into an active enzyme. This would not explain the increased synthesis of LDL cholesterol receptor.

31. **The correct answer is D.** Hypoparathyroidism can occur if all of the parathyroid glands are accidentally removed during total thyroidectomy. Hypoparathyroidism can lead to hypocalcemia and hyperphosphatemia. Symptoms of hypocalcemia include tingling of the lips and digits and muscle spasms. Additionally, individuals with hypocalcemia have positive Chvostek's sign (tapping of the facial nerve causes contraction of the facial muscles) and a positive Trousseau's sign (occlusion of the brachial artery in the upper arm causes a carpal spasm).

Answer A is incorrect. Acromegaly is caused by an excess of growth hormone in adults after growth plates have already been fused. It is not a side effect of thyroidectomy.

Answer B is incorrect. Cretinism is the term used for fetal hypothyroidism. Cretinism can be caused by either a defect in thyroxine formation or failure of thyroid development. It is most common in iodine-deficient regions, and remains common in China. Typical physical findings are a pot-bellied, pale, and puffy-faced child with protruding umbilicus and protuberant tongue.

Answer C is incorrect. Hypertension can occur from a variety of mechanisms; however, thyroidectomy is not a cause.

Answer E is incorrect. Renal osteodystrophy occurs in patients with renal failure. The failing kidney retains phosphate, leading to hyperphosphatemia and subsequent hypocalcemia; hypocalcemia causes a secondary hyperparathyroidism, which is the basis for the bone pathology.

32. **The correct answer is A.** δ-Aminolevulinic acid (δ-ALA) synthase irreversibly catalyzes the first reaction, glycine + succinyl-CoA → δ-ALA. This is the rate-limiting and committed step in heme synthesis. δ-ALA dehydratase catalyzes the second step in heme synthesis, 2δ-ALA → porphobilinogen. Since δ-aminolevulinic synthetases action is irreversible, only δ-ALA would accumulate.

Answer B is incorrect. Uroporphyrinogen decarboxylase acts on uroporphyrinogen III to synthesize coproporphyrinogen. It would also be deficient in a δ-ALA hydrase deficiency.

Answer C is incorrect. Glycine would not accumulate because δ-ALA cannot be converted back to succinyl-CoA and glycine.

Answer D is incorrect. Porphobilinogen is made from the action of alanine dehydrase on δ-ALA. In this case porphobilinogen levels would decrease.

Answer E is incorrect. Succinyl-CoA would not accumulate because δ-ALA cannot be converted back to succinyl-CoA and glycine.

33. **The correct answer is E.** The drug's action is during metaphase of the cell cycle and thus most likely serves to disrupt the mitotic spindle. Paclitaxel is a chemotherapeutic agent that prevents microtubule depolymerization. This stabilizes the mitotic spindle and disallows the migration of chromatids to their respective ends of the cell. Mitosis remains incomplete, leading to cell death. Paclitaxel is primarily used to treat advanced ovarian cancer and metastatic breast cancer.

Answer A is incorrect. Bleomycin intercalates DNA during the G_2 phase of the cell cycle and causes scission of DNA by an oxidative process. Bleomycin is used in the treatment of testicular tumors, lymphomas, and squamous cell carcinomas. The adverse effects are pulmonary related, including rales, cough, and infiltration leading to fibrosis of the lung.

Answer B is incorrect. Cyclophosphamide is a DNA alkylator that is activated by cytochrome P450. It induces apoptosis by crosslinking DNA at any stage of the cell cycle. Its oncologic uses include leukemias, lymphomas, and testicular and gynecologic cancers. The adverse effects of this drug include hemorrhagic cystitis, which can be prevented through adequate hydration and intravenous injection of mesna before the administration of cyclophosphamide.

Answer C is incorrect. 5-Fluorouracil (5-FU) arrests the cell cycle in S phase, resulting in impaired DNA synthesis. 5-FU is a pyrimidine analog with a stable fluorine atom in place of a hydrogen atom at position 5 of the uracil ring. The fluorine interferes with the conversion of deoxyuridylic acid to thymidylic acid. 5-FU is used to treat slow-growing solid tumors such as breast, ovarian, pancreatic, colorectal, and gastric carcinomas.

Answer D is incorrect. Methotrexate acts in the S phase of the cell cycle, impairing DNA synthesis by inhibiting the enzyme dihydrofolate reductase. Dihydrofolate reductase converts folic acid to tetrahydrofolic acid, the coenzyme required for synthesis of thymidine. Methotrexate is effective against acute lymphocytic leukemia, choriocarcinoma, Burkitt's lymphoma, breast cancer, and head and neck carcinomas.

34. The correct answer is G. This woman gave birth to a child with phenylketouronia (PKU). Patients with PKU are unable to convert phenylalanine to tyrosine due to a deficiency of phenylalanine hydroxylase or tetrahydrobiopterin. Phenylalanine crosses the placenta and harmful levels can accumulate in a phenylketouronic fetus. Artificially sweetened products such as diet soda often contain phenylalanine. As a result of the child's disease, the phenylalanine will accumulate with minimal production of tyrosine.

Answer A is incorrect. Alanine would not be deficient as a result of PKU.

Answer B is incorrect. Cysteine would not be deficient as a result of PKU.

Answer C is incorrect. Glutamine would not be deficient as a result of PKU.

Answer D is incorrect. Phenylalanine would accumulate, not be deficient, in this case.

Answer E is incorrect. Proline would not be deficient as a result of PKU.

Answer F is incorrect. Serine would not be deficient as a result of PKU.

35. The correct answer is D. Vitamin B_{12} is a necessary cofactor in the regeneration of folate for methyl group donation in DNA synthesis. For this reason, vitamin B_{12} and folate deficiencies each present with megaloblastic anemia (as seen in the image) and hypersegmented neutrophils, as all blood cell lines are affected by the defect in DNA synthesis. However, only vitamin B_{12} deficiency increases serum methylmalonic acid levels and impairs myelin synthesis. This myelin defect primarily impacts the posterior and lateral spinal columns, causing paresthesias and impaired proprioception.

Thus, neurologic abnormality in the context of megaloblastic anemia is a USMLE-favorite hint that vitamin B_{12}, rather than folate, is deficient.

Answer A is incorrect. Confusion, confabulation, and ataxia are typical of Wernicke-Korsakoff syndrome, a disorder of thiamine (vitamin B_1) deficiency typical in alcoholics.

Answer B is incorrect. Folate and vitamin B_{12} deficiencies present similarly, but folate deficiency does not manifest with an elevated methylmalonic acid level or neurologic problems. In the absence of increased serum methylmalonate levels, therefore, the physician would diagnose folate deficiency, and no neurologic symptoms would be expected.

Answer C is incorrect. Concurrent onset of dysarthria (defective articulation) and diplopia may indicate that a transient ischemic episode or cerebrovascular accident has occurred. These symptoms are not typical of any vitamin deficiency.

Answer E is incorrect. Syncope may be a sign of vasovagal stimulation, low blood pressure, arrhythmia, and other cardiovascular disorders. Lethargy is a sign of decreased consciousness. Neither of these symptoms is typically associated with a vitamin deficiency.

36. The correct answer is D. Microtubules are involved in the transport of vesicles down the axons of neurons. Microtubules are made of polymerized tubulin. The microtubule is made up of two subunits, α and β, that polymerize to form a hollow tubule. Two attachment proteins, dynein and kinesin, attach to membranous organelles and move along the tubules toward and away from the cell center.

Answer A is incorrect. Intermediate filaments of muscle cells are made up primarily of desmin.

Answer B is incorrect. Intermediate filaments are cytoskeletal elements that are prominent in cells that withstand stress. Intermediate filaments of epithelial cells are composed primarily of keratin.

Answer C is incorrect. Titin, also known as connectin, is a protein that is important in the contraction of striated muscle tissues. In the sarcomere, titin connects the M line to the Z line.

Answer E is incorrect. Vimentin is polymerized to form intermediate filaments that are found in cells of mesodermal origin, such as fibroblasts.

37. **The correct answer is C.** I-cell disease is caused by a failure of addition of mannose-6-phosphate, an intracellular signal sequence, to lysosomal proteins, leading to an inappropriate release of those proteins into the extracellular space. Thus, lysosomal enzymes, including hexosaminidase, iduronate sulfatase, and arylsulfatase A, will be found in the extracellular space, but not intracellularly. I-cell disease is characterized by skeletal abnormalities, restricted joint movement, coarse facial features, and severe psychomotor impairment. Death usually occurs by the age of 8 years.

    Answer A is incorrect. Apolipoprotein B-48 mediates the extracellular secretion of chylomicrons.

    Answer B is incorrect. Collagen is an extracellular molecule. Procollagen has a specific extracellular signal sequence at its N-terminal end. Faulty collagen synthesis can lead to many diseases including scurvy, osteogenesis imperfecta, and Ehlers-Danlos syndrome.

    Answer D is incorrect. Rough endoplasmic reticulum (RER) typically translates proteins meant for extracellular use. The RER in I-cell disease is not abnormal.

    Answer E is incorrect. Sphingomyelinase is a lysosomal enzyme that is deficient in Niemann-Pick disease. This is an autosomal recessive disease characterized by progressive neurodegeneration, hepatosplenomegaly, and cherry red spot on macula.

38. **The correct answer is E.** Congenital albinism is often due to a deficiency in tyrosinase, the enzyme needed for converting tyrosine to melanin. Hereditary forms can be autosomal dominant or autosomal recessive. Albinism can also result from altered neural crest migration, but this is not an option included among the answer choices. Albinos are at increased risk for skin cancer because the melanin pigment that normally absorbs ultraviolet radiation is lacking.

    Answer A is incorrect. Acetaldehyde dehydrogenase converts acetaldehyde to acetate. A person lacking this enzyme will get very sick from the build-up of acetaldehyde following ethanol consumption. This plays no role in pigmentation.

    Answer B is incorrect. A dietary deficiency is not an established cause of congenital albinism.

    Answer C is incorrect. Although phenylalanine can be converted to tyrosine, decreased dietary phenylalanine does not have a substantial effect on melanin levels, as tyrosine itself can be obtained by dietary means. This is also not a congenital cause of albinism.

    Answer D is incorrect. Tryptophan hydroxylase converts tryptophan to serotonin and is not related to pigmentation.

39. **The correct answer is B.** Obstructive liver disease refers to the obstruction of intrahepatic and/or extrahepatic bile ducts with subsequent cholestasis and liver injury. This entity commonly presents with jaundice, conjugated hyperbilirubinemia, increased urine bilirubin, and decreased urine urobilinogen. The majority of bilirubin results from the breakdown of heme groups in senescent erythrocytes. After cellular release, bilirubin binds to albumin, which delivers the molecule to the liver. Hepatocellular uptake and glucuronidation in the endoplasmic reticulum generate conjugated bilirubin, which is water-soluble and excreted in the bile. Gut bacteria deconjugate the bilirubin and degrade it to urobilinogens. The urobilinogens are excreted in the feces, with some reabsorption and excretion into urine. Based on this metabolic schema, the laboratory values in obstructive liver disease become evident. Failed excretion of conjugated bilirubin leads to a direct bilirubinemia and failure of production of urobilinogen by gut flora. Thus, urine urobilinogen levels are low. The urine bilirubin level is elevated secondary to

the increased plasma concentrations of direct bilirubin, which undergoes renal excretion.

Answer A is incorrect. Conjugated hyperbilirubinemia, increased urine bilirubin, and normal urine urobilinogen can be seen in patients with hepatocellular jaundice. The urine urobilinogen level is normal because, unlike in obstructive jaundice, gut bacteria have the opportunity to synthesize urobilinogen.

Answer C is incorrect. Unconjugated hyperbilirubinemia, increased urine bilirubin, and decreased urine urobilinogen can occur with hepatocellular disease if there is also concurrent conjugated hyperbilirubinemia. However, a purely obstructive condition is not characterized by unconjugated hyperbilirubinemia.

Answer D is incorrect. Unconjugated hyperbilirubinemia, decreased urine bilirubin, and increased urine urobilinogen is a classic pattern seen in hemolytic jaundice. In this case, the bilirubin level rises due to increased heme turnover and may overwhelm the liver's ability to conjugate it. However, none of these changes is consistent with obstructive liver disease.

Answer E is incorrect. Unconjugated hyperbilirubinemia, decreased urine bilirubin, and decreased urine urobilinogen are very unlikely to occur simultaneously in any given condition.

40. **The correct answer is E.** The calcium-calmodulin complex activates myosin light chain kinase, which phosphorylates myosin and allows it to bind to actin, leading to contraction and shortening of the muscle fiber.

Answer A is incorrect. In smooth muscle, unlike skeletal muscle, there is no troponin. Instead, calcium is the regulator of myosin on the thick filament.

Answer B is incorrect. Actin is not phosphorylated or dephosphorylated in the contraction and relaxation cycle of smooth muscle.

Answer C is incorrect. The calcium-calmodulin complex activates myosin light chain kinase, which phosphorylates myosin. Myosin light chain phosphatase removes the phosphate group from myosin.

Answer D is incorrect. Actin is not phosphorylated or dephosphorylated in the contraction and relaxation cycle of smooth muscle.

41. **The correct answer is C.** Symptoms of severe epigastric pain radiating to the back, nausea, and vomiting, combined with risk factors such as chronic alcohol use and gallstones, are suggestive of acute pancreatitis. Increases in serum lipase and amylase confirm the diagnosis. Pathologically, acute pancreatitis is marked by necrosis and inflammation of the pancreatic tissue. Based on anatomic evidence of pancreatic injury, the most likely mechanism leading to acute pancreatitis is thought to be an inappropriate activation of pancreatic enzymes. There is evidence for three possible pathways by which activation of pancreatic enzymes is initiated. One possibility is pancreatic duct obstruction resulting from cholelithiasis, ampullary obstruction, or chronic alcoholism. Acinar cell injury caused by alcohol, drugs, trauma, ischemia, or viruses can also result in enzymatic activation. Finally, defective intracellular transport secondary to alcohol, duct obstruction, or metabolic injury is another possible cause of inappropriate enzyme activation.

Answer A is incorrect. Exhaustion of enzyme reserve may be a consequence of multiple injuries to the pancreas, sometimes seen in patients with chronic pancreatitis. However, this would lead to pancreatic insufficiency, not acute pancreatitis.

Answer B is incorrect. A hyperactive renin-angiotensin system commonly occurs in congestive heart failure or prerenal azotemia; however, it is not a mechanism responsible for acute pancreatitis.

Answer D is incorrect. Inappropriate pancreatic enzyme deactivation is not a mechanism responsible for acute pancreatitis. In fact, enzymes must be activated to cause damage.

Answer E is incorrect. pH alteration of the surrounding milieu is not a mechanism responsible for acute pancreatitis. This occurs in the gastrointestinal lumen to allow digestion of food.

42. **The correct answer is D.** This child has PKU due to a defect of tetrahydrobiopterin metabolism, due to a deficiency of either phenylalanine hydroxylase or (less frequently) tetrahydrobiopterin cofactor. Patients therefore cannot convert phenylalanine to tyrosine. If the defect is a tetrahydrobiopterin deficiency, the patient needs supplementation with tetrahydrobiopterin in addition to a low-phenylalanine, high-tyrosine diet. Excess phenylalanine leads to a build-up of phenylketones. Children with untreated PKU display mental and growth retardation, fair skin, eczema, and a musty body odor.

Answer A is incorrect. A diet free of branched-chain amino acids is used to treat maple syrup urine disease (MSUD). MSUD is caused by a deficiency of α-ketoacid dehydrogenase. Untreated patients present with lethargy, seizures, failure to thrive, mental retardation, and urine that smells like maple syrup.

Answer B is incorrect. Low-fructose diets are used to treat hereditary fructose intolerance, an autosomal recessive inherited disease due to a deficiency of aldolase B, causing an accumulation of fructose-1-phosphate. This accumulation decreases the available phosphate, leading to inhibition of gluconeogenesis and glycogenolysis. Patients present with jaundice, cirrhosis, and hypoglycemia after ingestion of fructose.

Answer C is incorrect. A ketogenic diet will not help this patient with PKU. Diets high in ketogenic nutrients (high in fats) are used as treatment for pyruvate dehydrogenase deficiency.

Answer E is incorrect. Low-tyrosine diets are used for the treatment of type II tyrosinemia, a disorder in which patients are unable to completely metabolize tyrosine. Patients present with mental retardation and eye and skin lesions.

43. **The correct answer is A.** This child suffers from severe combined immunodeficiency (SCID). In 3 months, she has been diagnosed with a number of severe infections with unusual pathogens common in immunocompromised individuals (*Pneumocystis jiroveci and*

Candida albicans). She also demonstrates failure to thrive, as evidenced by her growth charts. There are a variety of genetic causes of SCID; however, approximately 20% of cases (1 in 200,000 live births) are attributed to a deficiency of adenosine deaminase. The enzyme is a component of the purine salvage system, and its absence ultimately leads to an inability to complete DNA synthesis in B and T cells.

Answer B is incorrect. Aldolase B is an enzyme involved in fructose metabolism. It is needed to convert fructose-1-phosphate into glyceraldehydes and dihydroxyacetone phosphate. Individuals who are deficient in aldolase B have fructose intolerance and can experience severe hypoglycemia, vomiting, jaundice, and hemorrhage as a result of intracellular trapping of fructose-1-phosphate.

Answer C is incorrect. Arylsulfatase A is involved in lysosomal storage and converts sulfatides to galactocerebroside. Arylsulfatase A deficiency causes metachromic leukodystrophy, an autosomal recessive disorder associated with central and peripheral demyelination, ataxia, and dementia.

Answer D is incorrect. B-cell tyrosine kinase is needed for pre-B cells to mature. The gene is located on the X chromosome (Xq21.22). It is mutated in patients with X-linked agammaglobulinemia of Bruton. The disease typically manifests in male infants >6 months old, who present with recurrent respiratory infections caused by *Haemophilus influenzae*, *Streptococcus pneumoniae*, and *Staphylococcus aureus*.

Answer E is incorrect. HGPRTase is another enzyme in the purine salvage system. It is responsible for converting hypoxanthine to IMP and guanine to GMP. HGPRTase deficiency is X-linked recessive and causes Lesch-Nyhan syndrome, characterized by excess uric acid production, gout, mental retardation, self-mutilation, and aggressive behavior.

44. **The correct answer is E.** Steroid hormones enter cells and bind to receptor proteins. The receptor-hormone complex binds to specific response elements, or the regulatory region of DNA, and activates gene transcription.

Answer A is incorrect. Steroid hormones do not regulate the initiation of protein synthesis.

Answer B is incorrect. Steroid hormones do not regulate mRNA degradation.

Answer C is incorrect. Steroid hormones do not regulate mRNA processing.

Answer D is incorrect. Steroid hormones regulate gene transcription, not translation.

45. **The correct answer is A.** This patient has factor V Leiden thrombophilia, an inherited condition that predisposes patients to thromboses, especially those in unusual locations (eg., the mesenteric veins), and repeated thrombotic events (superficial and/or deep). Many patients have their first thrombotic event at <50 years old. Heterozygous patients have a slightly increased risk of thrombotic events, while homozygous individuals are at a significantly increased risk.

Answer B is incorrect. Familial hypercholesterolemia leads to increased levels of low-density lipoprotein cholesterol, thereby increasing the risk of atherosclerosis, myocardial infarction, and stroke.

Answer C is incorrect. People with Fanconi's anemia have a pancytopenia that causes increased incidence of infections, anemia, fatigue, and bleeding.

Answer D is incorrect. von Hippel-Lindau disease is characterized by abnormal blood vessel growth leading to angiomas and hemangioblastomas in the retina, brain, and spinal cord as well as in other regions of the body.

Answer E is incorrect. von Willebrand's deficiency causes a prolonged bleeding time, which manifests as increased bleeding after trauma or surgery, nosebleeds, and hematomas.

46. **The correct answer is D.** Fructose-1-phosphate is metabolized to dihydroxyacetone-phosphate + glyceraldehyde. This reaction is catalyzed by aldolase B. If there is a deficiency in aldolase B, the reactant fructose-1-phosphate accumulates in the liver. This depletes the liver's stores of free phosphate, which is necessary for the creation of ATP. Thus, aldolase B deficiency causes a fall in ATP production. Fructokinase deficiency produces an elevation of fructose in the body and does not affect essential processes such as ATP production.

Answer A is incorrect. ATP will not be increased, because much of the free phosphate needed to combine with adenosine diphosphate to form ATP is already bound to fructose.

Answer B is incorrect. Phosphate will be sequestered as fructose-1-phosphate, and the amount of free circulating phosphate will fall.

Answer C is incorrect. This occurs with fructokinase deficiency.

Answer E is incorrect. If aldolase B is deficient, the end product of the fructokinase pathway will be great, and this will feedback-inhibit the activity of fructokinase.

47. **The correct answer is B.** This patient suffers from methemoglobinemia, which is characterized by a high blood level of methemoglobin in which the oxygen-caring iron is present in the oxidized (Fe^{3+}) state instead of the normal (Fe^{2+}) reduced state. The oxidized form of hemoglobin (Fe^{3+}) does not bind oxygen effectively. Thus, signs and symptoms of methemoglobinemia reflect decreased blood oxygen content and subsequent cellular hypoxia, including headache, dizziness, and nausea, and at higher levels, shortness of breath, confusion, seizures, and coma. Cyanosis that is worst in the fingernails, ears, and lips may be present on physical exam. Because oxygen diffusion is not impaired, the arterial partial pressure of oxygen will be normal. However, blood may have a characteristic muddy color secondary to the oxidization state of iron. Methemoglobinemia may occur as an adverse effect of oxidizing agents such as sulfonamides, from hereditary hemoglobin abnormalities, or secondary to a hereditary deficiency of NADH. Methylene blue has been shown to increase the conversion of Fe^{3+} back to Fe^{2+}.

Answer A is incorrect. Hyperbaric oxygen is used to treat carbon monoxide poisoning. Carbon monoxide binds to hemoglobin with significantly higher affinity than oxygen, thus displacing oxygen from hemoglobin and decreasing the oxygen carrying capacity of blood. Further mechanisms of carbon monoxide toxicity may include inhibition of cytochrome oxidase and binding to myoglobin. Like methemoglobinemia, signs and symptoms include headache, dizziness, and nausea, and at higher levels, confusion, seizures, and coma. Death may occur. Although the arterial partial oxygen pressure may be normal as in methemoglobinemia, carbon monoxide poisoning is characterized by cherry-red skin color due to the presence of carboxyhemoglobin. Hyperbaric oxygen aids in the displacement of carbon monoxide from hemoglobin, thus improving its elimination.

Answer C is incorrect. N-Acetylcysteine is used to treat acetaminophen toxicity, most likely by reducing the effects of toxic metabolites. Signs and symptoms of acetaminophen overdose include anorexia, nausea, or vomiting, followed by elevation of aspartate aminotransferase and alanine aminotransferase within 48 hours of ingestion. Fulminant hepatic failure and death may occur. Muddy blood and cyanosis is characteristic of methemoglobinemia, not cyanide poisoning.

Answer D is incorrect. Protamine is used to reverse the effects of heparin. Heparin overdose can lead to excessive anticoagulation and bleeding. Protamine is a positively charged molecule that works by binding to negatively charged heparin.

Answer E is incorrect. Sodium thiosulfate and sodium and amyl nitrites are used to treat hydrogen cyanide toxicity. Cyanide is a toxic gas that binds irreversibly and inhibits the function of the enzyme cytochrome c oxidase, thus impairing the electron transport chain and aerobic respiration. Like methemoglobinemia, signs and symptoms include headache, dizziness, and nausea, and at higher levels, shortness of breath, confusion, seizures, and coma. However, muddy blood and cyanosis is characteristic of methemoglobinemia, not cyanide

poisoning. The nitrites oxidize hemoglobin, inducing methemoglobinemia. Cyanide binds more tightly to methemoglobin than to cytochrome c oxidase, resulting in the formation of cyanmethemoglobin. Sodium thiosulfate converts this product into thiocyanate, an excretable product.

48. **The correct answer is C.** This baby was born prematurely, and therefore his lungs have not fully developed. Type II pneumocytes in the lungs are responsible for secreting surfactant (dipalmitoyl phosphatidylcholine). Additionally, a lecithin:sphingomyelin ratio <2.0 is associated with a greater risk of neonatal respiratory distress syndrome. This baby is showing signs of neonatal respiratory distress syndrome due to the lack of surfactant.

Answer A is incorrect. Angiotensin-converting enzyme (ACE) is found primarily in the lungs but is also present throughout the body. ACE is a key enzyme involved in the renin-angiotensin system and converts angiotensin I to angiotensin II, a potent vasoconstrictor. However, it is not associated with neonatal distress syndrome.

Answer B is incorrect. Collagen is an important part of the connective tissues in lungs. However, it is not associated with neonatal respiratory distress syndrome.

Answer D is incorrect. Elastase is an endogenous proteolytic enzyme in the lung that is normally broken down by α_1-antitrypsin. In patients with α_1-antitrypsin deficiency, however, there is an increased level of elastase, which leads to lung tissue destruction and emphysema.

Answer E is incorrect. Cilia dysfunction may result in decreased mucus clearance from lungs and predispose patients to recurrent respiratory infections that can cause increased respiratory distress.

Answer F is incorrect. Myelin is synthesized by Schwann cells. It is layered onto nerves and helps speed up the transmission of electrical impulses down a nerve. Destruction of myelin has been implicated in neurodegenerative diseases such as multiple sclerosis.

49. **The correct answer is B.** A cell with the shortest G_1 phase is a cell that is rapidly dividing, as is the case with a mucosal cell of the intestine. Neurons and myocytes replicate relatively slowly as compared to mucosal cells. The oocyte in the adult female does not undergo mitosis at all, nor does the RBC.

Answer A is incorrect. Hepatocytes do not ordinarily replicate rapidly unless part of the liver is removed, prompting hepatic regeneration.

Answer C is incorrect. Neurons replicate extremely slowly and would have a long G_1 phase.

Answer D is incorrect. Oocytes of the adult female do not undergo mitosis. Spermatocytes of the adult male do.

Answer E is incorrect. RBCs do not divide.

50. **The correct answer is F.** This question describes a Southwestern blot. In a Southwestern blot procedure, protein is separated by electrophoresis and labeled DNA is used as a probe. This technique can be used to detect protein-DNA interactions such as those with transcription factors.

Answer A is incorrect. ELISA is an immunologic technique used in laboratories to determine whether a particular antibody is present in a patient's blood. Labeled antibodies are used to detect whether serum contains antibodies against a specific antigen precoated on an ELISA plate. This is not the technique described above.

Answer B is incorrect. Northern blots are similar to Southern blots except that in Northern blotting, mRNA is separated by electrophoresis instead of DNA. This is not the technique described above.

Answer C is incorrect. PCR is a laboratory technique used to produce many copies of a segment of DNA. In this procedure, DNA is mixed with two specific primers, deoxynucleotides and a heat-stable polymerase. The solution is heated to denature the DNA and is then cooled to allow synthesis. Twenty cycles of heating and cooling amplify the DNA more than a million times. This is not the procedure described above.

Answer D is incorrect. Sequencing is a laboratory technique that utilizes dideoxynucleotides to randomly terminate growing strands of DNA. Gel electrophoresis is used to separate the varying lengths of DNA. The DNA sequence can then be read based on the position of the bands on the gel. This is not the technique described above.

Answer E is incorrect. In a Southern blot procedure, DNA is separated with electrophoresis, denatured, transferred to a filter, and hybridized with a labeled DNA probe. Regions on the filter that base-pair with the labeled DNA probes can be identified when the filter is exposed to film that is sensitive to the radiolabeled probe. This is not the procedure described above.

Answer G is incorrect. In a Western blot procedure, protein is separated by electrophoresis and labeled antibodies are used as a probe. This technique can be used to detect the existence of an antibody to a particular protein.

CHAPTER 3

Embryology

1. A physician is asked to evaluate a 5-year-old girl who has developed a mass in her neck. During the interview, he learns that the mass appeared within the past few months and has been enlarging; however, it causes no pain or discomfort. The mass is in the midline of the neck just below the hyoid bone. Laboratory tests reveal a triiodothyronine level of 150 ng/dL, a thyroxine level of 8.0 μg/dL, and a thyroid-stimulating hormone level of 1 μU/mL. A CT scan of the neck is performed and the doctor recommends surgery. What is the most likely diagnosis?

   (A) Branchial cleft cyst
   (B) Dermoid cyst
   (C) Ectopic thyroid gland
   (D) Enlarged pyramidal lobe of the thyroid
   (E) Lipoma
   (F) Thyroglossal duct cyst

2. A 5-year-old girl is brought to her pediatrician because her mother says she is frequently bumping into stationary objects while playing. Visual field examination shows bilateral peripheral vision defects. CT of the head reveals calcifications in the pituitary fossa. Which of the following is the most likely origin of this child's brain tumor?

   (A) Adenohypophyseal lactotrophs
   (B) Fourth ventricle neuroectoderm
   (C) Rathke's pouch
   (D) Vascular endothelium
   (E) Ventricular lining

3. A newborn infant is found to have a congenital urethral abnormality in which the urethral meatus opens on the ventral side of the penis, resulting in difficulty directing the urine stream and ventral curvature of the penis. Which of the following is the cause of this malformation?

   (A) Failure of urethral fold fusion
   (B) Failure of urethrorectal septum formation
   (C) Maldevelopment of the urinary sphincters
   (D) Short urethra
   (E) Urethral stricture

4. A neonate is found to have strong, bounding pulses in both upper extremities and carotids, but her femoral pulses are very weak. She is diagnosed with coarctation of the aorta and is taken to surgery to correct the defect. Subsequent follow-up examinations show no further heart abnormalities. Sixteen years later, the patient is noted to have poorly developed secondary sexual characteristics, including persistent, nonprogressive Tanner stage 2 breast and pubic hair development. She has not experienced menarche. Which of the following would most likely be found in this patient?

   (A) Decreased estrogen levels
   (B) Normal ovaries
   (C) Patent ductus arteriosus
   (D) Simian crease
   (E) 46,XY karyotype

5. A newborn boy is brought to the pediatrician for further evaluation of an extensive skin rash. Physical examination shows that this child has microcephaly, hearing loss, and a petechial skin rash. The abdominal examination reveals hepatosplenomegaly. Further questioning of the infant's mother reveals that she had "the flu" early in her pregnancy. A tissue sample from the infant is sent for culture, which confirms the diagnosis. Which of the following is the correct diagnosis?

   (A) Congenitally acquired cytomegalovirus
   (B) Congenitally acquired Epstein-Barr virus
   (C) Congenitally acquired herpes simplex virus
   (D) Congenitally acquired HIV
   (E) Congenitally acquired syphilis

6. A 13-month-old child is brought to the emergency department after his parents found blood in his stool. They state that he did not appear distressed at the time, although he now displays some tenderness to abdominal pressure. Other than this tenderness, there are no significant findings on physical examination. After performing radionuclide imaging using 99mTc pertechnetate, the doctor makes a diagnosis

and recommends surgery to correct the problem. What is the probable source of this child's condition?

(A) Blockage of the intestine due to folding of the distal ileum into the proximal colon
(B) Breakdown of the stomach mucosal barrier with erosion of the underlying mucosa
(C) Damage to the intestinal epithelium due to ingestion of coins
(D) Ectopic gastric epithelium in a persistent omphalomesenteric duct
(E) Incomplete bowel rotation resulting in obstruction of the superior mesenteric artery

7. The accompanying image shows the x-ray findings in a congenital condition. Which of the following is the most common cause of death in infants with this condition?

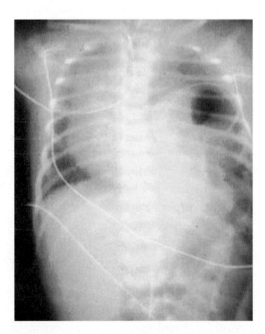

Reproduced, with permission, from PEIR Digital Library (http://peir.net).

(A) Cardiac tamponade
(B) Mediastinal shift
(C) Pulmonary hypoplasia
(D) Renal agenesis
(E) Small bowel obstruction

8. An infant girl presents with cyanosis 4 hours after birth. A physician diagnoses her with a con-

dition that develops due to a failure of neural crest cell migration that results in a nonspiraling aorticopulmonary septum. A careful interview of the mother reveals that she has a disease that predisposed her child to this congenital condition. Which of the following collections of symptoms is this infant's mother most likely experiencing?

(A) Arachnodactyly, hyperextensible joints, and aortic aneurysm
(B) Cold intolerance, delayed reflexes, constipation
(C) Megaloblastic anemia without neurologic symptoms
(D) Mild fever with a descending maculopapular rash and clear buccal mucosa
(E) Polydipsia, polyuria, and blurred vision

9. Spermatogenesis, the process of forming spermatozoa, occurs in the seminiferous tubules. As the cells proceed through the different stages of spermatogenesis, they contain varying numbers of chromosomes and varying amounts of DNA. Spermiogenesis describes a particular stage of spermatogenesis. When the cells are going through spermiogenesis, which of the following is the amount of DNA and the number of chromosomes that exist in those cells?

(A) 23, 1n
(B) 23, 2n
(C) 46, 1n
(D) 46, 2n
(E) 46, 4n

10. A 1-week-old infant presents with a urachal fistula, which occurs when the allantois fails to regress. Normally, the allantois and urachus regress to form a specific structure in the fully matured neonate. Which of the following is the mature structure derived from the fetal allantois and urachus?

(A) Ligamentum arteriosum
(B) Ligamentum teres hepatis
(C) Ligamentum venosum
(D) Medial umbilical ligament
(E) Median umbilical ligament
(F) Nucleus pulposus

11. The pancreas is derived from two elements of the foregut: the ventral pancreatic bud and the dorsal pancreatic bud. The ventral bud is responsible for part of the head, the uncinate process, and one other structure. Which of the following is the additional structure formed from the ventral pancreatic bud?

    (A) Body of the pancreas
    (B) Isthmus of the pancreas
    (C) Main pancreatic duct
    (D) Pancreatic acinar cells
    (E) Pancreatic islet cells
    (F) Tail of the pancreas

12. A full-term neonate presents to the pediatrician with failure to pass meconium. Digital examination of the rectum results in a gush of retained fecal material. Which of the following is the most likely diagnosis in this infant?

    (A) Carcinoma of the colon
    (B) Chagas' disease
    (C) Hirschsprung's disease
    (D) Imperforate anus
    (E) Necrotizing enterocolitis

13. Immediately following delivery, a newborn is observed to have multiple abnormalities, including a small lower jaw, abnormal feet, and hands that are clenched into fists. Despite supportive therapy for a congenital heart condition, the baby dies before 1 year of age. What is the likely etiology of the patient's condition?

    (A) CAG tandem repeats
    (B) Deletion of chromosome 21
    (C) Trisomy of chromosome 13
    (D) Trisomy of chromosome 18
    (E) X chromosome fragility

14. A 5-year-old boy presents to his pediatrician with dyspnea on exertion. His mother says that when he exercises, he becomes slightly blue and breathes unusually heavily. When asked, the boy states that he becomes more comfortable when squatting. Which of the following embryologic defects underlies this condition?

    (A) Anterosuperior displacement of the aorticopulmonary septum

(B) Incomplete expansion and division of the bronchial tree
(C) Incomplete formation of the tracheoesophageal septum
(D) Incomplete fusion of the right bulbar ridge, the left bulbar ridge, and the AV cushions
(E) Nonspiral development of the aorticopulmonary septum

15. A 6-year-old boy who was born prematurely presents to his pediatrician because his mother says that he tires easily. She also notes that he has had several respiratory infections. On examination, the boy is noted to be below the fifth percentile in height; jugular venous pressure is elevated; lips are slightly cyanotic; and a continuous "machine-like" murmur is heard over the left upper sternal border. The congenital anomaly responsible for these signs and symptoms produces which of the following patterns of blood flow in fetal life?

    (A) It shunts blood from the inferior vena cava to the aorta
    (B) It shunts blood from the left pulmonary artery to the aorta
    (C) It shunts blood from the left ventricle to the right ventricle
    (D) It shunts blood from the portal vein to the inferior vena cava
    (E) It shunts blood from the right atrium to the left atrium

16. A baby boy dies 2 days after birth. He was born with wrinkled skin, deformed limbs, and abnormal facies. The mother's pregnancy was complicated by oligohydramnios. Which of the following embryologic processes most likely failed in this child?

    (A) Development of dermis
    (B) Development of the kidneys
    (C) Fusion of maxillary and medial nasal prominences
    (D) Migration of neural crest cells to the distal colon
    (E) Outgrowth of limb buds

17. As part of the routine physical examination, physicians typically evaluate palatal elevation by asking the patient to "say ah." The muscles used to perform palatal elevation are derived from which of the following embryologic structures?

    (A) Branchial arches 1 and 2
    (B) Branchial arches 3 and 4
    (C) Branchial arches 4 and 6
    (D) Branchial clefts 1 and 2
    (E) Branchial pouches 3 and 4

18. A 26-year-old woman learns she is pregnant shortly after discontinuing isotretinoin (13-cis-retoinic acid). During which period of development should this woman be most concerned about fetal teratogen exposure?

    (A) Conception
    (B) Weeks 1-2 of gestation
    (C) Weeks 3–8 of gestation
    (D) Weeks 8–10 of gestation
    (E) After the 10th week of gestation

19. A 3-week-old boy presents to his pediatrician because his mother has noticed that he "looks yellow." On questioning, she elaborates that the jaundice began several days after birth and has been associated with dark urine and acholic stools. Laboratory studies show a direct bilirubin level of 5.0 mg/dL and a total bilirubin level of 5.5 mg/dL. Which of the following is the most likely diagnosis?

    (A) Congenital extrahepatic biliary atresia
    (B) Crigler-Najjar syndrome type I
    (C) Gilbert syndrome
    (D) Hereditary spherocytosis
    (E) Physiological jaundice

20. Over the course of embryologic development, the predominant location of hematopoiesis changes several times. Where does this process take place during the 11th week of fetal life?

    (A) Bone marrow
    (B) Gastric fundus
    (C) Liver
    (D) Pancreas
    (E) Yolk sac

1. **The correct answer is F.** The thyroid gland originates as the thyroid diverticulum on the floor of the pharynx. It descends into the neck during development, but remains connected to the tongue by the thyroglossal duct. The thyroglossal duct eventually disappears, leaving a small cavity (the foramen cecum) at the base of the tongue. The pyramidal lobe of the thyroid can be thought of as the caudal part of the duct. Occasionally, part of the duct epithelium persists in the neck and may form cysts. Thyroglossal duct cysts are usually painless or slightly tender and appear in the midline of the neck. They often appear over or just below the hyoid, but may appear anywhere between the base of the tongue and the thyroid. If a normal thyroid gland is present, surgery to remove the thyroglossal duct cyst is recommended to prevent infection. In this case, the presence of a normal thyroid is demonstrated by normal triiodothyronine, thyroxine, and thyroid-stimulating hormone levels and is confirmed by CT scan.

Answer A is incorrect. Branchial cleft cysts can also occur in the neck but are not always in the midline. Unlike thyroglossal duct cysts, they are often associated with fistulas or sinus tracts.

Answer B is incorrect. Dermoid cysts are the second most common cause of midline neck masses, after thyroglossal duct cysts. They tend to be more superficial than thyroglossal duct cysts and more mobile relative to underlying structures.

Answer C is incorrect. Ectopic thyroid glands are often seen in the presence of a thyroglossal duct cyst. An ectopic thyroid gland occurs when the thyroid fails to descend during development; in contrast, ectopic thyroid tissue may occur along the path of the thyroglossal duct in the presence of a normal thyroid gland. Unlike this patient, who has normal thyroid levels, about one third of patients with an ectopic gland are hypothyroid. A CT scan is usually performed to confirm the presence of a normal

thyroid gland before surgery is performed on a thyroglossal duct cyst.

Answer D is incorrect. Hypertrophy of the pyramidal lobe of the thyroid is not the most likely cause of midline neck swelling in a young child. Furthermore, hypertrophic thyroid tissue would most likely alter thyroid hormone and thyroid-stimulating hormone levels.

Answer E is incorrect. Lipomas may cause neck swelling, but the location of this mass and the age of the patient make a thyroglossal duct cyst much more likely. Lipomas tend to be very superficial, with poorly defined edges.

2. **The correct answer is C.** The visual field defect described is a bitemporal hemianopia, typically caused by lesions in the sella turcica impinging on the optic chiasm. In children the most common tumor in this location is a craniopharyngioma, derived from the remnants of Rathke's pouch. This embryologic structure buds from the roof of the mouth to form the anterior pituitary. Bitemporal hemianopia is typically accompanied by severe headaches and poor pituitary function. Treatment includes surgery, radiotherapy, or both.

Answer A is incorrect. Pituitary adenomas, derived from secretory cells of the adenohypophysis, can cause bitemporal hemianopia and headaches, as they are also sella turcica tumors. However, they are more common in older patients, and are unlikely in a child. Also, pituitary adenomas tend to secrete pituitary hormones. The three most common forms of pituitary adenoma are prolactinomas (which are derived from lactotrophs and secrete prolactin, causing galactorrhea and amenorrhea), growth hormone-secreting tumors (somatotrophs, causing acromegaly), and ACTH-producing tumors (corticotrophs, causing Cushing's disease). In this case, the only data making this an incorrect answer are the patient's age and the lack of secretory action.

Answer B is incorrect. Medulloblastoma arises from primitive neuroectoderm in the fourth ventricle. It does not cause the visual symptoms seen in this patient, but the tumor may compress the fourth ventricle to cause hydrocephalus and symptoms consistent with increased intracranial pressure such as morning headache and vomiting. An additional, specific sign of this posterior fossa tumor is a head tilt. Treatment consists of surgery, chemotherapy, and radiation. When in doubt, remember that medulloblastoma is the most common malignant brain tumor in children.

Answer D is incorrect. Hemangioblastomas are vascular tumors of the central nervous system that usually occur in the cerebellum and spinal cord and thus would be unlikely to cause the visual field defects described in this case. Symptoms include cerebellar ataxia, motor weakness, and sensory dysfunction. Hemangioblastomas can occur sporadically or in patients with von Hippel-Lindau disease, which is an autosomal dominant disease in which patients develop cerebellar and retinal hemangioblastomas, pancreatic cysts, and pheochromocytomas.

Answer E is incorrect. Ependymomas form from the cells lining the ventricles and most often occur in the fourth ventricle. Like medulloblastomas, ependymomas can block the flow of cerebrospinal fluid and cause hydrocephalus. These patients, however, do not have the visual disturbances of the patient in this vignette.

3. **The correct answer is A.** The malformation described is hypospadias, resulting from incomplete union of the urethral folds. In the male, the urethral folds form the ventral aspect of the penis. In the female, the urethral folds develop into the labia minora.

Answer B is incorrect. Congenital failure of urethrorectal septum formation results in an abnormal communication between the urethra and the rectum. Clinical signs include feces in the urine. This is not a cause of hypospadias.

Answer C is incorrect. In males, the proximal portion of the urethra forms from the urogenital sinus. The distal urethra is formed by ectoderm that is canalized to form the navicular fossa. If the sphincters do not form properly,

urethral incompetence and incontinence result.

Answer D is incorrect. A short urethra causes chordee, or poorly developed penis with ventral curvature, without hypospadias.

Answer E is incorrect. Urethral stricture causes urethral obstruction and is the second most common cause of incontinence in older men. It is not a cause of hypospadias.

4. **The correct answer is A.** The patient has Turner's syndrome, which is associated with coarctation of the aorta. Turner's syndrome often presents in adolescence with amenorrhea, and a diagnostic work-up shows a 45,XO karyotype. Patients with Turner's syndrome have poor development of secondary sexual characteristics and are infertile.

Answer B is incorrect. Patients with Turner's syndrome have rudimentary ovaries; sexual ducts and external genital structures appear normal but are very immature. When examined histologically at or after birth, the ovaries are found to be long, pale streaks of tissue devoid of primordial follicles. Early in gestation the ovaries appear normal and contain primordial germ cells, but after the third month, numbers become severely reduced, and in most patients oocytes are not present after birth. These patients are therefore infertile and do not naturally progress through puberty.

Answer C is incorrect. Turner's syndrome is not associated with a patent ductus arteriosus (PDA). Furthermore, in the vignette the patient's cardiac examination is normal. With a PDA, the patient would have a continuous machinelike murmur.

Answer D is incorrect. A simian crease is commonly seen in Down's syndrome (trisomy 21). It is not seen in Turner's syndrome.

Answer E is incorrect. Patients with Turner's syndrome have a 45,XO karyotype. In androgen insensitivity syndrome (testicular feminization), a genetically male patient can be phenotypically female; however, this is not the case with Turner's syndrome.

5. **The correct answer is A.** This is a case of congenitally acquired cytomegalovirus (CMV) infection. Fetuses exposed to CMV during the first trimester may experience intrauterine growth retardation and be afflicted with central nervous system damage, with hearing and sight impairments. Mental retardation will occur along with microcephaly. A characteristic "blueberry muffin rash" is usually present.

Answer B is incorrect. Epstein-Barr virus, the cause of infectious mononucleosis, is a rare cause of congenital defects. These defects include cataracts, hypotonia, cryptorchidism, and micrognathia.

Answer C is incorrect. Herpes simplex virus can result in a variety of congenital defects, abortions, and neonatal encephalitis.

Answer D is incorrect. Congenital HIV results in neonatal AIDS.

Answer E is incorrect. Congenital syphilis can result in cranial nerve VIII deafness, mulberry molars, saber shins, saddle nose, and Hutchinson's teeth.

6. **The correct answer is D.** The child was diagnosed with a Meckel's diverticulum, which describes the persistence after birth of part of the omphalomesenteric duct (vitelline duct or yolk stalk). Meckel's diverticulum is usually found in the mid to distal ileum and may end blindly or connect to the umbilicus. It is described by the "**rule of 2's:**" it is about **2** inches long, **2** feet from the ileocecal valve, occurs in about **2**% of the population, is often presents before age **2** years (60% of cases), and may contain **2** types of epithelium (gastic or pancreatic). Ectopic gastric epithelium can cause ulcers and bleeding, but does not generally cause severe pain unless inflammation occurs. ^{99m}Tc pertechnetate is absorbed preferentially by gastric mucosa and thus may be used to detect ectopic gastric mucosa in the diverticulum.

Answer A is incorrect. Intussusception is the folding of the distal ileum into the proximal colon. It usually presents in the first two years of life and a Meckel diverticulum may predispose to this condition. However, it typically has an abrupt and severe presentation, with paroxysmal bouts of screaming, vomiting, diarrhea, and bloody bowel movements occurring within 24 hours of onset.

Answer B is incorrect. Breakdown of the mucosal barrier of the stomach and erosion of the underlying mucosal epithelium describes the pathology of a peptic ulcer. Peptic ulcers may present at any age, but are more common in patients 12–18 years old than in very young children. Additionally, it is not diagnosed by ^{99m}Tc pertechnetate scanning and is not treated surgically unless it perforates.

Answer C is incorrect. Ingestion of foreign objects occurs frequently in young children and may cause mechanical damage to the intestinal lining. However, they are not detected with ^{99m}Tc pertechnetate scanning and rarely require surgery.

Answer E is incorrect. Abnormal or incomplete rotation of the intestine as it returns to the abdomen after physiological herniation can trap and twist loops of bowel; twisting of these loops (volvulus) can result in obstruction of circulation and potentially lead to gangrene of the affected segment of intestine. Most affected infants present within the first 3 weeks of life with bile-containing vomit or bowel obstruction. Bloody stool is not a principal sign of malrotation or volvulus.

7. **The correct answer is C.** Pulmonary hypoplasia is the most common cause of death in infants born with congenital diaphragmatic hernia. When the pleuroperitoneal folds fail to fuse with the other components of the diaphragm during development, a hole is created that allows bowel into the thorax. The physical compression of the bowels on the lung buds then prevents full development of the respiratory system (pulmonary hypoplasia). This leads to a common presentation of dyspnea and cyanosis and, unless it can be repaired surgically, eventually leads to death.

Answer A is incorrect. Cardiac tamponade is most frequently associated with a pericardial effusion. This is not a common complication of congenital diaphragmatic hernia.

Answer B is incorrect. Mediastinal shift does occur in congenital diaphragmatic hernia, as the bowel invades the thorax and pushes the mediastinum to the right. However, this in itself is not a cause of death.

Answer D is incorrect. Renal agenesis is not associated with congenital diaphragmatic hernia.

Answer E is incorrect. Although it is theoretically possible for a volvulus to develop as the bowel herniates into the thorax, small bowel obstruction is not a common complication of congenital diaphragmatic hernia.

8. **The correct answer is E.** This question requires three steps to answer. First, the clinical scenario should be recognized as transposition of the great vessels. Early cyanosis is typically one of three conditions: Transposition, Tetralogy of Fallot, or Truncus arteriosus (the "3 T's"). Of these, only transposition is due to nonspiral development of the aorticopulmonary septum. Second, it must be known that maternal diabetes increases the risk of having a child with transposition. Finally, the common symptoms of diabetes must be known: polydipsia, polyuria, and blurred vision.

Answer A is incorrect. These are the symptoms seen in patients with Marfan's syndrome, a condition caused by a defect of connective tissue. This condition is not associated with transposition in the offspring of people with Marfan's syndrome.

Answer B is incorrect. These symptoms describe hypothyroidism, which does not increase the risk of congenital defects.

Answer C is incorrect. This describes the result of folate deficiency. This is associated with neural tube defects in the offspring but not with transposition of the great vessels.

Answer D is incorrect. These symptoms describe rubella, the result of infection by *Rubivirus*, a togavirus. Maternal rubella leads to many congenital defects, including patent ductus arteriosus, ventral septal defect, cataracts, and deafness, but it is not associated with transposition.

9. **The correct answer is A.** Spermiogenesis is the series of postmeiotic morphologic changes that mark the final maturation of the sperm. Spermatids are the 23, 1n cells that result from secondary spermatocyte meiosis II completion. They undergo morphologic changes to become mature sperm that include acrosome, head, neck, and tail formation.

Answer B is incorrect. Secondary spermatocytes are 23, 2n cells that result from primary spermatocytes completing meiosis I. Each primary spermatocyte forms two secondary spermatocytes.

Answer C is incorrect. At no point during male gametogenesis is there a haploid cell with 46 chromosomes.

Answer D is incorrect. Both primordial germ cells in the testes, which are dormant until puberty, and type A spermatogonia, which develop at puberty, are 46, 2n cell types. A type A spermatogonium perpetuates itself to provide a constant supply of sperm cells; it also differentiates into type B spermatogonia.

Answer E is incorrect. Primary spermatocytes are 46, 4n cells that result from type B spermatogonia DNA replication.

10. **The correct answer is E.** The allantois and urachus form the median umbilical ligament. Do not confuse this with the medial umbilical ligaments, which are remnants of the umbilical arteries. Even if one did not know the answer to this question immediately, it could be deduced from the fact that, of the answer choices, only the median umbilical ligament is related to the umbilical cord, through which the allantoic duct passes.

Answer A is incorrect. The ligamentum arteriosum is the derivative of the ductus arteriosus, which serves to shunt blood from the pulmonary artery to the aorta in fetal circulation.

Answer B is incorrect. The ligamentum teres hepatis is the derivative of the umbilical vein, which brings oxygenated blood from the maternal circulation to the fetus.

Answer C is incorrect. The ligamentum venosum is the derivative of the ductus venosus, which shunts blood from the portal vein to the inferior vena cava.

Answer D is incorrect. The medial umbilical ligaments are remnants of the umbilical arteries. This should not be confused with the median umbilical ligament, which is involved in the formation of a urachal fistula.

Answer F is incorrect. The nucleus pulposus is a remnant of the notochord.

11. **The correct answer is C.** The ventral pancreatic bud also forms the main pancreatic duct in addition to the uncinate process and a part of the head. The dorsal pancreatic duct is responsible for the rest of the structural components of the pancreas, including the portion of the head not formed by the ventral bud.

    Answer A is incorrect. The pancreatic body is formed by the dorsal pancreatic bud.

    Answer B is incorrect. The pancreatic isthmus is formed by the dorsal pancreatic bud.

    Answer D is incorrect. Pancreatic acinar cells, as well as duct epithelium, are formed from endoderm. In general, epithelium and glands of the gastrointestinal mucosa are formed from endoderm.

    Answer E is incorrect. Pancreatic islet cells, like pancreatic acinar cells, are derived from endoderm.

    Answer F is incorrect. The pancreatic tail is formed by the dorsal pancreatic bud.

12. **The correct answer is C.** This patient's inability to pass meconium, as well as the subsequent digital disimpaction, is consistent with Hirschsprung's disease, or congenital megacolon. This disorder is characterized by the absence of ganglion cells in the large bowel, leading to functional obstruction and colonic dilatation proximal to the affected segment. Signs and symptoms of the disease result from failure of neural crest cell migration into the bowel wall during development.

    Answer A is incorrect. Carcinoma of the colon can result in mechanical obstruction of the colon and present like acquired megacolon. However, colonic malignancies develop over time because the cells need to undergo multiple mutations before undergoing transformation. Thus, colon carcinoma would be unlikely in this infant.

    Answer B is incorrect. Chronic Chagas' disease, a result of *Trypanosoma cruzi* infection, can result in acquired megacolon, an unlikely possibility in a neonate.

    Answer D is incorrect. A neonate with imperforate anus will present with inability to pass meconium. However, digital examination of the rectum and subsequent disimpaction rule out this diagnosis.

    Answer E is incorrect. Necrotizing enterocolitis occurs in a preterm infant and not in a full-term one. This condition usually occurs secondary to bowel ischemia.

13. **The correct answer is D.** This newborn has Edwards' syndrome, or trisomy 18. Affected children are born with clenched fists, rocker-bottom feet, micrognathia (a small lower jaw), congenital heart disease, and mental retardation. The survival rate of less than 1 year is similar to that of trisomy 13 (Patau's syndrome), from which it should be distinguished.

    Answer A is incorrect. CAG tandem repeats are found in Huntington's disease, among others. Huntington's disease is characterized by degeneration of the caudate and putamen, leading to choreiform (dancelike) movements, but not the birth defects found in this patient.

    Answer B is incorrect. A deletion of chromosome 21 may cause physical deformity, but clenched fists and rocker-bottom feet are classic for trisomy 18.

    Answer C is incorrect. Trisomy of chromosome 13, or Patau's syndrome, is characterized by a constellation of findings including mental retardation, microphthalmia, microcephaly, cleft lip/palate, abnormal forebrain structures, polydactyly, and congenital heart disease.

Answer E is incorrect. This is fragile X syndrome. Associated with CGG tandem repeats, this syndrome is characterized by mental retardation, a large jaw, and large testes. Children with fragile X syndrome typically survive beyond 1 year of age.

14. **The correct answer is A.** **P**ulmonary valve stenosis (as evidenced here by the left upper sternal border systolic murmur), **R**ight ventricular hypertrophy, an **O**verriding aorta, and a **V**entricular septal defect are the four components of the tetralogy of Fallot (remember the mnemonic **PROVe**). This condition results from abnormal migration of neural crest cells and results in the aorticopulmonary septum being displaced anterosuperiorly. Life-threatening hypoxia may develop. The child will often squat in an effort to relieve hypoxia; squatting increases the systemic pressure, thereby reducing the right-to-left shunt and improving oxygenation. Treatment is corrective surgery.

Answer B is incorrect. Incomplete development of the bronchial tree leads to pulmonary hypoplasia. This may produce dyspnea but is otherwise inconsistent with this presentation.

Answer C is incorrect. A tracheoesophageal fistula is the result of incomplete formation of the tracheoesophageal septum. This produces gagging and possibly cyanosis on feeding but is not associated with any of the other findings in this vignette.

Answer D is incorrect. This describes the etiology of a pure ventricular septal defect (VSD). A VSD does not produce cyanosis unless it leads to Eisenmenger's syndrome, in which pulmonary hypertension transforms a left-to-right shunt into a right-to-left shunt. Moreover, a simple VSD does not cause any of the other findings of tetralogy of Fallot.

Answer E is incorrect. Nonspiral development of the aorticopulmonary septum results in transposition of the great vessels. This does cause dyspnea and cyanosis but it is evident much earlier in life and would not result in an echocardiogram showing tetralogy of Fallot.

15. **The correct answer is B.** The child is presenting with common signs and symptoms of a patent ductus arteriosus (PDA). In the fetus, the ductus arteriosus serves to shunt blood from the left pulmonary artery to the aorta, allowing the blood to avoid the high-resistance lungs and delivering more oxygenated blood to the rest of the body. Failure of the ductus arteriosus to close is common in premature babies, as in this case as well as in cases of maternal rubella during pregnancy. Indomethacin, a nonsteroidal anti-inflammatory drug, blocks the production of PGE_1 and can be used to close a PDA.

Answer A is incorrect. There is no fetal structure or congenital anomaly that shunts blood from the inferior vena cava to the aorta.

Answer C is incorrect. This pattern of blood flow is seen with a ventricular septal defect. This is not a normal feature of fetal circulation. After birth, this will also present with exercise intolerance but will produce a holosystolic murmur, not a continuous murmur. Also note that the question is asking about the blood flow in the fetus; because the pressure on the right side of the fetal heart is higher than the pressure on the left, blood will always be shunted from right to left, not left to right as this answer choice describes.

Answer D is incorrect. This is the pattern of blood flow of the ductus venosus. This does not lead to cardiac pathology.

Answer F is incorrect. In the fetus, the foramen ovale shunts blood from the right atrium to the left atrium, also bypassing the lungs. This typically closes at birth in response to the dramatic decrease in right atrial pressure and increase in left atrial pressure as the infant takes its first breath and opens the lungs. However, should it fail to close, a patent foramen ovale with left to right shunt results. This condition ranges in severity and may not become clinically apparent until the age of 30 or later. Signs and symptoms of a patent foramen ovale include a systolic ejection murmur (not a continuous murmur) and a widely split fixed S2.

16. **The correct answer is B.** The presentation described here is consistent with Potter's syndrome, or bilateral renal agenesis. The failure of both kidneys to develop leads to oligohydramnios because the fetus cannot excrete urine into the amniotic sac. This in turn allows compression of the fetus by the uterine wall, leading to limb deformities, abnormal facies, and wrinkly skin. Death occurs shortly after birth unless an appropriate donor is found.

Answer A is incorrect. A failure of development of the dermis would not present with oligohydramnios or deformed limbs, but rather with skin abnormalities.

Answer C is incorrect. This describes the etiology of cleft lip, which does not cause oligohydramnios or wrinkly skin and is compatible with life.

Answer D is incorrect. This describes the defect in Hirschsprung's disease, which results in failure to pass meconium and in constipation, but does not share any of the symptoms in this scenario.

Answer E is incorrect. A problem with limb bud growth would not produce abnormal facies or oligohydramnios.

17. **The correct answer is B.** The muscles that elevate the palate are derived from branchial arch 3 (the stylopharyngeus) and branchial arch 4 (the levator veli palatini). These are innervated by cranial nerves IX and X, respectively.

Answer A is incorrect. The first branchial arch generates "M" muscles: muscles of Mastication (teMporalis, Masseter, Medial and lateral pterygoids) and the Mylohyoid. The second arch gives rise to "S" muscles: Stapedius, Stylohyoid, and facial expression muscles. None of these muscles is involved in palatal elevation.

Answer C is incorrect. Although branchial arch 4 does give rise to the levator veli palatini, branchial arch 6 gives rise to the intrinsic muscles of the larynx (except the cricothyroid, which is a fourth arch derivative). These muscles are not involved in elevating the palate.

Answer D is incorrect. The first branchial cleft gives rise to the external auditory meatus, while the second, third, and fourth clefts are obliterated during development. The clefts are formed from ectoderm and could not give rise to muscles, which are derived from mesoderm.

Answer E is incorrect. Branchial pouch 3 gives rise to the thymus (ventral wings) and inferior parathyroid glands (dorsal glands), while the fourth branchial pouch gives rise to the superior parathyroids. These are obviously not involved in palatal elevation. Remember that pouches give rise to endoderm-derived tissue, while the arches give rise to mesoderm-derived tissue such as muscle.

18. **The correct answer is C.** Isotretinoin is commonly prescribed for severe acne vulgaris and is a dangerous teratogen that causes defects in fetal development. As a result, women at risk of pregnancy should undergo monthly pregnancy testing and be counseled to use two forms of contraception during treatment with isotretinoin. Like most other teratogens, exposure to isotretinoin during weeks 3–8 of fetal development is especially damaging since this is the period during which organogenesis occurs and developing fetal tissues are most susceptible to the effects of teratogens.

Answer A is incorrect. Teratogen exposure at the time of conception is less damaging and typically exerts an "all-or-nothing" effect resulting in either embryo-lethality, or no malformation at all as undifferentiated cells are simply replaced.

Answer B is incorrect. Teratogen exposure in early embryogenesis (weeks 1–2 of fetal development) normally produces an "all-or-nothing" effect on malformation and is less risky than exposure during organogenesis.

Answer D is incorrect. Teratogen exposure during weeks 8–10 of fetal development is generally less risky than exposure during weeks 3–8. However, severe birth defects are still possible as organogenesis sometimes lasts until the tenth week of fetal development.

Answer E is incorrect. Risk for malformation is less severe after the 10th week of fetal development as organogenesis is complete and most fetal structures have formed. However, teratogen exposure during this interval can lead to restrictions in fetal growth, low birth weight, and disorders of the central nervous system.

19. **The correct answer is A.** The patient is presenting with congenital extrahepatic biliary atresia. Vignettes that describe a pure elevation in direct (conjugated) bilirubin strongly suggest an obstructive etiology, as the liver is able to effectively conjugate bilirubin but fails to excrete it into the small intestine. The absence of bilirubin in the small bowel results in acholic stools while increased renal excretion of conjugated bilirubin causes a darkening of the urine. Congenital extrahepatic biliary atresia occurs when the developing bile ducts close completely and fail to recanalize. Appropriate therapy of biliary atresia involves anastomosis of the small bowel directly to intrahepatic bile ducts, a maneuver known as the Kasai procedure.

Answer B is incorrect. Crigler-Najjar syndrome type I is caused by a complete deficiency in UDP-glucuronosyltransferase, the hepatic enzyme necessary to conjugate bilirubin. This disorder produces a severe unconjugated (indirect) hyperbilirubinemia that causes death within the first few years of life. The patient in this case, however, has a conjugated hyperbilirubinemia, suggesting an obstructive cause and ruling out Crigler-Najjar syndrome.

Answer C is incorrect. Gilbert's syndrome is a benign disorder caused by a mutation in the promoter region of UDP-glucuronyltransferase, leading to diminished expression of the gene. Patients with this syndrome develop a mild unconjugated hyperbilirubinemia but are usually asymptomatic and have a normal life expectancy.

Answer D is incorrect. Hereditary spherocytosis can cause jaundice and hyperbilirubinemia secondary to hemolytic anemia. This autosomal dominant condition is due to mutations in spectrin or ankyrin causing RBC membrane defects that make the cells more fragile to hemolysis. Peripheral blood smears show small RBCs without central pallor and diagnosis can be confirmed with the osmotic fragility test. Unlike this patient, hereditary spherocytosis usually presents later in life with a mixed hyperbilirubinemia and normal stools.

Answer E is incorrect. Physiologic jaundice refers to the mild unconjugated (indirect) hyperbilirubinemia that affects nearly all newborns due to the greater turnover of neonatal RBCs and the decreased bilirubin clearance in the first few weeks of life. The peak total serum bilirubin occurs between 72 and 96 hours of age and resolves within the first few weeks of life. This patient has a severe conjugated hyperbilirubinemia that cannot be explained by normal neonatal physiological jaundice.

20. **The correct answer is C.** Until week 5, the yolk sac is solely responsible for hematopoiesis. By week 8, the liver has taken over as the predominant location. It remains so until the bone marrow takes over around week 28. The thymus and spleen also begin producing blood cells around week 12 but are never the predominant sites of hematopoiesis.

Answer A is incorrect. The bone marrow is the predominant site of hematopoiesis beginning around week 28 and remains so throughout adult life.

Answer B is incorrect. The gastric fundus is the site of parietal cells, which produce intrinsic factor and gastric acid. The stomach plays no role in hematopoiesis.

Answer D is incorrect. The pancreas produces insulin, glucagon, and digestive enzymes. It plays no role in hematopoiesis.

Answer E is incorrect. The yolk sac is the predominant site of hematopoiesis between fetal weeks 3 and 8.

CHAPTER 4

Microbiology

1. A 30-year-old sexually active woman presents with a painful vesicle on her external genitalia and bilateral inguinal lymphadenopathy. A Tzanck smear from the vesicle fails is negative, and polymerase chain reaction analysis of viral DNA is negative. A VDRL assay is also negative. Which of the following medications would be most helpful to this patient?

(A) Acyclovir
(B) Ceftriaxone
(C) Foscarnet
(D) Ribavirin
(E) Vancomycin

2. A hepatitis panel is ordered for a 27-year-old woman as part of a routine work-up for abdominal pain. Results of serologic testing are negative for HBeAg and HBsAg, but positive for HBsAb and IgG HBcAb. Which of the following is the appropriate conclusion?

(A) The patient has been exposed to hepatitis B and has completely recovered
(B) The patient has been exposed to hepatitis B and is in the acute disease phase
(C) The patient has been exposed to hepatitis B and is in the window phase
(D) The patient has been exposed to hepatitis B and is now chronically infected
(E) The patient has been exposed to hepatitis B but was never infected

3. A 43-year-old man living in Mexico presents to a clinic complaining of constipation and stomach pains for several months. On cardiac examination, the physician discovers a laterally displaced point of maximal impact. Radiological studies reveal pulmonary congestion, cardiomegaly, and megacolon. Sadly, the physician can only offer the patient symptomatic treatment. What insect is the most likely route of transmission for this patient's illness?

(A) *Anopheles* mosquito
(B) *Ixodes* tick
(C) Reduviid bug
(D) Sandfly
(E) Tsetse fly

4. A patient in the hospital develops pleuritic chest pain, shortness of breath, fever, chills, productive cough, and colored sputum after 3 days of being in the hospital for major surgery. Physical examination shows tenderness to palpation without any areas of increased tactile fremitus. Blood and sputum cultures confirm gram-negative rods that ferment lactose, have a large mucoid capsule, and form viscous colonies. The patient subsequently dies from her infection. Which of the following is most likely to be found at autopsy?

(A) Acute inflammatory infiltrates from bronchioles into adjacent alveoli
(B) Congestion, red hepatization, gray hepatization, and resolution
(C) Diffuse, patchy inflammation localized to the alveolar wall interstitium
(D) Intra-alveolar hyaline membranes without alveolar space exudates
(E) Predominantly intra-alveolar exudate resulting in consolidation

5. A homeless 37-year-old woman with HIV infection comes to the clinic with a 4-week history of worsening hemiparesis, visual field deficits, and cognitive impairment. She has gone 2 years without antiretroviral therapy. The patient's CD4+ cell count is 22/mm^3. MRI shows several hyperintensities on T2-weighted images that do not enhance with contrast and are not surrounded by edema. A lumbar puncture shows a normal opening pressure, and cerebrospinal fluid analysis shows a mildly elevated protein level and the presence of myelin basic protein, with a mild mononuclear pleocytosis. Which of the following entities is most likely responsible for this patient's clinical picture?

(A) Cytomegalovirus encephalitis
(B) JC virus
(C) Primary central nervous system lymphoma
(D) Toxoplasmosis

6. A sexually active 14-year-old boy comes to the physician because of a rash on his trunk and genital area. Physical examination reveals the

findings shown in the image. Which of the following types of virus most likely caused this patient's clinical findings?

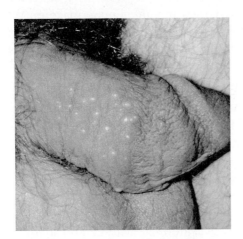

Reproduced, with permission, from Wolff K, Johnson RA, Suurmond D. *Fitzpatrick's Color Atlas & Synopsis of Clinical Dermatology*, 5th ed. New York: McGraw-Hill, 2005: Figure 25-2.

(A) Herpes simplex virus type 1
(B) Human herpesvirus 8
(C) Poxvirus
(D) Rubeola virus
(E) Varicella zoster virus

7. A 22-year-old man visits his college medical center complaining of flu-like symptoms that have persisted for about a week. He reports low-grade fevers, night sweats, a painful sore throat, headaches, and increasing fatigue. He used to exercise 5 days a week but is no longer able to because of a "lack of energy." Physical examination reveals enlarged cervical lymph nodes and a spleen that is palpable 2 inches below the left costal margin. What is the structure of the virus that has infected this patient?

(A) Linear, double-stranded, DNA virus with an envelope
(B) Linear, double-stranded, DNA virus without an envelope
(C) Linear, double-stranded, RNA virus with an envelope
(D) Partially circular, double-stranded, DNA virus with an envelope
(E) Segmented, linear, single-stranded, negative-polarity, RNA virus with an envelope

8. A 38-year-old man comes to the emergency department complaining of cyclic fevers and headaches. The fevers began about 1 week ago; 2 weeks ago the patient returned from a trip to Africa. Physical examination reveals splenomegaly, and brain imaging shows signs of significant cerebral involvement. Which of the following parasites most likely caused this patient's symptoms?

(A) *Babesia microti*
(B) *Plasmodium falciparum*
(C) *Plasmodium malariae*
(D) *Plasmodium ovale*
(E) *Plasmodium vivax*

9. A 32-year-old woman comes to the physician complaining of fever, fatigue, cough, headache, and shaking chills. Physical examination reveals an inflamed area on her right leg that, on closer examination, appears to be a tick bite. Blood samples are sent for laboratory examination, and the result of the blood smear is shown in the image. This patient is most likely infected with which of the following protozoa?

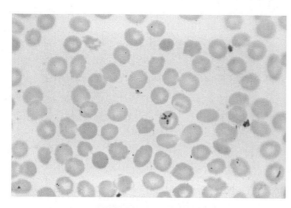

Image courtesy of the Centers for Disease Control and Prevention's Public Health Image Library; content provider Steven Glenn.

(A) *Acanthamoeba* species
(B) *Babesia* species
(C) *Leishmania donovani*
(D) *Naegleria fowleri*
(E) *Trypanosoma cruzi*

10. Oncogenic viruses act through a variety of mechanisms. Some introduce oncogenes directly into host cells, while others force cells to repeatedly undergo cycles of proliferation that eventually become unregulated. Still others introduce oncogenic potential by manipulating chromosomal structure through deletions or translocations. Which of the following viruses causes neoplasia by inactivating tumor suppressor genes such as *p53* and *Rb*?

(A) Epstein-Barr virus
(B) Hepatitis C virus
(C) HIV
(D) Human papillomavirus
(E) Human T-cell lymphotropic virus type 1

11. Influenza virus type A usually produces a mild, self-limited febrile illness in the general population. However, worldwide epidemics have occurred at different times in history due to rapid changes in viral genetic makeup. Which of the following is the most important reason why these sporadic worldwide epidemics occur?

(A) Antigenic drift
(B) Antigenic shift
(C) Hemagglutinin develops the ability to destroy a component of mucin, becoming more infectious
(D) Neuraminidase develops the ability to attach to sialic acid receptors, becoming more infectious
(E) RBCs agglutinate with certain strains

12. A 30-year-old woman comes to the physician because of a fever of 38.4°C (101.1°F) and a diffuse macular rash on her torso. Her blood pressure is 91/51 mm Hg. The physician obtains a culture from her vagina that shows catalase-positive, gram-positive cocci. Over the next few days, the rash on her torso desquamates. Which of the following organisms is most likely responsible for this patient's symptoms?

(A) *Actinomyces israelii*
(B) *Clostridium perfringens*
(C) *Proteus mirabilis*
(D) *Staphylococcus aureus*
(E) *Streptococcus pyogenes*

13. A young girl living in rural New Mexico is brought to her pediatrician with complaints of fever, cough, and fatigue for the past 2 weeks. The physician notices that the patient is having intermittent bouts of many coughs in a single breath followed by a deep inspiration. The parents report this pattern of cough had started in the past 2 days. The physician informs them that their daughter will most likely recover with only supportive care. However, he wants to confirm his diagnosis, so he sends a throat swab for culture. What type of medium should be used to grow the bacteria that are causing this patient's symptoms?

(A) Bordet-Gengou medium
(B) Charcoal yeast extract with iron and cysteine
(C) Chocolate agar with factor V and X
(D) Loffler's medium
(E) Thayer-Martin medium

14. A 40-year-old man comes to the emergency department because of diplopia and dysphagia that developed after he consumed homemade strawberry jam. While in the emergency department, he develops general muscle weakness and requires intubation due to sudden respiratory muscle paralysis. Which of the following pathogens is most likely responsible for this patient's condition?

    (A) *Bacillus cereus*
    (B) *Clostridium botulinum*
    (C) *Clostridium perfringens*
    (D) *Clostridium tetani*
    (E) Poliovirus

15. An elderly man returns to New York after spending the winter in Arizona. Over the course of the next several weeks, he develops breathing difficulty, productive cough, and joint pain. He visits his physician, who orders an x-ray of the chest, which reveals infiltrates in the lungs with evidence of granulomas. A PPD test is negative, but a tissue specimen from biopsy reveals a fungus with endospores containing spherules when grown at 37°C and branched hyphae when grown at 25°C. What is the most likely cause of his symptoms?

    (A) *Aspergillus fumigatus*
    (B) *Blastomyces dermatitidis*
    (C) *Candida albicans*
    (D) *Coccidioides immitis*
    (E) *Histoplasma capsulatum*

16. After a long camping trip in the woods, a 29-year-old man comes to the physician complaining of fever and general malaise. His physical examination is significant for a well-demarcated skin lesion with a black base on his arm. The patient recalls that earlier during his camping trip, there had been a small, itchy bump at the site of the lesion. Which of the

following organisms is most likely responsible for this patient's disease?

(A) *Borrelia burgdorferi*
(B) *Brucella melitensis*
(C) *Francisella tularensis*
(D) *Nocardia asteroides*
(E) *Yersinia pestis*

17. A 45-year-old man presents to the clinic complaining of several weeks of vague abdominal discomfort and early satiety. The physician orders upper gastrointestinal endoscopy as part of his work-up. During the study, mucosal rigidity and hyperplasia are seen in the stomach, and a biopsy is taken from the affected area. Microscopic analysis of the biopsy specimen shows sheets of atypical lymphocytes. The organism believed to be associated with this condition is best described by which set of laboratory results?

CHOICE	UREASE	CATALASE	OXIDASE
A	Negative	Negative	Negative
B	Negative	Negative	Positive
C	Negative	Positive	Negative
D	Negative	Positive	Positive
E	Positive	Negative	Negative
F	Positive	Positive	Negative
G	Positive	Positive	Positive

(A) A
(B) B
(C) C
(D) D
(E) E
(F) F
(G) G

18. A 36-year-old man comes to the physician because he is experiencing abdominal pain, vomiting, and a nonbloody diarrhea. He last ate chicken and rice about 6 hours ago at a Chinese restaurant. He has no other symptoms. Which of the following treatments should this man receive?

   (A) Bismuth subsalicylate, metronidazole, and amoxicillin
   (B) Ciprofloxacin
   (C) Erythromycin
   (D) Prompt replacement of water and electrolytes; tetracyclines shorten the disease's course
   (E) Supportive care only, without antibiotics

19. An 87-year-old man is hospitalized after falling and breaking his hip. After 6 days in the hospital, he develops burning on urination. Urinalysis shows leukocytosis and many gram-positive cocci. The patient is treated with trimethoprim-sulfamethoxazole, but his fever persists. Two days later, the patient has a low-grade fever and new onset of a diastolic murmur that radiates to the axilla. Which of the following is the first-line treatment for the probable cause of this patient's infection?

   (A) Ampicillin
   (B) Gentamicin
   (C) Piperacillin
   (D) Quinupristin/dalfopristin
   (E) Vancomycin

20. A neonate with purulent umbilical discharge for 1 day presents with fever, irritability, and diffuse flushing. One day later she is covered in large, fluid-filled blisters that rupture easily, leaving raw red areas beneath. Gram stain of a peripheral blood smear is shown in the image. This set of symptoms is due to separation at what layer of skin?

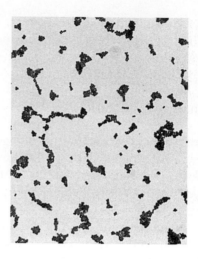

Reproduced, with permission, from Brooks GF, Carroll KC, Butel JS, Morse SA. *Jawetz, Melnick, & Adelberg's Medical Microbiology*, 24th ed. New York: McGraw-Hill, 2007: Figure 14-1.

   (A) Papillary dermis
   (B) Stratum basale
   (C) Stratum corneum
   (D) Stratum granulosum
   (E) Stratum lucidum

21. A 4-year-old boy presents to the pediatric emergency department with the classic meningitis triad of fever, headache, and nuchal rigidity. A lumbar puncture is performed and analysis of the fluid shows an increase in polymorphonuclear cells, an increased protein level, and a decreased glucose level. Which of the following is the most common cause of meningitis in a child of this age with this clinical picture?

   (A) Enteroviruses
   (B) Haemophilus influenzae type B
   (C) Herpes simplex virus
   (D) Listeria species
   (E) *Streptococcus pneumoniae*

22. A 32-year-old man presents to his doctor with painful urination and a purulent urethral discharge. The image shows cells that have been cultured from this discharge. Which of the following is the treatment of choice for this infection?

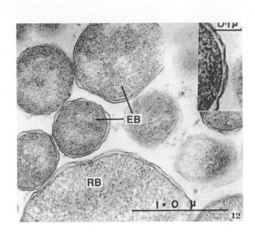

Reproduced, with permission, from Brooks GF, Carroll KC, Butel JS, Morse SA. *Jawetz, Melnick, & Adelberg's Medical Microbiology*, 24th ed. New York: McGraw-Hill, 2008: Figure 28-1.

(A) Azithromycin
(B) Ceftriaxone
(C) Fluconazole
(D) Penicillin
(E) Vancomycin

23. A 43-year-old man presents with flu-like symptoms, fevers, chills, and a productive cough. Physical examination is remarkable for pleuritic chest pain. On questioning, the patient says that he has just spent the last week on vacation in Central America. Cultures taken from the patient show a broad-based budding fungus. It is concluded that the man has systemic blastomycosis infection. Which of the following agents is the most appropriate treatment for this patient?

(A) Amphotericin B
(B) Fluconazole
(C) Itraconazole or potassium iodide
(D) Sodium stibogluconate only
(E) Topical miconazole or selenium sulfide

24. A 73-year-old woman steps on a rusty nail while gardening in her back yard. A neighbor drives her to the emergency department, where her wound is cleaned and bandaged. A complete history and review of her medical chart indicates that her vaccinations are not up to date, and she requires one vaccination and a shot of the appropriate immunoglobulin as

prophylaxis against infection. What is the mechanism of toxicity of the organism for which she was vaccinated?

(A) ADP-ribosylation of a G protein, increasing chloride secretion
(B) ADP-ribosylation of an elongation factor, causing disrupted protein synthesis
(C) Binding to the MHC II receptor and T-lymphocyte receptor, causing cytokine synthesis
(D) Blocking release of the inhibitory neurotransmitter glycine
(E) Blocking the release of acetylcholine
(F) Lysis of RBCs
(G) Stimulation of guanylate cyclase

25. A 50-year-old man develops nonbloody watery diarrhea while working as an aid worker in a refugee camp in Bangladesh. He arrived in the area 2 days ago. A stool smear shows no WBCs. He subsequently develops dehydration and electrolyte abnormalities leading to cardiac and renal failure. Which of the following organisms is the most likely cause of this man's enterocolitis?

(A) *Clostridium difficile*
(B) *Giardia lamblia*
(C) *Helicobacter pylori*
(D) *Salmonella* species
(E) *Vibrio cholerae*

26. Twenty-four hours after placement of a catheter, a hospitalized patient develops a fever and chills. Within 1 hour her systolic blood pressure falls 30 points and she develops swelling in her extremities. Despite valiant efforts by the hospital staff, the patient dies. X-ray of the patient's lungs taken only hours before she passed away shows pulmonary edema. Which of the following mediators of this patient's disease process is most likely responsible for the pathology described?

(A) C3a
(B) C5a
(C) Hageman factor
(D) γ-Interferon
(E) Interleukin-1
(F) Nitric oxide

27. A 31-year-old pregnant woman comes to the physician because of painful vesicular lesions that have recently appeared on her genitalia. A positive result on which of the following diagnostic tests would mean that her baby is at risk for congenital anomalies?

(A) Anti-hepatitis B surface antibody test
(B) Giemsa stain for cytoplasmic inclusions
(C) Monospot test
(D) Tzanck smear for multinucleated giant cells
(E) Weil-Felix test

28. A 13-year-old girl who returned a few days ago from a school camping trip in North Carolina is home ill from school. She tells her parents that she has a headache and the chills. Over the next few days, she develops a rash that begins on her palms and soles, but spreads inward to her wrists and ankles and then to her trunk. Her worsening condition leads her parents to take her to the emergency department, where a blood test reveals antibodies that react with the Proteus antigen. This patient is most likely infected with which of the following?

(A) *Borrelia burgdorferi*
(B) *Coxiella burnetti*
(C) Coxsackievirus A
(D) *Rickettsia rickettsii*
(E) *Rickettsia typhi*
(F) *Treponema pallidum*

29. A 53-year-old obese man with poorly controlled non-insulin-dependent diabetes mellitus presents with fever to 39.6° C (103.2° F), jaundice, hypotension, and acute onset of right upper quadrant pain. Right upper quadrant imaging shows multiple gallstones and cholecystitis. Urgent cholecystectomy is performed, and subsequent gall bladder fluid and blood cultures grow aerobic, non-lactose-fermenting, oxidase-positive, gram-negative rods. Blood tests show:

Hematocrit: 29%
WBC count: 14,700/mm³
Platelet count: 76,000/mm³
International Normalized Ratio: 3.2

D-dimer: 8500 ng/mL
Fibrinogen levels: low

Microscopic inspection of peripheral blood smear shows schistocytes and multiple helmet cells. Clinically, there is no evidence of active bleeding. What is the most appropriate treatment for this patient's coagulopathy?

(A) Amoxicillin
(B) Aztreonam
(C) Fresh frozen plasma
(D) Vancomycin
(E) Vitamin K

30. A 22-year-old woman presents to the physician with vaginal itching and burning. On examination, she has a foul-smelling greenish discharge. A swab sample is taken and a wet mount slide is prepared; results are shown in the image. Which of the following medications should be prescribed for this patient?

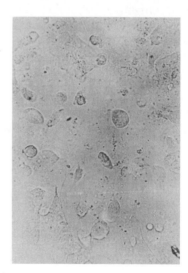

Reproduced, with permission, from Tintinalli JE, Kelen GD, Stapczynski JS, Ma OJ, Cline DM. *Tintinalli's Emergency Medicine: A Comprehensive Study Guide*, 6th ed. New York: McGraw-Hill, 2004: Figure 108-3.

(A) Metronidazole
(B) Nifurtimox
(C) Quinine
(D) Sodium stibogluconate
(E) Sulfadiazine and pyrimethamine

31. A 40-year-old man goes on a camping vacation with his family. One day after swimming in a freshwater lake near the camp site, he develops nausea and vomiting and starts to behave irrationally. His family takes him to the emergency department, where blood samples are taken and a spinal tap is performed. He is diagnosed with a rapidly progressing meningoencephalitis and dies shortly thereafter. Which of the following protozoa was most likely the cause of the man's illness?

(A) *Cryptosporidium* species
(B) *Entamoeba histolytica*
(C) *Leishmania donovani*
(D) *Naegleria fowleri*
(E) *Plasmodium falciparum*

32. A 54-year-old man presents to the clinic with scleral icterus, hepatosplenomegaly, ascites, and a history of episodes of jaundice over the past 3 years. He was involved in an auto accident when he was 21 years old, for which he required surgery and blood transfusions. Laboratory tests show:

Aspartate aminotransferase: 734 U/L
Alanine aminotransferase: 846 U/L
Direct bilirubin: 0.1 mg/dL
Indirect bilirubin: 7.6 mg/dL

Assuming a viral etiology, which of the following is the most likely cause of this patient's illness?

(A) Hepatitis A
(B) Hepatitis C
(C) Hepatitis D
(D) Hepatitis E
(E) Hepatitis G

33. A 19-year-old college student presents to his family physician with a 1-week history of fever, headache, and painful exudative pharyngitis. Physical examination shows significant lymphadenopathy of the cervical nodes and hepatosplenomegaly. Laboratory studies show a WBC count of 15,000/mm³ with 55% lymphocytes. A heterophile antibody test is positive. Which of the following is the most likely cause of this patient's symptoms?

(A) Cytomegalovirus
(B) Epstein-Barr virus
(C) HIV infection
(D) *Streptococcus pneumoniae*
(E) *Toxoplasma gondii*

34. A 36-year-old man comes to the physician complaining of an aching back, high fever, and vomiting of dark material. He is obviously ill and states that he has felt very poorly for approximately 1 week. Physical examination shows that the patient has a temperature of 39° C (102.2° F) and icteric sclera. The patient recently returned from a trip on safari in Africa. If a liver biopsy were done, it would show the following pathology. What are the names of the eosinophilic globules shown in this image?

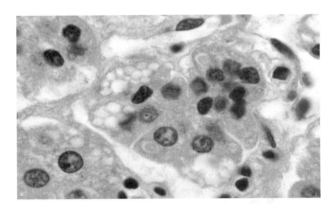

Reproduced, with permission, from PEIR Digital Library (http://peir.net).

(A) Councilman bodies
(B) Döhle bodies
(C) Negri bodies
(D) Pappenheimer bodies
(E) Weibel-Palade bodies

35. A 56-year-old man presents to the emergency department with sharp retrosternal pain radiating to his back and arms. The patient is sitting up and leaning forward. He states that the pain is less severe in this position and worsens when he lies down and takes a deep breath. He also indicates that he recently recovered from a fever and a cold. On physical examination a scratchy, leathery sound is heard at the lower left sternal border. An ECG is done and confirms the diagnosis. Which of the following microorganisms is the most likely cause of this condition?

(A) Coronavirus
(B) Coxsackievirus
(C) Cytomegalovirus
(D) Epstein-Barr virus
(E) *Staphylococcus aureus*

36. A 28-year-old man comes to the physician because of worsening muscle weakness that began in his legs and feet 3 days ago, and has now spread to his arms and hands. Other than having a flu-like illness 2 weeks ago, the patient has been in good health. Cerebrospinal fluid analysis shows an increased protein concentration, a normal cell count, and a normal glucose level. An infection with which of the following organisms is the most likely cause of the nervous system syndrome described in this patient?

(A) *Candida albicans*
(B) *Legionella pneumophila*
(C) *Mycoplasma pneumoniae*
(D) *Pseudomonas aeruginosa*
(E) *Streptococcus pneumoniae*

37. A 55-year-old man comes to his physician with a tender, swollen, and erythematous left knee. He has limited range of motion in his leg. On aspiration of the synovial fluid from his knee, the fluid is found to be yellow and cloudy and has 150,000 neutrophils/mm^3. Gram stain of the aspirate shows gram-positive cocci in clusters. The organism most likely responsible for this patient's symptoms has which of the following properties?

(A) Catalase-positive and coagulase-negative
(B) Catalase-positive and coagulase-positive
(C) Glycoprotein capsule
(D) α-Hemolysis
(E) Soluble in bile

38. A family who recently emigrated from Romania brings their 7-year-old child to the pediatrician with complaints of conjunctivitis and periorbital swelling. The child has had coughing with a runny nose and high fever for 3 days. Small lesions with blue-white centers are seen in his oral cavity. Which of the following is the most likely cause of this child's symptoms?

(A) Diphtheria
(B) Pertussis
(C) Roseola
(D) Rubella
(E) Rubeola

39. A 34-year-old woman newly diagnosed with HIV infection is unable to access antiretroviral medications. She is aware that if untreated, her disease will progress and make her susceptible to different infections. She inquires about the natural course her disease may take and the different infections she might acquire. Which of the following conditions is most likely to manifest only when the T cell count drops below 50/mm^3?

(A) Disseminated *Mycobacterium avium-intracellulare*
(B) Herpes simplex virus infection
(C) Herpes zoster infection
(D) Oral thrush
(E) Pneumonia due to *Pneumocystis jiroveci*
(F) Toxoplasmosis brain lesion

40. An 8-year-old boy is brought to his pediatrician by his parents because of a fever and a sore throat. On examination, he has tonsillar exudates and swollen, tender anterior cervical nodes. His parents report no history of cough. Gram stain of the tonsillar exudate reveals gram-positive cocci. Which of the following describes the organism most likely causing this patient's symptoms?

(A) Catalase-negative, α-hemolytic, optochin-resistant

(B) Catalase-negative, α-hemolytic, optochin-sensitive

(C) Catalase-negative, β-hemolytic, bacitracin-resistant

(D) Catalase-negative, β-hemolytic, bacitracin-sensitive

(E) Catalase-positive, coagulase-negative, no-vobiocin-resistant

(F) Catalase-positive, coagulase-negative, no-vobiocin-sensitive

ANSWERS

1. **The correct answer is B.** The differential diagnosis of a genital ulcer in a sexually active patient should include primary syphilis (though these ulcers are usually painless), genital herpes, and chancroid. Because the Tzanck smear (which looks for multinucleated giant cells typical of herpes infection), viral polymerase chain reaction (used to look for herpesvirus) are both negative, as is the VDRL to test for syphilis, chancroid becomes most likely. Chancroid is a bacterial infection caused by *Haemophilus ducreyi*, which presents typically as a painful genital ulcer with associated inguinal lymphadenopathy. It is typically treated with ceftriaxone, though azithromycin or ciprofloxacin can be used. Vancomycin is effective only for gram-positive organisms.

Answer A is incorrect. Acyclovir is used to treat herpes infections. It is activated by viral thymidine kinase, whereupon it inhibits the herpes viral polymerase. It can be used to treat herpes simplex virus (HSV) types 1 and 2, varicella-zoster virus (VSV), and Epstein-Barr virus (EBV) infections. It is not effective for bacterial organisms.

Answer C is incorrect. Foscarnet inhibits viral DNA polymerase without the need of activation by thymidine kinase. It is used to treat cytomegalovirus (CMV) retinitis, but it can also be used to treat acyclovir-resistant HSV.

Answer D is incorrect. Ribavirin is used to treat respiratory syncytial virus. It functions by inhibiting inosine monophosphate dehydrogenase, thus blocking the synthesis of guanine nucleotides.

Answer E is incorrect. Vancomycin is a bactericidal antibiotic used for multidrug-resistant gram-positive organisms such as *Staphylococcus aureus* and *Clostridium difficile*. It functions by binding to mucopeptide precursors, preventing formation of the bacterial cell wall.

2. **The correct answer is A.** This patient has been exposed to hepatitis B and has completely recovered, as is demonstrated by her serologic markers. She does not carry the hepatitis B surface antigen (HBsAg), which is found on the surface of the hepatitis B virus and indicates a carrier state. She does carry the surface antibody, which indicates that she was exposed to hepatitis B and made antibodies to convey immunity. The fact that she also has IgG antibody to the core antibody (HBcAb) shows that she has recovered. HBcAb is also positive in the chronic state, but in that case she would not also have HBsAb. To have both HBcAb and HBsAb without HBsAg is an indication of complete recovery.

Answer B is incorrect. The patient has completely recovered and is not in the acute disease phase.

Answer C is incorrect. The patient has completely recovered. In the window phase, HBsAg and HBsAb are both absent. The presence of HBsAb means she is not in the window phase.

Answer D is incorrect. The patient has completely recovered, and the absence of HBsAg confirms that she is not chronically infected.

Answer E is incorrect. The patient has completely recovered, but the presence of antibodies implies that she was once infected.

3. **The correct answer is C.** This patient is presenting with Chagas' disease, which is caused by infection with *Trypanosoma cruzi*. Acute symptoms include chagomas (small dermal granulomas caused by local multiplication of the pathogen), myocarditis, and congestive heart failure as a severe, but rare, complication of myocarditis. More chronic symptoms include arrhythmias, dilated cardiomyopathy, megacolon, and megaesophagus as *T. cruzi* infects cardiac tissue and colonic nerves. Treatment is mainly symptomatic, although nifurtimox is used during acute stages of infection. Another form of infection occurs when the organism enters the body through the conjunctiva. In that case, eye edema known as Romaña's sign occurs. Chagas' disease is mostly transmitted by the reduviid bug in Central and South America.

Answer A is incorrect. The *Anopheles* mosquito is responsible for transmission of the four *Plasmodia* species that cause malaria.

Answer B is incorrect. The *Ixodes* tick transmits *Borrelia burgdorferi* (the cause of Lyme disease) as well as *Babesia*.

Answer D is incorrect. The sandfly is responsible for transmission of *Leishmania donovani*, also known as "kala-azar" or visceral leishmaniasis. The clinical picture includes hepatosplenomegaly, anemia, and eventual leukopenia. Light-skinned patients may present with darkened skin.

Answer E is incorrect. The tsetse fly carries *Trypanosoma brucei gambiense* and *T. brucei rhodesiense*, the two causes of African sleeping sickness. In this disease, patients complain of repeatedly falling asleep in addition to headaches and dizziness. Other symptoms include recurrent fevers and lymphadenopathy. *T. brucei rhodesiense* causes a much more acute infection, while *T. brucei gambiense* causes a more indolent and progressive disease.

4. **The correct answer is A.** The characteristics of the microorganism indicate infection with *Klebsiella* species, while the physical exam points to a bronochopneumonia rather than a lobar pneumonia. *K. pneumoniae* is a gram-negative rod that ferments lactose and has a mucoid capsule. Bronchopneumonias are characterized by acute inflammatory infiltrates from bronchioles into adjacent alveoli. Pneumonia resulting from infection by this bacterium is often caused by aspiration, so that it is often seen in people with a loss of consciousness (ie, alcoholics). It is also more common in patients with diabetes.

Answer B is incorrect. Lobar pneumonia, most frequently due to *Streptococcus pneumoniae*, morphologically evolves through four stages without treatment: congestion, red hepatization, gray hepatization, and resolution. *S. pneumoniae* is an encapsulated gram-positive coccus. It is known for causing rust-colored sputum.

Answer C is incorrect. Interstitial pneumonias, from mycoplasma and viruses, are characterized by diffuse patchy inflammation localized to interstitial areas at alveolar walls.

Answer D is incorrect. Interstitial pneumonias, from mycoplasma and viruses, are characterized by diffuse patchy inflammation localized to interstitial areas at alveolar walls. They also have no exudates in alveolar spaces, but have intra-alveolar hyaline membranes.

Answer E is incorrect. Lobar pneumonia, most frequently due to *Streptococcus pneumoniae*, characteristically has predominantly intra-alveolar exudates, resulting in consolidation.

5. **The correct answer is B.** The clinical picture and imaging are consistent with progressive multifocal leukoencephalopathy secondary to reactivation of latent JC virus infection, which can occur with CD4+ cell counts <50/mm^3. It typically presents with rapidly progressive focal neurologic deficits without signs of increased intracranial pressure. Ataxia, aphasia, and cranial nerve deficits may also occur. Lumbar puncture is nondiagnostic and frequently demonstrates mild elevations in protein and white blood cells. Cerebrospinal fluid (CSF) analysis can reveal the presence of myelin basic protein, which is due to demyelination caused by the JC virus. Progressive multifocal leukoencephalopathy typically presents as multiple nonenhancing T2-hyperintense lesions. When it is suspected, stereotactic biopsy is required for definitive diagnosis, but a positive CSF polymerase chain reaction for JC virus is diagnostic in the appropriate clinical setting. Histology of the lesions shows nuclear inclusions in oligodendrocytes. Although there is no definitive treatment, clearance of JC virus DNA can be observed with response to highly active antiretroviral therapy.

Answer A is incorrect. CMV encephalitis can mimic the appearance of progressive multifocal leukoencephalopathy, but would be associated with enhancing periventricular white matter lesions in cortical and subependymal regions. CMV encephalitis is also typically associated with more systemic signs and symptoms. Polymerase chain reaction analysis of CSF would be positive for CMV, and histologic exam shows giant cells with eosinophilic inclusions in both the cytoplasm and the nucleus.

Answer C is incorrect. Central nervous system (CNS) lymphoma typically also affects those with CD4$^+$ cell counts under 50/mm^3. MRI will demonstrate one or more enhancing lesions (50% multiple; 50% single) that are typically surrounded by edema and can produce a mass effect. CNS lymphoma can present with polymerase chain reaction findings on CSF as positive for EBV.

Answer D is incorrect. Space-occupying lesions due to toxoplasmosis infection represent the most common cause of cerebral mass lesions in HIV-infected patients and typically present with multiple enhancing lesions on MRI. The lesions are typically located at the corticomedullary junction, and are surrounded by edema that frequently produces a mass effect and distinguishes its appearance from progressive multifocal leukoencephalopathy. Positive *Toxoplasma* serologies can assist in diagnosis, and clinical improvements will result from treatment with sulfadiazine and pyrimethamine or trimethoprim/sulfamethoxazole.

6. **The correct answer is C.** This is a classic case of molluscum contagiosum caused by the poxvirus. Physical examination is significant for pearly white or skin-colored nodules with central umbilication on the genitals and trunk. Molluscum contagiosum is a benign skin disease transmitted by sexual contact, clothes, or towels. It often resolves spontaneously but may require topical therapy or surgery in immunocompromised patients.

Answer A is incorrect. HSV type 1 affects mucosal surfaces, particularly oral mucosa. Erythema is the first sign of infection, followed by grouped vesicles that evolve to pustules. Pustules erode, then ulcerate, commonly producing a crust. Lesions resolve spontaneously without scar within 2–4 weeks.

Answer B is incorrect. Human herpesvirus 8 is thought to be the causative factor of Kaposi's sarcoma. These lesions are purple/red/blue and are most common in patients with AIDS.

Answer D is incorrect. Rubeola virus is another name for the RNA virus that causes measles, an exanthematous disease that begins as Koplik's spots on the oral mucosa and progresses to a maculopapular rash. Prodromal syndromes of malaise and fever are common.

Answer E is incorrect. VZV is the causative agent in chickenpox. It is a highly contagious DNA herpesvirus transmitted by respiratory droplets or by direct contact. The virus, characterized by recurrent crops of lesions classically described as "dew-drops on a rose petal," is commonly seen on the face and trunk. VZV infections are often accompanied by prodromal symptoms of fever and malaise.

7. **The correct answer is A.** The question stem describes classic symptoms of infection with EBV, including flu-like symptoms, increasing fatigue, lymphadenopathy, and splenomegaly. EBV is a member of the herpes viral family with linear double-stranded, enveloped DNA. Herpes viruses are unique in that it is the only virus that obtains its envelope via budding from the nuclear membrane.

Answer B is incorrect. Linear, double-stranded DNA without an envelope describes the adenoviruses. This virus is mostly known for conjunctivitis or "pink eye." It can also cause respiratory tract infections, hemorrhagic cystitis, and gastroenteritis.

Answer C is incorrect. The only double-stranded RNA viruses known to infect humans are the reoviruses. These includes coltivirus, which causes Colorado tick fever, and rotavirus, which causes gastroenteritis. Rotavirus infection is the principal cause of fatal diarrhea in children throughout the world. Colorado tick fever is transmitted via ticks carried by rodents and is found most commonly in hikers.

Answer D is incorrect. Partially circular, double-stranded DNA with an envelope describes the hepadnaviruses. The main infectious pathogen in this family is hepatitis B virus. Its main modes of transmission are blood and sexual contact. This patient does not present with signs of hepatitis.

Answer E is incorrect. The orthomyxoviruses are characterized by segmented, single-stranded RNA with negative polarity and an envelope. The principal disease caused by these viruses is influenza. Although this patient does have flu-like symptoms, lymphadenopathy and splenomegaly are not characteristic of the flu.

8. **The correct answer is B.** The *Plasmodium falciparum* parasite is responsible for causing malaria. It is spread by the *Anopheles* mosquito. Diagnosis of *P. falciparum* infection is made through a blood smear. The only species of *Plasmodium* that causes cerebral malaria is *P. falciparum*.

Answer A is incorrect. *Babesia microti* is a protozoan transmitted by the deer ticks that carry Lyme disease and granulocytic ehrlichiosis. Babesiae parasitize RBCs and cause fever and hemolytic anemia. The symptoms are mild except in debilitated or splenectomized individuals, who develop severe parasitemias. In blood smears, *Babesia* resembles *P. falciparum* ring stages. They form characteristic tetrads (Maltese cross), which are diagnostic. In fatal cases, findings are related to shock and hypoxia and include jaundice, hepatic necrosis, acute renal tubular necrosis, acute respiratory distress syndrome, hemolysis, and hemorrhages but no cerebral involvement.

Answer C is incorrect. *Plasmodium malariae* infection has a 72-hour cyclic fever. *P. malariae*, however, does not cause cerebral malaria.

Answer D is incorrect. *Plasmodium ovale* infection has a 48-hour cyclic fever. A unique feature of *P. vivax* and *P. ovale* organisms is that they can form hypnozoites that can remain dormant in the liver for long periods, only to resurface later. However, *P. ovale* does not cause cerebral malaria.

Answer E is incorrect. *Plasmodium vivax* infection has a 48-hour cyclic fever. A unique feature of both *P. vivax* and *P. ovale* organisms is that they can form hypnozoites that can remain dormant in the liver for long periods, only to resurface later. However, *P. vivax* does not cause cerebral malaria.

9. **The correct answer is B.** *Babesia* species infection presents with a malaria-like syndrome. Babesiosis is transmitted by the *Ixodes* tick. On microscopic examination, one observes the "tetrad" configuration (also known as a Maltese cross) of *Babesia* species and no RBC pigment. Trophozoites resemble *Plasmodium falciparum* but have distinguishing features: they vary more in shape and in size, and they do not produce pigment. Quinine is used to treat babesiosis.

Answer A is incorrect. *Acanthamoeba* species infection presents with meningoencephalitis in immunocompromised patients. It can also cause keratitis through contaminated contact lens solution. On histologic examination, spiky trophozoites are found in the CSF and brain tissue. Treatment is usually through multiple antibiotics and antifungals, and hospitalization is often needed.

Answer C is incorrect. *Leishmania donovani* infection presents with hepatomegaly and splenomegaly, malaise, anemia, and weight loss. *L. donovani* is transmitted via the sandfly. Microscopically, macrophages containing amastigotes are observed. Sodium stibogluconate is used to treat *L. donovani* infection.

Answer D is incorrect. *Naegleria fowleri* infection presents with meningoencephalitis that can progress to coma or death within 6 days. Other symptoms include nausea, vomiting, and irrational behavior. Transmission occurs through swimming in freshwater lakes. Microscopic analysis reveals amebas in the spinal fluid. Unfortunately, there is no treatment for *N. fowleri* infection.

Answer E is incorrect. *Trypanosoma cruzi* infection causes Chagas' disease, a condition in which the heart is enlarged and flaccid. *T. cruzi* is transmitted via the reduviid bug. Microscopic examination reveals flagellated trypomastigotes in the blood and nonmotile amastigotes in tissue culture. *T. cruzi* infection is treated with nifurtimox.

10. **The correct answer is D.** Human papillomavirus causes carcinoma (usually cervical) by inactivating tumor suppressor genes such as *p53* and *Rb* through the actions of viral proteins E6 and E7, respectively.

    Answer A is incorrect. EBV is associated with Burkitt's lymphoma (a B-lymphocyte lymphoma) and nasopharyngeal carcinoma. The t(8;14) translocation is consistently associated with Burkitt's lymphoma, but the translocation alone is not responsible for the neoplasm and is not found in nasopharyngeal carcinomas. The other factors that determine oncogenesis of EBV remain unclear.

    Answer B is incorrect. Both hepatitis C and hepatitis B virus infections are associated with an increased risk of developing hepatocellular carcinoma. The liver has a high regenerative potential, but if this process is overused, the chance of an oncogenic mutation occurring during the regeneration of cells increases.

    Answer C is incorrect. HIV as a direct oncogenic agent is being intensely researched, but it is already known that immune suppression and dysregulation caused by HIV infection give rise to lymphomas and Kaposi's sarcoma.

    Answer E is incorrect. Human T-cell lymphotropic virus causes adult T-cell leukemia, and although the mechanism of oncogenesis remains unclear, there is some evidence that integration into the host genome at locations near cellular growth genes may play a role.

11. **The correct answer is B.** Influenza virus has both hemagglutinin (HA) and neuraminidase (NA) molecules on its surface. These two molecules are responsible for the ability of the virus to be absorbed and penetrate the host cells. After a human is infected with the influenza virus, that person will be immune to infection by the same virus because of antibodies created against HA and NA. If either HA or NA is changed, as can be the case if two different influenza viruses infect the same cell and exchange RNA, antigenic shift can occur. This creates a new virus that has never been exposed to the human immune system before, with potentially catastrophic consequences. This type of mixing is most commonly thought to be between a human and an avian strain mixing in an intermediary porcine host, thus leading to the term "avian flu."

    Answer A is incorrect. Antigenic drift describes mutations that can occur in hemagglutinin and neuraminidase, making them less antigenic to the preexisting antibodies in the human host. Since this results in small changes in viral toxicity, it will lead to a slightly different strain, but it is not likely to lead to a global epidemic.

    Answer C is incorrect. Hemagglutinin has the ability to attach to sialic acid receptors, which activates fusion of the virus to the cell. All infectious influenza viruses have this molecule.

    Answer D is incorrect. Neuraminidase has the ability to destroy neuraminic acid, a component of mucin. This helps break down the barrier to the upper airways and aids in infectivity.

    Answer E is incorrect. RBCs agglutinate in the presence of hemagglutinin; hence the name. This does not affect the infection rate of the influenza virus.

12. **The correct answer is D.** *Staphylococcus aureus* is a gram-positive, catalase-positive coccus. It produces a superantigen called toxic shock syndrome toxin. The toxin causes a disease characterized by fever, hypotension, and a diffuse macular rash that desquamates after a few days.

    Answer A is incorrect. *Actinomyces israelii* is a filamentous organism that is part of the normal flora of the mouth and gastrointestinal tract. It does not cause toxic shock syndrome.

    Answer B is incorrect. *Clostridium perfringens* is the organism responsible for the development of gas gangrene. This organism is associated with contaminated wounds and not with toxic shock syndrome.

Answer C is incorrect. *Proteus mirabilis* is a common cause of urinary tract infections and is not associated with toxic shock syndrome.

Answer E is incorrect. *Streptococcus pyogenes*, a gram-positive coccus, can also cause toxic shock syndrome. Unlike *S. aureus*, it is catalase-negative.

13. **The correct answer is A.** This patient is presenting with a classic case of whooping cough caused by *Bordetella pertussis*. The initial phase is characterized by flu-like symptoms for the first 1–2 weeks. During this time, erythromycin is an effective treatment. The second phase, the paroxysmal stage, is marked by bouts of multiple coughs in a single breath followed by a deep inspiration (the classic whooping cough). Treatment during this phase does not change the disease course, so only supportive care is indicated and the infection ought to pass in otherwise healthy individuals. In the United States, the diptheria/tetanus/pertussis (DTaP) vaccine is supposed to be given to all infants and protects them against diphtheria, tetanus, and pertussis. Infants who are not vaccinated are at risk for infection. *B. pertussis* can only be cultured on Bordet-Gengou medium.

Answer B is incorrect. Charcoal yeast extract when buffered with increased levels of iron and cysteine is used to culture *Legionella pneumophila*.

Answer C is incorrect. Chocolate agar with factor V and X is used to culture *Haemophilus influenzae*.

Answer D is incorrect. Loffler's medium is needed to culture *Corynebacterium diphtheriae*.

Answer E is incorrect. Thayer-Martin medium is used to culture *Neisseria gonorrhoeae*.

14. **The correct answer is B.** Adult botulism is characterized by the development of diplopia and dysphagia. This is followed by the development of general muscle weakness, respiratory muscle failure, and even death. The organism responsible for this disease is *Clostridium botulinum*, and it can be found in contaminated homemade canned goods and smoked fish.

Answer A is incorrect. *Bacillus cereus* causes food poisoning, and the patient typically presents with vomiting and diarrhea. It is most often associated with eating reheated rice.

Answer C is incorrect. *Clostridium perfringens* is the organism responsible for the development of gas gangrene. This organism is associated with contaminated wounds.

Answer D is incorrect. *Clostridium tetani* causes tetanus, which presents with severe muscle spasms and not muscle weakness. The disease usually follows a puncture wound (as the bacteria involved are anaerobic) and is not associated with eating canned goods.

Answer E is incorrect. Poliovirus could cause muscle paralysis, but is unlikely given the acute onset of symptoms and the availability of vaccination.

15. **The correct answer is D.** The patient presents with a pneumonia. The presence of a single-celled yeast endospore containing spherules is indicative of *Coccidioides immitis* infection. *Coccidioides* is characterized by endospores containing spherules when cultured at 37° C and branched hyphae when the organism is cultured at 25° C. *Coccidioides* infection is most commonly seen in immunocompromised patients or the elderly, and is most prevalent in the southwest United States. While normal hosts are susceptible to infection, they usually do not present with symptoms. This patient's recent travel to Arizona makes *C. immitis* the most likely candidate.

Answer A is incorrect. *Aspergillus* infection is also seen almost exclusively in the immunocompromised patient; exceptions include allergic bronchopulmonary aspergillosis, an allergic disease that occurs in otherwise healthy individuals. *Aspergillus* most often causes fever, hemoptysis, and pneumonia. A tissue biopsy will show branching hyphae with septae, but a sputum culture will show radiating chains of spores.

Answer B is incorrect. *Blastomyces* grows as thick-walled budding yeasts at 37° C and hyphae with small conidia at 25° C. It is mostly seen along the Mississippi River and in Central America. It also causes a pneumonia that can progress to disseminated granulomatous disease.

Answer C is incorrect. *Candida* is the cause of thrush and is seen most often in the immunocompromised patient, such as those with HIV infection. In a tissue biopsy it will be seen as pseudohyphae and budding yeast. Candidal infection, however, is more likely to affect the esophagus than the airways and lungs.

Answer E is incorrect. *Histoplasma* grows as branched hyphae at 25° C and as full yeast cells at 37° C that are 2–5 μm in diameter and live within macrophages. *Histoplasma* infection causes both a pulmonary disease similar to a pneumonia and a severe granulomatous disease throughout the body, especially in the adrenals, liver, and spleen. It is prevalent in the Mississippi and Ohio River valleys.

16. **The correct answer is C.** One of the diseases caused by the gram-negative coccobacillus *Francisella tularensis* is ulceroglandular tularemia. This disease is characterized by a well-demarcated skin lesion with a black base following a tick or deerfly bite, contact with the body fluids or fur of an infected rabbit, or less frequently, from infected food or water. Over the next few days, systemic symptoms including fever, headache, and malaise develop and the local lymph nodes may become swollen and painful. *F. tularensis* can also be transmitted through inhalation of aerosols, and there is concern for its potential use as an agent of bioterrorism.

Answer A is incorrect. *Borrelia burgdorgeri* is a spirochete that causes Lyme disease. The organism is transmitted through the bite of the *Ixodes* tick. In the first stage of infection, usually within a month of the bite, a flat, erythematous rash with central clearing forms at the site of the bite; this lesion is called erythema migrans. Associated symptoms are fevers, chills, headache, and myalgias. The sec-

ond stage of infection, which occurs weeks to months later, is characterized by arthralgias, arthritis, neurologic manifestations such as meningitis and facial nerve palsy, and cardiac disease including myopericarditis. Months to years later the third stage occurs, with chronic joint, nervous system, and skin symptoms. However, infection does not result in ulcers with lack bases.

Answer B is incorrect. *Brucella* species enter the body after the ingestion of contaminated milk products or following direct contact with contaminated livestock. It is an intracellular bacterium that causes undulating fever, weakness, aches, and loss of appetite. The undulating fever of brucellosis is characterized by fever that peaks in the evening and falls at nighttime. Infection is not associated with ulcers with black bases.

Answer D is incorrect. *Nocardia asteroides* is an acid-fast aerobe found in soil. This organism causes pulmonary infections, primarily in immunocompromised individuals.

Answer E is incorrect. *Yersinia pestis* is a gram-negative rod that causes the plague. Humans are infected with the organism after being bitten by a flea that has previously bitten an infected rodent. After the bite, high fever and buboes may developed within 1 week. Buboes are painful, enlarged lymph nodes usually found in the groin and armpits. *Y. pestis* can then enter the bloodstream, resulting in sepsis and later, disseminated intravascular coagulation. Pneumonia and meningitis may also occur.

17. **The correct answer is G.** This patient is likely presenting with a mucosa-associated lymphoid tissue lymphoma. This type of indolent lymphoma is believed to be associated with infection by the organism *Helicobacter pylori*. *H. pylori* is commonly identified by the presence of urease, catalase, and oxidase. Eradication of the infection with antibiotics and proton-pump inhibitors is often sufficient to cause regression of the lymphoma.

Answer A is incorrect. This pattern is seen in benign flora such as the lactobacilli.

Answer B is incorrect. This pattern would be commonly seen in streptococcal species such as *Streptococcus pneumoniae*.

Answer C is incorrect. This pattern of results is commonly seen in facultative anaerobes such as *Escherichia coli*.

Answer D is incorrect. This pattern represents *Pseudomonas aeruginosa*, an opportunistic lung pathogen.

Answer E is incorrect. This represents a pattern common of true anaerobes in the *Bacteroides* family.

Answer F is incorrect. This pattern is seen in *Proteus mirabilis*, a common cause of urinary tract infection.

18. **The correct answer is E.** Food poisoning is the major cause of illness in this patient, and the most likely cause in this case is *Bacillus cereus*. In general, food poisoning is caused by preformed exotoxins secreted into the gastrointestinal tract by pathogenic bacteria. These exotoxins are fast acting, so the symptoms of food poisoning (nausea, vomiting, diarrhea) are usually rapid in onset (within 6–8 hours). Other major causative organisms of food poisoning include *Staphylococcus aureus*, *Clostridium perfringens*, and enterotoxigenic *Escherichia coli*, which causes traveler's diarrhea. Since the food poisoning in *B. cereus* infection is caused by preformed enterotoxins, antibiotic treatment will not help.

Answer A is incorrect. Bismuth subsalicylate, metronidazole, and amoxicillin are used in the treatment of *Helicobacter pylori* infection.

Answer B is incorrect. Fluoroquinolones can be used in the treatment of severe *Shigella* species infection.

Answer C is incorrect. *Campylobacter jejuni* enterocolitis can be treated with erythromycin or ciprofloxacin. Infection with this organism is not associated with eating reheated rice.

Answer D is incorrect. *Vibrio cholerae* causes large-volume, watery diarrhea. Treatment involves prompt replacement of water and electrolytes. Although antibiotics are not needed

for treatment, tetracyclines have been shown to reduce the course of the disease.

19. **The correct answer is A.** Enterococci are a common cause of nosocomial urinary tract infection and subacute endocarditis. Ampicillin is the standard treatment for susceptible enterococcal infections. For those strains that are not susceptible, vancomycin is the treatment of choice. For vancomycin-resistant strains, other therapies (such as quinupristin/dalfopristin) are available, but extensive knowledge of the indications for each is beyond the scope of knowledge necessary for the USMLE Step 1 examination.

Answer B is incorrect. Gentamicin is an aminoglycoside antibiotic. It inhibits the 30S subunit by inhibiting the formation of the initiation complex. It is not an effective monotherapy for enterococci, but it can be used in combination with other therapies to increase efficacy.

Answer C is incorrect. Piperacillin is an extended-spectrum penicillin agent. In addition to gram-positive organisms, it is particularly active against *Pseudomonas aeruginosa* and the Enterobacteriaceae viruses. It is not first-line therapy for enterococcal infections.

Answer D is incorrect. Quinupristin/dalfopristin (Syncrcid) is a new therapy that may be effective for vancomycin-resistant enterococcal endocarditis. It is not first-line treatment for enterococcal infections.

Answer E is incorrect. Vancomycin is an antibiotic that is effective only against gram-positive cocci. It binds tightly to a cell wall precursor containing the amino acid sequence D-ala D-ala, preventing cell wall synthesis. It is indicated for ampicillin-resistant enterococcal infection.

20. **The correct answer is D.** The image shows gram-positive cocci in clusters. Staphylococcal scalded skin syndrome is caused by the release of two exotoxins (epidermolytic toxins A and B) from *Staphylococcus aureus*. Desmosomes are cell structures specialized for cell-to-cell adhesion. The exotoxins that are released bind to a molecule within the desmosome called desmoglein 1, thereby disrupting cell adhesion.

In staphylococcal scalded skin syndrome, the epidermis separates at the stratum granulosum due to the binding of exotoxins to desmosomes in this layer. Clinically, this results in bullous lesions and a positive Nikolsky's sign.

Answer A is incorrect. The papillary dermis is the more superficial of the two layers of the dermis. Its papillae interdigitate with the epidermis. It is composed of loose connective tissue containing capillaries, elastic fibers, reticular fibers, and some collagen.

Answer B is incorrect. The stratum basale (also called the stratum germinativum) is the deepest layer of the epidermis, immediately superficial to the dermoepidermal junction. It is composed of a single row of cuboidal or columnar keratinocytes attached to the basement membrane via hemidesmosomes. The cells of this basal layer are stem cells, and they allow the epidermis to regenerate after the more superficial layers exfoliate in staphylococcal scalded skin syndrome.

Answer C is incorrect. The stratum corneum is the outer layer of the epidermis, consisting of several layers of flat keratinized nonnucleated cells.

Answer E is incorrect. The stratum lucidum is a layer just deep to the stratum corneum that is present only in the thick, hairless skin of the palms and soles.

21. **The correct answer is E.** The results of the fluid analysis are consistent with a bacterial meningitis (increased polymorphonuclear cells, high protein, low glucose). The most common cause of meningitis in children aged 6 months to 6 years is *Streptococcus pneumoniae*.

Answer A is incorrect. Results of the fluid analysis are not consistent with a viral meningitis. One would expect to see increased lymphocyte counts, normal protein levels, and normal sugar levels in this type of infection.

Answer B is incorrect. *Haemophilus influenzae* meningitis is a less common cause of meningitis in children of this age group. Since the

introduction of the *Haemophilus* flu vaccine, the incidence of this cause of meningitis has greatly decreased.

Answer C is incorrect. The clinical picture does not fit with a viral meningitis. In a viral meningitis, one would expect the fluid analysis to come back with increased lymphocytes, normal protein, and normal sugar.

Answer D is incorrect. *Listeria* species is not a common cause of meningitis in this age group. It is much more commonly seen in newborns age 0–6 months and in the elderly.

22. **The correct answer is A.** These symptoms are typical of urethritis. The most common causes of urethritis in males are *Chlamydia trachomatis* and *Neisseria gonorrhoeae*. The image shows intracellular inclusions that indicate that this man is infected with *C. trachomatis*; in the image, *EB* indicates the elementary body particles within cell walls and *RB* indicates the reticular body. While they may be difficult to differentiate, *C. trachomatis* infection induces a predominantly immunologic reaction with only some polymorphonuclear leukocytes (PMNs), while *N. gonorrhoeae* induces predominantly nonimmunologic inflammation with a PMN-rich infiltrate. The treatment of choice for *Chlamydia* urethritis is azithromycin (macrolide family antibiotic) or doxycycline (tetracycline family antibiotic).

Answer B is incorrect. Ceftriaxone is an effective treatment for gonorrhea, but the cephalosporin class of antibiotics is relatively ineffective against *Chlamydia trachomatis*.

Answer C is incorrect. Fluconazole inhibits fungal steroid synthesis. It is used in the treatment of fungal infections, such as *Candida albicans*.

Answer D is incorrect. Penicillin has been shown to suppress chlamydial multiplication. However, it does not eradicate the organism and thus is not the best treatment for this type of infection. Penicillin is the treatment of choice for syphilis.

Answer E is incorrect. Vancomycin has not been shown to be effective in the treatment of chlamydial infection. It is used to treat drug-resistant *Staphylococcus aureus* and *Clostridium difficile*.

23. **The correct answer is A.** Blastomycosis can present with flu-like symptoms, fevers, chills, productive cough, myalgia, arthralgia, and pleuritic chest pain. Some patients will fail to recover from an acute infection and progress to develop chronic pulmonary infection or widespread disseminated infection. Fluconazole or ketoconazole is used for the treatment of local blastomycosis infections, and amphotericin B is used for the treatment of systemic infections.

Answer B is incorrect. Fluconazole or ketoconazole are effective treatments for local blastomycosis infections but are ineffective if the infection is systemic. Systemic infections require amphotericin B.

Answer C is incorrect. Itraconazole or potassium iodide is used for the treatment of *Sporothrix schenckii*. *S. schenckii* is the cause of sporotrichosis. When *S. schenckii* is introduced into the skin, usually by a thorn prick, it causes a local pustule or ulcer with nodules along draining lymphatics (ascending lymphangitis). *S. schenckii* is a dimorphic fungus that has cigar-shaped budding yeast visible in pus.

Answer D is incorrect. Sodium stibogluconate is used to treat *Leishmania donovani* infection. *L. donovani* presents with hepatomegaly and splenomegaly, malaise, anemia, and weight loss. *L. donovani* is transmitted via the sandfly. Microscopically, macrophages containing amastigotes are observed.

Answer E is incorrect. Topical miconazole or selenium sulfide (Selsun) is used to treat *Malassezia furfur*. *M. furfur* is the cause of tinea versicolor. Symptoms of this infection include hypopigmented skin lesions that occur in hot and humid conditions.

24. **The correct answer is D.** The penetrating wound from the rusty nail puts this patient at risk for infection with *Clostridium tetani*, whose symptoms are caused by the tetanus toxin. This toxin blocks the release of glycine from Renshaw cells in the spinal cord and results in "lockjaw" and other similar symptoms. Tetanus re-vaccination is required approximately every 10 years to ensure adequate blood levels of protective antibodies.

Answer A is incorrect. The *Vibrio cholera* toxin ADP-ribosylates a G protein in the intestine, increasing adenylate cyclase activity and causing pumping of water and chloride ions into the gut lumen. Its most characteristic symptom is voluminous "rice water" diarrhea. The heat-labile toxin of *Escherichia coli* has the same mechanism of action.

Answer B is incorrect. The *Corynebacterium diphtheriae* toxin inactivates the elongation factor EF-2 by ADP ribosylation, disrupting protein synthesis. It causes pharyngitis and "pseudomembrane" in the throat. Although the patient's prior vaccinations most likely included vaccination for diphtheria as well, this infection is less likely than tetanus to occur with a penetrating wound.

Answer C is incorrect. Superantigens such as the *Staphylococcus aureus* toxin and the *Streptococcus pyogenes* erythrogenic toxin bind to the MHC class II receptor and the T-lymphocyte receptor, resulting in cytokine release and sometimes toxic shock syndrome.

Answer E is incorrect. The *Clostridium botulinum* toxin inhibits the release of acetylcholine, resulting in anticholinergic symptoms and even CNS. *C. botulinum* is most often found in canned food and honey (resulting in "floppy baby" syndrome when consumed by young children).

Answer F is incorrect. The streptolysin O toxin of *Streptococcus pyogenes* is a hemolysin.

Answer G is incorrect. The heat-stable toxin of *Escherichia coli* stimulates guanylate cyclase.

25. **The correct answer is E.** *Vibrio cholerae* causes watery stools, often called rice-water stool. This illness is not accompanied by abdominal pain, but the symptoms are due to de-

hydration leading to electrolyte imbalances. Cholera toxin causes uncontrolled stimulation of adenylate cyclase; the resulting excess of cAMP causes uncontrolled secretion of chloride and water (due to the osmotic gradient), resulting in extremely watery diarrhea accompanied by electrolyte imbalances.

Answer A is incorrect. *Clostridium difficile* causes severe nonbloody diarrhea associated with pseudomembranes. Diarrhea may be bloody when very severe mucosal ulceration occurs. *C. difficile* infection is associated with previous antibiotic treatment.

Answer B is incorrect. *Giardia lamblia* is a protozoan parasite that is a frequent cause of nonbloody diarrhea. The stools are usually foul-smelling and contain fat (steatorrhea). It is less severe than the diarrhea caused by *Vibrio cholerae*.

Answer C is incorrect. *Helicobacter pylori* infection causes gastritis and would not cause the symptoms described in this patient.

Answer D is incorrect. *Salmonella* species invade the mucosa to cause bloody diarrhea and can be acquired from poultry, meat, and eggs.

26. **The correct answer is A.** This patient suffered from shock, most likely endotoxic shock due to gram-negative bacteremia. The endotoxin lipopolysaccharide (LPS) is found in the cell wall of gram-negative bacteria. LPS activates the alternative pathway of the complement cascade. The patient's pulmonary edema contributes to the acute respiratory distress syndrome that accompanies septic shock. The C3a component of the complement cascade contributes to the hypotension and edema seen in endotoxic shock.

Answer B is incorrect. The C5a component of the complement cascade, activated by endotoxin, functions in neutrophil chemotaxis.

Answer C is incorrect. Endotoxin can directly activate Hageman factor, activating the coagulation cascade and leading to disseminated intravascular coagulation.

Answer D is incorrect. γ-Interferon is produced by T lymphocytes and, among other functions, activates tumoricidal macrophages.

Answer E is incorrect. The cytokine interleukin-1, released by macrophages activated by endotoxin, causes fever.

Answer F is incorrect. Nitric oxide, released by macrophages activated by endotoxin, causes hypotension (shock).

27. **The correct answer is D. ToRCHeS** is an acronym for organisms that can cross the placenta and cause congenital anomalies: **To**xoplasmosis, **R**ubella, **C**ytomegalovirus, **H**IV/ **H**erpes, and **S**yphilis. Genital lesions suggest a sexually transmitted disease. The Tzanck test is a smear of an opened skin vesicle that detects multinucleated giant cells, indicative of HSV types 1 and 2 or VZV. HSV-1, HSV-2, and VZV may all be transmitted vertically to the fetus. Remember: "**Tzanck** heaven I don't have **herpes!**" In the United States today, CMV is the most common cause of congenital abnormalities.

Answer A is incorrect. The presence of anti-HB surface antibody indicates immunity to the hepatitis B virus, either by previous exposure or by vaccination. While active or chronic hepatitis B can be vertically transmitted to the fetus, it does not cause congenital anomalies. Furthermore, hepatitis B is not associated with genital lesions.

Answer B is incorrect. Cytoplasmic inclusions seen on Giemsa or fluorescent antibody-stained smear suggest *Chlamydia trachomatis*. Although *Chlamydia* can be vertically transmitted to the fetus at delivery, it is not associated with congenital anomalies or with painful vesicular lesions. It can, however, cause blindness and pneumonia in the newborn and should be treated during pregnancy.

Answer C is incorrect. The monospot test detects heterophile antibodies by the agglutination of sheep RBCs, indicative of EBV infection. While EBV can cause mononucleosis and Burkitt's lymphoma, it is not one of the ToRCHeS organisms and does not transmit vertically to the fetus. Moreover, EBV does not produce genital lesions.

Answer E is incorrect. The Weil-Felix test uses *Proteus* antigen to test for antirickettsial antibodies, indicative of typhus or Rocky Mountain spotted fever. *Rickettsia* species can cause headache, fever, and rash; however, they do not produce genital lesions.

28. **The correct answer is D.** This patient most likely has Rocky Mountain spotted fever, as indicated by the rash on her palms and soles and the inward, "centripetal" pattern of spread. Other supporting evidence are the accompanying headache and fever, and a positive Weil-Felix reaction, which is a cross-reaction of certain anti-rickettsial antibodies with the Proteus antigen. Rocky Mountain spotted fever is caused by the rickettsial organism *Rickettsia rickettsii*, and is endemic to the east coast of the United States. It is transmitted by the *Ixodes* tick, thus the patient probably acquired it during her recent camping trip.

Answer A is incorrect. *Borrelia burgdorferi* causes Lyme disease. The rash of Lyme disease is typically a bull's-eye type rash, with negative Weil-Felix reaction.

Answer B is incorrect. *Coxiella burnetti* is also a rickettsial organism. It is transmitted by aerosols, causes Q fever, and has no associated rash or positive Weil-Felix reaction.

Answer C is incorrect. Coxsackie A is an RNA virus that causes hand, foot, and mouth disease, which can also present with a rash on the palms and soles, in addition to oral and occasionally genital lesions. However, the positive Weil-Felix reaction in this case and recent history of a camping trip point to *Rickettsia rickettsiae* as a more likely causative organism in this case.

Answer E is incorrect. *Rickettsia typhi* causes endemic typhus, and is transmitted by fleas. The rash of typhus is centrifugal; it spreads outward, not inward as in this case.

Answer F is incorrect. *Treponema pallidum* is the spirochete that causes syphilis, a sexually transmitted disease. Although syphilis can also present with a rash on the palms and soles, this patient has no history of a sexual encounter that would put her at risk for this disease.

29. **The correct answer is B.** This patient has leukocytosis and Charcot's triad (fever, jaundice, right upper quadrant pain), along with the ominous sign of hypotension, a clear clinical picture of cholecystitis. In addition, he has *Pseudomonas aeruginosa* sepsis and disseminated intravascular coagulation (DIC). Gram-negative rod sepsis is the clear cause of this patient's DIC, and antipseudomonal coverage with aztreonam is most appropriate. Aztreonam is a β-lactamase-resistant monobactam that interferes with cell wall biosynthesis by binding to penicillin-binding protein 3. Aztreonam is a potent antipseudomonal agent indicated for pseudomonal sepsis.

Answer A is incorrect. Amoxicillin is an aminopenicillin antibiotic that interferes with cell wall synthesis. Although amoxicillin has an extended spectrum compared with penicillin (covering *Haemophilus influenzae*, *Escherichia coli*, *Listeria*, *Proteus*, *Salmonella*, and *Enterococci*), it does not provide antipseudomonal coverage.

Answer C is incorrect. Use of fresh frozen plasma (FFP) is reserved for patients with coagulopathy and signs of active, life-threatening bleeding. Although provision of FFP will temporarily reverse some of this patient's laboratory signs of DIC (elevated International Normalized Ratio, decreased fibrinogen), treatment of the underlying cause (ie, *Pseudomonas* sepsis) is most important.

Answer D is incorrect. Vancomycin is an antibiotic used for serious multidrug-resistant, gram-positive infections. Major uses are for methicillin-resistant *Staphylococcus aureus* and moderate to severe *Clostridium difficile* infections. Its mechanism of action is to inhibit cell wall mucopeptide formation by binding the D-ala-D-ala portion of cell wall precursors.

Answer E is incorrect. Coagulopathy caused by warfarin overdose is reversed by pharmacologic administration of vitamin K. This patient's coagulopathy is caused by *Pseudomonas sepsis*, so vitamin K therapy plays no role here.

30. **The correct answer is A.** *Trichomonas vaginalis* is the cause of vaginitis. Symptoms of vaginitis include a foul-smelling greenish discharge, itching, and burning. *T. vaginalis* is transmitted sexually. On microscopic wet mount, one finds trophozoites. Metronidazole is used to treat *T. vaginalis* infection.

    Answer B is incorrect. Nifurtimox is used to treat *Trypanosoma cruzi*. *T. cruzi* infection causes Chagas' disease, a condition in which the heart is enlarged and flaccid. *T. cruzi* is transmitted via the reduviid bug. Microscopic examination reveals flagellated trypomastigotes in the blood and nonmotile amastigotes in tissue culture.

    Answer C is incorrect. Quinine is used to treat babesiosis. *Babesia* species present with a malaria-like syndrome. Babesiosis is transmitted by the *Ixodes* tick. On microscopic examination, one observes no red blood cell pigment and the Maltese cross-appearing parasite.

    Answer D is incorrect. Sodium stibogluconate is used to treat *Leishmania donovani* infection. *L. donovani* presents with hepatomegaly and splenomegaly, malaise, anemia, and weight loss. *L. donovani* is transmitted via the sandfly. Microscopically, macrophages containing amastigotes are observed.

    Answer E is incorrect. Sulfadiazine and pyrimethamine are used to treat toxoplasmosis. *Toxoplasma gondii* infection presents with brain abscesses in HIV-positive patients and with birth defects. *T. gondii* is transmitted via cysts in raw meat or cat feces. The definitive stage (sexual stage) occurs in cats. Microscopically, acid-fast staining cysts are found.

31. **The correct answer is D.** *Naegleria fowleri* presents with a rapidly progressing meningoencephalitis that can progress to coma or death within 6 days. Other symptoms include nausea, vomiting, and irrational behavior. Transmission occurs through swimming in freshwater lakes. Microscopic analysis will reveal amebas in the spinal fluid. Unfortunately, there is no treatment for *N. fowleri*.

    Answer A is incorrect. *Cryptosporidium* species infection presents with severe diarrhea in HIV-positive patients and mild watery diarrhea in HIV-negative patients. *Cryptosporidium* species are transmitted via cysts in water (fecal-oral transmission). Microscopically, acid-fast staining cysts are found. Unfortunately, there is no treatment available for *Cryptosporidium* species Infection; however, in healthy patients, cryptosporidiosis is self-resolving.

    Answer B is incorrect. *Entamoeba histolytica* infection presents with bloody diarrhea (dysentery), abdominal cramps with tenesmus, and pus in the stool. It can also cause right upper quadrant pain and liver abscesses. *E. histolytica* is transmitted via cysts in water (fecal-oral transmission). On microscopy, one observes amebas with ingested RBCs. Treatment for *E. histolytica* infection includes metronidazole and iodoquinol.

    Answer C is incorrect. *Leishmania donovani* infection presents with hepatomegaly and splenomegaly, malaise, anemia, and weight loss. *L. donovani* is transmitted via the sandfly. Microscopically, macrophages containing amastigotes are observed. Sodium stibogluconate is used to treat *L. donovani* infection.

    Answer E is incorrect. The *Plasmodium falciparum* parasite is responsible for causing malaria. It is spread by the *Anopheles* mosquito. Diagnosis of *Plasmodium falciparum* infection is made through a blood smear.

32. **The correct answer is B.** This is a classic presentation of chronic hepatitis C infection. It is a common cause of post-transfusion viral hepatitis. Hepatitis C is a blood-borne pathogen that can ultimately cause cirrhosis of the liver.

    Answer A is incorrect. Hepatitis A is transmitted via the fecal-oral route and does not cause chronic infection.

    Answer C is incorrect. Hepatitis D is transmitted parenterally and can cause infection only if its host is coinfected with hepatitis B.

Answer D is incorrect. Hepatitis E is transmitted via the fecal-oral route and does not cause chronic infection.

Answer E is incorrect. Hepatitis G is a transmissible flavivirus that has not been shown to cause liver disease.

33. **The correct answer is B.** EBV causes infectious mononucleosis and is a member of the Herpesviridae family. Mononucleosis typically presents with high fever, elevated WBC count, painful pharyngitis, and enlarged lymph nodes. There are two significant clinical differences between EBV mononucleosis and that of CMV: exudative pharyngitis and cervical lymphadenopathy are commonly seen with EBV, but not with CMV. A positive heterophile antibody test is specific for EBV infection.

    Answer A is incorrect. CMV causes a mononucleosis syndrome that is very similar to the one caused by EBV; however, one rarely sees an exudative pharyngitis or cervical lymphadenopathy when CMV is the cause. CMV can also cause pneumonia and, if transmitted congenitally, birth defects. After infection with CMV, most healthy individuals are asymptomatic, but CMV can reactivate in the immunocompromised and cause a variety of illnesses in various organ systems.

    Answer C is incorrect. HIV is the virus that causes AIDS. AIDS is a syndrome characterized by a decline in CD4$^+$ cell count <200/mm^3 and a variety of opportunistic infections due to the corresponding immunosuppression. An acute HIV prodrome would present in a very similar fashion to EBV mononucleosis and can result in either an elevated or a depressed WBC. It would not, however, have a positive heterophile test.

    Answer D is incorrect. *Streptococcus pneumoniae* is a gram-positive diplococcus and the most common cause of lobar pneumonia worldwide. It is unlikely to be causing the constellation of symptoms seen in our patient, which are more indicative of an infectious mononucleosis. *S. pneumoniae* infection would not result in a positive heterophile antibody test.

    Answer E is incorrect. *Toxoplasma gondii* is the protozoa that causes toxoplasmosis and is transmitted by ingestion of undercooked meat or food contaminated by cat feces. It is usually asymptomatic in immunocompetent individuals but can present as a brain lesion with focal neurologic deficits in immunocompromised patients. Infection with *Toxoplasma* does not typically present as a mononucleosis syndrome and would not result in a positive heterophile antibody test.

34. **The correct answer is A.** The disease described is yellow fever, caused by a member of the Flaviviridae family. It presents with symptoms of jaundice, aching pain, and high fever. Its vector is the mosquito. Liver biopsy can reveal Councilman bodies, which are eosinophilic globules believed to be the result of apoptosis of individual hepatocytes.

    Answer B is incorrect. Döhle bodies are oval bodies found in the neutrophils of patients with infections, trauma, pregnancy, or cancer.

    Answer C is incorrect. Negri bodies are pathognomonic for the rabies virus. They are eosinophilic inclusion bodies found in the cytoplasm of nerve cells of infected individuals.

    Answer D is incorrect. Pappenheimer bodies are found in RBCs in sideroblastic anemia and sickle cell disease. They are phagosomes containing ferruginous granules.

    Answer E is incorrect. Weibel-Palade bodies can be seen by electron microscopy in vascular endothelial cells. They are collections of microtubules.

35. **The correct answer is B.** This patient presents with classic signs and symptoms of pericarditis. Pericarditis frequently follows an upper respiratory viral infection most commonly due to coxsackie B virus, which causes inflammation of the pericardial membrane. Auscultation of the

chest would reveal a pericardial friction rub that accounts for the scratchy, leathery sound heard during both systole and diastole. On ECG there would be diffuse ST segment elevation and a depression of the PR segment unique to pericarditis.

Answer A is incorrect. Coronavirus is a common virus that causes a self-limiting cold. SARS-CoV, however, has been identified as the cause of severe acute respiratory syndrome

Answer C is incorrect. CMV causes a mononucleosis syndrome in young adults similar to that caused by EBV, which is characterized by fever and pharyngitis. It can also cause a severe infection in immunocompromised patients, which is characterized by retinitis, pneumonia, and even death.

Answer D is incorrect. EBV causes heterophil-positive mononucleosis with symptoms of fever, fatigue, lymphadenopathy, and lymphocytosis. In cases of suspected EBV infection, the peripheral blood smear should be evaluated for atypical lymphocytes and a heterophile antibody test should be performed.

Answer E is incorrect. *Staphylococcus aureus* is a common cause of acute bacterial endocarditis in intravenous drug users, and rarely causes pericarditis.

36. **The correct answer is C.** The syndrome described is Guillain-Barré syndrome, a common cause of acute peripheral neuropathy that results in progressive weakness over a period of days. Although one-third of patients report no history of an antecedent infection, the other two-thirds have recently experienced an acute gastrointestinal or influenza-like illness prior to developing the neuropathy. The most common epidemiologic associations involve infections with *Campylobacter jejuni*, *Haemophilus influenzae*, CMV, EBV, *Mycoplasma pneumoniae*, and VZV. Laboratory abnormalities associated with Guillain-Barré syndrome include elevated gamma-globulin, decreased nerve conduction velocity indicative of demyelination, and albuminocytologic dissociation (CSF shows increased protein concentration with normal cell

count in the setting of normal glucose). Although the organisms listed frequently precede the syndrome, there has never been any consistent demonstration of any single infectious agent in the peripheral nerves of these patients, and the cause of the disease is thought to be mediated by hypersensitive T lymphocytes.

Answer A is incorrect. Although immunocompromised patients may be at greater risk for the organisms that are commonly associated with Guillain-Barré syndrome, there is no indication this patient has a weak immune system. Furthermore, *Candida albicans* does not have any association with the syndrome.

Answer B is incorrect. While Legionnaire's disease has been at least anecdotally associated with Guillain-Barré syndrome, an otherwise healthy 28-year-old man would not be expected to develop an infection with *Legionella pneumophila*.

Answer D is incorrect. *Pseudomonas aeruginosa* is not an organism associated with Guillain-Barré syndrome.

Answer E is incorrect. Pneumococcal pneumonia is not associated with the development of Guillain-Barré syndrome.

37. **The correct answer is B.** This man is suffering from septic arthritis, commonly characterized by a swollen, tender, and erythematous joint. The organism most commonly responsible for this infection is *Staphylococcus aureus*. The infection results from the invasion of the bacteria into the synovial fluid. The diagnosis of septic arthritis requires aspiration of the synovial fluid, which appears yellow and turbid with a predominance of neutrophils. When *Staphylococcus* is the causative agent, Gram stain and culture of the synovial fluid show gram-positive cocci in clusters. *S. aureus* is catalase-positive and coagulase-positive.

Answer A is incorrect. While *S. aureus* is indeed catalase-positive, it is not coagulase-negative. This answer instead describes the properties of *S. epidermidis*.

Answer C is incorrect. *S. aureus* does not possess a glycoprotein capsule. *S. pneumoniae* is a gram-positive cocci that does possess a glycoprotein capsule.

Answer D is incorrect. *S. aureus* displays a β-hemolytic pattern, not an α-hemolytic pattern.

Answer E is incorrect. Bile solubility is not a characteristic property of *S. aureus*; instead, it is a property of *S. pneumoniae*.

38. **The correct answer is E.** Rubeola, also called measles, is a relatively rare illness in the United States because of the ubiquity of the measles/mumps/rubella (MMR) vaccine. It presents with the prodrome described in this patient. The rash that spreads from head to toe over a 3-day period develops 1 or 2 days after the appearance of Koplik's spots, which are red oral lesions with blue-white centers.

Answer A is incorrect. Diphtheria is an illness virtually unknown in the United States because of the prevalence of the DTaP vaccine. It is caused by *Corynebacterium diphtheriae* and is characterized by a membranous pharyngitis.

Answer B is incorrect. Pertussis, or whooping cough, is also rare due to widespread vaccinations. It is a respiratory infection of children that characteristically produces coughing spasms followed by a loud inspiratory whoop.

Answer C is incorrect. Roseola is a febrile disease of very young children that begins with a high fever and progresses to a rash similar to measles. Infants and young children are most at risk. It is believed to be caused by human herpesvirus 6.

Answer D is incorrect. Rubella, also known as German measles, is a less severe viral exanthem. Many infections are subclinical, but rubella can cause severe birth defects when infection occurs during the prenatal period.

39. **The correct answer is A.** Disseminated *Mycobacterium avium-intracellulare* commonly infects birds and other animals. It can infect humans when their T lymphocyte count is below approximately 50/mm³. It presents as a chronic

wasting illness as the bacteria proliferate throughout the body. Prophylaxis is with azithromycin. This is the only answer choice whose development requires a T lymphocyte count <50 cells/mm³.

Answer B is incorrect. HSV infection often occurs severely with a T lymphocyte count <400/mm³ or earlier. While herpes simplex can affect individuals with a normal immune system, infection in immunocompromised patients will be more severe, with more oral and genital ulcers.

Answer C is incorrect. Herpes zoster infection can present when the T lymphocyte count is <400/mm³ or earlier. It is characterized as a painful collection of vesicles in a dermatomal pattern.

Answer D is incorrect. Oral thrush can present when the T lymphocyte count is <400/mm³ or earlier. It presents with white patches and plaques on the oral mucosa.

Answer E is incorrect. *Pneumocystis jiroveci* pneumonia is one of the most common opportunistic infections, commonly seen when the T lymphocyte count is <200/mm³. The disease commonly presents with fever, malaise, dyspnea on exertion, and a nonproductive cough. Physical exam is notable for scattered rales and x-ray of the chest may reveal diffuse interstitial infiltrates or may be completely normal if the infection is new. Prophylaxis is with trimethoprim-sulfamethoxazole.

Answer F is incorrect. Toxoplasmosis brain lesions usually present with focal neurologic deficits. CT scan will show a ring-enhancing lesion. Toxoplasmosis prophylaxis is started when the T lymphocyte count is <100/mm³.

40. **The correct answer is D.** This patient has a classic presentation (fever, sore throat, anterior cervical lymphadenopathy, lack of cough) of streptococcal pharyngitis, or strep throat. Strep throat is caused by *Streptococcus pyogenes*, or group A streptococcus. Diagnosis is confirmed with a rapid strep test or with throat swab culture. The treatment of choice is penicillin. To differentiate this organism from other gram-

positive organisms, several tests can be performed in the lab. For example, when cultured on blood agar, *S. pyogenes* creates a clear halo (β-hemolysis) around the colonies due to damage of the RBCs. To further differentiate streptococcal species, sensitivity to different antibiotics is measured. *S. pyogenes* is sensitive to bacitracin.

Answer A is incorrect. Catalase-negative, α-hemolytic, optochin-resistant describes the viridans streptococci. *Streptococcus mutans* is associated with the formation of dental caries.

Answer B is incorrect. Catalase-negative, α-hemolytic, optochin-sensitive describes *Streptococcus pneumoniae*. This organism causes pneumonia and otitis media. Rates of *S. pneumoniae* meningitis have decreased with the advent of the pneumococcal vaccine.

Answer C is incorrect. Catalase-negative, β-hemolytic, bacitracin-resistant describes *Streptococcus agalactiae*, or group B streptococcus. *S. agalactiae* is a significant cause of serious bacterial infection in neonates.

Answer E is incorrect. Catalase-positive, coagulase-negative, novobiocin-resistant describes *Staphylococcus saprophyticus*. This is the second most common cause of urinary tract infection in young, healthy women.

Answer F is incorrect. Catalase-positive, coagulase-negative, novobiocin-sensitive describes *Staphylococcus epidermidis*. Infection with *S. epidermidis* is associated with skin penetration by implanted prosthetic devices such as prosthetic heart valves, intravenous lines, and intraperitoneal catheters.

CHAPTER 5

Immunology

1. A 48-year-man with chronic renal failure undergoes a cadaveric renal transplant. One week later, the patient has an elevated creatinine level. The surgical team is concerned about the possibility of acute transplant rejection. The cell type shown in the image is believed to be an important mediator of this process. In which of the following locations does this cell type complete maturation?

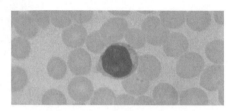

Reproduced, with permission, from Berman I. *Color Atlas of Basic Histology*, 3rd ed. New York: McGraw-Hill, 2003: 83.

(A) Bone marrow
(B) Lung
(C) Spleen
(D) Thymus
(E) Yolk sac

2. A 23-year-old man comes to the physician with a bacterial infection. On questioning the patient reveals a history of recurrent bacterial, fungal, and viral infections. Blood is drawn and sent for laboratory analysis, which reveals all levels of immune cells (eg., T lymphocytes, B lymphocytes) are low. Which of the following conditions is most likely to have caused the patient's symptoms?

(A) Ataxia-telangiectasia
(B) Chédiak-Higashi disease
(C) Common variable immunodeficiency
(D) Job's syndrome
(E) Severe combined immunodeficiency
(F) Wiskott-Aldrich syndrome
(G) X-linked agammaglobulinemia

3. A 13-year-old boy is diagnosed with a hyperactive immune system. Normally an antigen will activate the immune system to trigger a proinflammatory response. Following the proinflammatory response, anti-inflammatory signals then dampen the immune response to prevent it from causing damage. This patient has trouble dampening the immune response after it is no longer needed. Decreased activity in which of the following anti-inflammatory cytokines is most likely the basis for this boy's condition?

(A) Interferon-γ
(B) Interleukin-1
(C) Transforming growth factor-β
(D) Tumor necrosis factor-α
(E) Tumor necrosis factor-β

4. A 19-year-old man comes to the physician with a bacterial infection. Without treatment, the patient's immune system will most likely be able to fight off the infection within a few days. One of the tools the patient's body uses against the organism is the membrane attack complex. The membrane attack complex functions as which of the following?

(A) A chemoattractant for neutrophils
(B) An anaphylactic signal causing degranulation of mast cells
(C) An opsonization molecule, facilitating phagocytosis
(D) A proteinaceous pore in the plasma membrane
(E) A scaffold on cell membranes to which antibodies can bind

5. To assess the risk of erythroblastosis fetalis occurring during the future pregnancy of an Rh-negative woman, a clinician sends a sample of serum for detection of anti Rh-blood group antibodies. The laboratory performs an indirect Coombs' test by mixing the patient's serum with Rh-positive RBCs and then adding an anti-IgG antibody. In doing so, the laboratory technician observes agglutination of the RBCs. After receiving this test result, the clinician would be correct to conclude which of the following?

(A) The Coombs' test yielded a negative result, and therefore the mother does not have anti-Rh antibodies

(B) The laboratory performed the test incorrectly; they should have mixed the patient's serum with Rh-negative rather than Rh-positive RBCs

(C) The patient has had previous pregnancies and all of her children are Rh-negative

(D) The patient is currently pregnant with an Rh-positive fetus

(E) The presence of anti-Rh antibodies in the patient's serum suggests that she has been pregnant with an Rh-positive fetus

6. A newborn child is exposed to *Streptococcus agalactiae* and subsequently develops meningitis. Which of the following could have contributed to this child's bacterial infection?

(A) A defect in DNA repair enzymes with associated IgA deficiency

(B) An X-linked recessive defect in a tyrosine kinase gene

(C) Improper development of the thymus and parathyroid glands

(D) Improper transfer of IgG from the mother to the fetus

(E) Improper transfer of IgM from the mother to the fetus

7. *Haemophilus influenzae* and *Neisseria meningitidis* both possess a polysaccharide outer capsule. Effective vaccination against these species results in the generation of antibodies that recognize this polysaccharide capsule. Which of the following best explains why the childhood vaccines for *H. influenzae* type B and *N. meningitidis* serogroup C are composed of a polysaccharide coat conjugated to a protein carrier?

(A) The protein carrier increases the half-life of the vaccine

(B) The protein carrier increases the production of IgE immunoglobulins, which confer protection

(C) The protein carrier is added to recruit T lymphocyte help and increase antibody production

(D) The protein carrier makes the vaccine less virulent and thus decreases the risk of a child developing disease from the immunization

(E) The protein carrier plays no role and is included only for ease of preparation

8. A type B blood group, Rh-positive recipient is mistakenly transplanted with a kidney from a type A blood group, Rh-negative donor. Which of the following best describes the mechanism of transplant rejection that is most likely to ensue in this recipient?

(A) Acute rejection mediated by preformed recipient antibodies

(B) Acute rejection mediated by recipient T lymphocytes

(C) Graft-versus-host disease mediated by donor T lymphocytes

(D) Hyperacute rejection mediated by preformed donor antibodies

(E) Hyperacute rejection mediated by preformed recipient antibodies

9. A 12-year-old girl is brought to the pediatrician by her mother because of a fever. The physician notes that the girl has features of albinism and the mother states that her daughter has always looked the way she does. The physician diagnoses the girl with a staphylococcal infection and prescribes a course of antibiotics. Three months later, the child returns to the pediatrician with another streptococcal infection. The patient's medical records indicate that she has had repeated bouts of staphylococcal and streptococcal infections for her entire life. This patient most likely has which of the following types of immune deficiency?

(A) Chédiak-Higashi disease

(B) Chronic granulomatous disease

(C) Hyper-IgM syndrome

(D) Selective IgA deficiency

(E) Severe combined immunodeficiency

10. A 60-year-old post-menopausal woman presents with fatigue, mild jaundice, and tingling in the lower extremities. Laboratory studies show elevated serum levels of homocysteine and methyl malonic acid, and complete blood cell count shows a mild thrombocytopenia. Which of the following findings would be expected on a peripheral blood smear from this patient?

(A) A megaloblastic anemia with hypersegmented polymorphonuclear leukocytes
(B) A microcytic anemia with hypersegmented polymorphonuclear leukocytes
(C) A microcytic hypochromic anemia with decreased serum iron and increased total iron-binding capacity
(D) A normochromic normocytic anemia with decreased serum iron and decreased total iron-binding capacity
(E) Normal peripheral blood smear with normal serum iron and normal total iron-binding capacity

11. Antigen processing and presentation within the context of a major histocompatibility complex (MHC) class I molecule is essential to generating a CD8+ T-lymphocyte response. In which of the diagramed subcellular locations is the self-peptide loaded onto MHC class I molecules?

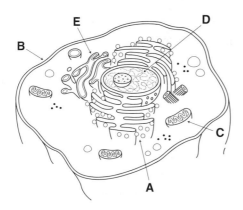

Reproduced, with permission, from USMLERx.com.

(A) A
(B) B
(C) C
(D) D
(E) E

12. A 7-year-old boy presents to the clinic with a staphylococcal infection. He is well known at the clinic because he has had recurrent staphylococcal infections for most of his life. He is started on an antibiotic regimen and the infection subsides. Three weeks later, the boy is diagnosed with pruritic papulovesicular dermatitis. Which of the following immune deficiency syndromes would account for this patient's recurrent staphylococcal infections and pruritic papulovesicular dermatitis?

(A) Ataxia-telangiectasia
(B) Bruton's agammaglobulinemia
(C) Job's syndrome
(D) Thymic aplasia
(E) Wiskott-Aldrich syndrome

13. Hyper-IgM syndrome usually presents with severe pyogenic infections. The typical immunoglobulin profile in a patient with this disease shows an elevated level of IgM in contrast to the other immunoglobulin isotypes. Which of the following is the etiology behind the increased level of IgM in a patient with hyper-IgM syndrome?

(A) A defect in DNA repair enzymes
(B) A defect in LFA-1 adhesion proteins on phagocytes
(C) A defect in the CD40 ligand on CD4 T helper cells
(D) Failure of interferon-γ production
(E) Failure of the thymus and parathyroid glands to develop

14. A 40-year-old man presents to his physician with numbness and tingling on the dorsal surface of his right hand and forearm and raised "varicose veins" that are firm to the touch along the same distribution. He also complains of weight loss. His serum creatinine level is 2.0 mg/dL. He has no previous medical history of significance. An immune complex disease is suspected, and assays for autoantibodies in neutrophils are conducted. What diseases are associated with the identification of anti-myeloperoxidase and anti-proteinase-3 antibodies, respectively?

(A) Kawasaki's disease, Buerger's disease
(B) Microscopic polyangiitis, Wegener's granulomatosis
(C) Polyarteritis nodosa, Buerger's disease
(D) Takayasu's arteritis, Wegener's granulomatosis
(E) Temporal arteritis, Wegener's granulomatosis

15. A 32-year-old man with Hodgkin's lymphoma is scheduled to undergo a bone marrow transplant. HLA typing of his immediate family shows that his identical twin brother is a suitable match for harvesting an allogenic bone marrow graft. This type of graft can be classified as which of the following?

(A) Autologous
(B) Combination graft
(C) Heterograft
(D) Syngeneic
(E) Xenogeneic

16. Patients sharing similar clinical symptoms and disease pathology may nevertheless present differently based upon age at disease onset. Adult-onset rheumatoid arthritis (RA) and juvenile rheumatoid arthritis (JRA) are both the result of inflammatory processes. How does the presentation of JRA differ from the presentation of adult-onset RA?

(A) JRA is simply the presence of RA that begins before the age of 21 years
(B) Patients with JRA are less likely to have systemic symptoms, but the likelihood of high levels of serum rheumatoid factor is the same
(C) Patients with JRA are more likely to have large joint involvement, but the likelihood of concurrent systemic symptoms is the same
(D) Patients with JRA are more likely to have systemic symptoms and high levels of serum rheumatoid factor
(E) Patients with JRA are more likely to have systemic symptoms and large joint involvement

17. A 37-year-old man comes to the physician with recurrent viral infections. Blood studies show normal levels of circulating lymphocytes and neutrophils. A deficiency in which of the following cytokines would most likely lead to this man's condition?

(A) Interleukin-2
(B) Interleukin-3
(C) Interleukin-4
(D) Interleukin-5
(E) Interleukin-8

18. Cluster of differentiation (CD) antigens are glycoproteins present on the cell surface of many cell types involved in the immune system. They are recognized by monoclonal antibodies and aid in the identification of various cell types. Which of the following glycoproteins is present on the cell surface of all thymocytes: helper T-cells, cytotoxic T-cells, and natural killer cells?

(A) B7
(B) CD2
(C) CD3
(D) CD4
(E) CD19
(F) T-cell receptor

19. A 2-year-old girl with a lifelong history of malabsorptive and foul-smelling diarrhea, weakness, and general failure to thrive has just undergone a small intestine biopsy (see image). Her parents believe her problems began at 6 months of age, when she started eating solid foods, but have significantly worsened over the past few months. The only recent change in her diet is that she eats a bowl of cereal every morning with her parents before they go to work. She tried a dairy-free diet a month ago, but it did not improve her symptoms. Which of the following is the most likely diagnosis?

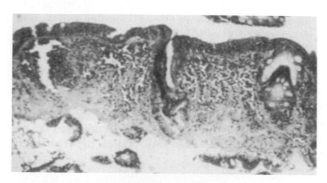

Reproduced, with permission, from Chandrasoma P, Taylor CR. *Concise Pathology*, 3rd ed. New York: McGraw-Hill, 1998: Figure 39-3.

(A) Abetalipoproteinemia
(B) Celiac sprue
(C) Lactase deficiency
(D) Viral enteritis
(E) Whipple's disease

20. A pediatrician becomes concerned after learning the family and medical history of an infant who is currently suffering from pneumonia, with a presumed diagnosis of *Streptococcus pneumoniae* infection. Over the past year, the patient has suffered from erysipelas as well as a previous bout of pneumococcal pneumonia; both were treated successfully with antibiotics. The patient's mother says that her son's maternal uncle also suffered from repeated bacterial infections and was successfully treated with antibiotics. On physical examination, it appears that the patient does not have tonsils. His mother denies a previous tonsillectomy. Analy-

sis of the boy's serum would most likely yield which of the following results?

(A) Absence of T lymphocytes
(B) <200 CD4$^+$ T lymphocytes/mm^3
(C) IgA, IgG, and IgM levels normal
(D) IgG and IgM levels markedly decreased, no IgA
(E) IgG and IgM levels normal, IgA markedly decreased

21. A 25-year-old man presents to his doctor with a 2-day history of blood in his urine. A kidney biopsy is obtained. When the tissue is stained with fluorescent anti-IgG antibodies, the staining reveals a linear pattern. Which of the following is the most likely diagnosis?

(A) Acute poststreptococcal glomerulonephritis
(B) Alport's syndrome
(C) Goodpasture's syndrome
(D) IgA nephropathy
(E) Membranous glomerulonephritis

22. A clinician is concerned that an Rh-negative mother may be pregnant with an Rh-positive fetus. The potential pathology that the clinician is concerned about is classified as which of the following immune reactions?

(A) Graft-versus-host disease
(B) Type I hypersensitivity
(C) Type II hypersensitivity
(D) Type III hypersensitivity
(E) Type IV hypersensitivity

23. A 14-year-old boy presents to the physician with recurrent pyogenic infections. Physical examination shows that the boy has pruritic papulovesicular dermatitis. Blood is drawn and sent for laboratory evaluation of platelets and immunoglobulin levels. The results show a markedly low platelet count, a low serum IgM level, and an elevated IgA level. This patient most likely has which of the following conditions?

(A) Bruton's agammaglobulinemia
(B) Chédiak-Higashi disease
(C) Job's syndrome
(D) Thymic aplasia
(E) Wiskott-Aldrich syndrome

24. A 32-year-old woman comes to the emergency department complaining of sudden blindness. On obtaining a thorough history, it is learned that the patient's right leg has "given out" from time to time, causing the patient to have episodes of weakness and falling. Periventricular white matter plaques are found on MRI. Which of the following cells are primarily damaged in this disease?

   (A) Astrocytes
   (B) Ependymal cells
   (C) Oligodendrocytes
   (D) Schwann cells
   (E) T cells

25. Women have about a 2.7 times greater lifetime risk of developing at least one autoimmune disease than men. Which of the following statements, if true, would support the higher rate of systemic lupus erythematosus in women than in men?

   (A) Androgens such as testosterone have an inhibitory role in the process of clearing immune complexes
   (B) Both estrogens and androgens have the same potency in inhibiting the clearing of immune complexes
   (C) Estrogen has an inhibitory role in the process of antibody production of B cells
   (D) Estrogen has an inhibitory role in the process of clearing immune complexes
   (E) Estrogen has a stimulatory role in the process of clearing immune complexes

26. A 2-year-old boy is brought to the physician by his parents because of recurrent sinus infections. The parents also state that the boy has had multiple lung infections. Which of the following results would most likely be found on further testing?

   (A) A deficit in IgA level
   (B) A low IgM level, with increased IgA
   (C) A negative nitroblue tetrazolium dye test
   (D) An increase in IgE level
   (E) A normal Ig level for all isotypes

27. A 50-year-old man presents to his clinician because of bilateral itching, burning, and redness of the lower extremities. He states that he wore shorts while gardening outside his house recently and could have come in contact with poison ivy. Which of the following statements regarding this patient's immune response is most correct?

   (A) Goodpasture's syndrome is a disease with a similar reaction pathogenesis
   (B) Histamine is the primary mediator leading to this type of reaction
   (C) The pathogenesis implicates previously sensitized B lymphocytes
   (D) The patient has never been exposed to poison ivy
   (E) The patient is suffering from a type I hypersensitivity reaction
   (F) The patient must have been exposed to a poison ivy plant prior to this instance

28. Antibodies are one of the major players in the adaptive immune response. All antibody molecules consist of two heavy chains and two light chains, and the specific type of heavy and light chain will determine the antigen binding site. In all antibodies, the two heavy chains and the two light chains are identical. Like most proteins, much of their functional capabilities and antigen binding characteristics stem from their three-dimensional structure. Which of the following holds the heavy and light chains together to make the three-dimensional structure of the antibody?

   (A) Disulfide bonds
   (B) Hydrogen bonds
   (C) Ionic bonds
   (D) Triple covalent bonds
   (E) Van der Waals forces

29. A 23-year-old woman comes to the physician for a routine checkup. She has generally been well over the past year, although she notes that she has "had a few falls lately." On physical examination, the lesion shown in the image is found on her skin. Blood is drawn for laboratory evaluation. The results show that the woman has very low levels of IgA. Based on her presentation, this patient will most likely also present with which of the following symptoms?

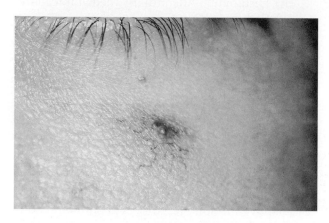

Reproduced, with permission, from Wolff K, Johnson RA, Suurmond D. *Fitzpatrick's Color Atlas & Synopsis of Clinical Dermatolgy*, 5th ed. New York: McGraw-Hill, 2005: Figure 9-22.

(A) Cerebellar problems
(B) Granulomas
(C) Low levels of all other immunoglobulin isotypes
(D) Tetany
(E) Visual hallucinations

30. A 50-year-old man comes to the physician with hemoptysis and diffuse joint pain. He states that both his father and cousin had similar symptoms and were diagnosed with microscopic polyangiitis, a disease affecting medium- to small-sized arteries that is believed to have an autoimmune component to its pathogenesis. Which of the following autoantibodies might be present in this patient?

(A) Anticentromere antibodies
(B) Antineutrophil cytoplasmic autoantibodies
(C) Anti-Smith antibodies
(D) Anti-SS-A (Ro) antibody
(E) Anti-SS-B (La) antibody

ANSWERS

1. **The correct answer is D.** Acute rejection is one complication of kidney transplantation. In acute rejection, the principal mediator is believed to be the cytotoxic T lymphocyte. Activated cytotoxic lymphocytes invade the tubular interstitium of the transplanted kidney, leading to tubulitis. In contrast, chronic rejection is mediated by antibody complex formation. Elevated creatinine levels allow early detection of acute rejection in the absence of clinical signs, which may include graft tenderness, oliguria, and fever. T lymphocytes mature in the thymus, where they undergo positive and negative selection. Thus, the correct answer is the thymus.

Answer A is incorrect. B lymphocytes mature in the bone marrow. B lymphocytes are not the principal mediators of acute rejection, since B lymphocytes are involved in antibody production, which would occur over a longer time frame.

Answer B is incorrect. T lymphocytes do not undergo maturation in the lung.

Answer C is incorrect. T lymphocytes are found in the periarterial lymphatic sheath in the white pulp of the spleen, but maturation occurs in the thymus, not in the spleen.

Answer E is incorrect. The yolk sac, the liver, and the spleen are important in RBC formation in utero but are not relevant in T-lymphocyte development.

2. **The correct answer is E.** Severe combined immunodeficiency is a defect in early stem cell differentiation that can have many causes and leads to a total lack of a cellular immune system. The typical presentation of this disease includes recurrent bacterial, viral, protozoal, and fungal infections.

Answer A is incorrect. Ataxia-telangiectasia is a defect in DNA repair enzymes. The disease is associated with an IgA deficiency. The typical presentation of the disease is given away by the name, as symptoms include cerebellar problems (ataxia) and spider angiomas (telangiectasia).

Answer B is incorrect. Chédiak-Higashi disease is an autosomal recessive disease that presents with recurrent streptococcal and staphylococcal infections. A defect in lysosomal emptying of phagocytic cells due to microtubular dysfunction is the underlying cause of the disease.

Answer C is incorrect. Common variable immunodeficiency is characterized by low IgM, IgG, and IgA levels but normal B and T lymphocyte levels.

Answer D is incorrect. Job's syndrome involves the failure of helper T lymphocytes to produce interferon-γ (INF-γ). Since the latter is a potent activator of phagocytic cells, a decrease in its production leads to a failure of neutrophils to respond to chemotactic stimuli.

Answer F is incorrect. Wiskott-Aldrich syndrome is an X-linked defect associated with elevated IgA levels, elevated IgE levels, and low IgM levels. It involves a defect in the body's ability to mount an IgM response to bacteria. Recurrent pyogenic infections, eczema, and thrombocytopenia are the typical triad of symptoms that present with this disease.

Answer G is incorrect. X-linked agammaglobulinemia is characterized by decreased IgM, IgG, IgA, and B lymphocyte levels, but normal T lymphocyte levels.

3. **The correct answer is C.** Mounting a strong immune response is crucial for the body to be able to fight off infections. However, reducing this response once the infection has been warded off is critical in order for the body to maintain its normal balance. Transforming growth factor-β is the cytokine that is responsible for dampening the immune response after it is no longer needed.

Answer A is incorrect. IFN-γ is secreted by helper T lymphocytes and helps stimulate macrophages.

Answer B is incorrect. Interleukin (IL)-1 is secreted by macrophages and serves as one of the main cytokines involved in mounting an acute phase response.

Answer D is incorrect. Tumor necrosis factor-α is one of the main cytokines involved in mounting an acute-phase response; it is secreted by macrophages.

Answer E is incorrect. Tumor necrosis factor-β has functions similar to tumor necrosis factor-α in that it helps mount an acute-phase response. However, it is secreted by activated T lymphocytes instead of macrophages.

4. **The correct answer is D.** The C5b, 6, 7, 8 complex guides the polymerization of C9 molecules in lipid bilayer of the target cell's plasma membrane. C9 polymers form pores in the membrane, allowing the passage of ions and small molecules into the cell, causing the cell to lyse.

Answer A is incorrect. This answer choice refers to C5a, which is involved in neutrophil chemotaxis.

Answer B is incorrect. C3a and C5a are the molecules that are involved in anaphylaxis, not the membrane attack complex.

Answer C is incorrect. This answer choice refers to C3b, which is involved in opsonization.

Answer E is incorrect. This is not the function of the membrane attack complex.

5. **The correct answer is E.** When an Rh-negative mother gives birth to an Rh-positive fetus, fetal RBCs may enter the mother's circulation, and the body may recognize the Rh antigen as foreign and produce antibodies against it. As maternal IgG freely crosses the placenta, any subsequent Rh-positive fetus is at risk for hemolytic disease. Thus, the indirect Coombs' test is an important laboratory tool to monitor for Rh incompatibilities that may complicate fetal health. The test result given in this question indicates that the patient possesses anti-Rh antibodies in her serum. Therefore, it would be logical for the clinician to suspect previous pregnancy with an Rh-positive fetus.

Answer A is incorrect. The test yielded a positive result. Agglutination occurs when the anti-IgG antibody binds to the anti-Rh antibodies that are already bound to the Rh-positive RBCs.

Answer B is incorrect. The laboratory protocol described in the question stem is correct. Rh-positive RBCs must be added because the test is assaying for the presence anti-Rh antibodies, which will bind the Rh antigen on the RBCs.

Answer C is incorrect. The presence of anti-Rh antibodies within the patient's serum suggests that she has been exposed to the blood of at least one Rh-positive fetus.

Answer D is incorrect. The results of the test cannot be used to determine the Rh status of a current fetus; only direct typing of fetal blood can determine its Rh status.

6. **The correct answer is D.** Circulating IgG that is passed from the mother to the newborn through the placenta protects the newborn from many microorganisms for the first 6 months of life. Thus, improper transfer of IgG from the mother to the fetus can leave the newborn susceptible to infections. While IgA is found in breast milk, a neonate will have access only to antenatal antibodies, and IgG is the only antibody isotype that can cross the placenta.

Answer A is incorrect. Ataxia-telangiectasia is caused by a defect in DNA repair enzymes with associated IgA deficiency. This usually presents with cerebellar problems (ataxia) and spider angiomas (telangiectasia). It would not cause a neonate to be immunocompromised, because for the first 6 months of life the infant relies on IgG from the mother.

Answer B is incorrect. An X-linked recessive defect in a tyrosine kinase gene is seen in Bruton's agammaglobulinemia. This is associated with low levels of all classes of immunoglobulins. However, with Bruton's agammaglobulinemia, bacterial infections tend to occur after 6 months of age, when levels of maternal IgG antibody start to decline to levels insufficient to provide host defense.

Answer C is incorrect. Improper development of the thymus and parathyroid glands is seen in thymic aplasia (DiGeorge's syndrome). This leads to recurrent viral and fungal infections due to a T lymphocyte deficiency. It would not have any effect on susceptibility to bacterial infections.

Answer E is incorrect. The only antibody isotype that can cross the placenta is IgG. Therefore, IgM would not play a role in an infant's immunity until an infant can produce it themselves, at the age of 6 months.

7. **The correct answer is C.** Helper T lymphocytes can assist in the activation of B cells as long as the epitopes they recognize are linked (they do not have to be identical). Polysaccharides are very poor T-lymphocyte epitopes and thus do not by themselves elicit a T lymphocyte response. Because the polysaccharides are T lymphocyte-independent antigens, they do not elicit effective immunity in infants. Conjugating the polysaccharide to a protein carrier links the two epitopes and allows a B lymphocyte that recognizes the polysaccharide to be activated by a T-helper cell that recognizes epitopes present within the protein carrier.

Answer A is incorrect. Even if the protein carrier does increase the half-life of the vaccine, it is not the reason the vaccine is conjugated to a protein carrier.

Answer B is incorrect. IgE mediates allergic and type I hypersensitivity responses. It is not expected to be an important immunoglobulin isotype produced in response to this vaccination.

Answer D is incorrect. The polysaccharide coat is not capable of causing disease. It is not a live or attenuated bacterium.

Answer E is incorrect. The protein carrier is essential to eliciting an effective immune response involving T cells that leads to immunization against the bacteria.

8. **The correct answer is E.** This clinical scenario would result in hyperacute rejection (within minutes of transplantation; clinical presenta-

tion within minutes to hours) mediated by preformed recipient antidonor antibodies in the recipient. The recipient would possess antitype A antibodies, which react to the A antigen present not only on RBCs but on most other cell types. Hyperacute rejection occurs almost immediately, as the antidonor antibodies bind directly to vascular endothelial cells, initiating complement and clotting cascades and resulting in hemorrhage and necrosis of the transplanted kidney. It should be noted that it is not only ABO blood group mismatches but any antidonor antibodies possessed by the recipient that can lead to hyperacute rejection; thus it is important to carefully cross-match donor and recipient.

Answer A is incorrect. Acute rejection is cell-mediated and occurs within weeks following major histocompatibility complex (MHC)-mismatched transplant as a result of cytotoxic T lymphocytes reacting to foreign MHC molecules. It is reversible with cyclosporine.

Answer B is incorrect. Acute rejection is cell-mediated and occurs within weeks following MHC-mismatched transplant as a result of cytotoxic T lymphocytes reacting to foreign MHC molecules. In this scenario, hyperacute rejection would be expected to occur first (within the first few hours after transplant).

Answer C is incorrect. Graft-versus-host disease (GVHD) is a serious side effect of bone marrow transplantation mediated by donor-derived T lymphocytes. Acute GVHD usually occurs within the first 3 months following an allogeneic bone marrow transplantation, whereas chronic GVHD usually develops after the third month posttransplant.

Answer D is incorrect. Hyperacute rejection is typically mediated by preformed antidonor antibodies that are possessed by the recipient.

9. **The correct answer is A.** Chédiak-Higashi disease is an inherited autosomal recessive disease. It is caused by a deficiency in lysosomal emptying of phagocytic cells due to a defect in microtubular function. Therefore, patients with Chédiak-Higashi disease often present with recurrent streptococcal and staphylococ-

cal infections. Partial albinism may be present, as melanosomes are derivatives of lysosomes.

Answer B is incorrect. Chronic granulomatous disease presents with an increased susceptibility to infections by microbes that produce their own catalase (eg., *Staphylococcus* and *Candida*). It results from defective neutrophil phagocytosis due to a lack of NADPH oxidase (or similar enzymes) activity. A negative nitroblue tetrazolium dye reduction test confirms the diagnosis of chronic granulomatous disease.

Answer C is incorrect. Hyper-IgM syndrome is caused by a defect in the CD40 ligand on $CD4^+$ T helper cells. This defect leads to an inability to class switch between the different immunoglobulin isotypes. Since IgM is initially produced and subsequently switched to the other isotypes, an inability to do so leads to elevated IgM levels and low levels of all other isotypes.

Answer D is incorrect. Selective immunoglobulin deficiency is a deficit in a specific class of immunoglobulins. IgA deficiency is the most common of these diseases. Since IgA is the most prominent immunoglobulin found in mucous membranes, patients suffering from a deficiency of it often present with sinus and lung infections.

Answer E is incorrect. Severe combined immunodeficiency is a defect in early stem cell differentiation that can have many causes. The typical presentation of this disease includes recurrent bacterial, viral, protozoal, and fungal infections.

10. **The correct answer is A.** The symptoms and laboratory findings suggest a chronic progressive anemia caused by a failure to absorb vitamin B_{12} due to a lack of available intrinsic factor (IF). Autoimmune gastritis/pernicious anemia is associated with two forms of auto-antibodies: (1) antibodies directed against the transmembrane proton pumps of parietal cells (the cells that secrete gastric acid and intrinsic factor), and (2) antibodies directed against IF itself. The latter antibodies can prevent either the binding of vitamin B_{12} to IF, or the binding of

the vitamin B_{12}-IF complex to its receptor in the distal ileum (where absorption takes place). Antiparietal cell antibodies lead to parietal cell destruction and selective atrophy of the fundus and corpus of the stomach (the portions of the stomach where parietal cells are located), while both anti-parietal and anti-IF antibodies can contribute to a lack of available IF. Symptoms of this autoimmune disease are generally due to the resultant vitamin B_{12}-deficiency anemia. They can include fatigue, pallor, mild to moderated jaundice, glossitis (a painful, beefy tongue), neuropathies (particularly of the lower extremities), and atrophy of the posterior columns in the spinal cord. Serum levels of homocysteine and methyl malonic acid can be elevated, and complete blood cell count can show a thrombocytopenia. Vitamin B_{12} deficiency anemia is a megaloblastic anemia and is associated with hypersegmented neutrophils. In the past, pernicious anemia was often diagnosed with the Schilling test, in which patients were given radiolabeled vitamin B_{12} orally, and absorption was monitored by the amount of radioactivity appearing in the urine. Currently serological tests directed against IF antibodies are more commonly used.

Answer B is incorrect. The findings in this answer choice are not consistent with pernicious anemia, the condition described in the question stem. Microcytosis with hypersegmented neutrophils could be seen in iron-deficiency anemia or the anemia of chronic disease. Hypersegmented neutrophils, however, are most classically associated with vitamin B_{12} deficiency, which is strictly megaloblastic.

Answer C is incorrect. The findings in this choice are often found in iron deficiency anemia, not pernicious anemia.

Answer D is incorrect. The findings in this choice are often found in anemia of chronic disease, not pernicious anemia, the condition described in the question stem.

Answer E is incorrect. The findings in this answer choice are not consistent with pernicious anemia, the condition described in the question stem.

11. **The correct answer is A.** Self- and virally-derived cytosolic proteins are targeted for degradation by the proteasome. After degradation, peptides enter the rough endoplasmic reticulum (RER) by ATP-dependent transport via TAP (transporters associated with antigen processing) proteins. These peptides may then bind within the peptide-binding groove of a newly folded MHC class I molecule. The MHC class I molecule can now exit the RER and travel via the Golgi apparatus to the cell surface, where it may interact with the T-lymphocyte receptor and CD8 coreceptor.

Answer B is incorrect. Self-peptide is loaded onto class I in the rough endoplasmic reticulum. The MHC molecule does not travel to the cell surface unless peptide is bound within the peptide-binding groove.

Answer C is incorrect. Mitochondria are not directly involved in antigen processing or presentation.

Answer D is incorrect. The nucleus is not directly involved in antigen processing or presentation.

Answer E is incorrect. The Golgi apparatus is not the site of self-peptide loading onto the MHC molecule.

12. **The correct answer is C.** Job's syndrome involves the failure of helper T lymphocytes to produce IFN-γ. Since IFN-γ is a potent activator of phagocytic cells, a decrease in its production leads to a failure of neutrophils to respond to chemotactic stimuli. Job's syndrome presents with recurrent staphylococcal abscesses, eczema, and high levels of IgE.

Answer A is incorrect. Ataxia-telangiectasia is caused by a defect in DNA repair enzymes. The disease is associated with an IgA deficiency. The typical presentation of the disease is given away by the name, as symptoms include cerebellar problems (ataxia) and spider angiomas (telangiectasia).

Answer B is incorrect. Bruton's agammaglobulinemia is an X-linked defect and therefore presents in males. It is caused by a defect in tyrosine kinase associated with low levels of all

classes of immunoglobulins. After 6 months of age, when the levels of maternal antibodies have declined, patients with the disease tend to present with recurrent bacterial infections.

Answer D is incorrect. The third and fourth pharyngeal pouches, and thus the thymus and parathyroid glands, fail to develop in patients with thymic aplasia (DiGeorge's syndrome). The disease often presents with many congenital defects, such as cardiac abnormalities, cleft palate, and abnormal facies. Thymic aplasia can also present with tetany due to hypocalcemia.

Answer E is incorrect. Wiskott-Aldrich syndrome is an X-linked defect associated with elevated IgA levels, elevated IgE levels, normal IgG levels, and low IgM levels. It involves a defect in the body's ability to mount an IgM response to bacteria. Recurrent pyogenic infections, eczema, and thrombocytopenia are the typical triad of symptoms. It does not present with any specific enzyme abnormality.

13. **The correct answer is C.** Hyper-IgM syndrome is caused by a defect in the CD40 ligand on CD4 T helper cells. This defect leads to an inability to class switch between the different immunoglobulin isotypes. Since IgM is initially created and subsequently switched to the other isotypes, an inability to do so leads to elevated IgM levels and low levels of all other isotypes.

Answer A is incorrect. Ataxia-telangiectasia is caused by a defect in DNA repair enzymes. The disease is associated with an IgA deficiency. The typical presentation of the disease is given away by the name, as symptoms include cerebellar problems (ataxia) and spider angiomas (telangiectasia).

Answer B is incorrect. Leukocyte adhesion deficiency syndrome is caused by a defect in the LFA-1 adhesion protein on the surface of neutrophils. The disease usually presents with marked leukocytosis and localized bacterial infections that are difficult to detect until they have progressed to an extensive life-threatening level. Since neutrophils are unable to adhere to the endothelium and transmigrate into tissues, infections in patients with leukocyte adhesion deficiency syndrome act similarly to those observed in neutropenic patients.

Answer D is incorrect. Job's syndrome involves the failure of helper T lymphocytes to produce IFN-γ. Since IFN-γ is a potent activator of phagocytic cells, a decrease in its production leads to a failure of neutrophils to respond to chemotactic stimuli. Job's syndrome presents with recurrent staphylococcal abscesses, eczema, and high levels of IgE.

Answer E is incorrect. In thymic aplasia (DiGeorge's syndrome), the third and fourth pharyngeal pouches, and thus the thymus and parathyroid glands, fail to develop. The disease often presents with many congenital defects, such as cardiac abnormalities, cleft palate, and abnormal facies. Thymic aplasia can also present with tetany due to hypocalcemia.

14. **The correct answer is B.** Patients suffering from microscopic polyangiitis often have autoantibodies against the enzyme myeloperoxidase, which stains in a perinuclear pattern and is therefore commonly called P-ANCA (perinuclear-antineutrophil cytoplasmic antibody). Wegener's granulomatosis is a vasculitis characterized by necrotizing granuloma formation in the lung and kidneys. These patients often have autoantibodies specific for proteinase-3, which stains in a cytoplasmic distribution and is therefore commonly called C-ANCA (cytoplasmic-antineutrophil cytoplasmic antibody). In both of these diseases, the patient's autoantibody titer is usually a good indicator of disease severity, particularly in Wegener's granulomatosis, where specificity and sensitivity of antibody testing are both >90%.

Answer A is incorrect. Kawasaki's disease is not associated with serum P-ANCA, and Buerger's disease is not associated with serum C-ANCA.

Answer C is incorrect. "Classic" polyarteritis nodosa is not associated with P-ANCA, and Buerger's disease is not associated with C-ANCA.

Answer D is incorrect. Takayasu's arteritis is not associated with serum P-ANCA.

Answer E is incorrect. Temporal arteritis is not associated with serum P-ANCA.

15. **The correct answer is D.** Allogenic grafts, or homografts, are harvested from another individual of the same species. An allogenic graft from a patient's identical twin sibling is called a syngeneic graft.

Answer A is incorrect. An autologous bone marrow graft, or self-graft, would be a transplantation from the patient's own tissue.

Answer B is incorrect. A combination graft is usually composed of a mixture of autogenous and allogenic tissue.

Answer C is incorrect. A heterograft (also called a xenogeneic graft) is a graft taken from a different species.

Answer E is incorrect. A xenogeneic graft, or heterograft, is a graft taken from a different species.

16. **The correct answer is E.** JRA may appear with a different presentation than adult-onset RA. By definition, JRA begins before age 16 years and must include arthritis in at least one joint for at least 6 weeks. Additionally, the morphologic joint pathology is similar to that of adult-onset RA. However, there are several signs and symptoms that occur more commonly in JRA than in adult-onset RA; these include increased likelihood of systemic onset (with symptoms including high fevers, lymphadenopathy, and hepatomegaly), increased likelihood of large joint involvement, and increased likelihood of antinuclear antibody seropositivity. Furthermore, JRA patients are less likely to have rheumatoid nodules and rheumatoid factor.

Answer A is incorrect. There are several signs and symptoms that occur more commonly in JRA than in adult-onset RA, including increased likelihood of systemic onset, increased likelihood of large joint involvement, and increased likelihood of antinuclear antibody seropositivity.

Answer B is incorrect. Systemic symptoms are more likely, but high levels of serum rheumatoid factor are less likely, in patients with JRA.

Answer C is incorrect. Both systemic symptoms and large joint involvement are more likely in patients with JRA.

Answer D is incorrect. Systemic symptoms are more likely, but high levels of serum rheumatoid factor are less likely, in patients with JRA.

17. **The correct answer is A.** Recurrent viral infections are a sign of T lymphocyte dysfunction. Particularly important in the response to viral infections are cytotoxic (CD8) T lymphocytes. IL-2 is a cytokine secreted by helper T lymphocytes that stimulates the growth of helper and cytotoxic T lymphocytes. Therefore, even though this patient may have an adequate number of T lymphocytes, a deficiency in IL-2 could lead to impaired cytotoxic T lymphocyte differentiation and activation. This would result in an increased susceptibility to viral infections.

Answer B is incorrect. IL-3 is secreted by activated T lymphocytes and has functions similar to granulocyte macrophage colony-stimulating factor.

Answer C is incorrect. IL-4 is secreted by helper T lymphocytes and promotes the growth of B lymphocytes.

Answer D is incorrect. IL-5 is secreted by helper T lymphocytes and promotes the differentiation of B lymphocytes.

Answer E is incorrect. IL-8 is the major chemotactic factor for neutrophils.

18. **The correct answer is B.** CD2 is a marker present in all lymphocytes of thymic origin, and is in the Ig superfamily of adhesion molecules. In T lymphocytes, it precedes either CD4 or CD8 expression and is present throughout the cell's life. It is also expressed by natural killer cells.

Answer A is incorrect. B7 is a protein complex consisting of CD80 and CD86 glycoproteins that is present on antigen presenting cells, including B lymphocytes. CD80/86 serves as a ligand for the costimulatory receptor CD28 present on T lymphocytes; a dual CD28-TCR signal is a potent activator of T lymphocytes.

Answer C is incorrect. CD3 is a pan-T-lymphocyte marker that complexes with T-cell receptor and CD4 or CD8 to convey activation signals to the T lymphocytes. CD3 is not present on natural killer cells.

Answer D is incorrect. CD4 is present on the surfaces of helper (rather than cytotoxic) T lymphocytes, while CD8 is present on the surfaces of cytotoxic (rather than helper) T lymphocytes.

Answer E is incorrect. CD19 is present on B lymphocytes, CD8 is present on cytotoxic T lymphocytes, and CD4 is present on helper T lymphocytes.

Answer F is incorrect. T-cell receptor (TCR) is an α/β heterodimer encoded by genes undergoing V(D)J recombination. Each clone of T lymphocytes therefore binds a wide range of antigens owing to the specificity of this receptor. Natural killer cells do not express TCR.

19. **The correct answer is B.** Celiac sprue is also known as gluten-sensitive enteropathy, nontropical sprue, and celiac disease. It is due to a sensitivity to gluten, which is found in wheat, grains, and many cereals. Biopsy shows marked atrophy, total loss, or flattening of the villi of the small bowel.

Answer A is incorrect. Abetalipoproteinemia is an autosomal recessive disease that causes a defect in the synthesis and export of lipids by mucosal cells because of the inability to synthesize apolipoprotein B. These patients usually have acanthocytes (or spur cells, RBCs that have spiny projections) and do not have any characteristic features of the intestine found in celiac disease.

Answer C is incorrect. Lactase deficiency causes osmotic diarrhea from the inability to break down lactose into glucose and galactose.

Answer D is incorrect. Viral enteritis, usually caused by a rotavirus, is common in children and can cause diarrhea. However, the clinical time course, suggested gluten sensitivity, and findings on biopsy make viral enteritis unlikely.

Answer E is incorrect. Whipple's disease usually presents in middle-aged men who have malabsorptive diarrhea, and the hallmark is the presence of periodic acid-Schiff-positive macrophages in the intestinal mucosa. Rod-shaped bacilli of the causal agent, *Tropheryma whippelii*, are found on electron microscopy.

20. **The correct answer is D.** The infant's family history is suggestive of a trait with X-linked inheritance, and the preponderance of bacterial infections suggests a defect in the humoral (antibody-mediated) immune response. These two clues are most suggestive of a diagnosis of Bruton's X-linked agammaglobulinemia. The molecular defect occurs in a signaling molecule named Btk (Bruton's tyrosine kinase), leading to maturing arrest of developing B cells at the pre-B-cell stage. Arrest at the pre-B-cell stage would result in an inability to produce immunoglobulins, and thus the patient would have very low levels of all immunoglobulins in his serum. Indeed, it should be noted that these patients are particularly susceptible to extracellular pyogenic bacterial infections with organisms such as *Haemophilus influenzae*, *Streptococcus pyogenes*, *Staphylococcus aureus*, and *Streptococcus pneumoniae*.

Answer A is incorrect. Absence of T lymphocytes would result in a defect in cell-mediated immunity, and the patient would be more highly susceptible to viral and intracellular bacterial pathogens.

Answer B is incorrect. A CD4+ T-lymphocyte count <200/mm^3 suggests a diagnosis of AIDS, not an inherited genetic defect, and one that results in a defect in cell-mediated immunity.

Answer C is incorrect. The physical examination and family and patient history are all highly suggestive of an immunoglobulin deficiency.

Answer E is incorrect. Low serum IgA levels are suggestive of selective IgA deficiency, the most common inherited immunodeficiency in the European population and, interestingly enough, one that appears to have no striking disease associations.

21. **The correct answer is C.** Goodpasture's syndrome is characterized by autoantibodies forming against the glomerular basement membrane. Forming against a tissue, as opposed to something in the blood, constitutes a type II sensitivity reaction. This produces linear immunofluorescent staining. Renal involvement in Goodpasture's syndrome leads to hematuria, anemia, and crescentic glomerulonephritis. Along with the kidney, this syndrome may include pulmonary involvement, leading to hemoptysis.

Answer A is incorrect. Acute poststreptococcal glomerulonephritis occurs 1–4 weeks after a β-hemolytic streptococci infection; it is classified as a type III sensitivity reaction in which deposits of IgG, IgM, and C3 form in the mesangium along the basement membrane. On immunofluorescent staining, a granular pattern is seen, rather than a linear one.

Answer B is incorrect. Alport's syndrome is not an immune reaction against the glomerular basement membrane. It is an X-linked disorder characterized by absent or mutated collagen IV, affecting kidney, nerve, and ocular function.

Answer D is incorrect. IgA nephropathy, also known as Berger's disease, produces mesangial deposits of IgA antibodies. It does not produce a linear pattern, and the staining will require anti-IgA antibodies rather than IgG.

Answer E is incorrect. Membranous glomerulonephritis is an immune-mediated kidney disease that leads to sub-epithelial deposits of IgG and complement. With immunofluorescent staining, it produces a granular pattern along the glomerular basement membrane.

22. **The correct answer is C.** This clinician is concerned that the fetus may have erythroblastosis fetalis (hemolytic disease of the newborn). This disease is mediated by maternally derived IgG anti-Rh antibodies developed in Rh-negative mothers that are directed at the Rh antigen present on the fetal RBCs of a Rh-positive fetus in a previous pregnancy. If the mother possesses the antibodies developed from a previous exposure to an Rh-positive fetus, they may cross

the placenta (antibodies of the IgG isotype readily cross the placenta) and coat the fetal RBCs of a Rh-positive fetus if the mother is now pregnant with another Rh-positive child. Antibody coating of the RBCs leads to phagocytosis of RBCs (via Fc receptors) and/or destruction of the RBCs by the complement system and potentially fatal anemia. This antibody-mediated cytotoxic reaction is an example of a type II hypersensitivity reaction.

Answer A is incorrect. GVHD is a potentially lethal side effect of bone marrow transplantation.

Answer B is incorrect. Type I hypersensitivity reactions are antibody-mediated but require antigen binding to IgE, which is prebound to the surface of mast cells. Mast cell degranulation then ensues. Examples include anaphylaxis, asthma, hives, and local wheal and flare.

Answer D is incorrect. Type III hypersensitivity reactions are immune complex-mediated. Examples include polyarteritis nodosa, glomerulonephritis, rheumatoid arthritis, and systemic lupus erythematosus.

Answer E is incorrect. Type IV hypersensitivity reactions are a group of T-cell-mediated pathologies. Examples include the tuberculin skin test, transplant rejection, and contact dermatitis.

23. **The correct answer is E.** Wiskott-Aldrich syndrome is an X-linked defect associated with elevated IgA levels, elevated IgE levels, normal IgG levels, and low IgM levels. It involves a defect in the body's ability to mount an IgM response to bacteria. Recurrent pyogenic infections, eczema, and thrombocytopenia are the typical triad of symptoms. It does not present with any specific enzyme abnormality.

Answer A is incorrect. Bruton's agammaglobulinemia is an X-linked deficit and therefore presents in males. It is a defect in a tyrosine kinase associated with low levels of all classes of immunoglobulins. After 6 months of age, when the levels of maternal antibodies have declined, patients with the disease tend to present with recurrent bacterial infections.

Answer B is incorrect. Chédiak-Higashi disease is an autosomal recessive disease that presents with recurrent streptococcal and staphylococcal infections. A defect in lysosomal emptying of phagocytic cells due to microtubular dysfunction is the underlying cause of the disease.

Answer C is incorrect. Job's syndrome involves the failure of helper T lymphocytes to produce IFN-γ. Since IFN-γ is a potent activator of phagocytic cells, a decrease in its production leads to a failure of neutrophils to respond to chemotactic stimuli.

Answer D is incorrect. The third and fourth pharyngeal pouches, and thus the thymus and parathyroid glands, fail to develop in patients with thymic aplasia (DiGeorge's syndrome). The disease often presents with congenital defects such as cardiac abnormalities, cleft palate, and abnormal facies. Thymic aplasia can also present with tetany due to hypocalcemia.

24. **The correct answer is C.** Multiple sclerosis is a central nervous system (CNS) demyelinating disorder characterized by lesions that are separated by both time and anatomic location in the CNS. The exact etiology is unknown, but there is evidence supporting a role of autoimmune antibody attack to the CNS myelin-secreting oligodendrocytes. Oligodendrocytes, which are found in the CNS, are involved in myelination of axons.

Answer A is incorrect. Astrocytes are found in the central nervous system and are involved in regulating the metabolic and structural environment of neurons, including repair and scar formation. Astrocytes are not the primary cells affected in multiple sclerosis, but they may proliferate in areas of multiple sclerosis lesions in an effort to repair inflammatory damage.

Answer B is incorrect. Ependymal cells line the ventricles. Disruptions in this cell barrier can cause proliferation of astrocytes nearby, but is not thought to be related to multiple sclerosis.

Answer D is incorrect. Schwann cells are found in the peripheral nervous system and are involved in myelination of axons. Schwann cells are not the primary cells affected in multiple sclerosis. The morphologic changes in this disease are limited to the central nervous system.

Answer E is incorrect. T cells are the primary cells responsible for cellular immunity. It is likely that they are involved in the putative autoimmune attack on the central nervous system in multiple sclerosis, but they are not the cells primarily damaged in this disease.

25. **The correct answer is D.** This statement supports the notion that there is a higher occurrence of systemic lupus erythematosus (SLE) among women than among men. SLE is a type III hypersensitivity disease. Autoantibodies bind to self-antigens to form immune complexes that activate complement, leading to the activation of neutrophils. Since estrogen plays an inhibitory role on the process of clearing immune complexes, women have a higher risk than men of developing pathologically high levels of immune complexes, a number of which can lead to autoimmune diseases such as SLE.

Answer A is incorrect. If this statement were true, then men, who have higher levels of androgens than women, would be at an increased risk of developing pathologically high levels of immune complexes (see the explanation of the correct answer). Note that androgens actually accelerate the clearance of circulating immune complexes.

Answer B is incorrect. This statement does not support the epidemiologic phenomenon that women have a higher occurrence of SLE than men.

Answer C is incorrect. This statement does not support the higher occurrence of SLE in women than in men. As stated in the explanation of the correct answer choice, antibodies (particularly certain antibodies against self-antigens) are needed to form immune complexes. Estrogen actually stimulates the process of antibody production by B cells, which contributes to the higher risk of developing SLE among women than among men.

Answer E is incorrect. This statement is the exact opposite of the correct answer choice.

26. **The correct answer is A.** Selective immunoglobulin deficiency is a deficit in a specific class of immunoglobulins. IgA deficiency is the most common of these diseases. Since IgA is the most prominent immunoglobulin found in mucous membranes, patients suffering from a deficiency of it can present with sinus and lung infections.

Answer B is incorrect. A low IgM level with an elevated IgA level and a normal IgG level is characteristic of Wiskott-Aldrich syndrome. Wiskott-Aldrich syndrome involves a defect in the body's ability to mount an IgM response to encapsulated bacteria. The triad of symptoms consists of recurrent pyogenic infections, eczema, and thrombocytopenia.

Answer C is incorrect. Normal immunoglobulin levels and a negative nitroblue tetrazolium dye reduction test indicate a diagnosis of chronic granulomatous disease. Chronic granulomatous disease involves a defect in the phagocytic ability of neutrophils and does not present with low levels of immunoglobulins. The definitive test for this disorder is a negative nitroblue tetrazolium dye reduction test.

Answer D is incorrect. A very high IgE level and normal levels of all immunoglobulins are characteristics of Job syndrome. Job syndrome is a disorder of the immune system that involves the failure of helper T lymphocytes to produce INF-γ. It presents with multiple "cold," or non-inflamed, skin lesions and high IgE levels.

Answer E is incorrect. Normal immunoglobulin levels can be seen in thymic aplasia (DiGeorge's syndrome). Thymic aplasia presents with recurrent viral and fungal infections. It results from a congenital problem with the migration of the pharyngeal pouches that form the thymus and parathyroid glands. It results in a total lack of T lymphocytes and tetany due to hypocalcemia. It often presents with disorders of the great vessels and heart.

27. **The correct answer is F.** The contact dermatitis that erupts following re-exposure to a poison ivy plant is a type IV hypersensitivity reaction, also known as delayed-type hypersensitivity. This reaction can only occur if an individual has had a prior exposure to the antigen, which triggers the differentiation of CD4$^+$ T lymphocytes into T-helper type 1 lymphocytes. When these differentiated cells are reexposed to that antigen, they are quickly activated to secrete cytokines, which mediate the local inflammatory response that takes place in the skin.

Answer A is incorrect. Goodpasture's syndrome is a type II hypersensitivity reaction and usually affects the lungs and kidneys.

Answer B is incorrect. Histamine is one of the primary mediators released, together with leukotriene and prostaglandin, during a type I hypersensitivity reaction.

Answer C is incorrect. Type IV hypersensitivity reactions are mediated by previously sensitized T lymphocytes, not B lymphocytes.

Answer D is incorrect. The patient must have been previously exposed in order to activate the cytokines to mediate the dermatitis.

Answer E is incorrect. Contact dermatitis is a type IV hypersensitivity reaction, not a type I hypersensitivity reaction.

28. **The correct answer is A.** Antibody molecules consist of two heavy chains and two light chains. Interchain disulfide bonds connect both the heavy chains and the light chains.

Answer B is incorrect. Hydrogen bonds are weaker than disulfide bonds and do not connect the antibody chains.

Answer C is incorrect. Ionic bonds are found in chemicals such as sodium chloride but are not responsible for holding antibody chains together.

Answer D is incorrect. Triple covalent bonds are seen between some atoms, such as nitrogen, but are not responsible for holding the chains of antibody molecules together.

Answer E is incorrect. Van der Waals forces are weak attraction forces and do not hold antibody chains together.

29. **The correct answer is A.** Ataxia-telangiectasia involves a defect in DNA repair enzymes. The image shows spider angiomas, which are a common symptom in patients with this condition. Ataxia-telangiectasia is associated with an IgA deficiency and cerebellar problems leading to ataxia and, in this case, multiple falls.

Answer B is incorrect. Granulomas are collections of cells seen in (among other things) chronic granulomatous disease. This disease is caused by an inability of neutrophils to kill bacteria once they have phagocytosed them.

Answer C is incorrect. Bruton's agammaglobulinemia is an X-linked deficit and therefore presents in males. It is a defect in a tyrosine kinase associated with low levels of all classes of immunoglobulins. After 6 months of age, when the levels of maternal antibodies have declined, patients with the disease tend to present with recurrent bacterial infections. Patients also presents with uniformly low antibody titers of all classes.

Answer D is incorrect. The third and fourth pharyngeal pouches, and thus the thymus and parathyroid glands, fail to develop in patients with thymic aplasia (DiGeorge's syndrome). The disease often presents with many congenital defects such as, cardiac abnormalities, cleft palate, and abnormal facies. Thymic aplasia can also present with tetany due to hypocalcemia.

Answer E is incorrect. Visual hallucinations are not a symptom of any of the known immune deficiencies.

30. **The correct answer is B.** Microscopic polyangiitis is one of the trio of diseases (with Wegener's granulomatosis and Churg-Strauss syndrome) that are referred to as the ANCA (antineutrophil cytoplasmic antibody)-associated vasculitides. Over 80% of patients with this disease have ANCA, usually the perinuclear pattern of staining (P-ANCA) type. In-

HIGH-YIELD PRINCIPLES

Immunology

flammation of the pulmonary capillaries, which can lead to hemoptysis, is common in these patients, and 90% of patients have necrotizing glomerulonephritis (leading to hematuria). Other common symptoms include intestinal pain/bleeding, muscle pain, and weakness. The pathologic lesions are similar to those found in classic polyarteritis nodosa (PAN), but unlike PAN, large and muscular arteries as well as those in the pulmonary circulation are spared. The term "classic" is now often added to the term PAN to differentiate classic polyarteritis nodosa from other small-vessel vasculitides (such as microscopic polyangiitis), which are now thought to represent distinct entities. Classic polyarteritis nodosa has little association with ANCA.

Answer A is incorrect. Anticentromere antibodies, which are found in 90% of patients with the CREST variant of scleroderma, are not particularly associated with microscopic polyangiitis. Anticentromere antibodies are more specific for the CREST variant of scleroderma.

Answer C is incorrect. Anti-Smith antibodies are found in 20%–30% of patients with systemic lupus erythematosus and are not particularly associated with microscopic polyangiitis. "Smith antigen" describes certain core proteins of small nuclear ribonucleoprotein particles. Nonspecific antinuclear antibodies and/or rheumatoid factor may be found in patients with microscopic polyangiitis, but anti-Smith antibodies are more specific for systemic lupus erythematosus.

Answer D is incorrect. Anti-ribonucleoprotein (anti-RNP) antibody SS-A (Ro), which is present in 70%–95% of patients with Sjögren's syndrome, is not particularly associated with microscopic polyangiitis. Anti-RNP SS-A is more specific for Sjögren's syndrome.

Answer E is incorrect. Anti-ribonucleoprotein (anti-RNP) antibody SS-B (La), which is present in 60%–90% of patients with Sjögren's syndrome, is not particularly associated with microscopic polyangiitis. Anti-RNP SS-B is more specific for Sjögren's syndrome.

CHAPTER 6

Pathology

1. A 57-year-old man is brought to the emergency department because of blurry vision, difficulty standing, and mental confusion. On physical examination the patient appears malnourished, he had diffuse crackles bilaterally, and on standing his gait is wide-based and unsteady. The patient's friend, who accompanies him, says the patient "hasn't been himself lately," and is having difficulty remembering to do everyday tasks. Which neuropathologic findings are most consistent with this patient's symptoms?

(A) Atrophy of the caudate nucleus
(B) Depigmentation within the substantia nigra pars compacta
(C) Neurofibrillary tangles and widening of ventricles
(D) No neuropathologic findings
(E) Symmetric lesions in the paraventricular regions of the thalamus and hypothalamus, mammillary bodies, and periaqueductal region of the midbrain

2. A 41-year-old man visits his physician because of increasingly painful headaches. CT of the head is shown in the image. If a biopsy of this tumor were obtained, what would the pathologist likely see under the microscope?

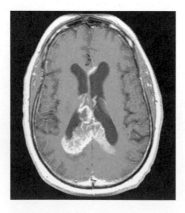

Reproduced, with permission, from Kantarjian HM, Wolff RA, Koller CA. *The MD Anderson Manual of Medical Oncology*. New York: McGraw-Hill, 2006: Figure 30-4.

(A) Densely packed cells with halos of cytoplasm surrounding large round nuclei
(B) Perivascular pseudorosettes with tumor cells surrounding vessels
(C) Pseudopalisading tumor cells surrounding necrotic regions
(D) Sharply demarcated areas of tumor cells located at the grey-white matter junction
(E) Whorled pattern of concentrically arranged spindle cells with psammoma bodies

3. After a 63-year-old man with a progressive, chronic movement disorder dies, the family requests an autopsy. On gross inspection of the patient's brain, the pathologist notes the presence of a deep brain stimulator electrode. The pathologist then obtains a tissue specimen of the basal ganglia for histologic analysis (see image) that stains positive for α-synuclein. From which disease did the decedent most likely suffer?

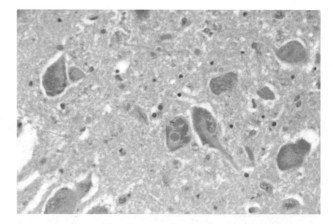

Reproduced, with permission, from PEIR Digital Library (http://peir.net).

(A) Guillain-Barré syndrome
(B) Huntington's disease
(C) Parkinson's disease
(D) Pick's disease
(E) Werdnig-Hoffmann disease

4. A newborn girl is diagnosed as dysmorphic by a pediatrician in the newborn nursery. On physical examination the girl has a broad neck, wide-spaced nipples, and a systolic ejection murmur. An echocardiogram is performed and demonstrates coarctation of the aorta. The echocardiography technologist also runs his transducer across the patient's abdomen and notices a renal abnormality associated with this patient's syndrome. The most likely observed renal abnormality increases this patient's risk for developing which disease?

(A) Neuroblastoma
(B) Ovarian cancer
(C) Transitional cell carcinoma
(D) Uterine cancer
(E) Wilms' tumor

5. A 65-year-old man presents to the office with complaints regarding his urine. He states that he has recently had bloody urine, but does not have any urinary pain, hesitation, dribbling, or increased frequency. He also says he has lost 4.5 kg (10 lb) over the past 2 months. A biopsy of the patient's bladder wall is shown in the image. Which of the following risk factors has the strongest association with this patient's disease?

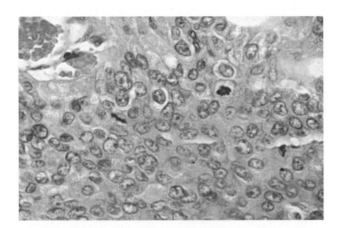

Reproduced, with permission, from PEIR Digital Library (http://peir.net).

(A) History of aniline dye exposure
(B) History of cyclophosphamide treatment
(C) History of heavy cigarette smoking
(D) History of pelvic irradiation
(E) History of schistosomiasis infection

6. A 2-year-old girl is brought to the ED because of fevers that have been occurring daily for 3 weeks. Physical examination reveals a 1.2-kg (2.6-lb) weight loss since her last doctor's visit 1 month earlier. She also has pallor, hepatomegaly, and splenomegaly. She is admitted to the hospital and undergoes bone marrow aspiration; results are shown in the image. Which of the following is the most likely diagnosis?

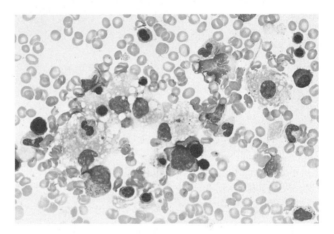

Image courtesy of Armed Forces Institute of Pathology.

(A) Acute lymphoblastic leukemia
(B) Ewing's sarcoma
(C) Hemophagocytic lymphohistiocytosis
(D) Neuroblastoma
(E) Wilms' tumor

7. Following a course of chemotherapy, a 5-year-old male oncology patient develops altered mental status, tachycardia, decreased blood pressure, flushing of the extremities, and decreased urine output. After 48 hours in the pediatric intensive care unit, the patient dies from complications secondary to overwhelming gram-negative sepsis. At autopsy, the pathologist notes the abnormal appearance of the decedent's kidneys, as shown in the image. What process most likely caused the findings demonstrated in the image?

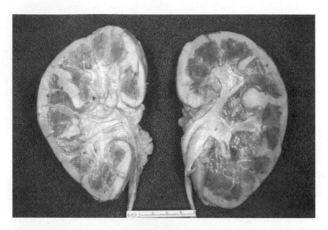

Reproduced, with permission, from PEIR Digital Library (http://peir.net).

(A) Acute pyelonephritis
(B) Diffuse cortical necrosis
(C) Obstructive uropathy
(D) Papillary necrosis
(E) Renal infarction

8. A 26-year-old woman visits her physician with complaints of vaginal bleeding after sexual intercourse. She started menses at age 14 years and has 32-day cycles. She acknowledges having unprotected sex with multiple partners. Cytologic specimens are taken from the cervix and vagina. On microscopy, cervical cells have large nuclei with open chromatin; several cells have mitotic figures. What would most likely be present in the specimens that account for these findings?

(A) Double-stranded DNA virus
(B) Gram-negative diplococci
(C) Gram-positive cocci

(D) Single-stranded RNA
(E) Squamous cells covered with bacteria

9. A 36-year-old woman with a family history of hereditary nonpolyposis colon cancer (HN-PCC) presents to her gastroenterologist for her annual examination. Because of a strong family history of colon cancer, she undergoes yearly colonoscopy. However, she has shown no signs and symptoms of HNPCC and has no significant past medical history. Other than colorectal carcinoma, what is another condition for which she is at increased risk given a family history of HNPCC?

(A) Carcinoma of the endometrium
(B) Cholelithiasis causing cholecystitis
(C) Melanin spots of the buccal mucosa
(D) Pseudopolyps of the small or large bowel
(E) Vitamin B_{12} deficiency due to malabsorption

10. A 35-year-old woman presents with dull, persistent flank and abdominal pain, polyuria, nocturia, and frequent urinary tract infections. Physical examination is notable for blood pressure of 150/90 mm Hg and multiple bilateral abdominal masses. Urinalysis is notable for microscopic hematuria and 1+ protein. CT of the abdomen reveals multiple cysts in the kidneys. The patient notes that she was adopted and knows nothing about her family medical history. What is the most likely etiology of this patient's illness?

(A) A mutation on chromosome 3
(B) A mutation on chromosome 6
(C) A mutation on chromosome 9
(D) A mutation on chromosome 16

11. A 3-year-old developmentally delayed girl presents to the pediatric neurologist for evaluation of new onset seizures. The parents are also concerned because the child frequently exhibits inappropriate outbursts of laughter. Physical examination is significant for abnormal facies marked by microcephaly, deep-set eyes, and a large mouth with a protruding tongue. The child's gait is unstable. The most likely diagnosis is an example of which of the following genetic phenomena?

(A) Anticipation
(B) Heteroplasmy
(C) Imprinting
(D) Locus heterozygosity
(E) Mosaicism

12. A mother brings her 5-year-old son to his pediatrician's office. The boy has been experiencing frequent falls as well as progressive difficulty with walking, jumping, and hopping. Laboratory testing reveals a creatine kinase level of 2840 U/L. Muscle biopsy reveals variation in fiber diameter, an increased number of internalized nuclei, and muscle fiber degeneration and regeneration. Western blot analysis will most likely reveal the complete absence of which of the following?

(A) Cystic fibrosis transmembrane conductance regulator
(B) Dystrophin
(C) Phenylalanine hydroxylase
(D) Spectrin
(E) Type II collagen

13. A 55-year-old recent immigrant from Taiwan presents to the clinic with a 3-month history of worsening nasal congestion, epistaxis, and recurrent ear infections. Physical examination reveals painless firm lymph node enlargement in the neck. CT of the head reveal a large mass situated in the upper nasopharynx. Biopsy of the lesion shows large epithelioid cells intermixed with numerous infiltrating lymphocytes. The infectious agent directly associated with this patient's pathology is best described by which category?

(A) DNA virus
(B) *Eubacterium*
(C) Fungus
(D) *Mycobacterium*
(E) RNA virus

14. A 65-year-old male immigrant from Africa presents to the emergency department after an episode of gross hematuria. He states that he has seen small amounts of blood in his urine from time to time over the past several months. His physical examination is remarkable only for mild hepatosplenomegaly. A urology consult is called, and the urologist performs a bedside cystoscopy. A large fungating mass is seen adherent to the superior part of the bladder. Results of a biopsy are shown in the image. What is the most likely environmental exposure associated with this disease in the patient?

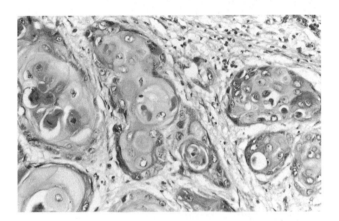

Image courtesy of Armed Forces Institute of Pathology.

(A) Cigarette smoking
(B) Exposure to aniline dyes
(C) Helminth infection
(D) Infection with a papovavirus
(E) Long-term indwelling catheter

15. A patient with AIDS and a CD4+ cell count <50/mm³ is suffering from an infection that affects his lungs, eyes, gastrointestinal tract, and central nervous system. Results of a biopsy are shown in the image. With what is the patient most likely infected?

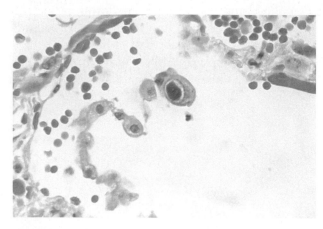

Image courtesy of the Centers for Disease Control and Prevention's Public Health Image Library; content provider Dr. Edwin P. Ewing, Jr.

(A) *Candida albicans*
(B) *Cryptococcus neoformans*
(C) Cytomegalovirus
(D) Herpes simplex virus
(E) *Mycobacterium avium*
(F) *Pneumocystis jiroveci*

16. A 66-year-old woman has an autosomal recessive disease with multiple sequelae, including diabetes mellitus and arthritis. Physical examination reveals hepatomegaly and skin hyperpigmentation. A biopsy of her liver is shown in the image. What is the most likely explanation for her health problems?

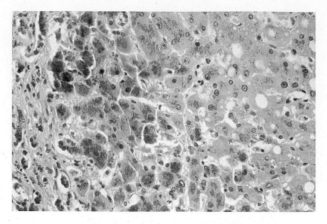

Reproduced, with permission, from PEIR Digital Library (http://peir.net).

(A) Chronic ingestion of alcohol
(B) Genetic deficiency in the synthesis of β-globin chains
(C) Inappropriately high iron absorption
(D) Mutation in RBC membrane protein

17. A 37-year-old HIV-positive man presents for evaluation of anogenital lesions. He states that the lesions have been present for years, but have recently grown in size and become pruritic and tender. On examination he is circumcised and has multiple hyperkeratotic papules on his penis shaft, perineum, and anal area. He also has a palpable rectal mass with guaiac-positive stool and conjunctival pallor. On further questioning, he admits to recent unintentional weight loss, constipation, and bloating. His CD4+ cell count is 150/mm³ and his hematocrit is 26%. CT scan of the abdomen shows a 3 × 4-cm rectal mass with multiple metastatic lesions in his liver. What tumor-suppressor protein is targeted by the virus causing this patient's rectal cancer?

(A) APC
(B) BRCA1
(C) MSH2
(D) NF1
(E) p53

18. A 5-year-old boy presents with an unsteady gait and severe vertigo and nausea. A brain lesion is seen on CT scan; a biopsy of the lesion is shown in the image. Where in the brain is the patient's lesion?

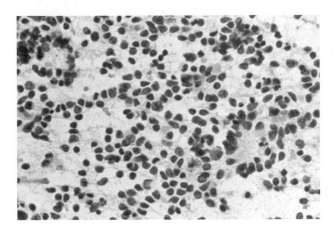

Reproduced, with permission, from PEIR Digital Library (http://peir.net).

(A) Cerebellar vermis
(B) Intermediate section of the cerebellar hemisphere
(C) Lateral section of the cerebellar hemisphere
(D) Occipital cortex
(E) Postcentral gyrus of the parietal lobe

19. A 64-year-old retired shipyard worker has been experiencing shortness of breath, a cough, and chest pain for 5 months. In that time he has lost 14.5 kg (32 lb). He develops progressive ascites, and ultimately dies due to a pulmonary embolus. Autopsy results are shown in the image. Exposure to which substance is a risk factor for this patient's disorder?

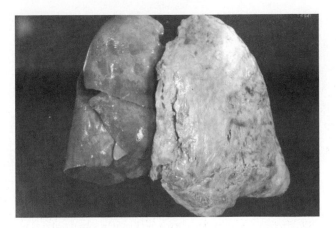

Reproduced, with permission, from PEIR Digital Library (http://peir.net).

(A) Aflatoxin B
(B) Asbestos
(C) Benzene
(D) Cadmium
(E) Silica

20. A 59-year-old man is hospitalized after suffering a severe myocardial infarction. He is initially treated with nitrates, β-blockers, and aspirin, and subsequently undergoes cardiac catheterization with placement of two stents. Following the procedure he is hemodynamically stable without recurrence of chest pain. However, 5 days after admission his heart rate is 134/min, blood pressure is 72/35 mm Hg, and respiratory rate is 29/min. Physical examination reveals distant heart sounds and an elevated jugular venous pressure. Which of the following complications is most likely causing this patient's symptoms?

(A) Aneurysm formation
(B) Cardiac arrhythmia
(C) Fibrinous pericarditis
(D) Rupture of the papillary muscle
(E) Rupture of the ventricular free wall

1. The correct answer is E. This patient presents with signs and symptoms of Wernicke's encephalopathy (confusion, ophthalmoplegia, and ataxia) and Korsakoff's psychosis (personality change, confabulation, and memory loss). This syndrome is secondary to thiamine deficiency and commonly seen in malnourished alcoholics. On postmortem examination, patients suffering from Wernicke-Korsakoff syndrome commonly present with symmetric lesions in the paraventricular regions of the thalamus and hypothalamus, mammillary bodies, and periaqueductal region of the midbrain.

Answer A is incorrect. Atrophy of the caudate nucleus is found in Huntington's disease, a disease of autosomal dominance associated with chorea and dementia.

Answer B is incorrect. Depigmentation within the substantia nigra pars compacta is commonly seen in Parkinson's disease, not thiamine deficiency.

Answer C is incorrect. Neurofibrillary tangles, composed of abnormally phosphorylated tau protein, are commonly found in the frontal and temporal lobes of patients with Alzheimer's disease.

Answer D is incorrect. Thiamine deficiency is associated with neuropathologic changes observed on postmortem examination.

2. The correct answer is C. This patient has a lesion consistent with glioblastoma multiforme (GBM), which is the most common primary brain tumor and is characterized on CT by a serpentine border and central areas of necrosis. The diagnosis should be confirmed by MRI with and without contrast. The lesion consists of highly malignant astrocyte tumor cells that surround areas of necrosis; this is known as pseudopalisading. GBM has been associated with genetic alterations, including loss of *p53* function, increased activity of the epidermal growth factor receptor gene (*EGFR*), and loss of heterozygosity on chromosome arm 10q. GBM has a poor prognosis, with a mean sur-

vival of 8–10 months after diagnosis; most patients die within 2 years.

Answer A is incorrect. Densely packed cells with halos of cytoplasm surrounding large round nuclei are characteristic of oligodendrogliomas, which are slow-growing tumors originating in the cerebral hemispheres. These lesions have a better prognosis than astrocytomas, with a mean patient survival of 5–10 years.

Answer B is incorrect. Perivascular pseudorosettes with tumor cells surrounding vessels are characteristic of ependymomas, which are tumors located in the periventricular space or in the spinal cord that may obstruct the flow of cerebrospinal fluid.

Answer D is incorrect. Sharply demarcated areas of tumor cells located at the grey-white matter junction are characteristic of secondary metastatic lesions from a primary tumor elsewhere in the body, most commonly the breast, lung, thyroid, skin, kidney, and gastrointestinal tract.

Answer E is incorrect. A whorled pattern of concentrically arranged spindle cells with calcified psammoma bodies is characteristic of meningiomas, which are the second most common primary intracranial neoplasm. Meningiomas are benign, slow-growing tumors of the meninges.

3. The correct answer is C. The tissue section shown demonstrates the presence of a Lewy body, which is a cytoplasmic inclusion consisting of aggregated α-synuclein, ubiquitin, tubulin, and neurofilament proteins. The Lewy body is believed to result from disrupted proteasomal activity, leading to the accumulation of cellular proteins, which results in the disruption of normal cellular processes. Lewy bodies present in the substantia nigra, in the context of a movement disorder (evidenced by this patient's history and the presence of a deep brain stimulator), are highly suggestive of Parkinson's disease.

Answer A is incorrect. Guillain-Barré syndrome is a demyelinating disease of the peripheral nervous system. Lewy bodies are not present.

Answer B is incorrect. Huntington's disease is an autosomal dominant disease involving atrophy of the caudate nucleus. It is a progressive, terminal neurodegenerative disorder characterized by chorea and dementia. Lewy bodies are not present.

Answer D is incorrect. Pick's disease is a neurodegenerative disease characterized by progressive dementia, aphasia, and parkinsonism. Pick bodies (intracellular inclusions of aggregated tau protein), not Lewy bodies, are present in affected patients.

Answer E is incorrect. Werdnig-Hoffmann disease (also known as spinal muscular atrophy) is an autosomal recessive disease involving progressive degeneration of the anterior spinal horns. Lewy bodies are not present.

4. **The correct answer is E.** This patient has classic findings associated with Turner's syndrome, a genetic disorder resulting from a 45,XO complement of chromosomes. Approximately 25%–30% of patients will have associated renal anomalies, including horseshoe kidney, pelvic kidney, or duplicated collecting systems. Patients with horseshoe kidneys are approximately four times more likely to develop Wilms' tumor when compared to the general population.

Answer A is incorrect. Although it has been suggested that patients with Turner's syndrome are at increased risk of developing malignancy, they do not have a specific increased risk of developing neuroblastoma.

Answer B is incorrect. Although it has been suggested that patients with Turner's syndrome are at increased risk of developing malignancy, they do not have a specific increased risk of developing ovarian cancer. Familial *BRCA* gene mutations or no history of childbirth each increases the risk of ovarian cancer.

Answer C is incorrect. Although it has been suggested that patients with Turner's syndrome

are at increased risk of developing malignancy, they do not have a specific increased risk of developing transitional cell carcinoma. Smoking greatly increases the risk of transitional cell carcinoma.

Answer D is incorrect. Although it has been suggested that patients with Turner's syndrome are at increased risk of developing malignancy, they do not have a specific increased risk of developing uterine cancer. Unopposed estrogen secretion (eg., hormone replacement therapy without progesterone) increases the risk of uterine cancer.

5. **The correct answer is C.** This patient has transitional cell carcinoma of the bladder, as evidenced by his painless hematuria and absent signs of prostate cancer. Histology confirms the diagnosis with the presence of invasive transitional cells and prominent, atypical nuclei and mitotic spindles. Numerous factors increase the risk of developing transitional cell carcinoma, the most significant of which is an extensive history of cigarette smoking. Cigarette smoking increases a patient's risk by three- to sevenfold. Treatment of transitional cell carcinoma largely depends on the stage of disease, although these tumors have a tendency to recur regardless of disease stage. Low-grade lesions may be treated with excision, whereas higher-grade lesions require a combination of excision and chemotherapy.

Answer A is incorrect. Aniline dye exposure (eg., in a textile mill worker) is a risk factor for the development of transitional cell carcinoma; however, smoking is the most significant risk factor.

Answer B is incorrect. Cyclophosphamide therapy (eg., in a patient with a history of treated Ewing's sarcoma) is a risk factor for the development of transitional cell carcinoma; however, smoking is the most significant risk factor.

Answer D is incorrect. Pelvic irradiation (eg., in a patient treated for prostatic cancer) is a risk factor for the development of transitional cell carcinoma; however, smoking is the most significant risk factor.

Answer E is incorrect. Schistosomiasis infection (eg, in a patient with travel to an endemic area, including the Middle East) is a risk factor for the development of transitional cell carcinoma; however, smoking is the most significant risk factor.

6. **The correct answer is C.** This patient has symptoms consistent with hemophagocytic lymphohistiocytosis (HLH), and bone marrow aspiration (demonstrating macrophages engulfing RBCs) confirms the diagnosis. Familial-type HLH is an autosomal recessive defect in several genes, including perforin-related genes; the secondary type is frequently due to infection with Epstein-Barr virus. HLH involves the abnormal activation and proliferation of lymphohistiocytes leading to hemophagocytosis and the upregulation of proinflammatory cytokines. Treatment consists of a combination of etoposide, corticosteroids, and methotrexate, although stem cell transplant is often required.

Answer A is incorrect. Acute lymphoblastic leukemia frequently presents with constitutional symptoms (fever, weight loss, pallor, hepatosplenomegaly). Bone marrow aspiration would not demonstrate hemophagocytosis.

Answer B is incorrect. Ewing's sarcoma frequently presents in the second decade of life with constitutional symptoms (fever, weight loss), bone tenderness, and pathologic fractures. Bone marrow aspiration would not demonstrate hemophagocytosis.

Answer D is incorrect. Neuroblastoma frequently presents with constitutional symptoms (fever, weight loss, pallor, hepatosplenomegaly). It is the most common malignancy of infancy. A bone marrow aspirate would not demonstrate hemophagocytosis.

Answer E is incorrect. Wilms' tumor frequently presents with an asymptomatic flank mass and/or gross hematuria. It is the most common primary renal tumor in children. Bone marrow aspiration would not demonstrate hemophagocytosis.

7. **The correct answer is B.** This patient died from complications secondary to septic shock.

The patient had evidence of early end-organ failure as demonstrated by his decreased urine output. Patients suffering from septic shock can develop diffuse cortical necrosis (shown in the image) of the kidneys, which is believed to result from a combination of hypoperfusion, microangiopathic thrombosis, and infarction; thromboses may be present in the arterioles, capillaries, and glomeruli. The areas of necrosis are generally confined to the cortex and, on gross examination, are sharply demarcated from the rest of the kidney. In cases where the underlying sepsis is quickly treated with fluid resuscitation and antibiotics, some function of the kidneys may be preserved; otherwise, overwhelming cortical necrosis usually culminates in death.

Answer A is incorrect. Acute pyelonephritis results from hematogenous or ascending infection of the kidneys. On gross pathologic examination the kidney typically demonstrates patchy areas of abscess formation, but not diffuse, sharply demarcated areas of cortical necrosis as seen in the image.

Answer C is incorrect. Obstructive uropathy results from a blockage distal to the collecting system of the kidneys. On gross pathologic examination the kidney typically demonstrates dilation of the renal pelvis and calyces, but not sharply demarcated areas of cortical necrosis as seen in the image.

Answer D is incorrect. Papillary necrosis can result from infection, analgesic overuse, sickle cell disease, and a number of other conditions. On gross pathologic examination the kidney typically demonstrates yellow-white areas of necrosis limited to the papillae, but not sharply demarcated areas of cortical necrosis as seen in the image.

Answer E is incorrect. Renal infarction results from thromboembolic disease involving the renal vasculature. On gross pathologic examination the kidney typically demonstrates wedge-shaped areas of yellow-white infarction extending from the medulla to the cortex, but not diffuse, sharply demarcated areas of cortical necrosis as seen in the image.

8. **The correct answer is A.** The findings on microscopy indicate a malignant transformation of normal cells. Increased nuclear-to-cytoplasm ratio, open chromatin, and mitotic figures indicate that cells are actively dividing. Given the patient's history of multiple sexual partners and postcoital bleeding, these cells likely indicate the presence of cervical cancer. Cervical cancer is commonly linked to human papillomavirus infection. The virus can be isolated during cytology through various methods. It is a double-stranded DNA virus.

Answer B is incorrect. Gram-negative diplococci are not associated with cervical cancer. However, they can be found in gonorrhea cervicitis.

Answer C is incorrect. There are no gram-positive cocci associated with cervical cancer.

Answer D is incorrect. There is no single-stranded virus associated with cervical cancer.

Answer E is incorrect. Squamous cells covered with bacteria can be found in bacterial vaginosis, which causes foul-smelling discharge. There is no known association between bacterial vaginosis and cervical cancer.

9. **The correct answer is A.** HNPCC, also known as Lynch's syndrome, is a rare autosomal dominant disorder associated with an increased incidence of colorectal cancer. Generally, the syndrome is associated with mismatch repair. Approximately 70% of people with the syndrome will develop colorectal cancer, typically at 40–45 years of age. Also, there is a high risk of extracolonic cancer, including endometrial, ovarian, urinary tract, small intestinal, stomach, and biliary cancer. As a result, high-risk patients begin annual screening colonoscopies at age 20–25 years, or 10 years before the age of the youngest diagnosed family member. Women >35 years old typically undergo annual endometrial biopsy due to the high risk of endometrial carcinoma.

Answer B is incorrect. Cholecystitis is secondary to gallstones in 90% of cases. Increased gallstone formation related to HNPCC may be plausible if the patient had undergone resection of the ileum for extracolonic cancer of the small bowel. Gallstones are known to occur in such patients after ileal resection due to disturbed bilirubin metabolism. Moreover, although HNPCC can be associated with biliary cancer, the patient in this case has yet to show signs of HNPCC, and biliary cancer does not cause cholelithiasis. Thus, the patient presumably has no increased risk of gallstones or cholecystitis.

Answer C is incorrect. Melanin spots of the buccal mucosa and lips can be seen in Peutz-Jeghers syndrome. This syndrome involves multiple polyps of the small bowel, although the large bowel and rectum can be involved. The polyps are generally considered to be non-malignant hamartomas, but cancer can occasionally develop. Peutz-Jeghers syndrome is not associated with HNPCC.

Answer D is incorrect. Pseudopolyps, also known as inflammatory polyps, are areas of regenerating, normal mucosa around which the mucosa has been lost. This typically occurs in the setting of inflammatory bowel disease but may be seen in colitis related to amebic and schistosomal infection or bowel ischemia. Although these "polyps" are not premalignant, they resemble adenomatous polyps on gross examination and should thus be removed and examined histologically. Pseudopolyps are not associated with HNPCC and are unlikely in this patient with no significant past medical history.

Answer E is incorrect. Although vitamin B_{12} deficiency is most commonly associated with pernicious anemia, abdominal surgery secondary to cancer might lead to vitamin B_{12} deficiency. For example, if the patient underwent gastrectomy for gastric cancer caused by HNPCC, intrinsic factor would not be produced. Furthermore, if the patient underwent bowel resection, including the ileum for small bowel cancer related to HNPCC, B_{12} could not be absorbed because absorption occurs in the ileum. However, the patient in this case has yet to show signs of HNPCC and presumably has normal vitamin B_{12} levels.

10. The correct answer is D. The patient's symptoms are consistent with adult polycystic kidney disease (APKD), a disease most commonly caused by mutation of the polycystin 1 gene located on chromosome 16. APKD can also be caused by a mutation in polycystin 2 located on chromosome 4, although this is less common. APKD is characterized by the growth of renal cysts, which are believed to lead to renal failure by compressing adjacent normal parenchyma. The disease often presents in the third or fourth decade of life, and symptoms and signs include abdominal discomfort, frequent urinary tract infections, hematuria, polyuria, and nocturia. Cystic kidneys are often seen on imaging. Mild proteinuria is common. Hepatic cysts, as seen in the image, are also common. The disease is also associated with berry aneurysms and mitral valve prolapse.

Answer A is incorrect. A mutation on chromosome 3 is associated with von Hippel-Lindau disease, which can not only cause renal cysts but also retinal angiomas and central nervous system hemangioblastomas.

Answer B is incorrect. A mutation on chromosome 6 is associated with recessive polycystic kidney disease, which is associated with a much younger age of onset.

Answer C is incorrect. A mutation on chromosome 9 is associated with tuberous sclerosis, which can not only cause renal cysts, but also presents with adenoma sebaceum and central nervous system hamartomas.

11. The correct answer is C. This child most likely has Angelman's syndrome. Individuals with this phenotype have a characteristic facies with microcephaly, maxillary hypoplasia, deep-set eyes, and a large mouth with tongue protrusion. Their gait is jerky and "puppet-like," and their behavior is marked by frequent paroxysms of inappropriate laughter. Severe mental retardation and speech impairment are usually present, and 80%–90% of patients have epilepsy. Angelman's syndrome, along with Prader-Willi syndrome, is a classic example of imprinting, which occurs when the phenotype differs depending on whether the mutation is of paternal or maternal origin. Deletions in Prader-Willi syndrome, a phenotypically distinct disorder, occur exclusively on the paternal chromosome 15, whereas deletions at the same site of chromosome 15 on the maternal chromosome result in Angelman's syndrome.

Answer A is incorrect. Anticipation is the phenomenon in which the severity of a disease worsens in succeeding generations. This occurs, for example, in triplet repeat diseases such as Huntington's disease, wherein the triplet repeat tends to lengthen, age of onset decreases, and disease severity increases with successive generations. This does not occur in Angelman's syndrome.

Answer B is incorrect. Heteroplasmy describes the presence of both normal and mutated mitochondrial DNA. This phenomenon is responsible for the variable expression of mitochondrial inherited diseases.

Answer D is incorrect. Locus heterozygosity describes the phenomenon by which mutations at different loci can result in the same phenotype. An example of this is albinism, which can be caused by a number of different mutations.

Answer E is incorrect. Mosaicism occurs when cells in the body have different genetic makeup. This sometimes occurs, for example, in Turner's syndrome. This does not occur in Angelman's syndrome.

12. The correct answer is B. Duchenne's muscular dystrophy (DMD) is the most common form of muscular dystrophy, affecting 1 in 3500 live male births. Symptoms become evident by the age of 5 years and include delayed walking, clumsiness, weakness in the pelvic girdle muscles, and enlargement of the calf muscles (termed pseudohypertrophy). Laboratory testing reveals an elevated creatine kinase level. DMD is caused by an abnormality of Xp21, the region that codes for dystrophin, a myocyte anchoring protein.

Answer A is incorrect. Cystic fibrosis transmembrane conductance regulator (CFTR) transports chloride ions across epithelial cell membranes. Mutations of the *CFTR* gene lead to cystic fibrosis, which is associated with symptoms such as difficulty breathing, frequent pneumonias, and pancreatic insufficiency.

Answer C is incorrect. Phenylalanine hydroxylase (PAH) is an enzyme that catalyzes the conversion of phenylalanine to tyrosine. Deficiency of PAH leads to phenylketonuria, characterized by problems with brain development, mental retardation, and seizures.

Answer D is incorrect. Spectrin is a cytoskeletal protein important in maintaining RBC plasma membrane structure. Absence of spectrin leads to hereditary spherocytosis, whose symptoms include anemia, splenomegaly, and jaundice.

Answer E is incorrect. Type II collagen is the building block of articular and hyaline cartilages. Deficiency of type II collagen leads to a severe form of osteogenesis imperfecta that is usually lethal in the perinatal period.

13. **The correct answer is A.** This patient has developed nasopharyngeal carcinoma, a condition common in certain parts of the world, including Asia and Africa. Development of this tumor is always associated with infection by Epstein-Barr virus (EBV), a DNA virus in the herpesvirus family. Development of this tumor is believed to be related to a synergistic interaction between EBV and a diet high in carcinogenic nitrosamines (common in foods that has been smoked or preserved). Common symptoms include nasal congestion, epistaxis, ear infections (due to tumor-induced blockage of the Eustachian tubes), and headache.

Answer B is incorrect. Many bacteria are capable of infecting the nasopharynx; however, none are directly associated with malignancy.

Answer C is incorrect. Nasopharyngeal zygomycosis is a condition that could present with these symptoms in an immunocompromised patient. However, biopsy would show filamentous nonseptate hyphae and a granulomatous response.

Answer D is incorrect. Although a tuberculoma in the nasopharynx can be confused with a nasopharyngeal tumor, biopsy would show caseating granulomas with multinucleated giant cells.

Answer E is incorrect. Although a retrovirus such as HIV can create an immunocompromised state favoring the development of a malignancy, it is not the direct cause of tumor formation. Lymphomas can be associated with the retrovirus human T-cell lymphoma virus; however, biopsy would show sheets of malignant T lymphocytes typical of this lymphoma. Other RNA viruses are not associated with malignancy.

14. **The correct answer is C.** This patient is suffering from squamous cell carcinoma of the bladder. Although this condition is rare in the United States, it is the most common type of bladder cancer in the world. The most common cause is chronic irritation by the eggs of the helminth *Schistosoma haematobium*, which lodge in the bladder wall. Squamous cell carcinoma can be distinguished from transitional cell carcinoma pathologically by its appearance. This specimen shows keratin pearl formation, a common finding in squamous cell cancers.

Answer A is incorrect. Cigarette smoking is the most common risk factor associated with transitional cell bladder carcinoma. In this case, however, the patient's presentation and pathology are more suggestive of squamous cell carcinoma.

Answer B is incorrect. Aniline dyes are associated with transitional cell carcinoma, the most common type of bladder cancer in the United States. They are not associated with squamous cell carcinoma of the bladder.

Answer D is incorrect. Papovaviridae such as human papilloma virus are responsible for genital warts and cervical carcinoma. They are not associated with bladder cancers.

Answer E is incorrect. Long-term catheterization is associated with the development of squamous cell carcinoma of the bladder. Based on the patient's history, however, there is no reason to assume this patient has had an indwelling catheter at any time.

15. The correct answer is C. The image shows the typical large, round intranuclear inclusion with perinuclear halo seen in cells affected by cytomegalovirus (CMV) infection. This Cowdry type A bodies are typically referred to as "owl's eyes" due to their microscopic appearance. In immunocompromised patients, CMV infection can present as retinitis, pneumonitis, inflammation along the gastrointestinal tract, polyradiculopathy, transverse myelitis, and focal encephalitis. In patients with HIV/AIDS, these sequelae occur most prominently when the $CD4^+$ cell count is $<100/mm^3$ or when the HIV viral load is $>10,000$ copies/mm^3. CMV can cause further immunosuppression, leading to other opportunistic infections such as *Pneumocystis* and *Aspergillus* pneumonia.

Answer A is incorrect. Candida is a fungus that produces a wide spectrum of diseases, ranging from superficial mucocutaneous disease in immunocompetent hosts to invasive illnesses in immunocompromised hosts. Histology reveals round or ovoid yeast cells, hyphae, or pseudohyphae.

Answer B is incorrect. *Cryptococcus neoformans* causes meningitis and meningoencephalitis in patients with AIDS. This fungus is difficult to observe with routine hematoxylin and eosin stains, so methenamine silver or periodic acid-Schiff stains are used to identify the characteristic narrow-based buds and round-to-oval yeast, surrounded by a polysaccharide capsule.

Answer D is incorrect. Herpes simplex virus in HIV-infected individuals can cause recurrent orolabial, genital, and perianal lesions. A Tzanck smear is positive for multinucleated epithelial giant cells. It does not cause the large intranuclear inclusion body shown.

Answer E is incorrect. *Mycobacterium avium* causes lung disease in immunocompromised hosts and is subsequently spread via the blood to the liver, spleen, bone marrow, and other sites. Histology of mycobacterium is not consistent with this image. Rather, acid-fast staining would show organisms in foamy macrophages, granulomas, giant cells, and cells with eosinophilic necrosis.

Answer F is incorrect. *Pneumocystis jiroveci* (formerly *carinii*) causes pneumonia in immunocompromised individuals.

16. The correct answer is C. Hereditary hemochromatosis is an autosomal recessive adult onset disorder characterized by inappropriately high iron absorption that leads to progressive iron overload. The organs damaged by iron deposition include the liver, heart, pancreas, pituitary, joints, and skin. Cirrhosis results from progressive iron deposition in the liver parenchyma of patients with hemochromatosis. In the image, hepatocellular iron deposition is seen as granular brown cytoplasmic pigment. Microscopic evidence of cirrhosis includes an increased quantity of connective tissue extending from the portal areas. Cirrhosis, which simply means fibrosis, is the result of past or chronic tissue destruction. Acute destruction would be evidenced by the presence of inflammatory cells in the portal areas, as is seen in hepatitis.

Answer A is incorrect. Alcoholic liver disease occurs in patients who are heavy drinkers. Liver biopsy in these patients may show cirrhosis. However, in contrast to patients with hemochromatosis, the hepatic iron levels are relatively normal, and iron stores are usually <4 g.

Answer B is incorrect. β-Thalassemia is caused by a mutation in the β-globin gene, resulting in reduced or absent β-globin. In the more severe form of the disease, patients must receive periodic RBC transfusions throughout their lives. This, paired with enhanced iron absorption in reaction to the anemia, results in iron overload. The resulting clinical picture is similar to that observed in primary hemochromatosis (eg., endocrine dysfunction, liver dysfunction, cardiac dysfunction).

Answer D is incorrect. Iron overload may be due to chronic anemia, with increased effective erythropoiesis and increased iron absorption. Examples of conditions that can result in chronic anemia include hereditary spherocytosis and acquired sideroblastic anemia. In patients with hereditary spherocytosis, RBCs have a membrane protein defect, resulting in cytoskeleton instability and increased RBC turnover.

17. **The correct answer is E.** This HIV-positive patient has multiple anogenital warts, or condylomata acuminata, which are commonly caused by human papilloma virus (HPV) types 6 and 11. A feared complication of condylomata acuminata is anorectal cancer, as seen here. Immunodeficiency predisposes to the development of HPV-induced transformation. The mechanism of HPV-induced transformation involves the production of a viral protein, E6, which binds to a cellular ubiquitin ligase E6AP. On binding to E6, E6AP polyubiquitinates the tumor suppressor p53, leading to dysregulated cell proliferation and, eventually, oncogenesis.

Answer A is incorrect. *APC* is a tumor suppressor gene mutated in certain hereditary forms of colon cancer. The APC protein normally degrades the transcription factor β-catenin, which is involved in colonic epithelial cell proliferation. In the absence of APC, increased levels of β-catenin accumulate, eventually leading to oncogenesis.

Answer B is incorrect. *BRCA1* is a tumor suppressor gene commonly mutated in hereditary forms of breast and ovarian cancers. The BRCA1 protein functions in DNA repair processes, and inherited mutations in BRCA1 interfere with DNA repair, leading to the accumulation of mutations and, eventually, oncogenesis.

Answer C is incorrect. The *MSH2* gene regulates a mismatch repair enzyme and is mutated in certain hereditary forms of colon cancer. In the absence of MSH2, increased levels of DNA mutations accumulate, leading to eventual cellular transformation.

Answer D is incorrect. *NF1* is a tumor suppressor gene mutated in neurofibromatosis type 1. The NF1 protein functions as a GTPase activating protein for the small G protein Ras. Because Ras is only active when it is GTP-bound, NF1-mediated GTP hydrolysis leads to inactivation of Ras. In the absence of NF1, Ras is hyperactive, leading to enhanced growth factor signal transduction and, eventually, oncogenesis.

18. **The correct answer is A.** The boy's brain biopsy demonstrates medulloblastoma. This is a poorly differentiated neuroectodermal tumor that occurs predominantly in children and exclusively in the cerebellum. The cerebellar vermis is the medial section of the cerebellum and is responsible for proximal muscle coordination, balance, and vestibulo-ocular reflexes. As seen in this patient, lesions of the vermis lead to vertigo, nausea, and difficulties in coordinating movement of trunk and proximal limb muscles. The presence of medulloblastoma commonly leads to obstruction of the outflow of cerebrospinal fluid and the potential for hydrocephalus, a life-threatening condition.

Answer B is incorrect. Medulloblastomas arise in the midline of the cerebellum in children. The intermediate section of the cerebellar hemisphere is more lateral than the vermis. Lesions in the intermediate section would cause deficits in coordinating movements of the ipsilateral distal extremities, not the vertigo and proximal limb problems seen in this patient.

Answer C is incorrect. Medulloblastomas arise in the midline of the cerebellum in children. Lesions of the lateral hemisphere would likely cause deficits in planning movements of the ipsilateral distal extremities, not the vertigo and proximal limb problems seen in this patient.

Answer D is incorrect. Medulloblastomas arise in the midline of the cerebellum in children, not in the occipital cortex. Occipital cortex lesions could lead to defects in vision, not the vertigo and proximal limb problems seen in this patient.

Answer E is incorrect. Medulloblastomas arise in the midline of the cerebellum in children, not in the parietal cortex. The postcentral gyrus of the parietal lobe is the primary somatosensory cortex. Lesions of this area would cause sensory deficits, not the vertigo and proximal limb problems seen in this patient.

19. **The correct answer is B.** This image demonstrates an advanced case of mesothelioma, in

which the entire left lung is encased with tumor. The clinical history supports this diagnosis. Asbestos is present in certain building materials and fire-resistant materials, and exposure to asbestos is a risk factor for the development of mesothelioma.

Answer A is incorrect. Aflatoxin B is produced by *Aspergillus* and is a common contaminant of cereals, spices, and nuts. It has been associated with carcinoma of the liver.

Answer C is incorrect. Long-term exposure to high levels of benzene can lead to leukemia and Hodgkin's lymphoma. Benzene is the main component of light oil, and is found in gasoline and other fuels.

Answer D is incorrect. Cadmium is a carcinogen associated with the development of prostate cancer. It can be found in batteries and in metal coatings.

Answer E is incorrect. Exposure to silica may occur in the manufacturing of several materials, such as glass, ceramics, and electronics. Silicosis is characterized by bilateral, fine nodularity in the upper lung lobes. It is slowly progressive. Its role as a carcinogen is controversial.

20. **The correct answer is E.** This patient is in shock due to cardiac tamponade secondary to the rupture of the ventricular free wall, which usually occurs 4–10 days after the initial myocardial infarction (MI). It usually presents with sudden shock with signs of cardiac tamponade, such as the hypotension, distant heart sounds, and elevated jugular venous pressure observed in this patient. Survival depends primarily on the rapid recognition of myocardial rupture and the provision of immediate therapy, such as urgent pericardiocentesis or surgery. Unfortunately, this complication of an MI is often a fatal one.

Answer A is incorrect. Aneurysm formation may occur post-MI due to a lack of contractility that results in the infarcted area. Sequelae of ventricular aneurysm formation include decreased cardiac output, increased risk of arrhythmias, and potential mural thrombus formation with risk of embolization.

Answer B is incorrect. Cardiac arrhythmias are a common cause of death in the first few days after an MI. However, this patient's clinical picture is more consistent with a diagnosis of cardiac tamponade secondary to ventricular free wall rupture.

Answer C is incorrect. Fibrinous pericarditis is a complication that usually occurs 3–5 days post-MI. This condition usually presents with chest pain that is relieved when the patient leans forward; often a pericardial friction rub can be auscultated on cardiac examination. However, this patient's clinical picture is more consistent with a diagnosis of cardiac tamponade secondary to ventricular free wall rupture.

Answer D is incorrect. Papillary muscle rupture is another complication of MI that usually occurs 4–10 days post-MI. However, patients with papillary muscle rupture usually present with acute mitral regurgitation, causing the abrupt onset of heart failure in the setting of a new systolic murmur. Emergent surgical intervention is the treatment of choice for this condition.

CHAPTER 7

Pharmacology

1. A 37-year-old man who is HIV-positive recently started on a highly active antiretroviral regimen. The patient's CD4$^+$ cell count subsequently fell below 200/mm^3. Over the course of the next 3 months, he develops diarrhea and notices a redistribution of fat on his body. Which of the following agents is most likely causing this patient's symptoms?

(A) Fusion inhibitor
(B) Non-nucleoside reverse transcriptase inhibitor
(C) Nucleoside reverse transcriptase inhibitor
(D) Nucleotide reverse transcriptase inhibitor
(E) Protease inhibitor

2. A patient is being treated with β-blockers for hypertension. Which of the following describes the effects of β-blockers on end-diastolic volume (EDV), blood pressure (BP), contractility, heart rate (HR), and ejection time?

CHOICE	EDV	BP	CONTRACTILITY	HR	EJECTION TIME
A	No effect or ↓	↓	Little/no effect	↓	Little/no effect
B	↓	↓	↓	↑	↓
C	↓	↓	↓	↓	↓
D	↑	↓	↓	↓	↑
E	↓	↓	↑	↑	↓

(A) A
(B) B
(C) C
(D) D
(E) E

3. A 68-year-old woman with type 2 diabetes mellitus and a 13.6-kg (30-lb) weight loss over the past 2 months presents to the physician with a history of nausea and bloating. Symptoms are most prominent following a meal. An outpatient gastric emptying study shows esophageal dysmotility. Which of the following is the best treatment for this patient?

(A) Esophageal resection
(B) Metoclopramide
(C) Omeprazole
(D) Ondansetron
(E) Vagotomy

4. A 33-year-old woman with a history of Graves' disease is brought to the emergency department unresponsive following a bout of confusion and agitation. On physical examination her temperature is 39.2° C (102.5° F), her blood pressure is 100/70 mm Hg, and her pulse is 165/min. A systolic ejection murmur is heard at the apex, and the patient has 3+ pitting edema at the ankles. Following primary stabilization, which of the following would constitute appropriate pharmacotherapy for this patient's underlying condition?

(A) Aspirin
(B) Dobutamine
(C) Iodine
(D) Levothyroxine
(E) Propylthiouracil

5. A 36-year-old man who works at an explosives factory comes to the clinic for an annual check-up. He is concerned about long-term exposure to industrial chemicals. He reports that although he is in excellent health otherwise, he experiences headaches, dizziness, and palpitations every Monday. Laboratory tests show:

Na$^+$: 137 mEq/L
K$^+$: 3.4 mEq/L
Cl$^-$: 102 mEq/L
HCO$_3^-$: 24 mEq/L
Blood urea nitrogen: 12 mg/dL
Creatinine: 1.0 mg/dL
WBC count: 8000/mm^3
Platelet count: 310,000/mm^3
Hematocrit: 46%
Hemoglobin: 15 g/dL

An ECG shows normal sinus rhythm with no Q wave changes. Which of the following is the most likely serious complication that can occur as a result of his exposure?

(A) Anemia
(B) Atherosclerosis
(C) Cardiac arrest
(D) Congestive heart failure
(E) Dementia

6. A 32-year-old woman presents to her primary care physician complaining of overwhelming fear and apprehension. The patient states that for the past 8 months she has been feeling anxious and worried about many things. She has difficulty concentrating and difficulty sleeping because she "can't seem to keep [her] mind off of the everyday issues of life." She also says she often feels tense and restless. She denies past substance abuse. Which of the following drugs would be considered first-line treatment for her illness?

(A) Amitriptyline
(B) Buspirone
(C) Diazepam
(D) Flumazenil
(E) Midazolam

7. A 64-year-old man develops chronic renal failure. He has an extensive medical history, and also complains of increasingly poor vision in his right eye. After a kidney biopsy is taken (see image), his physician immediately starts him on a new medication. What pharmacologic treatment has been shown to most effectively delay the progression of the pathology shown in this photomicrograph?

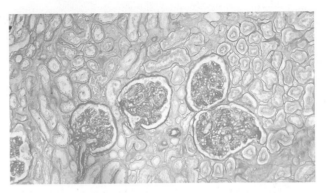

Reproduced, with permission, from PEIR Digital Library (http://peir.net).

(A) Angiotensin-converting enzyme inhibitors
(B) β-Blockers
(C) Cyclophosphamide
(D) Gold therapy
(E) Prednisone

8. A 5-year-old boy presents to the physician's office for treatment of chronic recurrent pulmonary infections and bronchitis. The boy's history is significant for ileus as a newborn and chronic floating, foul-smelling diarrhea. Analysis of the child's sweat reveals an increased concentration of chloride ions. A mutation in which chromosome is responsible for this patient's disease process?

(A) Chromosome 3
(B) Chromosome 5
(C) Chromosome 7
(D) Chromosome 12
(E) Chromosome 15

9. A 70-year-old man presents to his cardiologist with shortness of breath, crackles along both lung bases, and 1+ pitting edema in his lower extremities. His cardiologist diagnoses him with mild congestive heart failure and places him on a thiazide diuretic. Two days later, the patient comes to the emergency department obtunded and oliguric, with a highly elevated creatinine level of 8.3 mg/dL. His wife reports that the only medication that he took besides his diuretic was "some ibuprofen for his headache." Which of the following is the most likely reason for this patient's sudden renal failure?

(A) Decrease of prostaglandin E_2 production in both arterioles of the kidney
(B) Decrease of prostaglandin E_2 production in the afferent arterioles of the kidney
(C) Decrease of prostaglandin E_2 production in the efferent arterioles of the kidney
(D) Increase of prostaglandin E_2 production in the afferent arterioles of the kidney
(E) Increase of prostaglandin E_2 production in the efferent arterioles of the kidney

10. A 74-year-old man comes to the physician complaining of increased urinary frequency along with difficulty starting and stopping urination. Assuming a benign underlying cause, which of the following is the mechanism of action of a common medication used to treat this condition?

(A) Formation of superoxide radicals that attack DNA bonds
(B) Gonadotropin-releasing hormone analog
(C) Inhibition of cyclic guanosine monophosphate–specific phosphodiesterase type 5
(D) Inhibition of cytochrome P450 enzymes
(E) Inhibition of 5α-reductase
(F) Inhibition of testosterone's negative feedback on gonadotropin secretion

11. A 56-year-old male stabbing victim has been in the hospital for 4 days with an infected wound that presented with crepitus and exquisite tenderness on palpation. Following tissue débridement and the initiation of intravenous antibiotics, the wound has started to heal, but on hospital day 5, the patient develops a fever, an increased WBC count, and watery diarrhea. The patient's new symptoms most likely resulted from the use of which of the following therapeutic agents?

(A) Amantadine
(B) Clindamycin
(C) Metronidazole
(D) Tetracycline
(E) Vancomycin

12. The targets of multiple lipid-lowering agents are labeled in the image. Which of the targets corresponds to the therapy associated with the most significant decrease in triglyceride levels?

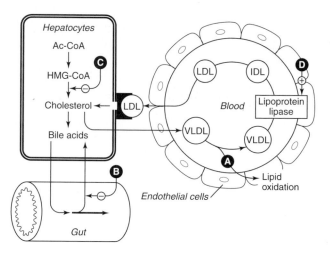

Reproduced, with permission, from USMLERx.com.

(A) A
(B) B
(C) C
(D) D

13. A 72-year-old man comes to the emergency department because of shortness of breath and dyspnea on exertion for the past few days. Physical examination reveals pitting edema bilaterally in the lower extremities. The patient is given a combination drug therapy for his condition. Which of the following therapies, while effective, may lead to dangerous physiological sequelae when used in combination?

(A) Acetylsalicylic acid and a thiazide diuretic
(B) Acetylsalicylic acid and nitroprusside

(C) β-Blocker and a thiazide diuretic
(D) β-Blocker and spironolactone
(E) Digoxin and furosemide
(F) Digoxin and spironolactone

14. A 68-year-old man comes to the emergency department because of a 5-hour history of palpitations and light-headedness. He states that he has experienced shorter episodes of palpitations before, but nothing so severe. After admission to the hospital, the patient receives a full cardiac work-up and is diagnosed with rapid atrial fibrillation, most likely secondary to a moderately stenosed mitral valve. Medical treatment to convert him to sinus rhythm is unsuccessful. However, his heart rate is well controlled with various atrioventricular node blocking agents. The patient is prescribed a regimen of daily medications including drugs to control potentially disastrous complications of atrial fibrillation. Which of the following drugs is most likely prescribed long-term to prevent such complications?

(A) Aspirin
(B) Protamine sulfate
(C) Streptokinase
(D) Unfractionated heparin
(E) Warfarin

15. The plasma concentration of drug Y is 50 mg/L, and it is eliminated at a rate of 2 mg/min. Which of the following is the clearance rate of drug Y?

(A) 0.01 L/min
(B) 0.04 L/min
(C) 4 L/min
(D) 10 L/min
(E) 400 L/min

16. A 33-year-old immigrant from Peru comes to a women's health clinic because she has missed her period for the past 2 months. Already a mother of four, she explains that she can't afford to have another child. When her preg-

nancy test comes back positive, she becomes obviously distraught, saying that she has been on the pill for the past year and has not missed a single dose. As she starts to cry, her tears are noted to have an orange tint. The physician tells her that the most likely reason her oral contraceptives were ineffective was an interaction with one of her other medications. For which condition is this patient most likely being treated?

(A) Breast cancer
(B) Epilepsy
(C) *Giardia* infection
(D) Refractory atrial fibrillation
(E) Tuberculosis

17. A 43-year-old man with a 7-year history of chronic renal disease comes to the emergency department with a 5-day history of productive cough and shortness of breath. On physical examination, he is found to have rales in the middle lobe of his right lung. An x-ray film of the chest shows consolidation in the same area, and he is started on levofloxacin. Which of the following indicates how the dosing of the levofloxacin would be different in this patient as compared to an otherwise healthy patient?

(A) Higher loading dose, higher maintenance dose
(B) Higher loading dose, same maintenance dose
(C) Lower loading dose, lower maintenance dose
(D) Lower loading dose, same maintenance dose
(E) Same loading dose, higher maintenance dose
(F) Same loading dose, lower maintenance dose
(G) Same loading dose, same maintenance dose

18. A 40-year-old man has been diagnosed with glioblastoma multiforme. The patient's neurologist must choose an appropriate cancer drug to treat this tumor. Which of the following can cross the blood–brain barrier for effective treatment of brain tumors?

    (A) Cytarabine
    (B) Etoposide
    (C) Nitrosoureas
    (D) Selective estrogen receptor modulators
    (E) Vinca alkaloids

19. A 24-year-old law student has been experiencing frequent headaches for which he has been taking increasingly large doses of aspirin for 3 months. One night he takes a particularly large dose, becomes confused, and falls into a seizure. He presents to the emergency department with a serum salicylate level of 130 mg/dL. Which of the following is the most appropriate treatment?

    (A) Bicarbonate
    (B) Glucagon
    (C) N-acetylcysteine
    (D) Protamine
    (E) Vitamin K

20. A 29-year-old man with a 3-year history of hip and lower back pain complains of morning stiffness of his back that improves with exercise. He is otherwise healthy and currently not taking any medications. His physical examination is unremarkable except for a decrease in chest expansion. X-ray of the spine is shown in the image. To prevent potential serious adverse effects associated with the preferred treatment, which test should be administered first?

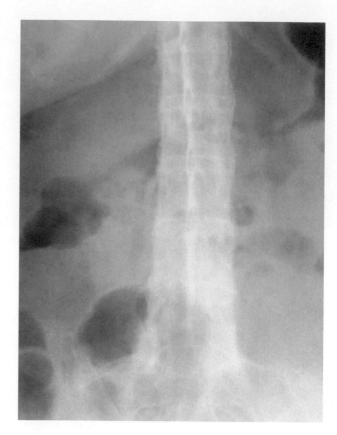

Reproduced, with permission, from Chen MYM, Pope TL Jr, Ott DJ. *Basic Radiology*. New York: McGraw-Hill, 2004: Figure 7-45.

    (A) Blood pressure
    (B) Erythrocyte sedimentation rate
    (C) *Neisseria gonorrhoeae* nucleic acid hybridization test
    (D) Pulmonary function test
    (E) Purified protein derivative skin test

21. A 4-year-old girl is brought to the emergency department with abdominal pain after eating 10–15 sugar-coated iron tablets. Soon after arriving she begins to vomit, and the emesis has blood in it. Physical examination shows hypotension and tachycardia. Which of the following is the best treatment for this patient's elevated blood iron levels?

    (A) Aminocaproic acid
    (B) Deferoxamine
    (C) Dimercaprol
    (D) Oral bicarbonate
    (E) Penicillamine

22. A 52-year-old man with end-stage renal disease presents to his renal clinic with a hemoglobin concentration of 8 g/dL and an absolute reticulocyte count of <25,000 cells/mm^3. His WBC count is 11,000/mm^3 and the differential is within normal limits. A peripheral blood smear shows hypochromic, microcytic RBCs. Iron staining of a bone marrow aspirate shows macrophages positive and RBCs negative for iron within the cytoplasm. Which of the following is the most likely cause of this patient's condition?

(A) An overdose of tacrolimus
(B) Anti-Rh D immunoglobulin
(C) Iron deficiency
(D) Low erythropoietin
(E) Myelodysplastic syndrome
(F) Tissue plasminogen activator

23. The following illustration contains the dose-response curves for drug X as well as two other agents. Which of the following curves represents drug X plus a noncompetitive antagonist?

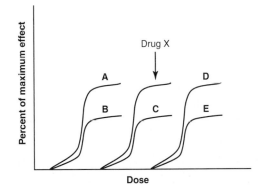

Reproduced, with permission, from USMLERx.com.

(A) Curve A
(B) Curve B
(C) Curve C
(D) Curve D
(E) Curve E

24. Class I antiarrhythmics are Na$^+$ channel blockers that slow or block cardiac conduction, especially in depolarized cells. Which of the following class I antiarrhythmics will increase both the action potential and the effective refractory period?

(A) Encainide
(B) Mexiletine
(C) Procainamide
(D) Propafenone
(E) Tocainide

25. A 40-year-old man with a long history of medically managed Crohn's disease presents with shortness of breath. He complains of repeated incidents of bruising following minor trauma and increasing weakness. Laboratory tests show:

Hemoglobin: 5.5 g/dL
Hematocrit: 13%
WBC count: 2200/mm^3
Platelet count: 39,000/mm^3

A bone marrow biopsy is shown in the image. A detailed history reveals that the patient had an acute episode of gout 3 months ago and was prescribed a medicine to prevent future attacks. Adverse interactions of which two drugs most likely caused this patient's condition?

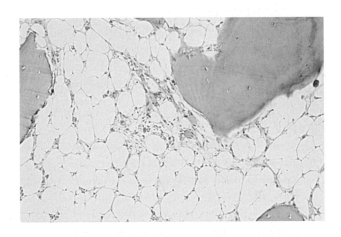

Reproduced, with permission, from Fauci AS, Braunwald E, Kasper DL, Hauser SL, Longo DL, Jameson JL, and Loscalzo J, eds. *Harrison' Principles of Internal Medicine*, 17th ed. New York: McGraw-Hill, 2008; Figure 102-1, C.

(A) Azathioprine and allopurinol
(B) Azathioprine and colchicine
(C) Infliximab and colchicine
(D) Prednisone and allopurinol
(E) Prednisone and colchicine

1. **The correct answer is E.** Protease inhibitors such as lopinavir/ritonavir (Kaletra), amprenavir, nelfinavir, indinavir, and saquinavir can cause gastrointestinal intolerance and fat redistribution. Lopinavir/ritonavir is one of the main combinations forming the basis of highly active antiretroviral therapy. Two nucleotide reverse transcriptase inhibitors are added to form the backbone.

Answer A is incorrect. The only fusion inhibitor currently available, enfuvirtide, is not recommended for inclusion in the initial highly active antiretroviral therapy regimen. It is associated with reactions at the injection site, but not fat distribution.

Answer B is incorrect. Non-nucleoside reverse transcriptase inhibitors such as nevirapine, delavirdine, and efavirenz cause a variety of adverse effects such as rash and hepatitis, but they do not cause fat redistribution.

Answer C is incorrect. Some of the nucleoside reverse transcriptase inhibitors (zidovudine, stavudine, didanosine, zalcitabine, abacavir, and lamivudine) can cause peripheral neuropathies, gastrointestinal intolerance, and pancreatitis, but they are not known to cause fat redistribution.

Answer D is incorrect. The nucleotide reverse transcriptase inhibitor tenofovir is usually well tolerated. It is recommended that it be taken with meals. The Department of Health and Human Services recommends that it be used in one of its treatment regimens.

2. **The correct answer is D.** β-Blockers decrease contractility and heart rate (resulting in decreased oxygen consumption) by inhibiting β-receptors in the heart. A decrease in heart rate will then allow more time for diastolic filling (increasing EDV) and systolic ejection (increasing ejection time). In addition, β-blockers will decrease the secretion of renin, thus diminishing the renin-angiotensin cascade.

Answer A is incorrect. Answer A does not reflect the effects of β-blockers.

Answer B is incorrect. Answer B does not reflect the effects of β-blockers.

Answer C is incorrect. Answer C does not reflect the effects of β-blockers.

Answer E is incorrect. Answer E is compatible with the effects of nitrates. These drugs serve to decrease the afterload on the heart by vasodilation. However, vasodilation produces a reflex increase in both contractility and heart rate. An increase in heart rate causes a decrease in EDV and ejection time.

3. **The correct answer is B.** This patient presents with gastroparesis, specifically esophageal dysmotility, secondary to her diabetes. Other causes of esophageal dysmotility include diabetic gastroparesis, Chagas' disease, lupus, and other collagen vascular diseases. Initial treatment consists of promotility agents, with metoclopramide being first-line therapy.

Answer A is incorrect. Esophageal resection is the treatment for squamous cell carcinoma or adenocarcinoma of the esophagus or for high-grade Barrett's esophagus.

Answer C is incorrect. Omeprazole is a proton pump inhibitor used to treat gastroesophageal reflux disease, peptic ulcer disease, and acid hypersecretion.

Answer D is incorrect. Ondansetron is a 5-HT_3 receptor antagonist used to treat refractory or severe nausea and vomiting.

Answer E is incorrect. Vagotomy is a treatment option for peptic ulcer disease or acid hypersecretion states such as in Zollinger-Ellison syndrome.

4. **The correct answer is E.** This patient is presenting with a medical emergency: an extreme form of thyrotoxicosis known as "thyroid storm." The symptoms of this syndrome are due primarily to increased β-adrenergic outflow stimulated by thyroid hormones. After primary stabilization (airway, breathing, and circulation), propylthiouracil or methimazole is

the most appropriate pharmacologic treatment for this condition. These agents inhibit the endogenous synthesis of thyroxine, which can cause or worsen this condition.

Answer A is incorrect. Aspirin displaces thyroxine from thyroid-binding globulin and can thus worsen the symptoms of thyrotoxicosis. In contrast, acetaminophen is useful as an antipyretic in the treatment of thyrotoxicosis and thyroid storm.

Answer B is incorrect. Dobutamine is a β-adrenergic agonist that is useful in the treatment of acute congestive heart failure but would exacerbate the adrenergic effects of high-output congestive heart failure secondary to thyrotoxicosis. A β-adrenergic antagonist such as propranolol would be more appropriate in the treatment of thyrotoxicosis.

Answer C is incorrect. Iodine, which decreases the release of preformed thyroxine, can be used as an adjunct to propylthiouracil or methimazole but should not be used until one of these agents is allowed to take effect. Iodine can stimulate the endogenous synthesis of thyroxine and thus exacerbate this condition.

Answer D is incorrect. Levothyroxine, a synthetic form of thyroid hormone, is contraindicated in the treatment of thyrotoxicosis. The addition of more thyroid hormone to a patient with a condition of symptomatic hyperthyroidism would only worsen the condition.

5. **The correct answer is C.** This patient's symptoms suggest that he is experiencing nitroglycerine withdrawal. Nitroglycerine is a vasodilator. Chronic industrial exposure leads to tolerance for vasodilatation on work days and a compensatory vasoconstriction on weekends when the exposure is removed, thus resulting in the "Monday disease." The most severe consequence is when the compensatory vasoconstriction is unopposed in critical areas such as the coronary vessels, leading to non-atherosclerotic-related ischemia.

Answer A is incorrect. Anemia can be a result of lead or other heavy metal poisoning, but not nitroglycerine.

Answer B is incorrect. Atherosclerosis is formed by fatty streak deposition, which along with endothelial damage results in plaque formation over time. It is not linked to nitroglycerine exposure.

Answer D is incorrect. Congestive heart failure can be a complication of long-term coronary artery disease or a myocardial infarction, but not of nitroglycerine exposure.

Answer E is incorrect. Dementia can be a result of neurotoxin exposures (eg., mercury). Nitroglycerine exposure does not cause dementia.

6. **The correct answer is C.** This patient suffers from generalized anxiety disorder (GAD), which is marked by symptoms of excessive worry and anxiety about every aspect of one's life. *The Diagnostic and Statistical Manual of Mental Disorders*, Fourth Edition, Text Revision (DSM-IV-TR) criteria for generalized anxiety disorder include: (1) At least 6 months in which the person experiences a majority of the days feeling anxious and apprehensive; (2) the anxiety and apprehension impair functioning in areas such as work and social life; (3) there are ≥3 associated symptoms including restlessness, difficulty concentrating, irritability, decreased energy, muscle tension, and/or sleep disturbance; and (4) the anxiety and apprehension are not associated with another medical or psychiatric disorder. Benzodiazepines are first-line agents in the treatment of GAD due to their sedative properties. However, patients with polydrug or alcohol use, chronic pain disorders, and severe personality disorders probably should not be prescribed benzodiazepines in light of the high potential in such patients for benzodiazepine dependence.

Answer A is incorrect. Amitriptyline, a tricyclic antidepressant, may be effective for the treatment of GAD but is not considered a first-line agent. Agents in this class are better suited for the treatment of endogenous depression.

Answer B is incorrect. Buspirone appears to be as effective as the benzodiazepines for the treatment of GAD, but the onset of action can take 1-2 weeks. Buspirone is prescribed instead of benzodiazepines mainly because of its lack of abuse potential; however, abuse of benzodiazepines is quite rare in practice. Most abusers of benzodiazepines have a history of polydrug or alcohol abuse; these patients should not be prescribed benzodiazepines, especially on a long-term basis.

Answer D is incorrect. Flumazenil is a competitive γ-aminobutyric acid–receptor antagonist that is used to reverse the effects of benzodiazepines; it is indicated for use in cases of acute benzodiazepine overdose.

Answer E is incorrect. Midazolam is a short-acting benzodiazepine that should not be used as a first-line medication for long-term use (ie., treatment of GAD) since it can easily cause dependence, rebound anxiety, and withdrawal symptoms.

7. **The correct answer is A.** The photomicrograph shows Kimmelstiel-Wilson nodules, which are pathognomonic for diabetic nephropathy. Even without recognizing this specific histopathology, however, one should be reminded of diabetes due to the combination of renal and visual findings (diabetic nephropathy and retinopathy). Angiotensin-converting enzyme (ACE) inhibitors are the drugs of choice in the control of diabetes-induced renal disease because they reduce systemic blood pressure, reduce the effects of angiotensin II (AT II) on efferent arterioles, and attenuate the stimulatory effect of AT II on glomerular cell growth and matrix production. ACE inhibitors have been conclusively shown to delay the time to end-stage renal disease by 50% in type 1 diabetics and to significantly delay progression of renal disease in type 2 diabetics. All diabetics should begin ACE inhibitor therapy at the onset of microalbuminuria, even in the absence of hypertension.

Answer B is incorrect. β-Blockers are used to control essential hypertension, not diabetic nephropathy.

Answer C is incorrect. Cyclophosphamide is often used in conjunction with prednisone to treat immunologically mediated kidney disease.

Answer D is incorrect. Gold therapy, used in the treatment of rheumatoid arthritis, is known to cause glomerular disease.

Answer E is incorrect. Prednisone is used in the treatment of immune-mediated nephropathy, not diabetic nephropathy.

8. **The correct answer is C.** This is the classic presentation of a child with cystic fibrosis, an autosomal recessive defect in the cystic fibrosis transmembrane conductance regulator (*CFTR*) gene on chromosome 7. This results in a defective chloride channel, leading to the secretion of abnormally thick mucus in the lungs, pancreas, and liver.

Answer A is incorrect. The *CFTR* gene is located on chromosome 7, not chromosome 3.

Answer B is incorrect. The *CFTR* gene is located on chromosome 7, not chromosome 5.

Answer D is incorrect. The *CFTR* gene is located on chromosome 7, not chromosome 12.

Answer E is incorrect. The *CFTR* gene is located on chromosome 7, not chromosome 15.

9. **The correct answer is B.** Renal failure is a very dangerous adverse event associated with nonsteroidal anti-inflammatory drugs (NSAIDs). The patient was in congestive heart failure when he first presented. His cardiologist consequently treated him with a diuretic, intending to reduce his total body fluids. When the amount of fluids in the body contracts, the body attempts to compensate by releasing angiotensin II, a potent vasoconstrictor. In order to protect the kidney from losing its perfusion due to this vasoconstriction, the kidney simultaneously releases prostaglandins at both the afferent and efferent arterioles, where they act as vasodilators. By taking an NSAID like ibuprofen and inhibiting the cyclooxygenase (COX)-1 and COX-2 enzymes, this patient blocked the pathway producing the prostaglandins that were keeping the afferent arterioles

dilated and thus keeping his kidneys perfused. His renal failure is prerenal in origin, resulting from the constriction of these arterioles.

Answer A is incorrect. NSAIDs will block the production of prostaglandin E_2 at both arterioles, but the constriction of the afferent arteriole is the primary cause of this man's renal failure.

Answer C is incorrect. While NSAIDs would also have blocked the production of prostaglandin E_2 at the efferent arteriole, this would not cause renal failure, it would actually increase glomerular filtration rate (blocking the outflow without blocking the inflow will increase filtration). This would not cause the patient to present with oliguria or a rising creatinine level.

Answer D is incorrect. Ibuprofen blocks the synthesis of prostaglandins, and thus a decrease in the prostaglandin level would be seen, not an increase.

Answer E is incorrect. Ibuprofen blocks the synthesis of prostaglandins, and thus a decrease in the prostaglandin level would be seen, not an increase.

10. **The correct answer is E.** This man has the symptoms of benign prostatic hypertrophy, which include difficulty starting and maintaining a urine stream, feeling as though the bladder is never emptied, having the urge to urinate again soon after voiding, and pain on urination or dysuria. Finasteride is most commonly used to treat this condition. Finasteride acts by inhibiting the conversion of testosterone to dihydrotestosterone by inhibiting 5α-reductase. This leads to a reduction in the size of the prostate, providing symptomatic relief.

Answer A is incorrect. Bleomycin acts by chelating mechanisms to attack the phosphodiester bonds of DNA. It is used to treat testicular tumors and lymphomas (especially Hodgkin's), not benign prostatic hypertrophy.

Answer B is incorrect. Leuprolide is a gonadotropin-releasing hormone analog that binds the luteinizing hormone-releasing hormone receptor in the pituitary. This leads to desensitization of the receptor and, subsequently, to reduced release of luteinizing hormone. Leuprolide is used to treat metastatic carcinoma of the prostate, not benign prostatic hypertrophy.

Answer C is incorrect. Sildenafil inhibits cGMP-specific phosphodiesterase type 5, resulting in increased concentrations of cGMP, which increases vasodilation leading to increased blood flow to the corpus cavernosum. Sildenafil is used primarily to treat erectile dysfunction.

Answer D is incorrect. Ketoconazole is an antifungal with antiandrogenic properties that acts by inhibiting cytochrome P450 enzymes. It is not used in the treatment of benign prostatic hypertrophy.

Answer F is incorrect. Flutamide is a potent androgen receptor antagonist that has limited efficacy when used alone because the increased luteinizing hormone secretion stimulates higher serum testosterone levels. This drug is used primarily in conjunction with a gonadotropin-releasing hormone analog in the treatment of metastatic prostate cancer.

11. **The correct answer is B.** The finding of crepitus suggests that the patient initially had a wound infection from a gas-producing anaerobic organism, most likely *Clostridium perfringens*, which responds well to clindamycin. Unfortunately, one of the adverse effects of clindamycin is superinfection (ie., an infection on top of another infection) caused by destruction of the colon's normal flora and allowing an overgrowth of *Clostridium difficile*, which is resistant to clindamycin. *C. difficile* causes pseudomembranous colitis, one of the most common nosocomial infections. Endoscopy reveals areas of colonic mucosa covered by a "membrane" of necrotic tissue produced by *C. difficile* exotoxin. Though the danger of pseudomembranous colitis exists with the use of any antibiotic, the risk is substantially higher with clindamycin, penicillins, and cephalosporins.

Answer A is incorrect. Amantadine is an antiviral agent associated with ataxia, dizziness, and slurred speech.

Answer C is incorrect. Metronidazole is associated with a disulfiram-like reaction with alcohol. It is frequently used to treat pseudomembranous colitis.

Answer D is incorrect. Tetracycline is associated with tooth discoloration in children.

Answer E is incorrect. Vancomycin is associated with "red man" syndrome when given rapidly through an intravenous line. Given orally, it can be used to treat pseudomembranous colitis.

12. **The correct answer is D.** Fibrates like gemfibrozil act at point D. They are ligands for the peroxisome proliferator-activated receptor-α (PPAR-α) protein, a receptor that regulates the transcription of genes involved in lipid metabolism. Increased expression of the PPAR-α protein results in increased expression of lipoprotein lipase on endothelial cells and thus increased clearance of triglyceride-rich lipoproteins. Fibrates have been shown to decrease triglyceride levels by as much as 35%–50%.

Answer A is incorrect. There are no lipid-lowering drugs that act at point A.

Answer B is incorrect. Bile acid sequestrants such as cholestyramine act at point B by blocking the reabsorption of bile acids. The liver must then metabolize more cholesterol to replace the bile acids, thereby primarily lowering LDL-cholesterol levels.

Answer C is incorrect. 3-Hydroxy-3-methylglutaryl coenzyme A (HMG-CoA) reductase inhibitors act at point C by competitively inhibiting the synthesis of mevalonate by HMG-CoA reductase, an essential step in the production of cholesterol in the liver. Serum LDL cholesterol levels are, in turn, decreased as the liver upregulates LDL receptor expression to compensate for diminished capacity to endogenously synthesize cholesterol.

13. **The correct answer is E.** This patient has congestive heart failure. Decreased cardiac contractility results in a back-up of the cardiac circuit, leading to pulmonary edema followed by peripheral edema. Digoxin and diuretics are often given to increase cardiac output and reduce edema, respectively. Diuretics such as thiazides, furosemide, or ethacrynic acid can cause hypokalemia, and hypokalemia can worsen digoxin toxicity.

Answer A is incorrect. Acetylsalicylic acid (aspirin) and thiazides together do not constitute an effective therapy for congestive heart failure and do not result in a drug interaction.

Answer B is incorrect. Acetylsalicylic acid (aspirin) and nitroprusside together do not constitute an effective therapy for congestive heart failure and do not result in a drug interaction.

Answer C is incorrect. β-Blockers and thiazides may interact to produce an increased β-blocker effect, but this would not necessarily lead to an adverse effect.

Answer D is incorrect. β-Blockers and spironolactone together do not cause a drug interaction.

Answer F is incorrect. Digoxin and spironolactone may result in reduced digoxin effectiveness due to hyperkalemic states caused by potassium-sparing diuretics, but this would not be as dangerous as the interaction of digoxin and furosemide.

14. **The correct answer is E.** Chronic atrial fibrillation is a risk factor for clot formation and systemic embolization. This man needs ongoing anticoagulation to prevent possible complications, such as cerebrovascular accidents or mesenteric infarction. Warfarin inhibits gamma-carboxylation of vitamin K-dependent clotting factors and is used for chronic anticoagulation. It is taken orally and has a long half-life. The degree of anticoagulation must be followed by measuring the International Normalized Ratio.

Answer A is incorrect. Aspirin works by irreversibly inhibiting cyclooxygenase, thereby preventing the conversion of arachidonic acid to prostaglandins. The four effects of aspirin are antiplatelet (thereby inhibiting thrombus formation), antipyretic, analgesic, and anti-inflammatory. Aspirin is not used to prevent clot formation in the setting of atrial fibrillation, but rather to prevent myocardial infarction. In the setting of atrial fibrillation, the patient needs a drug that prevents activation of the clotting cascade, whereas aspirin acts only on platelet aggregation.

Answer B is incorrect. Protamine sulfate is used for rapid reversal of heparinization in the setting of overzealous anticoagulation.

Answer C is incorrect. Streptokinase is a thrombolytic used to break down existing clots. This could be used in the setting of a myocardial infarction. It would not be used prophylactically to prevent clot formation in atrial fibrillation.

Answer D is incorrect. Heparin is taken parenterally and is used for immediate, not long-term, anticoagulation. This patient was likely given heparin on admission to the hospital and was then converted to warfarin for chronic anticoagulation before his discharge.

15. **The correct answer is B.** Clearance is calculated as: (rate of drug elimination / plasma drug concentration) = (2 mg/min) / (50 mg/L) = 0.04 L/min.

    Answer A is incorrect. Calculation error.

    Answer C is incorrect. Calculation error.

    Answer D is incorrect. Calculation error.

    Answer E is incorrect. Calculation error.

16. **The correct answer is E.** Rifampin is an antibiotic used to treat tuberculosis. It works by suppressing RNA synthesis. One major adverse effect of rifampin is that it is metabolized by and induces the cytochrome P450 system; thus drugs such as oral contraceptives, warfarin, and ketoconazole may need to be given in higher concentrations in order to be therapeutic. This is probably the reason why this woman's oral contraceptive pills failed. Another well-known adverse effect that can be frightening to patients is that rifampin turns all bodily fluids (tears, sweat, and urine) orange.

Answer A is incorrect. Chemotherapeutic agents used to treat breast cancer have a number of adverse effects, but are not associated with orange body fluids. Chronic pain often associated with cancer is a difficult entity to treat. Frequently patients depend on NSAIDs to help control their pain. Chronic use of NSAIDs can cause epigastric distress and even ulcers. NSAIDs also decrease platelet aggregation ability and can cause bleeding problems, thus they should be discontinued before surgery.

Answer B is incorrect. Phenytoin is one of the drugs used to treat epilepsy, particularly tonic-clonic and partial seizures. It has many adverse effects, including induction of the P450 cytochrome system, and thus would interact with oral contraceptive pills. However, phenytoin does not cause red-orange body fluids. Some other adverse effects of phenytoin include gingival hyperplasia, megaloblastic anemia secondary to folate deficiency, and central nervous system depression. Phenytoin is also teratogenic and causes fetal hydantoin syndrome (prenatal growth deficiency, mental retardation, and congenital malformations).

Answer C is incorrect. *Giardia* infection is treated with metronidazole, an antibiotic effective against amoebae and anaerobes. One of metronidazole's famous adverse effects is a disulfiram-like reaction with ethanol. Metronidazole is also highly teratogenic and should not be given to pregnant women.

Answer D is incorrect. Amiodarone is an antiarrhythmic drug that has properties of both class I and class III antiarrhythmics and is most often used to treat refractory atrial fibrillation and ventricular tachyarrhythmias. Amiodarone is infamous for its many adverse effects including interstitial pulmonary fibrosis, thyroid dysfunction (both hyper- and hypothyroidism), and hepatocellular necrosis. Amiodarone and other antiarrhythmic drugs do not cause orange bodily fluids.

17. **The correct answer is F.** The most important concept in this answer is that the loading dose is independent of renal or liver disease; the

loading dose has more to do with volume of distribution, since excretion and metabolism have not yet occurred. The maintenance dose will be lower, since this patient has a history of renal disease and levofloxacin is excreted in the urine.

Answer A is incorrect. A higher loading dose is unnecessary and may lead to elevated drug levels, which can cause elongated QT intervals. A higher maintenance dose would also lead to elevated drug levels.

Answer B is incorrect. A higher loading dose is unnecessary and may lead to elevated drug levels, which can cause elongated QT intervals. Keeping the maintenance dose the same may also lead to elevated drug levels.

Answer C is incorrect. A lower loading dose would lead to subtherapeutic drug levels; however, adjusting for the compromised renal excretion and lowering the maintenance dose would be appropriate.

Answer D is incorrect. A lower loading dose would lead to subtherapeutic drug levels; keeping the maintenance dose the same may also lead to elevated drug levels.

Answer E is incorrect. Keeping the same loading dose is the correct choice; however, a higher maintenance dose would lead to elevated drug levels.

Answer G is incorrect. Keeping the same loading dose is the correct choice; however, keeping the maintenance dose the same may also lead to elevated drug levels.

18. **The correct answer is C.** The lipophilic nitrosoureas, such as carmustine and lomustine, are alkylating agents that can penetrate the blood–brain barrier, making them excellent drugs for the treatment of brain tumors. The nitrosoureas are metabolized to active products and excreted in the urine.

Answer A is incorrect. Cytarabine inhibits DNA polymerase and is used in the treatment of acute myelogenous leukemia. Cytarabine cannot penetrate the blood–brain barrier.

Answer B is incorrect. Etoposide is noted for poor penetration into the cerebrospinal fluid.

Answer D is incorrect. Selective estrogen receptor modulators, such as raloxifene, block estrogen from binding to estrogen receptors on estrogen receptor-positive cells. These drugs do not penetrate the blood–brain barrier.

Answer E is incorrect. Vinca alkaloids, given intravenously, are concentrated in the liver and excreted through bile in the feces. Vinca alkaloids do not cross the blood–brain barrier.

19. **The correct answer is A.** Administration of bicarbonate will alkalinize the urine, thereby allowing the acidic toxin to be excreted and not reabsorbed. Alkalinization of the urine will lead to ionization of acids (such as salicylates) within the renal tubules. In general, charged molecules cannot be reabsorbed, while uncharged molecules are easily reabsorbed from the tubules. Thus, bicarbonate administration is indicated because it promotes "trapping" and hence excretion of salicylate molecules. Note that the concept can only be applied in reverse order to promote excretion of basic drugs: the goal is to acidify the urine so as to promote retention of the charged basic drug molecules within the urine.

Answer B is incorrect. Glucagon is used to treat β-blocker toxicity.

Answer C is incorrect. N-acetylcysteine is used to treat acetaminophen toxicity.

Answer D is incorrect. Protamine is used to treat heparin toxicity.

Answer E is incorrect. Vitamin K is used to treat warfarin toxicity.

20. **The correct answer is E.** This patient has ankylosing spondylitis; the image shows the "bamboo spine" characteristic of this disease. An effective treatment is infliximab, an anti-tumor necrosis factor-α monoclonal antibody that relieves symptoms and slows the progression of the disease. However, due to its immunosuppressive properties, a rare but serious adverse effect is opportunistic infection, especially

flare-up of dormant tuberculosis. A purified protein derivative skin test should be conducted prior to treatment. If results are positive, the patient should be sent for an x-ray of the chest and treated with anti-tubercular medications prior to initiating treatment with infliximab.

Answer A is incorrect. Increase or decrease of blood pressure may occur after infusion of infliximab, but is a common and temporary reaction that usually resolves quickly.

Answer B is incorrect. A high erythrocyte sedimentation rate is a nonspecific finding in inflammatory processes and is seen in other processes as well (i.e., malignancy, aging). While the erythrocyte sedimentation rate may be elevated in a patient with ankylosing spondylitis, it does not confirm the diagnosis and does not indicate potential adverse effects.

Answer C is incorrect. Many patients with *Neisseria gonorrhoeae* infection experience arthritis-like joint pain, most commonly in the knees. This patient's long history of back pain does not suggest gonorrhea infection. In addition, infliximab treatment does not increase the risk of gonorrheal infection.

Answer D is incorrect. The use of infliximab is associated with an increased incidence of pneumonia. Pulmonary function tests, however, would not be predictive of the likelihood of this adverse effect. Infliximab does not otherwise commonly affect lung function.

21. **The correct answer is B.** Symptoms of iron overdose include onset of nausea, vomiting (including hemorrhagic gastroenteritis), and abdominal pain within 4 hours of ingestion. Other symptoms may include hyperglycemia, leukocytosis, shock, and coma. Deferoxamine is a chelating agent specific for iron and will reduce effective blood iron levels.

Answer A is incorrect. Aminocaproic acid is used in the treatment of tissue plasminogen activator or streptokinase overdose.

Answer C is incorrect. Dimercaprol is used to treat poisoning by arsenic, mercury, and gold.

Answer D is incorrect. Bicarbonate would be used to inactivate iron in the gastrointestinal tract. Although this treatment may prevent iron from entering the blood from the gastrointestinal tract, it will do nothing to inactivate iron already in the bloodstream.

Answer E is incorrect. Penicillamine is used to treat lead and arsenic toxicity, not iron poisoning.

22. **The correct answer is D.** Erythropoietin is a hormone produced in the kidney, and hence low levels are seen in the setting of kidney failure. Low levels of erythropoietin could cause anemia, which this patient is experiencing. Erythropoietin acts by increasing RBC proliferation and differentiation in the bone marrow. Lack of erythropoietin causes a microcytic anemia with iron sequestration in the bone marrow, as shown on the slide. Human recombinant erythropoietin (epoetin) is used in patients with severe anemias (hemoglobin <11 g/dL), which often occur in the setting of renal failure.

Answer A is incorrect. Tacrolimus is an immunosuppressive agent used in organ transplant recipients. It does not cause microcytic anemia.

Answer B is incorrect. Anti-Rh D immunoglobulin is administered to Rh-negative mothers with Rh-positive fetuses to prevent the development of erythroblastosis fetalis (fetal hydrops). It does not cause anemia and in fact prevents the development of the immune-mediated fetal anemia that can occur in the context of Rh-incompatibility.

Answer C is incorrect. Although iron deficiency causes a microcytic hypochromic anemia as seen in this patient, analysis of bone marrow biopsies in iron deficiency anemia shows reduced iron in all cells, unlike in this scenario.

Answer E is incorrect. Patients with myelodysplastic syndrome typically present with a pancytopenia, not an isolated anemia, as is seen in this case. Isolated anemia in the context of chronic renal failure is much more likely to be due to erythropoietin deficiency than to a concurrent myelodysplastic syndrome.

Answer F is incorrect. Tissue plasminogen activator is a thrombolytic agent that produces fibrinolysis and is utilized in thromboembolic disease. It does not cause anemia.

23. **The correct answer is C.** A noncompetitive antagonist, or an irreversible antagonist, can bind to the active site of the receptor or to other sites on the receptor. However the binding occurs, it results in the same potency, but with a decreased maximum response, or efficacy, that cannot be overcome by the addition of more agonist.

Answer A is incorrect. Curve A represents a dose-response curve with the same efficacy but increased potency. The addition of any antagonist would be unlikely to cause this response.

Answer B is incorrect. Curve B represents a drug with a lower efficacy but a greater potency than drug X. This could occur with the addition of a partial agonist.

Answer D is incorrect. Curve D represents a drug with a decreased potency but the same efficacy. This could occur with the addition of a competitive antagonist.

Answer E is incorrect. Curve E represents a drug with a lower efficacy and potency. This could occur with the addition of a partial antagonist.

24. **The correct answer is C.** Class IA antiarrhythmics, such as procainamide, affect both atrial and ventricular arrhythmias. They block sodium channels and thus slow conduction velocity in the atria, ventricles, and Purkinje fibers. This decreased conduction velocity slows phase 0 of the action potential (AP) and is manifested as an increased QRS duration on ECG. In addition to blocking sodium channels, Class IA antiarrhythmics also block potassium channels and thus increase the AP duration and ERP.

Answer A is incorrect. Encainide is a class IC antiarrhythmic.

Answer B is incorrect. Mexiletine is a class IB antiarrhythmic.

Answer D is incorrect. Class IC antiarrhythmics, such as propafenone, slow phase 0 of the AP, but have no effect on the AP duration. These antiarrhythmics have no affect on the effective refractory period.

Answer E is incorrect. Class IB antiarrhythmics, such as tocainide, slow phase 0 of the AP, but decrease the AP duration. These antiarrhythmics affect ischemic or depolarized Purkinje and ventricular tissues. These antiarrhythmics have no affect on the effective refractory period.

25. **The correct answer is A.** Azathioprine is a common treatment for Crohn's disease; its metabolite, 6-mercaptopurine, is normally inactivated by xanthine oxidase. Allopurinol is a xanthine oxidase inhibitor used to prevent repeat gout attacks. When these two are used concomitantly, allopurinol interferes with the metabolism of azathioprine's toxic metabolite, which can lead to fatal hematologic disorders, such as aplastic anemia, as in this case.

Answer B is incorrect. Colchicine can be used to treat acute gout. It binds to tubulin and prevents microtubule polymerization. It does not interfere with azathioprine metabolism and is not known to cause pancytopenia. Colchicine can, however, cause cytopenia.

Answer C is incorrect. Infliximab is an anti-tumor necrosis factor-α monoclonal antibody sometimes used to treat Crohn's disease. It is not known to interact with colchicine to cause pancytopenia.

Answer D is incorrect. Prednisone is a corticosteroid that can be used to manage Crohn's disease. It is not known to have fatally adverse interactions such as pancytopenia when used with allopurinol.

Answer E is incorrect. Although prednisone is a treatment for Crohn's disease and colchicine a treatment for gout, the two can be safely combined in treating primary sclerosing cholangitis.

Organ Systems

CHAPTER 8

Cardiovascular

1. A physician decides to place a patient on a calcium channel blocker for treatment of her angina. Calcium channel blockers can relax the smooth muscle of blood vessels and can also have various effects on cardiac contractility, conduction, and heart rate. Which of the following calcium channel blockers would be most effective in reducing heart rate and contractility?

(A) Dihydropyridine
(B) Diltiazem
(C) Nifedipine
(D) Nimodipine
(E) Verapamil

2. A 28-year-old African-American man presents to the physician with fever, weight loss, and abdominal pain. His blood pressure is 168/92 mm Hg, his pulse is 83/min, and his respiratory rate is 18/min. On physical examination, there is palpable purpura on his lower extremities; a fundoscopic examination reveals fluffy, white spots on his retina. His past medical history is significant for a previous hepatitis B infection. An arterial biopsy is shown in the image. Which of the following is the most prominent morphologic feature of the affected arteries in this patient's disease process?

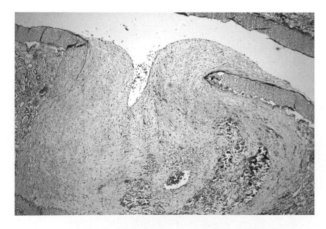

Reproduced, with permission, from PEIR Digital Library (http://peir.net).

(A) Caseating necrosis
(B) Eosinophilic infiltrate
(C) Fibrinoid necrosis
(D) Granulomatous inflammation
(E) Langhans' giant cells
(F) Onion skinning

3. A 50-year-old man with diabetes receives the results of a fasting lipid profile that reveals hypercholesterolemia. To reduce the patient's mortality risk, his physician recommends lifestyle changes and initiates therapy with a statin. Which of the following mechanisms describes the action of statins in reducing serum levels of LDL cholesterol?

(A) Competitive inhibition of 3-hydroxy-3-methylglutaryl coenzyme A reductase
(B) Inactivation of 3-hydroxy-3-methylglutaryl coenzyme A synthase
(C) Negative feedback to decrease thiolase activity
(D) Noncompetitive inhibition of citrate synthase
(E) Positive feedback to increase 3-hydroxy-3-methylglutaryl coenzyme A lyase activity

4. A 45-year-old man who takes spironolactone and digoxin for his congestive heart failure is admitted to the hospital because he is experiencing an altered mental status. The ECG changes shown in the image are noted on testing. Urinalysis would most likely reveal which of the following?

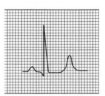

Reproduced, with permission, from USMLERx.com.

(A) High K⁺, high Na⁺, high-normal volume

(A) High K^+, high Na^+, high-normal volume
(B) High K^+, low Na^+, low volume
(C) High K^+, low Na^+, normal volume
(D) Low K^+, high Na^+, high-normal volume
(E) Low K^+, low Na^+, normal volume

·5. A medical student working in the emergency department sees a female baby, born 2 weeks ago, who is brought in by her anxious mother. The mother tells the student that her baby seems "purple," especially her fingers and toes, and looks extremely blue when crying. On physical examination the sleeping baby has mild cyanosis of the face and trunk, but moderate cyanosis of the extremities. Which of the following is the most common cause of cyanosis within the first few weeks of life?

(A) Atrial septal defect
(B) Patent ductus arteriosus
(C) Tetralogy of Fallot
(D) Transposition of the great vessels
(E) Ventricular septal defect

·6. A 55-year-old man with hypertension is prescribed an antiarrhythmic agent that alters the flow of cations in myocardial tissue. The image is a trace of a myocardial action potential. Each phase is associated with the opening and/or closing of various ion channels. Which of the following would be affected by an agent that affects phase 2 of the myocardial action potential?

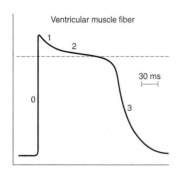

Reproduced, with permission, from USMLERx.com.

(A) Ligand-gated Ca^{2+} channels opening
(B) Ligand-gated Na^+ channels opening
(C) Voltage-gated Ca^{2+} channels opening
(D) Voltage-gated Na^+ channels closing
(E) Voltage-gated Na^+ channels opening

·7. A 48-year-old man presents to the emergency department 1.5 hours after the onset of severe substernal chest pain radiating to his left arm. The pain is accompanied by diaphoresis and shortness of breath. His blood pressure is 165/94 mm Hg, pulse is 82/min, and respiratory rate is 18/min. Which of the following tests is the most important tool in the initial evaluation of patients in whom acute myocardial infarction (MI) is suspected?

(A) Aspartate aminotransferase
(B) Creatine kinase-myocardial bound
(C) ECG
(D) Echocardiogram
(E) Lactate dehydrogenase

8. This image depicts the administration of drug X, which produces an increase in systolic, diastolic, and mean arterial pressure. Drug Y is then added, resulting in little or no change to the blood pressure. Drug X is then readministered, causing a net decrease in blood pressure. Which of the following drug combinations are drug X and drug Y, respectively?

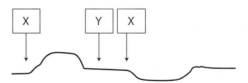

Reproduced, with permission, from USMLERx.com.

(A) Epinephrine, phentolamine
(B) Isoproterenol, clonidine
(C) Norepinephrine, propranolol
(D) Phenylephrine, metoprolol
(E) Phenylephrine, phentolamine

9. A 56-year-old woman arrives in the emergency department complaining of dizziness and headache. Her blood pressure is 210/140 mm Hg. She is currently not taking any medications and has not seen a doctor for several years. The physician decides to address her hypertension urgently. Which of the following drugs is contraindicated in this patient?

(A) Intravenous diltiazem
(B) Intravenous labetalol
(C) Intravenous metoprolol
(D) Oral captopril
(E) Sublingual nifedipine

10. A 65-year-old man presents to the emergency department with chest pain that he noticed after climbing a set of stairs. The emergency physician sends him for an exercise stress test. Which of the following physiologic mechanisms does the heart use to deal with increased work demand during an exercise stress test?

(A) Decreased coronary artery diameter
(B) Decreased metabolite production
(C) Decreased oxygen extraction
(D) Increased coronary blood flow
(E) Increased oxygen extraction

11. A 16-year-old Japanese exchange student presents to the physician with a history of fevers, joint pain, night sweats, and muscle pain. On physical examination, the patient has extremely weak pulses in her upper extremities. Laboratory abnormalities in which of the following parameters is most likely?

(A) Anti-IgG antibodies
(B) Antinuclear antibodies
(C) Cytoplasmic antineutrophil cytoplasmic antibody
(D) Erythrocyte sedimentation rate
(E) Perinuclear antineutrophil cytoplasmic antibody

12. A 72-year-old African-American man undergoes hip surgery. On his third hospital day he experiences chest pain, tachycardia, dyspnea, and a low-grade fever. The man goes into cardiac arrest, and efforts to resuscitate him are unsuccessful. On autopsy a massive pulmonary embolus is discovered. Which of the following, if present, would most likely predispose the patient to this event?

(A) Factor VIII deficiency
(B) Low serum homocysteine levels
(C) Mutation in the Factor V gene
(D) Overproduction of protein C
(E) von Willebrand factor deficiency

13. A 70-year-old woman with a history of type 2 diabetes mellitus, a body mass index of 30 kg/m^2, and an MI 10 years prior presents to the emergency department with crushing substernal chest pain radiating to her neck and jaw. Emergency cardiac catheterization with percutaneous coronary intervention (PCI) shows a 99% occlusion of her left anterior descending artery, and an ECG reveals an anterior wall ST segment elevation MI. The patient remains stable after PCI, and echocardiography shows a mildly impaired ejection fraction (EF) of 45%. Three days later, the patient becomes acutely hypotensive and dyspneic, and physical examination reveals a high-pitched holosystolic murmur, loudest at the apex and radiating to the axilla, that had not been heard on previous exams. An emergency echocardiogram shows an EF of 25%. This patient has developed which of the following?

(A) Aortic stenosis
(B) Dressler's syndrome
(C) Ruptured interventricular septum
(D) Ruptured left ventricular free wall
(E) Ruptured papillary muscle
(F) Ventricular aneurysm

14. A 67-year-old woman presents to the emergency department with dizziness, syncope, and palpitations. She states she is taking a medication for "heart troubles" but cannot remember its name. Results of an ECG are shown in the image. Which of this patient's current medications might have caused this abnormal ECG pattern?

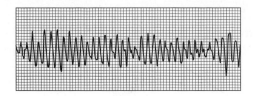

Reproduced, with permission, from USMLERx.com.

(A) Adenosine
(B) Bretylium
(C) Propranolol
(D) Quinidine
(E) Verapamil

15. A 35-year-old man with no significant medical history presents to his primary care physician with a 2-week history of progressive shortness of breath that occurs with activity. He previously exercised regularly and has never had symptoms like this before, but now he finds that he can walk only one block before becoming symptomatic. He has also noticed a 7-lb (3.2-kg) weight gain during this time. He does not smoke or use alcohol or illicit drugs and has not traveled recently. In addition, he has no family history of cardiac disease and does not have any sick contacts, but recalls having an upper respiratory infection about a month ago that improved on its own. Physical examination reveals crackles in his lungs bilaterally and an S3 gallop. X-ray of the chest reveals cardiomegaly. What is the most likely mechanism causing this patient's heart failure?

(A) Antibodies to a variety of cardiac proteins that cause immune-mediated damage to myocytes
(B) Direct cytotoxicity via receptor-mediated entry of virus into cardiac myocytes
(C) Granulomatous inflammation of myocytes
(D) Hyperadrenergic state leading to dilated cardiomyopathy
(E) Ischemic damage to cardiac myocytes

16. A 25-year-old pregnant woman goes to her gynecologist for her 36-week checkup. She complains of light-headedness when she goes to bed at night. In the office, her blood pressure is 120/70 mm Hg while sitting upright and 90/50 mm Hg while lying supine. Which of the following is the most likely cause of this hypotension?

(A) Cardiogenic shock
(B) Inferior vena cava compression
(C) Neurogenic shock
(D) Third spacing of fluid
(E) Vasodilation

17. A 48-year-old obese man presents to his primary care physician with complaints of lower leg pain that occurs after he walks a few city blocks and is relieved with rest. He has no other complaints. His blood pressure is 165/85 mm Hg, his pulse is 83/min, and his respiratory rate is 18/min. After further questioning, he admits to smoking two packs of cigarettes per day. Which of the following types of vessels is most likely involved in the pathologic process surrounding this patient's symptoms?

(A) Arteries
(B) Arterioles
(C) Capillaries
(D) Veins
(E) Venules

18. Jugular venous pressure (JVP) curves are designed to show the pressure changes that normally take place in the right atrium throughout the cardiac cycle. A JVP curve consists of two, or sometimes three, positive waves and two negative troughs. A normal JVP curve is shown in the image. Which of the following points on the normal jugular venous tracing in the image would be most prominently affected in tricuspid regurgitation?

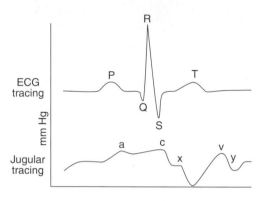

Reproduced, with permission, from USMLERx.com.

(A) A and C
(B) A and Y
(C) C and X
(D) V and Y

19. A 62-year-old breast cancer survivor visits her physician because of <u>weakness</u>, <u>fatigue</u>, <u>fever</u>, and weight gain 5 years following her radiation therapy. The physician also elicits complaints about abdominal discomfort and exertional dyspnea. Physical examination reveals hepatomegaly and jugular venous distention that fails to subside on inspiration, but shows no evidence of hypotension or pulsus paradoxus. An echocardiogram shows reduced end-diastolic volumes and elevated diastolic pressures in both ventricles. Which of the following is the most likely diagnosis?

(A) Cardiac tamponade
(B) Congestive heart failure
(C) Constrictive pericarditis
(D) Dilated cardiomyopathy
(E) Recurrence of breast cancer

20. The classic location for an abdominal aortic aneurysm is inferior to the renal arteries and extending to the bifurcation of the common iliac arteries. Repair involves resecting the diseased portion of the aorta and replacing it with a synthetic graft. Based on anatomic considerations, which of the following visceral arteries would likely be resected along with the diseased aortic tissue during the repair of an infrarenal abdominal aortic aneurysm?

(A) Gastroduodenal artery
(B) Hepatic artery
(C) Inferior mesenteric artery
(D) Left gastric artery
(E) Splenic artery
(F) Superior mesenteric artery

21. A 52-year-old African-American man is brought to the emergency department unresponsive, and efforts to resuscitate him are unsuccessful. On autopsy, it is found that he suffered from a ruptured aneurysm of the aortic root. His dilated aorta, as seen on autopsy, is shown in the image. In addition, inspection of the man's skin revealed several ulcerated lesions. Which of the following is most likely associated with the underlying etiology of this patient's aneurysm?

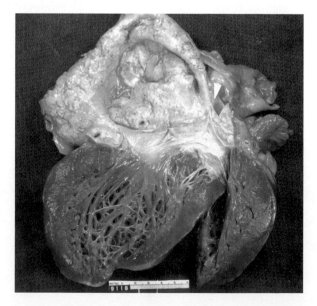

Reproduced, with permission, from PEIR Digital Library (http://peir.net).

(A) Atherosclerosis
(B) Congenital medial weakness
(C) Cystic medial necrosis
(D) Disruption of the vasa vasorum
(E) Hypertension

22. A baby is observed at birth to be noncyanotic. The mother is known to have been infected with rubella during the pregnancy. On physical examination the patient is found to have a continuous murmur that is present in both systole and diastole. A nonsteroidal anti-inflammatory drug is prescribed, and on follow-up the murmur has disappeared. Which of the following is the most likely congenital lesion?

(A) Patent ductus arteriosus
(B) Tetralogy of Fallot
(C) Transposition of the great vessels
(D) Truncus arteriosus
(E) Ventricular septal defect

23. A 25-year-old white woman with no past medical history presents to the emergency department for "a racing heartbeat." It is determined that she has paroxysmal supraventricular tachycardia. Which of the following is the drug of choice used for diagnosing and abolishing atrioventricular nodal arrhythmias by virtue of its effectiveness and its low toxicity?

(A) Adenosine
(B) Bretylium
(C) Encainide
(D) Lidocaine
(E) Sotalol

24. A 62-year-old man was admitted to the intensive care unit for overwhelming sepsis. The patient has received 4 L of normal saline bolus fluids. Empirical antibiotics were begun with no improvement in his condition. His blood pressure is 60/30 mm Hg, pulse is 112/min, temperature is 40.6° C (105° F), and respiratory rate is 23/min. The physician orders intravenous norepinephrine. Which of the following is a direct effect of norepinephrine in this clinical scenario?

(A) Bradycardia
(B) Bronchoconstriction
(C) Coronary vasodilation
(D) Decreased inotropy
(E) Periphearl vasodilation

25. An 85-year-old man dies from aspiration pneumonia as a complication of Alzheimer's disease. Autopsy reveals a small (230-g) heart that appears grossly dark brown in color. Hematoxylin and eosin staining of cardiac muscle cells reveals brownish perinuclear pigmentation. The pathologist determines this phenomenon to be a consequence of age and not a causative agent in the patient's death. Accumulation of which of the following substances is the most likely cause of the brown pigmentation seen most often in the heart, liver, or spleen of the elderly?

(A) Bilirubin
(B) Calcium
(C) Cholesterol
(D) Glycogen
(E) Iron
(F) Lipofuscin

26. A 72-year-old woman has a 1-month history of left-sided jaw pain when chewing food, headache, fever, and fatigue. Laboratory studies reveal an elevated erythrocyte sedimentation rate. Which of the following arteries is most likely involved?

(A) External carotid artery
(B) Facial artery
(C) Ophthalmic artery
(D) Postauricular artery
(E) Superficial temporal artery

27. A 67-year-old woman with a long history of poorly controlled diabetes mellitus and chronic renal failure is admitted to the hospital for treatment of cellulitis. Two days into her hospital stay she complains of chest pain that is relieved when she leans forward. An ECG shows diffuse ST segment elevations with PR depressions; her echocardiogram is normal. Which of the following is the most appropriate treatment at this time?

(A) Cardiac catheterization
(B) Dialysis
(C) Nonsteroidal anti-inflammatory drugs
(D) Pericardiocentesis
(E) Switch her to another antibiotic regimen

28. A 75-year-old woman arrives at the emergency department and states that her left arm is numb. She is diaphoretic. Laboratory studies show an elevated troponin I level and the patient is treated for an acute MI. A subsequent echocardiogram shows a wall motion abnormality of the posterior interventricular septum. Stenosis of which of the following arteries would most likely cause this condition?

(A) Acute marginal artery
(B) Circumflex artery
(C) Left anterior descending artery
(D) Posterior descending artery
(E) Right coronary artery

29. A 24-year-old man presents to the emergency department with a fever, chills, night sweats, malaise, and fatigue that started 3 days ago. In the past day he has also become short of breath. He admits to using intravenous drugs regularly. At presentation, the patient is shaking and appears pale. Physical examination is remarkable for a temperature of 39.4° C (103° F), hypoxia to 88% on room air, jugular venous distention, bilaterally decreased breath sounds at the bases with dullness to percussion at the bases, and a grade III/VI systolic murmur heard best at the lower left sternal border. The patient states that he never had anything wrong with his heart before. Which pathogen is most likely responsible for this patient's condition?

(A) *Enterococcus faecalis*
(B) *Haemophilus aphrophilus*
(C) *Staphylococcus aureus*
(D) *Streptococcus bovis*
(E) *Viridans* streptococci

30. Drugs such as cholestyramine and colestipol have been shown to decrease circulating serum LDL cholesterol and to slightly elevate triglycerides. These drugs work by which of the following mechanisms?

(A) Binding and excretion of bile-soluble lipids
(B) Decreased peripheral lipolysis
(C) Increased lipoprotein lipase activity
(D) Inhibition of cholesterol absorption at the small intestine brush border
(E) Inhibition of the rate-limiting enzyme of cholesterol formation
(F) Retention of bile acid resins in hepatocytes

31. A 30-year-old patient comes to an ophthalmologist with complaints of decreased vision. On examination, angiomatous lesions are visible in the retina. The patient also has documented cerebellar and spinal hemangioblastomas, bilateral renal cysts, and pancreatic microcystic adenomas. A previous chromosomal analysis on this patient showed a deleted tumor suppressor gene. A detailed family history shows similar problems in the patient's brother, father, aunt, and grandfather. Which of the following is the inheritance pattern of this patient's disease?

(A) Autosomal dominant
(B) Autosomal recessive
(C) Mitochondrial
(D) Spontaneous
(E) X-linked recessive

32. A 25-year-old Massachusetts college student presents to his primary care physician. He said he first started to notice problems a few months ago after returning from a hike in the woods. He originally had an expanding rash starting on his calf and flu-like symptoms that resolved spontaneously. Recently, he started having symptoms of dizziness, syncope, dyspnea, chest

pain, and palpitations for several weeks' duration. His physician obtains an ECG, as shown in the image. The vector that carries the organism responsible for the student's symptoms is also responsible for transmitting which of the following diseases?

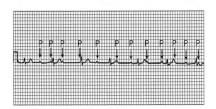

Reproduced, with permission, from USMLERx.com.

(A) Babesiosis
(B) Epidemic typhus
(C) Malaria
(D) Plague
(E) Rocky Mountain spotted fever

33. A 57-year-old white man presents to his primary care physician with dyspnea. He says that he likes to maintain his yard and garden, but that he has recently had trouble doing the work, and becomes short of breath even walking up the one flight of stairs in his house. On further questioning, he says that sometimes he wakes up short of breath in the middle of the night. Physical examination demonstrates pitting ankle edema. Which of the following findings would also be expected in this patient?

(A) Decreased sympathetic outflow
(B) Decreased venous pressure
(C) Increased aldosterone secretion
(D) Increased effective arterial blood volume
(E) Increased glomerular filtration rate

34. A number of tests are used to diagnose an MI. Measuring an elevation in the cardiac enzymes

aspartate aminotransferase (AST), creatine kinase-MB fraction (CK-MB), lactate dehydrogenase (LDH), and troponin is one indication that a MI has occurred. The image shown is a representation of the average length of time it takes to see an elevation in these four enzymes. What is the correct order of cardiac enzyme elevation after an MI?

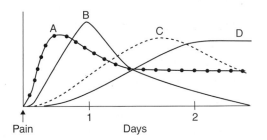

Reproduced, with permission, from USMLERx.com.

(A) AST, CK-MB, troponin, LDH
(B) AST, LDH, troponin, CK-MB
(C) CK-MB, AST, troponin, LDH
(D) CK-MB, troponin, AST, LDH
(E) LDH, CK-MB, troponin, AST
(F) Troponin, AST, CK-MB, LDH
(G) Troponin, CK-MB, AST, LDH

35. A 73-year-old man with a history of hypertension and type 2 diabetes mellitus presents with the sudden onset of right-sided paralysis. An ultrasound study shows significant atherosclerosis in a major artery that is embryologically derived from one of the aortic arches. The artery that is most likely involved in this patient's paralysis is derived from which of the following aortic arches?

(A) First aortic arch
(B) Second aortic arch
(C) Third aortic arch
(D) Fourth aortic arch
(E) Sixth aortic arch

36. A 76-year-old woman visits the emergency department complaining of increased fatigue. She states that she tires easily even with very low levels of activity. Her temperature is 36.7° C (98.1° F), heart rate is 123 beats/min, and blood pressure is 85/43 mm Hg. The woman has a history of coronary artery disease and diabetes. She also notes a recent traumatic episode when her grandson kicked her in the chest when she was picking him up. On physical examination, her doctor notices a disappearing arterial pulse on inspiration. The doctor orders an echocardiogram to confirm the diagnosis. What invasive procedure will be necessary to treat this patient?

(A) Angioplasty
(B) Aortic valve replacement
(C) Mitral valve replacement
(D) Pericardiocentesis
(E) Surgical reduction of an aortic aneurysm

37. A 60-year-old woman dies in a car accident. On autopsy, the cause of death is determined to be a massive brain hemorrhage due to a skull fracture. An additional abnormality, shown below in the image of the opened left atrium, is also found and determined to be unrelated to the cause of death. This abnormality could have led to which of the following physical examination findings when the woman was alive?

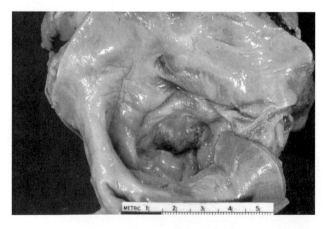

Reproduced, with permission, from PEIR Digital Library (http://peir.net).

(A) Continuous murmur throughout both diastole and systole, loudest at the end of ventricular systole
(B) Decrescendo murmur in early ventricular diastole
(C) Sharp, high-pitched sound in early ventricular diastole, followed by a decrescendo, crescendo murmur
(D) Sharp, high-pitched sound in early ventricular systole, followed by a crescendo, decrescendo murmur
(E) Sharp, high-pitched sound in mid ventricular systole, followed by a uniform murmur

38. A 3-year-old boy comes to the pediatrician with fever, conjunctivitis, erythema in the oral mucosa, and cervical lymphadenopathy. The boy suddenly becomes hypotensive and goes into cardiac arrest and dies shortly thereafter. Autopsy shows aneurysmal dilations of the left circumflex and right coronary arteries. The boy's disease is characterized as a self-limiting disease that most commonly affects the coronary arteries. Which of the following diseases is the correct diagnosis?

(A) Buerger's disease
(B) Kawasaki's disease
(C) Polyarteritis nodosa
(D) Takayasu's arteritis
(E) Wegener's granulomatosis

39. A 54-year-old woman comes to the physician 3 months after a undergoing a root canal because of persistent general malaise and fever. The symptoms developed slowly over the weeks following her root canal, but have not abated. On physical examination, the patient is found to have a temperature of 38.3° C (101° F). Ophthalmic examination reveals retinal hemorrhages with clear central regions. Examination of the extremities reveals painful red nodules on her digits and dark macules on her palms and soles. On cardiac examination, a click and a systolic murmur are auscultated over the mitral valve. She tells the physician that the click is due to a mechanical valve replacement done 4 years ago due to rheu-

matic fever as a child. Given this history, which of the following is the most appropriate treatment for this patient?

(A) Caspofungin
(B) Clindamycin
(C) Mebendazole
(D) Metronidazole
(E) Nafcillin
(F) Penicillin
(G) Pentamidine

40. A 67-year-old woman who has recently begun to take a new antihypertensive medication presents to her primary care physician with complaints of new-onset fatigue and depressed mood. Her physical examination is unremarkable except for a heart rate of 56/min. Laboratory tests show:

Na$^+$: 137 mEq/L
K$^+$: 4.0 mEq/L
Blood urea nitrogen: 12 mg/dL
Creatinine: 0.5 mg/dL
Glucose: 82 mg/dL

Which of the following is most likely the new medication that this patient has started?

(A) Furosemide
(B) Hydrochlorothiazide
(C) Losartan
(D) Metoprolol
(E) Nifedipine
(F) Prazosin

41. A dysfunctional myocardial endothelium underlies one form of heart disease. In patients with this common disease process, there is a lack of autoregulatory coronary artery vasodilation needed to provide increased blood flow in states of increased physical exertion or emotional stress. The pathogenesis is most often from severe narrowing of atherosclerotic coronary vessels and typically manifests as chest pain, relieved by rest or nitroglycerin tablets. Which of the following is a soluble metabolite

that mediates the compensatory coronary artery vasodilation during periods of increased myocardial oxygen demand?

(A) Acetylcholine
(B) Adenosine
(C) Carbon dioxide
(D) Lactate
(E) Norepinephrine

42. The image depicts the relationship of ventricular pressure and volume in the cardiac cycle. The various phases of the cardiac cycle are labeled I through IV. Which phase occurs between aortic valve closing and mitral valve opening?

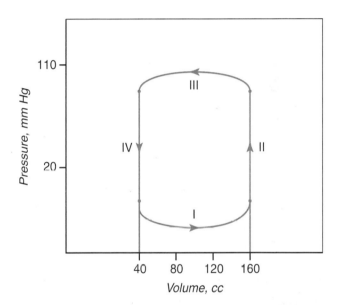

Reproduced, with permission, from USMLERx.com.

(A) Phase I
(B) Phase II
(C) Phase III
(D) Phase IV

43. A 32-year-old man with diabetes presents to his physician with orthostatic hypotension. This suggests a deficiency in the normal physiologic response carried out by arterial baroreceptors located in the aortic arch and the carotid sinus. What is the normal physiologic response to hypotension?

(A) Decreased baroreceptor afferent firing in the aortic arch leads to increased sympathetic efferent firing

(B) Decreased baroreceptor afferent firing in the carotid sinus leads to increased parasympathetic efferent firing

(C) Decreased baroreceptor afferent firing in the carotid sinus leads to increased sympathetic efferent firing

(D) Increased baroreceptor afferent firing in the aortic arch leads to increased parasympathetic efferent firing

(E) Increased baroreceptor afferent firing in the carotid sinus leads to increased parasympathetic efferent firing

44. A 56-year-old woman presents to her physician because of recent onset of chest pain and dyspnea. Six weeks earlier the patient suffered an MI. Her physical examination is remarkable for a friction rub over the fifth intercostal space in the midclavicular line together with an elevated jugular venous pressure. Which of the following myocardial complications is this individual most likely suffering from?

(A) Cardiac arrhythmia

(B) Dressler's syndrome

(C) Left ventricular failure

(D) Thromboembolism

(E) Ventricular rupture

45. A patient presents for treatment of his severe essential hypertension. He is being treated with numerous medications for high blood pressure, and hydralazine was recently added to his medication regimen. He explains that he has been experiencing flushing and headaches since his last visit, when hydralazine therapy was started. Which of the following is an adverse effect of hydralazine?

(A) Angina

(B) Cardiotoxicity

(C) First-dose orthostatic hypotension

(D) Nephrotoxicity

(E) Pulmonary embolism

46. A 76-year-old man receives a pacemaker to treat a dangerous form of heart block. This form of heart block is characterized by a constant PR interval with randomly blocked QRS complexes. The patient's ECG prior to treatment is shown in the image. Which of the following is the abnormality responsible for this type of heart block?

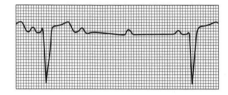

Reproduced, with permission, from USMLERx.com.

(A) Atrioventricular nodal abnormality

(B) Defect in the His-Purkinje system

(C) Independently contracting atria and ventricles

(D) Retrograde conduction

(E) Sinoatrial nodal abnormality

47. A 56-year-old white man is rushed to the emergency department with crushing substernal chest pain. He is morbidly obese, sweating profusely, breathing very rapidly, and clutching at his chest. The patient is stabilized and seems to be doing well when he suddenly goes into cardiac arrest and dies. Which of the following is the most likely cause of death in this patient?

(A) Fatal arrhythmia

(B) Mural thrombosis

(C) Myocardial failure

(D) Myocardial rupture

(E) Ruptured papillary muscle

48. A previously healthy 31-year-old woman is seen in the emergency department because of complete visual loss in her right eye. The patient's history is significant for a 3-day history of malaise, chills, and fatigue and some oral pain secondary to her recent wisdom tooth removal. Ophthalmologic examination reveals a graywhite retina with an associated cherry-red spot, two blot hemorrhages, and several segmented vessels with optic edema. Physical examination reveals a murmur consistent with mitral valve insufficiency. Which of the following is the most likely cause of this patient's loss of vision?

(A) Carotid artery stenosis
(B) Collagen vascular disease
(C) Diabetes mellitus
(D) Endocarditis
(E) Hypertensive crisis

49. Cardiac output is a function of stroke volume and heart rate. Stroke volume increases when contractility increases, preload increases, or afterload decreases. There are a number of factors that affect each of these components and ultimately cardiac output. Which of the following variations would increase cardiac output?

(A) β-Blocker treatment
(B) Aortic stenosis
(C) Cardiac glycoside administration
(D) Decreased intracellular calcium concentration
(E) Increased extracellular sodium concentration

50. A 54-year-old woman presents to her physician with swelling in her extremities. Palpation produces significant pitting. Which of the following conditions is the underlying physiologic basis of this physical finding?

(A) Decreased capillary permeability
(B) Decreased capillary pressure
(C) Increased interstitial fluid colloid osmotic pressure
(D) Increased interstitial fluid pressure
(E) Increased plasma protein levels

1. **The correct answer is E.** The calcium channel blockers verapamil and diltiazem are both effective in slowing the rate and contractility of the heart. Both drugs decrease the magnitude of inward calcium current through L type calcium channels and also decrease the rate of recovery of the channel. It is this latter effect that depresses the sinus node pacemaker and slows atrioventricular conduction. Verapamil is a stronger negative inotrope than diltiazem, and therefore is more effective in decreasing heart rate and contractility.

Answer A is incorrect. Dihydropyridines are the family of drugs to which nifedipine belongs. The dihydropyridines are more potent vasodilators than verapamil or diltiazem and in general have less potent effects on the heart.

Answer B is incorrect. Diltiazem is a calcium channel blocker but is not as effective as verapamil in reducing the rate and contractility of the heart.

Answer C is incorrect. Nifedipine is least effective in reducing the rate and contractility of the heart; conversely, it is most effective in evoking vasodilation. Although nifedipine has some negative inotropic effect on the heart, the decrease in arterial blood pressure secondary to vasodilation elicits sympathetic reflexes that result in increases in heart rate and inotropy.

Answer D is incorrect. Nimodipine is another member of the dihydropyridine family with similar properties, but it is approved only for the management of stroke with subarachnoid hemorrhage.

2. **The correct answer is C.** This individual is likely suffering from polyarteritis nodosa (PAN), which is characterized by necrotizing immune complex inflammation of small or medium-sized arteries. PAN is typically associated with fever, malaise, weight loss, abdominal pain, headache, myalgias, and hypertension. There are no diagnostic serologic tests specific for PAN. Patients with classic PAN are ANCA-negative and may have low titers of rheumatoid factor or antinuclear antibodies, both of which are nonspecific findings. In patients with PAN, appropriate serologic tests for active hepatitis B infection must be performed as up to 30% of patients with PAN are positive for hepatitis B surface antigen. Histologically, the intense inflammatory infiltrate in the arterial wall and surrounding connective tissue is associated with fibrinoid necrosis and disruption of the vessel wall.

Answer A is incorrect. Caseating necrosis is associated with tuberculosis infections. The granuloma of tuberculosis is referred to as a tubercle, and is characterized by central caseous necrosis and often by Langhans' giant cells. These lesions often coalesce and rupture into bronchi. The caseous contents may liquefy and be expelled, resulting in cavitary lesions.

Answer B is incorrect. Eosinophilic infiltrate is a more prominent feature in Churg-Strauss syndrome, a necrotizing vasculitis of small and medium-sized muscular arteries, capillaries, veins, and venules. Patients with Churg-Strauss syndrome often present with severe asthma attacks, pulmonary infiltrates, and mononeuritis multiplex, along with nonspecific symptoms such as weight loss, fever, malaise, and anorexia.

Answer D is incorrect. Granulomatous infiltrate is a more prominent feature in giant cell arteritis (also known as temporal arteritis), an inflammatory disease of medium and large-sized arteries. Patients with giant cell arteritis are usually >50 years old and present most commonly with fever, anemia, high erythrocyte sedimentation rate, and headaches.

Answer E is incorrect. Langhans' giant cells are associated with Wegener's granulomatosis, a granulomatous vasculitis of the upper and lower respiratory tracts together with glomerulonephritis. Many cases are associated with circulating anti-neutrophil cytoplasmic antibodies (C-ANCAs).

Answer F is incorrect. Onion skinning, seen in arteriolosclerosis, is the type of arteriosclerosis associated with malignant hypertension. Even though this patient meets the definition of being hypertensive, his blood pressure is not high enough to cause this pathology. Also, his physical exam consisting of palpable purpura and past medical history of hepatitis B point toward a different etiology, in this case, polyarteritis nodosa.

3. **The correct answer is A.** 3-Hydroxy-3-methylglutaryl coenzyme A reductase (HMG-CoA reductase) catalyzes the rate-limiting step in the synthesis of cholesterol. The enzyme converts 3-hydroxy-3-methylglutaryl coenzyme A (HMG-CoA) to mevalonic acid, a cholesterol precursor. Statins competitively inhibit HMGR by obstructing part of the enzyme's active site and preventing sufficient interaction with HMG-CoA to produce mevalonate. The consequent decrease in intrahepatic cholesterol causes up-regulation of hepatic LDL cholesterol receptors, ultimately lowering plasma LDL cholesterol levels. Diabetes mellitus is considered a cardiac heart disease equivalent, and by the ATP III recommendations, the target LDL cholesterol of a diabetic patient is <100 mg/dL, with pharmacotherapy initiated at levels >130 mg/dL.

Answer B is incorrect. HMG-CoA synthase is the enzyme that combines acetoacetyl-coenzyme A with acetyl-coenzyme A to form HMG-CoA. This is a preliminary step in cholesterol synthesis. It is not the site of action of statins.

Answer C is incorrect. Thiolase is an enzyme in the cholesterol synthesis pathway. It is responsible for combining two molecules of acetyl-coenzyme A to form acetoacetyl-coenzyme A. Statins do not affect thiolase activity.

Answer D is incorrect. Citrate synthase is the first enzyme of the Krebs cycle, which combines oxaloacetate with incoming acetyl-coenzyme A to form citrate. It is not involved in cholesterol synthesis and is not affected by statins.

Answer E is incorrect. HMG-CoA lyase is the enzyme that cleaves HMG-CoA into acetoacetate and acetyl-coenzyme A. It is involved in the breakdown of cholesterol, not the synthesis, and thus is unaffected by statins.

4. **The correct answer is D.** The key to answering this question is realizing that it asks for electrolyte levels in urine, not serum. The ECG shows peak T waves and widened QRS interval, which are classic changes seen in hyperkalemia. Spironolactone is the most likely medication to affect urinary electrolytes. As an inhibitor of aldosterone receptors in the collecting tubule and an inhibitor of Na^+ channels, spironolactone greatly decreases the excretion of K^+ and mildly increases the excretion of Na^+. Urine volume will be high-normal because the diuretic will increase saltwater wasting.

Answer A is incorrect. Spironolactone decreases K^+ excretion, so there will be decreased levels of K^+ in the urine sample.

Answer B is incorrect. Na^+ excretion will be increased with the use of spironolactone; also, diuretics will increase the amount of urine volume excreted.

Answer C is incorrect. Spironolactone will increase Na^+ excretion and decrease K^+ excretion so that K^+ concentrations will be decreased in the urine and Na^+ concentrations will be increased.

Answer E is incorrect. Spironolactone decreases K^+ excretion but increases Na^+ excretion; therefore, Na^+ concentrations will be elevated in the urine.

5. **The correct answer is C.** Tetralogy of Fallot is the most common cause of cyanosis within the first few weeks of life. The skin becomes bluish because of the malformed right-to-left shunt. Infants also have worsening cyanosis with agitation, difficulty feeding, and failure to gain weight. Patients may also have clubbing of the fingers and toes or even polycythemia. The four components of the teratology are (1) ventricular septal defect, (2) overriding aorta, (3) infundibular pulmonary stenosis, and (4) right ventricular hypertrophy.

Answer A is incorrect. Atrial septal defects typically are not clinically apparent until adulthood, when a patient experiences Eisenmenger's syndrome, a reversal of blood flow caused by pulmonary hypertension.

Answer B is incorrect. Patent ductus arteriosus typically is not clinically apparent until adulthood, when a patient experiences Eisenmenger's syndrome, a reversal of blood flow caused by pulmonary hypertension.

Answer D is incorrect. Transposition of the great vessels is a condition that leads to early cyanosis, but it is not as common as tetralogy of Fallot.

Answer E is incorrect. Ventricular septal defects (VSDs) are the most common cardiac congenital defects, but they do not present with early cyanosis. Infants with larger VSDs present with tachypnea, dyspnea, and feeding difficulties. In addition, they have other signs of breathing difficulties such as subcostal or intercostals retractions and a hyperdynamic precordium (brisk, quick movement of the thorax). A holosystolic murmur may be heard on auscultation.

6. **The correct answer is C.** Voltage-gated Ca^{2+} channels open slowly in response to the Na^+ upstroke as increasing K^+ conductance during phase 2 gradually depolarizes the cell. The result is a slow conduction velocity that prolongs the transmission from the atria to the ventricles.

Answer A is incorrect. Ion channels in the myocardium are voltage-gated.

Answer B is incorrect. Ion channels in the myocardium are voltage-gated.

Answer D is incorrect. Closing voltage-gated Na^+ channels would hyperpolarize the cell.

Answer E is incorrect. Nodal cells lack the voltage-gated Na^+ channels that are responsible for the upstroke in ventricular cells.

7. **The correct answer is C.** ECG is the gold standard for diagnosing MI within the first 6 hours of symptom onset. ECG changes will include ST-segment elevation (signifying transmural infarct), ST-segment depression (signifying subendocardial infarct), and Q waves (signifying transmural infarct).

Answer A is incorrect. Aspartate aminotransferase is a nonspecific protein that is found in cardiac, liver, and skeletal muscle cells. Levels peak around 2 days post-MI and are negative at 3 days post-MI.

Answer B is incorrect. Serial measurements of creatine kinase-myocardial bound (CK-MB) fraction along with troponin-I are made in every patient with suspected MI. However, since these enzymes take 4–6 hours to accumulate in the blood, and ECG results can be obtained faster, ECG is the initial test when triaging a patient with suspected MI. CK-MB levels peak around 24 hours and are negative at 3 days post-MI.

Answer D is incorrect. Echocardiography may indeed play an important role in the setting of MI but would not be the most cost- and time-efficient means of diagnosis. Echocardiograms are often ordered later in the work-up of MI to define the extent of infarction and assess the overall left ventricle and right ventricle function. Echocardiograms can also be useful in identifying complications of MI such as acute mitral regurgitation, left ventricular rupture, or pericardial effusion.

Answer E is incorrect. Lactate dehydrogenase was once the test of the choice for diagnosing MI. An increase in the blood concentration of LDH-1 (found in heart tissues) to a level greater than LDH-2 (found in the reticuloendothelial system) is highly suggestive of MI. The "flipped LDH" generally appears within 12–24 hours. LDH levels are elevated 2–7 days post-MI and peak around 3 days post-MI.

8. **The correct answer is A.** Epinephrine is a nonselective agonist of α and β adrenergic receptors. Administering a large dose of epinephrine causes an increase in blood pressure via an increased heart rate and contractility through stimulation of β_1 receptors (the β_2 effect is minimal) and increased systemic vascular resis-

tance through α_1-mediated vasoconstriction. Adding phentolamine blocks the α effects of epinephrine so readministration leaves only the β_1 receptor actions (increased contractility and heart rate) and the β_2-mediated increase in vasodilation, causing a net decrease in blood pressure.

Answer B is incorrect. Isoproterenol is an agonist of β and α adrenergic receptors, although its primary action is at the β receptor. Hence, adding isoproterenol would actually cause a decrease in pressure through β_2-mediated vasodilation. Clonidine is an α agonist at the α_2 receptor and would lead to decreased sympathetic outflow and possibly cause an additional decrease in pressure. Adding isoproterenol would lead to a further decrease in pressure.

Answer C is incorrect. Norepinephrine is an agonist at the β and α adrenergic receptors. It has a more potent α effect than β effect, leading to an increase in vasoconstriction through α_1 stimulation. Propranolol is a β-blocker, which would not block the effects of norepinephrine; readministration would cause an increase in pressure.

Answer D is incorrect. Phenylephrine is an α agonist that would cause an increase in pressure through α_1-stimulated vasoconstriction. Metoprolol is a β-blocker, which would not inhibit the effects of phenylephrine. Therefore, readministration of phenylephrine would cause another increase in pressure.

Answer E is incorrect. Phenylephrine is an α agonist, which would result in an increase in pressure through α_1-stimulated vasoconstriction. Phentolamine is a nonselective α blocker, which would block the increase in pressure caused by phenylephrine and cause no change in pressure.

9. **The correct answer is E.** Nifedipine is a dihydropyridine class calcium channel blocker that could be used in the long-term control of hypertension. However, in the case of a hypertensive emergency, nifedipine used sublingually can cause dangerous fluctuations in blood pressure that are difficult to control and can lead to more harm than good.

Answer A is incorrect. Diltiazem is a benzothiazepine class calcium channel blocker that reduces myocardial demand and also causes vasodilation. It is not contraindicated in this patient.

Answer B is incorrect. Labetalol is a combined α/β-blocker that has effects on both receptors. It can be used in a hypertensive situation as an emergent option for treatment. It is not contraindicated in this patient.

Answer C is incorrect. Metoprolol is a β-blocker used to treat angina by reducing heart rate and contractility. It also reduces the metabolic demand of the myocardium. It is often used to control hypertension, but is not contraindicated in this patient.

Answer D is incorrect. Captopril is an angiotensin-converting enzyme inhibitor used in the control of chronic hypertension. It is especially useful for patients who have signs of renal disease and can slow the progression of damage to the kidneys. It is not contraindicated in this patient.

10. **The correct answer is D.** An increase in myocardial contractility due to exercise leads to increased oxygen demand by the cardiac muscle and increased oxygen consumption, causing local hypoxia. This local hypoxia causes vasodilation of the coronary arterioles, which then produces a compensatory increase in coronary blood flow and oxygen delivery to meet the demands of the cardiac muscle. Oxygen extraction from heart muscle is maximized. Increased demand can be met only by increasing blood flow.

Answer A is incorrect. A decrease in the diameter of the coronary arteries (e.g., coronary artery constriction) will decrease, rather than increase, coronary blood flow and delivery of oxygen to the myocardium.

Answer B is incorrect. Blood flow through the coronary circulation is controlled almost entirely by local metabolites, with sympathetic innervation playing only a minor role. The most important local metabolic factors are hypoxia (decreased oxygen) and adenosine. During periods of exercise and increased contractility of the heart, the production of the metabolic factor adenosine would increase and oxygen levels would decrease.

Answer C is incorrect. The heart cannot increase or decrease its oxygen extraction. Even if this were the primary means of supplying the extra demand for oxygen, the heart would respond by increasing oxygen extraction, not decreasing.

Answer E is incorrect. Compared to most organs of the body, oxygen extraction of the heart is relatively high. It extracts optimal levels of oxygen at rest and therefore relies on increased coronary blood flow by vasodilation for further increases in oxygen supply. It does not have the ability to further increase its oxygen supply through extraction.

11. **The correct answer is D.** This individual is most likely suffering from Takayasu's arteritis, which is also known as "pulseless disease." It typically affects medium and large arteries, resulting in thickening of the aortic arch and/or proximal great vessels. Symptoms include fevers, arthritis, night sweats, myalgias, skin nodules, ocular disturbances, and weak pulses in the upper extremities. It is most common in young Asian females and is associated with an elevated erythrocyte sedimentation rate.

Answer A is incorrect. Anti-IgG antibodies, more commonly known as rheumatoid factors, are associated with rheumatoid arthritis (RA). RA manifests as an inflammatory polyarthritis classically associated with morning stiffness, rheumatoid nodules, and other features.

Answer B is incorrect. Antinuclear antibodies are associated with, but not specific for, systemic lupus erythematosus (SLE). While SLE is most common among young to middle-aged females, a classic pattern of rashes, renal disease, and other manifestations would be expected.

Answer C is incorrect. C-ANCA is associated with Wegener's granulomatosis, which is char-

acterized by pulmonary and renal focal necrotizing granulomatous vasculitis.

Answer E is incorrect. Perinuclear antineutrophil cytoplasmic antibody (P-ANCA) is commonly associated with microscopic polyangiitis and Churg-Strauss syndrome. Patients with either condition would not present with absent pulses.

12. **The correct answer is C.** A mutation in the Factor V gene, also known as Factor V Leiden, causes resistance to deactivation of Factor V by protein C. Uninhibited Factor V activity leads to a hypercoagulable state, which can lead to deep vein thrombosis and subsequent pulmonary embolism.

Answer A is incorrect. Factor VIII deficiency (hemophilia A) would actually predispose an individual to bleeding. Factor VIII is an integral part of the intrinsic coagulation cascade.

Answer B is incorrect. High, rather than low, homocysteine levels create a hypercoagulable state.

Answer D is incorrect. Proteins C and S act as negative regulators of the coagulation cascade. Therefore, a deficiency rather than an overproduction in either of these proteins will lead to a hypercoagulable state.

Answer E is incorrect. von Willebrand factor is a major factor in promoting blood clotting, and deficiency (von Willebrand disease) leads to bleeding complications.

13. **The correct answer is E.** This patient has suffered rupture of one of the two left ventricular papillary muscles, a complication that may occur 3–10 days after an acute MI, when the infarcted area of myocardium is replaced with granulation tissue and thus is the most weak. Without the anchor of the papillary muscle, there is severe acute mitral valve regurgitation, diagnosed by a new holosystolic "blowing murmur" that is loudest at the apex and radiates to the axilla, a severely reduced stroke volume (hypotension with EF of 25%), and evidence of pulmonary edema (dyspnea).

Answer A is incorrect. Aortic stenosis causes a crescendo-decrescendo systolic murmur, not a holosystolic murmur and would not be expected to develop acutely as a complication of an MI.

Answer B is incorrect. Dressler's syndrome is an uncommon form of acute pericarditis that occurs several weeks post-MI and is thought to be a result of autoimmune inflammation. Signs and symptoms of pericarditis include sharp, pleuritic chest pain, fever and a pericardial friction rub, not a holosystolic murmur.

Answer C is incorrect. Rupture of the interventricular septum may also occur 3–10 days after an acute MI and would also cause a holosystolic murmur. However, the murmur would be loudest over the left sternal border as blood flows from the left to right ventricle during systole. A murmur that is loudest at the apex and radiating to the axilla is characteristic of mitral regurgitation.

Answer D is incorrect. Rupture of the left ventricular (LV) free wall is another complication that can occur 3–10 days post-MI due to weakened myocardium; this development, however, would lead to cardiac tamponade, not to mitral regurgitation. In LV free wall rupture, blood accumulates in the pericardium and the constricted heart cannot pump effectively, causing a severely decreased stroke volume, systemic hypotension with pulsus paradoxus, jugular venous distension, and decreased heart sounds due to the insulating effects of the fluid around the heart. The holosystolic murmur loudest at the apex and radiating to the axilla detected in this patient is characteristic of mitral regurgitation.

Answer F is incorrect. While a ventricular aneurysm is a complication of an acute MI and could lead to a decreased EF, complications of ventricular aneurysm include thrombus formation with resulting emboli and ventricular arrhythmias, not the severe mitral regurgitation seen here.

14. **The correct answer is D.** The ECG shows torsades des pointes. Quinidine is a class IA antiarrhythmic agent used in the treatment of su-

praventricular arrhythmias. Quinidine slows conduction and can increase the QT interval, leading to torsades de pointes.

Answer A is incorrect. Adenosine is used both to diagnose and to treat supraventricular tachyarrhythmias. However, it is not associated with torsades des pointes.

Answer B is incorrect. Although the class III antiarrhythmics tend to be associated with torsades des pointes, especially sotalol, bretylium is an exception.

Answer C is incorrect. Propranolol is a class II antiarrhythmic but is not associated with torsades des pointes. β-Blockers such as propranolol are used to suppress abnormal pacemakers by decreasing the slope of phase 4 (slow diastolic depolarization in pacemaker cells).

Answer E is incorrect. Bepridil, not verapamil, is a calcium channel blocker and class IV antiarrhythmic associated with torsades des pointes. Verapamil and diltiazem are two calcium channel blockers used in the prevention of nodal arrhythmias (e.g., supraventricular tachycardia).

15. **The correct answer is B.** This patient is most likely experiencing congestive heart failure (CHF) secondary to dilated cardiomyopathy (DCM), which is characterized by dilation and impaired contraction of one or both ventricles. Symptoms of CHF include dyspnea (especially on exertion), orthopnea, paroxysmal nocturnal dyspnea, and peripheral edema with weight gain. DCM may also present with arrhythmias such as atrial fibrillation, or sudden cardiac death. DCM has a variety of etiologies including idiopathic, myocarditis, ischemic, drug-induced, hypertension, infiltrative disease, HIV infection, connective tissue disease, and the chemotherapeutic agent doxorubicin. In this case the most likely cause of the patient's DCM is viral myocarditis following his upper respiratory infection several weeks ago. Viruses known to cause myocarditis include coxsackievirus, influenza virus, adenovirus, echovirus, cytomegalovirus, and HIV. These viruses cause myocarditis with subsequent DCM by inflicting direct cytotoxicity via receptor-mediated

entry of the virus into cardiac myocytes. Patients with myocarditis may present initially with symptoms of chest pain or arrhythmias with ECG changes; in others, symptoms of heart failure may be the initial manifestation, as in this patient.

Answer A is incorrect. Antibodies to a variety of cardiac proteins causing immune-mediated damage to myocytes is the suspected mechanism of injury in familial DCM. This disorder is usually inherited in an autosomal dominant manner and therefore is associated with a significant family history of CHF. Given the patient's recent history of an upper respiratory infection and lack of a family history of cardiac disease, viral myocarditis leading to DCM is the more likely etiology of his CHF.

Answer C is incorrect. Granulomatous inflammation of myocytes is the mechanism of injury causing DCM in infiltrative diseases such as sarcoidosis. Cardiac sarcoidosis should be considered in an otherwise healthy young or middle-aged person with cardiac symptoms, or a patient with known sarcoidosis who develops arrhythmias, conduction disease, or CHF. Diagnosis depends upon evidence of the multisystem features of sarcoidosis, in addition to a biopsy of the myocardium showing noncaseating granulomas. In this patient, DCM secondary to viral myocarditis is a more likely etiology of his CHF given his history of a recent upper respiratory infection and lack of other systemic symptoms associated with sarcoidosis.

Answer D is incorrect. A hyperadrenergic state leading to DCM is the suspected mechanism of cardiac injury that occurs with cocaine use. Cocaine abuse is a known cause of both coronary ischemia and DCM with heart failure, and should be suspected in a young person with otherwise unexplained chest pain or heart failure. Abstinence from cocaine usually leads to a complete reversal of the myocardial dysfunction. This patient denies any drug use, and given his history of a recent upper respiratory infection, viral myocarditis leading to DCM is the more likely etiology of his CHF.

Answer E is incorrect. Coronary atherosclerosis is the most common cause of cardiomyopa-

thy in the United States, so it should definitely be considered in all patients who present with symptoms of heart failure. However, the patient is fairly young to have ischemic heart disease and does not have any known risk factors, such as hypertension, hyperlipidemia, a smoking history, or a family history of heart disease. Given the patient's history, DCM secondary to viral myocarditis is a more likely etiology of his CHF.

16. **The correct answer is B.** Inferior vena cava (IVC) compression is common in women during the third trimester of pregnancy. The large uterus compresses the IVC, decreasing venous return to the heart. This reduction in preload reduces stroke volume, thus reducing cardiac output. Recall that mean arterial pressure = cardiac output × total peripheral resistance; an acute decrease in either of these parameters will reduce blood pressure.

Answer A is incorrect. Cardiogenic shock can cause hypotension by decreasing the stoke volume and cardiac output, but it would not occur only in the supine position.

Answer C is incorrect. Neurogenic shock can cause hypotension by decreasing both cardiac output and peripheral resistance, but it does not typically occur in pregnant women only when they lie supine.

Answer D is incorrect. When fluid leaves the intravascular space and enters the interstitial space, it is referred to as third spacing. In pregnancy, there is a physiologic amount of third spacing, which causes dependent edema in the hands and feet. Some women may even experience pulmonary edema, which can be dangerous. Third spacing does cause hypertension if the intravascular volume is not replaced, but it would not cause isolated hypotension in the supine position.

Answer E is incorrect. Vasodilation will reduce blood pressure, and pregnant women do have a constant amount of vasodilation that is greater than that in nonpregnant women. However, there is no reason for all blood vessels to spontaneously vasodilate when changing from an upright to a supine position.

17. **The correct answer is A.** This patient is presenting with intermittent claudication. Combined with his history of smoking, this points to peripheral arterial disease, which is often the presenting sign of atherosclerosis. Peripheral atherosclerosis targets areas of high turbulence typically found at branching arterial sites; the most common sites are the abdominal aorta and iliac arteries, femoral and popliteal arteries (which is causing the calf pain in this patient), and tibial and peroneal arteries. Medical therapy with antiplatelet drugs such as aspirin has had moderate success, with surgical revascularization reserved for severe cases. Risk factors for atherosclerosis include smoking, hypertension, diabetes mellitus, hyperlipidemia, and a positive family history.

Answer B is incorrect. Arterioles help provide the dynamic regulation of blood flow through the capillary beds. Although they are the site of principle resistance in blood flow, they do not have the turbulence necessary to predispose to atherosclerotic formation. They, along with small muscular arteries, are the major site affected by hypertension.

Answer C is incorrect. Capillaries are the smallest form of blood vessel and represent the site of interchange of solutes and cells between the blood and extracellular fluid. They are not typically affected by atherosclerosis but play a major role in the pathophysiology of edema.

Answer D is incorrect. Veins are the vessels that return blood back to the heart and are not typically affected by atherosclerosis.

Answer E is incorrect. Venules are the first vessels to collect blood from the capillary beds and are not affected by atherosclerosis.

18. **The correct answer is C.** In tricuspid regurgitation, blood flows back into the atria during ventricular systole. This would affect the C and X waves, replacing them with a large positive deflection. This positive deflection joins the C wave and the V wave, creating the "CV wave." The C wave is thought to be due to pressure on the tricuspid valve during ventricular systole. If the valve allows backflow during ventricular systole, the pressure would drastically increase in the atria. The downward movement of the ventricle causes the X descent during ventricular systole. This would also be replaced by a positive deflection from blood regurgitating into the atria during ventricular systole.

Answer A is incorrect. These points are not the most likely to be affected in tricuspid regurgitation.

Answer B is incorrect. These points are not the most likely to be affected in tricuspid regurgitation.

Answer D is incorrect. These points are not the most likely to be affected in tricuspid regurgitation. The V wave is increased pressure because of right atrial filling against a closed tricuspid valve. With tricuspid regurgitation, not much change is seen with the V wave itself, but rather it is the end point for the new CV wave change.

19. **The correct answer is C.** Constrictive pericarditis interferes with the filling of the ventricles because of granulation tissue formation in the pericardium. It can follow purulent viral infections, trauma, neoplastic diseases, mediastinal irradiation, and other chronic diseases. Pericardial thickening and calcification are sometimes apparent on CT and MRI.

Answer A is incorrect. Cardiac tamponade is very similar in presentation to constrictive pericarditis. One defining characteristic of cardiac tamponade is the absence of Kussmaul's sign (failure of cervical venous distention to subside on inspiration). In addition, pulsus paradoxus (decrease in systolic pressure by ≥10 mm Hg during inspiration) is usually present. X-ray of the chest should reveal an enlarged cardiac silhouette with pericardial effusion.

Answer B is incorrect. CHF produces signs and symptoms similar to those of constrictive pericarditis. However, in CHF there would be significant enlargement and hypertrophy of the ventricles.

Answer D is incorrect. The echocardiogram results are not consistent with dilated cardiomyopathy, as diastolic volumes are reduced in this patient but end-diastolic volumes are increased in dilated cardiomyopathy.

Answer E is incorrect. Breast and lung carcinomas, lymphomas, and melanomas are the most common metastases to the pericardium and should therefore be considered in this case. However, metastasis causing constrictive pathology is much less common than pericarditis.

20. **The correct answer is C.** The inferior mesenteric artery originates from the aorta inferior to the renal arteries and superior to the bifurcation of the aorta into the common iliac arteries. This artery may sometimes be sacrificed during an infrarenal aortic aneurysm repair rather than being re-attached to a healthy segment of aorta. Usually, there is enough collateral flow to the hindgut from the superior mesenteric artery and the hypogastric arteries that the loss of the inferior mesenteric artery does not result in colonic ischemia.

Answer A is incorrect. The gastroduodenal artery is a branch of the hepatic artery, which is in turn a branch of the celiac trunk.

Answer B is incorrect. The hepatic artery is a branch of the celiac trunk and is found superior to the renal arteries.

Answer D is incorrect. The left gastric artery is a branch of the celiac trunk and is found superior to the renal arteries.

Answer E is incorrect. The splenic artery is a branch of the celiac trunk and is also found superior to the renal arteries.

Answer F is incorrect. The superior mesenteric artery is superior to the renal arteries and thus would not be disrupted in resection of the infrarenal aorta.

21. **The correct answer is D.** Syphilitic aortitis is characterized by obliterative endarteritis of the vasa vasorum of the media. This disruption of the vasa vasorum can lead to aneurysm, which typically involves the ascending aorta and is a manifestation of tertiary syphilis. Luetic (syphilitic) aneurysms favor the aortic root, where

they can be complicated by atherosclerosis. The patient's skin lesions are the gummas of tertiary syphilis.

Answer A is incorrect. Atherosclerosis is most frequently associated with a descending aortic aneurysm, especially one involving the abdominal aorta, and is rarely associated with ascending aortic aneurysms in the absence of underlying pathology, such as that of tertiary syphilis.

Answer B is incorrect. Congenital medial weakness is actually associated with the development of berry aneurysms, which typically occur along the circle of Willis. They are the most frequent cause of subarachnoid hemorrhage and are also associated with adult polycystic kidney disease.

Answer C is incorrect. Cystic medial necrosis (cystic degeneration of the tunica media of the aorta) is the most frequent preexisting histological lesion in aortic dissection, which is not usually associated with aortic dilation. It is also associated with dilation of the ascending aorta, and is commonly seen in connective tissue disorders such as Marfan's syndrome. Although this answer choice is possible, the skin lesions point to tertiary syphilis as the cause of the cardiac pathology.

Answer E is incorrect. Hypertension is often implicated in the etiology of dissecting aneurysms due to a longitudinal intraluminal tear. Dissection is usually not associated with aortic dilation.

22. **The correct answer is A.** A patent ductus arteriosus (PDA) rarely causes cyanosis. PDAs are associated with maternal rubella infection during pregnancy. During fetal development, the ductus arteriosus remains patent through the action of prostaglandin I_2 (PGI_2). PDAs at birth are closed with indomethacin, a nonsteroidal anti-inflammatory drug that inhibits PGI_2 formation. Remember that there are, in general, three congenital heart lesions that cause late cyanosis due to left to right shunt: ventricular septal defect, atrial septal defect, and PDA. The classic murmur heard with PDA is a continuous machinelike murmur.

Answer B is incorrect. Tetralogy of Fallot (TOF) is often associated with cyanosis at birth. In TOF, there is pulmonary stenosis, right ventricular hypertrophy (RVH), overriding aorta, and VSD. The early cyanosis is caused by a large right-to-left shunt across the VSD as the blood does not go through the high-resistance pulmonary artery. Babies can develop boot-shaped hearts on radiography due to RVH. Patients also suffer from "cyanotic spells."

Answer C is incorrect. Transposition of the great vessels is associated with cyanosis at birth. Surgery is often needed to correct this defect. Nonsteroidal anti-inflammatory drugs are contraindicated in transposition of the great vessels because left-to-right blood flow through the patent ductus arteriosus improves arterial oxygenation.

Answer D is incorrect. Truncus arteriosus is associated with cyanosis at birth. Truncus arteriosus is characterized by a large ventral septal defect in which a single great vessel arises. There is considerable mixing of oxygenated and deoxygenate blood and this results in cyanosis.

Answer E is incorrect. Ventricular septal defects are the most common congenital cardiac anomaly. They do not cause cyanosis at birth and do not close with nonsteroidal anti-inflammatory drug administration. Rubella can cause septal defects however. VSDs present with holosystolic murmurs.

23. **The correct answer is A.** Adenosine is extremely useful in abolishing atrioventricular (AV) nodal arrhythmias when given in high-dose intravenous boluses. Adenosine works by hyperpolarizing AV node tissue by increasing the conductance of potassium and by reducing calcium current. As a result, the conduction through the AV node is markedly reduced. In addition to this, adenosine's extremely short duration of action (15 seconds) limits the occurrence of its toxicities (i.e., hypotension, flushing, chest pain, and dyspnea).

Answer B is incorrect. Bretylium, a potassium channel blocker (class III), is used when other antiarrhythmics fail.

Answer C is incorrect. Encainide is used when ventricular tachycardia progresses to ventricular fibrillation; it is also used in intractable supraventricular tachycardia.

Answer D is incorrect. Lidocaine, a class Ib antiarrhythmic, is used in the treatment of acute ventricular arrhythmias such as post-MI arrhythmias.

Answer E is incorrect. Sotalol, which is both a β-adrenergic-receptor blocker (class II) and a potassium channel blocker (class III), is used when other antiarrhythmics fail.

24. **The correct answer is C.** Norepinephrine, a potent direct-acting α-agonist and a moderate β-agonist, can be useful in cases of septic shock because it stimulates peripheral vasoconstriction. However, the coronary vasculature expresses both α- and β-adrenergic receptors, with a net effect of vasodilation of the coronary vessels when catecholamines are present in high levels. Norepinephrine also exerts a mild inotropic effect as a β_1-agonist, but this effect may not be clinically relevant. Successful treatment of septic shock involves fluids, proper antibiotics, and pressors (i.e., norepinephrine) if the blood pressure is unresponsive to fluid resuscitation. Pressors are given to maintain tissue perfusion.

Answer A is incorrect. Norepinephrine itself is inotropic and chronotropic, but the potent vasoconstriction that it causes will increase blood pressures to stimulate the baroreceptors, resulting in a reflex bradycardia. However, this is not a direct function of the norepinephrine and is not the reason it would be given to a patient in septic shock.

Answer B is incorrect. Norepinephrine exerts no β_2 effects and thus has no effect on bronchial smooth muscle. If it were a β_2 agonist (epinephrine demonstrates moderate β_2 agonist activity but strong α_1 and β_2 activity), it would stimulate bronchodilation.

Answer D is incorrect. As a β_1 agonist, norepinephrine stimulates a mild increase in cardiac inotropy and increased blood flow to the cardiac muscle through vasodilation of the coronary vessels.

Answer E is incorrect. Norepinephrine is a peripheral vasoconstrictor, but it also induces vasodilation in the coronary vessels.

25. **The correct answer is F.** The combination of an atrophic heart and lipofuscin accumulation is referred to as brown atrophy. Lipofuscin is a "wear and tear" pigment that commonly deposits within hepatocytes, splenocytes, and myocardial cells in the elderly. It is comprised of oxidized and polymerized membrane lipids of autophagocytosed organelles accumulated slowly over years.

    Answer A is incorrect. Bilirubin can accumulate and stain internal organs, producing yellowish discoloration called jaundice. However, lack of clinical evidence of a hemolytic or obstructive process in this case makes this option highly unlikely.

    Answer B is incorrect. Age-related calcification is most often seen on heart valves. It would not appear brown in color, nor would it be associated with generalized cardiac atrophy.

    Answer C is incorrect. Cholesterol may accumulate as atheromatous plaques in the arteries; however, its accumulation is not associated with cardiac atrophy nor brown pigmentation.

    Answer D is incorrect. Glycogen storage diseases are inherited conditions that appear early in life. Glycogen does not appear pigmented on hematoxylin and eosin stain.

    Answer E is incorrect. Iron deposits within the heart could also appear as brownish granules. However, this would suggest that the patient suffers from hemochromatosis. The cardiac complications of hemochromatosis include cardiomyopathy and arrhythmia. The patient described in the question stem has an atrophic heart, making iron deposits a less likely option.

26. **The correct answer is E.** This individual is likely suffering from giant cell (temporal) arteritis (GCA), the most common systemic vasculitis in adults. GCA, which affects large to small arteries, typically presents in people >50 years old and is more common in women. Patients commonly present with constitutional symptoms (anorexia, fatigue, weight loss), unilateral temporal or occipital headache with overlying scalp tenderness, jaw claudication, and impaired vision. The superficial temporal artery is the most commonly affected artery in patients with GCA and is affected in this patient. On biopsy, affected arteries are characterized by nodular thickening that reduces the size of the lumen, granulomatous inflammation with mononuclear and giant cells, and fragmentation of the internal elastic membrane. GCA is treated with high-dose corticosteroids to reduce inflammation rapidly and prevent permanent blindness.

    Answer A is incorrect. GCA typically affects branches of the external carotid artery, such as the superficial temporal artery. It can also affect branches of the internal carotid artery, such as the ophthalmic artery. Unilateral vision loss can also be caused by a cholesterol embolus from a plaque on the common or internal carotid artery, but not the external carotid artery.

    Answer B is incorrect. The facial artery can be involved in GCA, but is not the likely cause of jaw claudication as seen in this patient.

    Answer C is incorrect. Sudden blindness is a serious complication of GCA, resulting from involvement of the ophthalmic artery.

    Answer D is incorrect. The postauricular artery supplies the skin behind the ear and is rarely involved in GCA. Involvement of this artery would present with ear pain, which is not observed in this patient.

27. **The correct answer is B.** The patient is experiencing pericarditis due to uremia secondary to chronic kidney disease in the setting of long-standing diabetes mellitus. Pericarditis presents with pleuritic, positional chest pain that is often relieved by sitting forward and with a pericardial friction rub on physical examination. Diffuse ST segment elevations may be found

on ECG, while an echocardiogram may be normal unless an effusion is also present. Pericarditis has multiple etiologies, including viral (coxsackievirus, echovirus, adenovirus, and HIV), bacterial (tuberculosis or *Streptococcus pneumoniae* or *Staphylococcus aureus* in the setting of endocarditis, pneumonia, or postcardiac surgery), neoplastic, autoimmune, uremic, cardiovascular, or idiopathic. Treatment of pericarditis secondary to uremia is dialysis.

Answer A is incorrect. Cardiac catheterization is indicated in patients who are experiencing acute coronary syndrome. While this patient is certainly at risk for ischemic heart disease given her age and history of diabetes, her symptoms and ECG findings of diffuse ST segment elevations are more indicative of pericarditis. In contrast, acute myocardial ischemia is more likely to present with chest pain that is not relieved by changes in position and ECG findings that show ST segment elevations in contiguous leads only.

Answer C is incorrect. Nonsteroidal anti-inflammatory drugs are the appropriate treatment for viral or idiopathic pericarditis. However, this patient is experiencing pericarditis due to uremia secondary to chronic kidney disease in the setting of long-standing diabetes mellitus, and therefore the most effective treatment for her is dialysis.

Answer D is incorrect. Pericardiocentesis would be indicated if this patient had evidence of a pericardial effusion, such as distant heart sounds on physical examination, electrical alternans on ECG, cardiomegaly on x-ray of the chest, or fluid in the pericardial space on echocardiogram. However, this patient does not have any of these findings, and therefore pericardiocentesis is not indicated.

Answer E is incorrect. Changing the patient's antibiotic regimen is indicated if she is suspected of having an allergic reaction (such as the development of a rash or anaphylaxis) to a particular medication. However, in this case her symptoms are not consistent with an allergic reaction, and therefore her antibiotic regimen does not need to be changed.

28. **The correct answer is D.** The posterior descending artery is a branch of the right coronary artery on the posterior surface of the heart. It courses along the posterior interventricular groove, extending toward the apex of the heart. It has posterior septal perforator branches that run anteriorly in the ventricular septum and supply the posterior one-third of the ventricular septal myocardium.

Answer A is incorrect. The acute marginal artery is a branch from the right coronary artery. It runs along the acute margin of the heart and supplies the anterior free wall of the right ventricle.

Answer B is incorrect. The circumflex artery is one of two main branches off the left main coronary artery and it courses along the left atrioventricular groove from the anterior to the posterior surface of the heart. In people who are left-dominant, it will give rise to the posterior descending artery and perfuse the atrioventricular node. Its main branches are the obtuse marginals, which supply blood to the lateral aspect of the left ventricular myocardium. It also has branches that supply blood to the left atrium and, in 40%–50% of people, the sinus node.

Answer C is incorrect. The left anterior descending artery supplies the anterior interventricular septum. One of two main branches off the left main coronary artery, it descends the left surface of the heart anteriorly and inferiorly in the anterior interventricular groove to the apex of the heart. Diagonal, septal perforating, and right ventricular branches come off of it, supplying portions of the anterior aspects of the left atrium, left ventricle, interventricular septum, and right ventricle. Although the left anterior descending artery is the artery that is most commonly occluded in coronary artery occlusion, the posterior descending artery supplies the posterior one-third of the intraventricular septum, which is the site of abnormality in this case.

Answer E is incorrect. The right coronary artery is one of the two main coronary arteries that take off from the aorta, just superior to the aortic valve leaflets. It courses from the aorta anterolaterally to descend in the right atrioventricular groove before curving posteriorly at the acute margin of the right ventricle. It supplies the sinoatrial and atrioventricular nodes, the right atrium, and portions of the right ventricle in addition to providing collaterals to the left anterior descending artery.

29. **The correct answer is C.** This patient is presenting with a classic case of acute bacterial endocarditis (ABE). Endocarditis is often characterized by constitutional symptoms (fever, malaise, chills), new-onset cardiac murmur, and a combination of other signs and symptoms (e.g., Janeway lesions, Osler nodes, and Roth spots). Acute and subacute endocarditis can be differentiated based on history, as the acute case will have a more severe and sudden onset, as in this patient. ABE is also most often seen in cases of intravenous drug use and indwelling catheters, and *Staphylococcus aureus* is the most common bacterial pathogen isolated in these cases because it is part of the skin flora and enters the blood at needle sites. This patient's history of intravenous drug abuse as well as auscultation of a murmur consistent with tricuspid regurgitation both point to a right-sided ABE infection. In right-sided endocarditis, septic emboli to the lungs leading to bilateral infiltrates are seen more often. This patient is manifesting signs of bilateral infiltrates with signs of hypoxia, decreased breath sounds, and dullness to percussion. It is important to note that many of the classic signs of endocarditis, such as Janeway lesions, Osler nodes, and Roth spots, are mostly seen as a complication of left-sided endocarditis, in which septic emboli leave the heart and enter the systemic circulation.

Answer A is incorrect. *Enterococcus faecalis* also causes subacute endocarditis. The classic picture is a slow onset of constitutional symptoms with low-grade fever. *Enterococcus* infection is not seen as frequently as viridans streptococci, but it is known to colonize damaged heart valves, especially in patients with a past history of rheumatic fever.

Answer B is incorrect. *Haemophilus aphrophilus* is part of the HACEK group of fastidious gram-negative bacilli that cause 5%–10% of cases of bacterial endocarditis that are not related to intravenous drug use. These organisms are slow growing and difficult to culture from blood samples, making diagnoses more complex.

Answer D is incorrect. *Streptococcus bovis* also causes subacute bacterial endocarditis with low-grade fever and insidious onset. It normally inhabits the lower gastrointestinal tract and lesions in the colon, such as those that occur in colon cancer, allow the bacteria access to the bloodstream. It most commonly affects the aortic valve.

Answer E is incorrect. *Viridans* streptococci are the most common cause of bacterial endocarditis overall. This group of bacteria is most often seen in subacute cases in which the onset of symptoms is more chronic and low-grade fevers are more common. *Viridans* streptococci commonly colonize heart valves previously damaged by rheumatic fever, thus causing left-sided infective endocarditis as opposed to the right-sided version seen more commonly with *Staphylococcus aureus*. One common source of infection is dental procedures during which normal flora of the oropharynx can enter the bloodstream.

30. **The correct answer is A.** Cholestyramine and colestipol are bile acid resins that promote binding and excretion of dietary fats that are bile-soluble. This prevents such fats from entering the blood stream effectively. They decrease serum LDL and total cholesterol levels.

Answer B is incorrect. Fibrates such as gemfibrozil and fenofibrate act by increasing lipoprotein lipase activity. HDL cholesterol and triglyceride levels subsequently improve after beginning treatment. These drugs have also been shown to assist in treating insulin resistance.

Answer C is incorrect. Niacin acts by decreasing lipolysis in adipose tissue. Its most significant result is an increase in serum HDL cholesterol. Adverse effects include flushing.

Answer D is incorrect. Ezetimibe is a newer lipid-lowering agent that acts by inhibiting cholesterol absorption at the small intestinal brush border. It is frequently given in combination with statins for greater overall LDL cholesterol reduction.

Answer E is incorrect. Statins inhibit the rate-limiting enzyme in cholesterol synthesis. They cause significant decreases in LDL cholesterol and modest increases in HDL cholesterol.

Answer F is incorrect. There is no available drug that retains and sequesters bile acid resins in hepatocytes.

31. **The correct answer is A.** This patient has von Hippel-Lindau syndrome, an autosomal dominant disorder characterized by abnormal blood vessel growth. The overgrowth of blood vessels leads to angiomas and hemangioblastomas in the retina, brain, and spinal cord, as well as in other regions of the body. Patients also show cystic growths in the kidneys and pancreas, phcochromocytomas, islet cell tumors, and clear cell renal carcinoma. The disease is due to deletion of the *VHL* tumor suppressor gene on the short arm of chromosome 3.

Answer B is incorrect. In autosomal recessive inheritance, a defective gene from each carrier parent is transmitted to the offspring. Disease is often seen in only one generation. Males and females are equally likely to be affected. Von Hippel-Lindau syndrome is not inherited in this manner.

Answer C is incorrect. In mitochondrial inheritance, children (male and female) of an affected mother may exhibit the disease. The disease is not transmitted from fathers to any of their children (only maternal transmission). Von Hippel-Lindau syndrome is not inherited in this manner.

Answer D is incorrect. Spontaneous mutations generally affect only one member of a family and are not seen in multiple generations. Von Hippel-Lindau syndrome is not inherited in this manner.

Answer E is incorrect. In X-linked recessive inheritance, affected males inherit a defective copy of the X chromosome from heterozygous (asymptomatic) mothers. There is no male-to-male transmission. Von Hippel-Lindau syndrome is not inherited in this manner.

32. **The correct answer is A.** This patient presents with symptoms consistent with Lyme disease. He had a characteristic expanding rash (erythema migrans) and resolving flu-like symptoms. Lyme disease can often lead to cardiac symptoms such as those described, as well as heart block that can require cardiac pacing. Lyme disease is carried by the *Ixodes* tick. *I. scapularis* is also the vector of disease for babesiosis, a malaria-like parasitic disease common in the northeastern corner of the United States.

Answer B is incorrect. Epidemic typhus is known as "louse-born typhus." The vector for transmission is *Pediculus corporis*. Epidemic typhus is unusual because the vector for disease feeds only on humans and not other animals. The bacterium responsible is *Rickettsia prowazekii.*

Answer C is incorrect. Malaria is a protozoan parasitic disease responsible for 1-3 million deaths per year worldwide. Its vector of transmission (and target for disease control) is the female *Anopheles* mosquito.

Answer D is incorrect. Plague is an infectious disease caused by the bacterium *Yersinia pestis*. It is mainly transmitted by fleas that live on infected rodents such as the oriental rat flea, or *Xenopsylla cheopis.*

Answer E is incorrect. Rocky Mountain spotted fever is caused by *Rickettsia rickettsii*, a species of bacteria spread to humans by the ticks of the *Dermacentor* family such as *D. variabilis.*

33. **The correct answer is C.** This individual is presenting with signs typical of CHF. In CHF, there is a decrease in effective arterial blood volume due to the inability of the heart to effectively pump blood, which stimulates the

renin-angiotensin-aldosterone axis to increase the tubular absorption of Na^+ to help increase intravascular volume.

Answer A is incorrect. Sympathetic outflow would be increased to counteract the diminished cardiac output of the failing heart.

Answer B is incorrect. The venous pressure would actually be increased due to the inability of the heart to effectively pump blood to the arterial system; this would lead to a passive congestion of blood in the venous circulation. This increased venous pressure can result in passive congestion of the liver known as a "nutmeg" liver.

Answer D is incorrect. The effective arterial blood volume would be decreased due to the decreased ability of the heart to pump blood through the arterial circulation.

Answer E is incorrect. Glomerular filtration rate would be decreased because of decreased renal blood flow secondary to decreased cardiac output.

34. **The correct answer is G.** Cardiac troponin I becomes elevated in the first 4 hours after an MI and remains elevated for 7–10 days. CK-MB peaks in the first 24 hours and then falls off. AST is the next to become elevated, as it gradually increases over the first 2 days and then slowly declines; however, it is not specific for damage to the heart. LDH is the last cardiac enzyme to become elevated (by day 2 post-MI) and it remains elevated for up to 7 days post-MI. Note that although troponin is a great enzyme to monitor for new infarcts, CK-MB is the enzyme of choice in the detection of reinfarction within the first week. If reinfarction occurs, the troponin level would still be elevated and thus not useful in detecting the new ischemic event. A final marker not mentioned here is myoglobin, which typically rises and falls within 6 hours pst-MI. However, like AST, it is nonspecific since it is found in skeletal muscle and is not used clinically to diagnose MI.

Answer A is incorrect. The correct order is troponin, CK-MB, AST, and then LDH.

Answer B is incorrect. The correct order is troponin, CK-MB, AST, and then LDH.

Answer C is incorrect. The correct order is troponin, CK-MB, AST, and then LDH.

Answer D is incorrect. The correct order is troponin, CK-MB, AST, and then LDH.

Answer E is incorrect. The correct order is troponin, CK-MB, AST, and then LDH.

Answer F is incorrect. The correct order is troponin, CK-MB, AST, and then LDH.

35. **The correct answer is C.** Given his age and his history of hypertension and diabetes, this patient is most likely presenting with a stroke. Part of the workup for stroke includes an ultrasound to evaluate the carotid arteries, which in this case showed significant atherosclerosis, the likely cause of the man's stroke. The common carotid arteries, as well as the proximal part of the internal carotids, have their embryologic origins in the third aortic arch. Remember this by noting that "C" is the **third** letter of the alphabet. The aortic arches are responsible for the major arteries in the head and neck regions, while the descending aorta is the origin for the arteries in the rest of the body.

Answer A is incorrect. The first aortic arch gives rise to the maxillary artery, which is not involved in the pathophysiology of stroke.

Answer B is incorrect. The second aortic arch gives rise to the stapedial (Second = Stapedial) and hyoid arteries, neither of which is involved in stroke.

Answer D is incorrect. The fourth aortic arch gives rise to the adult arch of the aorta on the left and the proximal part of the right subclavian artery on the right. In theory, it is possible for an embolus from an aortic arch thrombus to travel up the carotid and cause a stroke, but this is not a likely scenario and would not be evaluated by ultrasound. Similarly, a subclavian embolus may travel up the vertebral arteries to cause a posterior stroke, but this would not be evaluated by ultrasound.

Answer E is incorrect. The sixth arch gives rise to the proximal parts of the pulmonary arteries and, on the left, the ductus arteriosus. Note that the fifth aortic arch regresses.

36. The correct answer is D. This patient has cardiac tamponade. Although Beck's clinical triad of jugular venous distension, muffled heart sounds, and hypotension is more specific, the clinician must sometimes rely on other physical findings. Pulsus paradoxus (systolic blood pressure that drops >10 mm Hg during inspiration) is usually present. Pulsus paradoxus could also be detected by noting extra beats on cardiac auscultation while simultaneously palpating the radial pulse. Pericardiocentesis is required immediately and may be life-saving. The fluid that has filled the pericardial membrane is removed, thereby reversing the pressure levels that led to the elevated intracardiac pressure, limited ventricular filling, and reduced cardiac output that ultimately caused her symptoms of fatigue and pulsus paradoxus.

Answer A is incorrect. Angioplasty is required for a patient that has greater than 70% blockage of a coronary artery. This diagnosis could not be made by echocardiography.

Answer B is incorrect. Aortic valve replacement would be necessary in situations of valvular failure or rupture. Cardiac tamponade does not affect heart valves.

Answer C is incorrect. Mitral valve replacement would be necessary in situations of valvular failure or rupture. Cardiac tamponade does not affect heart valves.

Answer E is incorrect. Aortic aneurysms do not typically present with pulsus paradoxus or fatigue.

37. The correct answer is C. This image shows mitral stenosis, causing a classic "fish-mouth" appearance due to the fusion of the valve leaflets. Mitral stenosis often causes a sharp, high-pitched opening snap at the beginning of diastole, due to the opening of the stiffened mitral valve leaflets, followed by a decrescendo-crescendo murmur. The shape of the murmur of mitral stenosis is unique and occurs because the pressure gradient between the left atrium and left ventricle is the greatest when the mitral

valve opens and decreases during rapid and slow ventricular filling (decrescendo) and then intensifies slightly during atrial contraction at the end of ventricular diastole (crescendo). The murmur of mitral stenosis is low-pitched and is best heard at the apex of the heart. This woman may have had rheumatic heart disease, which is the most common cause of mitral stenosis.

Answer A is incorrect. A patent ductus arteriosus causes a continuous murmur as blood flows from the higher-pressure aorta to the lower-pressure pulmonary artery during both diastole and systole. The murmur increases during ventricular systole as the pressure in the aorta increases, reaches a maximum at the end of ventricular systole, and decreases throughout diastole, as the pressure in the aorta decreases. This patient, however, has a stenotic mitral valve, not a patent ductus arteriosus.

Answer B is incorrect. Aortic or pulmonic regurgitation, not mitral stenosis, would cause a decrescendo murmur that would be loudest in early diastole, when the pressure gradient between the aorta and the left ventricle is the greatest, and would decrease throughout diastole as the left ventricular pressure increases.

Answer D is incorrect. Aortic stenosis leads to a crescendo-decrescendo murmur best heard at the right sternal border during ventricular systole, as the pressure gradient between the left ventricle and the aorta increases to a maximum during midsystole and then decreases in late ventricular systole. The characteristic murmur of aortic stenosis may be preceded by a sharp ejection click due to the opening of the stiffened aortic valve leaflets. This patient had a stenotic mitral valve, not a stenotic aortic valve.

Answer E is incorrect. Mitral valve prolapse characteristically causes a sharp, high-pitched click during mid to late systole followed by the continuous murmur of mitral regurgitation as blood flows from the higher-pressure left ventricle to the lower-pressure left atrium. While the stenotic mitral valve, seen in this patient, could lead to a systolic murmur of mitral regurgitation in addition to the diastolic murmur of mitral stenosis, the murmur of mitral regurgitation due to a stenotic valve would be a holosystolic, continuous murmur. The mid-systolic click followed by a continuous murmur is unique to mitral valve prolapse, which is most commonly caused by enlarged, floppy, and myxomatous mitral valve leaflets.

38. **The correct answer is B.** This is Kawasaki's disease, which typically affects infants and children under 5 years old is self-limiting. It involves the mouth, skin, and lymph nodes at first, but if left untreated the patient may have arrhythmias due to inflammation of the outer membranes of the heart. The most common histopathologic sign of Kawasaki's disease is acute necrotizing vasculitis of small and medium-sized vessels.

Answer A is incorrect. Buerger's disease is characterized as an idiopathic, segmental thrombosing vasculitis with intermittent claudication, superficial nodular phlebitis, and cold sensitivity. Patients are usually young men (20–40 years old) who are also heavy smokers.

Answer C is incorrect. PAN is characterized by cotton-wool spots, microaneurysms, and palpable purpura. This condition most often arises in the fourth or fifth decades of life, and is twice as likely to occur in men. It is also associated with hepatitis B. The cardinal histopathologic sign is inflammation throughout the entire arterial wall. PAN predominantly affects the kidneys, peripheral nervous system, and gastrointestinal tract and can lead to symptoms such as renal failure, mononeuritis multiplex, and bowel infarction. Up to 80% of patients with PAN have P-ANCA, an antibody against myeloperoxidase.

Answer D is incorrect. Takayasu's arteritis is characterized by weak pulses in the upper extremities, fever, arthritis, and night sweats. The condition most often arises in women under the age of 40 years (9:1 female predominance). The classic pulselessness is a result of chronic inflammation and subsequent narrowing of the aorta and its branches, making it a large-vessel vasculitis.

Answer E is incorrect. Wegener's granulomatosis is characterized by necrotizing granulo-

mas in the lung and upper airways together with glomerulonephritis; however, it can occur in any organ. There is a nearly equal gender distribution in incidence, and the condition typically occurs in middle age. Histopathological diagnosis is critical, even though C-ANCA testing is positive in most patients.

39. **The correct answer is F.** This woman is likely suffering from prosthetic valve endocarditis. She may not have taken appropriate prophylactic antibiotics before her root canal procedure, and her susceptible mitral valve after rheumatic fever has been exposed to transient bacteremia. Her symptoms, including low-grade persistent fever, new-onset murmur, and insidious onset, suggest subacute bacterial endocarditis. This is further supported by her physical examination, which reveals the presence of Roth spots (retinal hemorrhages), Osler's nodes (painful red nodules on digits), and Janeway lesions (dark macules on palms and soles). Given her clinical history and symptoms, the bacterium most likely to have caused this episode is *Streptococcus sanguis*, part of the viridans group. The most appropriate treatment for such an infection is penicillin G.

Answer A is incorrect. Caspofungin is an antifungal used to treat aspergillosis. It would not treat a gram-positive cocci infection.

Answer B is incorrect. Clindamycin, the treatment for several important anaerobic infections, works by blocking peptide bond formation at the 50S ribosomal subunit. This is not an anaerobic infection.

Answer C is incorrect. Mebendazole is an antiparasitic drug used to treat roundworm infections such as pinworm and whipworm. Mebendazole is not used to treat bacterial endocarditis.

Answer D is incorrect. Metronidazole is a bactericidal agent used to treat protozoal infections, specifically *Giardia*, *Entamoeba*, and *Trichomonas* species, as well as anaerobes, specifically *Bacteroides* and *Clostridium* species. Gram-positive cocci are not within metronidazole's spectrum.

Answer E is incorrect. Nafcillin works like penicillin but is used clinically to treat *Staphylococcus aureus*, the cause of acute bacterial endocarditis, among other infections. Nafcillin is used for *S. aureus* because it is penicillinase-resistant due to a bulkier R group. Because of this special property, nafcillin is reserved for suspected *S. aureus* cases, which is not the cause of this patient's condition.

Answer G is incorrect. Pentamidine is an antiparasitic drug used for prophylaxis against *Pneumocystis carinii* pneumonia. Pentamidien is not used to treat bacterial endocarditis.

40. **The correct answer is D.** The patient's primary complaints are fatigue and depression that began after she started a new medication. Her physical examination and laboratory studies are within normal limits and reveal no additional side effects of this new medication. Mild sedation and depression are common adverse effects of β-blockers; diarrhea, pruritis, disturbance of the sleep cycle, exercise intolerance, and a diminished hypoglycemic response can also occur with the use of β-blockers. Of all the medications listed, metoprolol is the only one that may cause depression.

Answer A is incorrect. Furosemide is a loop diuretic and thus can cause electrolyte abnormalities such as hypokalemia and metabolic alkalosis. It is not associated with sedation.

Answer B is incorrect. Hydrochlorothiazide, a diuretic, has side effects such as hypokalemia and hyperglycemia. It is not associated with sedation or changes in mood.

Answer C is incorrect. Losartan is an angiotensin receptor blocker; its use can result in hyperkalemia, but it is not associated with sedation.

Answer E is incorrect. Nifedipine is a calcium channel blocker that functions primarily on the vasculature. It can be associated with edema, flushing, and dizziness, but is not usually sedating.

Answer F is incorrect. Prazosin, an α-antagonist, can be associated with dizziness, headache, and orthostasis, but is not considered sedating.

41. **The correct answer is B.** The question describes the pathology associated with stable angina. Autoregulation is the process whereby blood flow is altered to meet demands of tissue. The principle factors determining autoregulation of blood flow to the heart are local metabolites including adenosine, oxygen, and nitric oxide.

Answer A is incorrect. Parasympathetic innervation to the heart via acetylcholine is not a mediator of autoregulation of coronary blood flow. Parasympathetic discharge will decrease heart rate, decrease atrioventricular nodal conduction velocity, and decrease atrial contractility with little or direct effect on coronary blood flow.

Answer C is incorrect. Carbon dioxide is more important for autoregulation of cerebral blood flow.

Answer D is incorrect. Lactate, a solute produced by skeletal muscle during nonoxidative metabolism, is a mediator of the autoregulation of blood flow to skeletal muscle.

Answer E is incorrect. Sympathetic innervation to the heart via norepinephrine is not a mediator of autoregulation of coronary blood flow. Sympathetic discharge will increase heart rate, increase atrioventricular nodal conduction velocity, and increase myocardial contractility, thus increasing oxygen demand with little direct effect on coronary blood flow.

42. **The correct answer is D.** Isovolumetric relaxation (phase IV in the image) is the period in which both the aortic and mitral valves are closed, thus keeping ventricular volume constant. Ventricular muscle relaxes from its prior contraction to allow for filling.

Answer A is incorrect. Ventricular filling (phase I in the image) is the period between mitral valve opening and closing.

Answer B is incorrect. Isovolumetric contraction (phase II in the image) is the period between mitral valve closing and aortic valve opening.

Answer C is incorrect. Ventricular ejection (phase III in the image) is the period between aortic valve opening and closing.

43. **The correct answer is C.** The carotid sinus baroreceptor sends an afferent signal via the glossopharyngeal nerve to the medulla, which in turn responds with a sympathetic efferent signal that causes vasoconstriction, increased heart rate, increased contractility, and increased blood pressure.

Answer A is incorrect. The baroreceptor located in the aortic arch responds only to an increase in blood pressure.

Answer B is incorrect. The correct efferent response to a decreased baroreceptor afferent firing rate would be increased sympathetic activity and decreased parasympathetic activity.

Answer D is incorrect. The baroreceptor located in the aortic arch responds only to an increase in blood pressure.

Answer E is incorrect. The afferent firing rate would decrease, not increase, with hypotension.

44. **The correct answer is B.** Dressler's syndrome is an autoimmune phenomenon that results in fibrinous pericarditis. This delayed pericarditis typically develops 2–10 weeks post-MI and presents clinically as chest pain and a pericardial friction rub. It is generally treated with nonsteroidal antiinflammatory agentes or corticosteroids.

Answer A is incorrect. Cardiac arrhythmia is a common cause of post-MI death and typically occurs 2 days post-MI. It does not typically present with a friction rub.

Answer C is incorrect. Left ventricular failure occurs in 60% of people who suffer from MI and can present as CHF or cardiogenic shock.

Answer D is incorrect. Thromboemboli are typically systemic emboli that originate from mural thrombi and can lead to cerebrovascular accidents, transient ischemic attacks, and renal artery thrombosis.

Answer E is incorrect. Ventricular rupture is a cause of post-MI death that typically occurs 4–10 days post-MI. It often presents with persistent chest pain, syncope, and distended jugular veins.

45. **The correct answer is A.** At toxic levels of hydralazine, the body may compensate with severe reflex tachycardia as well as with salt and water retention. Because of these compensations, a patient with cardiac disease may experience angina as a result of increased oxygen demand secondary to increased cardiac output or increased heart rate. Hydralazine works by increasing cyclic guanosine monophosphate, which induces smooth muscle relaxation. This smooth muscle relaxation occurs more in the arterioles than in the veins and thus reduces the afterload on the heart.

Answer B is incorrect. Hydralazine does not have any direct cardiotoxic effects. Many other drugs do, such as digoxin or theophylline, if given out of their therapeutic range.

Answer C is incorrect. Prazosin, an α-blocker, may cause first-dose orthostatic hypotension.

Answer D is incorrect. Hydralazine does not directly cause nephrotoxicity. The most common drug classes associated with nephrotoxicity include penicillins, cephalosporins, sulfonamides, and nonsteroidal anti-inflammatory drugs.

Answer E is incorrect. Pulmonary embolism (PE) typically occurs in the setting of preexisting risk factors such as surgery, extended periods of venous stasis in the lower extremities, pregnancy, or disease states such as malignancy or autoimmunity. Hydralazine treatment alone does not increase the risk for PE.

46. **The correct answer is B.** This is a Mobitz type II second-degree heart block. A defect in the His-Purkinje system is responsible for this type of heart block defect.

    Answer A is incorrect. In contrast to this patient's findings, atrioventricular nodal abnormalities lengthen the PR interval and are responsible for first-degree heart block and Mobitz type I second-degree heart block.

    Answer C is incorrect. Independently contracting atria and ventricles occur in the complete absence or ablation of the His-Purkinje system, not simply a defect in the system.

    Answer D is incorrect. Retrograde conductions would result in an increase in the number of P waves and a decrease in the PR interval.

    Answer E is incorrect. Sinoatrial nodal abnormalities are responsible for problems in automaticity and would not result in randomly dropped QRS complexes.

47. **The correct answer is A.** Fatal arrhythmias following an MI, also known as sudden cardiac death, are the most common cause of death in the first few hours following an infarction. Arrhythmias arc due to disruption of the conduction system and myocardial irritability following injury.

    Answer B is incorrect. Following MI, thrombus formation over the infarcted area of endocardium can lead to a left-sided embolism; however, this is not the most common cause of sudden cardiac death.

    Answer C is incorrect. Myocardial failure can lead to further complications, such as CHF and cardiogenic shock following an infarction. However, these complications rarely cause immediate death.

    Answer D is incorrect. Myocardial rupture is a complication that most commonly occurs 3–7 days after an infarction, due to the weakened wall strength of the damaged area. The ventricular free wall is the most likely site of rupture; this can lead to bleeding into the pericardial space, causing fatal cardiac tamponade. However, death due to myocardial rupture is unlikely to occur within hours of the ischemic episode.

    Answer E is incorrect. A ruptured papillary muscle is a possible complication of an infarction, but it most commonly occurs 3–7 days after the ischemic event. Thus, papillary muscle rupture would not cause immediate death.

48. **The correct answer is D.** Individuals with central retinal artery occlusion typically present with the acute onset of painless monocular visual loss that is usually the result of thromboembolic phenomena relating to vascular disease. However, since this patient is young and has no consistent prior medical history, one must consider other causes, which in this patient would almost certainly relate to her recent dental procedure, which can lead to bacteremia. In the setting of a murmur and bacteremia, the most likely cause of this patient's symptoms is a septic embolism that originated in the heart and has lodged in the central retinal artery. Unfortunately, even with treatment, <25% of patients regain useful vision in the affected eye.

    Answer A is incorrect. A large proportion of central retinal artery occlusions is secondary to thromboembolic phenomena originating from stenosed, atherosclerotic carotid arteries. However, given the history and this patient's lack of macrovascular disease, this is a less likely cause of the patient's occlusion.

    Answer B is incorrect. Central retinal artery occlusion may result from sequelae of collagen vascular disease, but this is a relatively infrequent cause and is unlikely given the lack of any history consistent with such a diagnosis.

    Answer C is incorrect. Although diabetes is a leading cause of microvascular disease, it is a rare cause of central retinal artery occlusion.

    Answer E is incorrect. Hypertensive crises would be more likely to result in bleeding than thromboembolic phenomena or other causes of central retinal artery occlusion.

49. **The correct answer is C.** Cardiac glycosides such as digoxin inhibit the Na^+-K^+-ATPase transport system to increase intracellular sodium concentration, which then increases intracellular calcium concentration via the sodium-calcium exchange carrier mechanism. This increased calcium level augments the calcium released to the myofilaments during excitation, resulting in a positive inotropic effect. Increased contractility of the heart directly increases cardiac output. Glycosides are largely not used today because of the advent of newer drugs that have fewer adverse effects; the outstanding exception is digoxin, which is still widely used to treat heart failure and atrial fibrillation.

Answer A is incorrect. β-Blockers inhibit sympathetic cardiac activation by blocking the activity of catecholamines on the heart, which causes a decrease in heart rate and a decreased cardiac output. These agents are specifically used in CHF to decrease myocardial energy use and oxygen demand.

Answer B is incorrect. Aortic stenosis increases afterload and causes the heart to work harder to produce optimum cardiac output, but would not increase it above normal ranges.

Answer D is incorrect. A decreased intracellular calcium level would decrease the contractility of the heart, resulting in decreased cardiac output.

Answer E is incorrect. Increased extracellular sodium levels would not increase cardiac output. Increasing cardiac output would require an increase in intracellular calcium levels released from the sarcoplasmic reticulum. This is done by increasing the calcium influx triggered by sodium channel activation. Increasing extracellular sodium concentrations would not affect sodium influx and thus would not lead to increase cardiac output.

50. **The correct answer is C.** Net filtration pressure is governed by the equation $P_{net} = [(P_c - P_i) - (p_c - p_i)]$, where P_c is capillary pressure, P_i is interstitial fluid pressure, p_c is plasma colloid osmotic pressure, and p_i is interstitial fluid colloid osmotic pressure. Increasing P_c, p_i, or the permeability of the capillaries will lead to a net flow of fluid from the capillaries to the interstitium. Likewise, decreasing p_c and P_i will also lead to net outward flow and edema.

Answer A is incorrect. Decreasing capillary permeability would result in fluid being trapped in the vascular space.

Answer B is incorrect. Decreased capillary pressure would decrease the amount of fluid in the interstitial space.

Answer D is incorrect. Increased interstitial fluid pressure would increase fluid flow back into the vascular space.

Answer E is incorrect. Increased plasma protein levels would cause an increase in fluid retention in the vascular space.

CHAPTER 9

Endocrine

1. A 42-year-old woman with a history of pernicious anemia comes to the physician complaining of increased anxiety, heart palpitations, heat intolerance, unexplained weight loss, and multiple daily bowel movements. She has not had a period in 4 months. On physical examination, the patient is found to have a goiter, a thyroid bruit, and mild exophthalmos. Laboratory studies show elevated triiodothyronine and free thyroxine levels, and an undetectable thyroid-stimulating hormone. Which of the following is the most likely etiology of this patient's disease?

(A) Autoimmune stimulation of thyroid-stimulating hormone receptors
(B) Idiopathic replacement of thyroid tissue with fibrous tissue
(C) Thyroid adenoma
(D) Thyroid hormone-producing ovarian teratoma
(E) Viral infection leading to destruction of thyroid tissue

2. A certain endocrine disorder can lead to an elevated blood pressure, decreased potassium levels, sodium and water retention, and decreased renin activity. Which of the following is the most likely diagnosis?

(A) Addison's disease
(B) Hyperthyroidism
(C) Pheochromocytoma
(D) Primary hyperaldosteronism
(E) Secondary hyperaldosteronism

3. A 59-year-old man with no prior medical history presents to the physician with marked hyperglycemia, diarrhea, and weight loss. A CT scan of the abdomen reveals a pancreatic mass. A trial period on an oral hypoglycemic agent has not helped reduce his glucose levels. His physical examination is significant for the rash shown in the image. Which of the following is the most likely diagnosis?

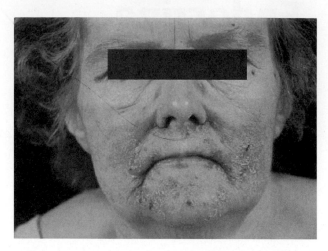

Reproduced, with permission, from Wolff K, Johnson RA, Suurmond D. *Fitzpatrick's Color Atlas & Synopsis of Clinical Dermatolgy*, 5th ed. New York: McGraw-Hill, 2005: Figure 17-12.

(A) Corticosteroid therapy
(B) Glucagonoma
(C) Insulinoma
(D) Type 1 diabetes mellitus
(E) VIPoma

4. A 5-year-old girl is brought to the pediatrician by her mother because she has noticed a single soft, nontender mass underneath her daughter's tongue. The physician reassures the mother that it is a common congenital ectopic anomaly that does not affect the function of the mass or the hormone it secretes. Hypersecretion of this hormone can cause which of the following conditions?

(A) Amenorrhea
(B) Cold intolerance
(C) Constipation
(D) Hyperlipidemia
(E) Weight gain

5. A 60-year-old patient from an underserved indigent family sees a physician and complains of years of polydipsia, polyuria, polyphagia, and

worsening fatigue and weight loss. Urinalysis reveals severe proteinuria, and a renal biopsy is ultimately performed, with a typical histologic section shown in the image. Which of the following histological findings is apparent in the renal tissue?

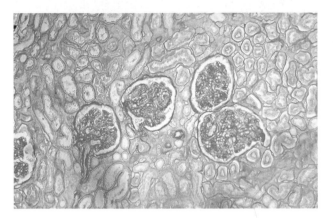

Reproduced, with permission, from PEIR Digital Library (http://peir.net).

(A) Bence Jones proteins
(B) Crescent formation
(C) Hyaline arteriolosclerosis
(D) Nodular glomerulosclerosis
(E) Wire loop abnormality

6. A 34-year-old man with moderately severe ulcerative colitis has been taking oral prednisone for 4 months. Which of the following symptoms is the most likely adverse effect of this drug?

(A) Diabetes insipidus
(B) Diabetes mellitus
(C) Hyperpigmentation of the skin
(D) Hypotension
(E) Muscle hypertrophy
(F) Sodium wasting

7. A 45-year-old man with type 2 diabetes mellitus undergoes a neurologic examination. The patient is unable to sense the vibration produced by a tuning fork placed on his big toe. Which of the following receptors is most likely affected in this patient?

(A) Krause end bulbs
(B) Meissner's corpuscle
(C) Merkel nerve endings
(D) Pacinian corpuscle
(E) Ruffini corpuscle

8. A 53-year-old woman with newly diagnosed type 2 diabetes presents to the emergency department complaining of vomiting, severe headache, dizziness, blurry vision, and difficulty breathing. She says that she had been at a cocktail party when the symptoms began. Her skin is notably flushed on physical examination. Which of the following medications is responsible for this reaction?

(A) Acarbose
(B) Glipizide
(C) Glyburide
(D) Metformin
(E) Tolbutamide
(F) Troglitazone

9. A 25-year-old man comes to the emergency department after experiencing tremors. He appears visibly anxious and relates a recent history of sweats, nausea, vomiting, and lightheadedness. Laboratory studies show a blood glucose level of 50 mg/dL. An abdominal CT scan shows a 1.5-cm mass in the head of the pancreas. Surgical resection of this mass will necessitate ligation of branches from which of the following vascular structures?

(A) The gastroduodenal and inferior mesenteric arteries
(B) The gastroduodenal and superior mesenteric arteries
(C) The left gastric and inferior mesenteric arteries
(D) The left gastric and superior mesenteric arteries
(E) The proper hepatic and inferior mesenteric arteries
(F) The proper hepatic and superior mesenteric arteries

10. A 36-year-old woman presents to the physician with amenorrhea. She reports an increase in her ring and shoe sizes over the past year, increased sweating, and increased fatigue. Physical examination shows a blood pressure of 150/90 mm Hg and coarse facial features with mild macroglossia. Which of the following is most appropriate for this patient?

(A) Finasteride
(B) Leuprolide
(C) Octreotide
(D) Recombinant growth hormone
(E) Somatrem

11. A 23-year-old man comes to the physician because of intermittent severe headaches, anxiety, and heart palpitations. While he has no significant medical history, his uncle had similar symptoms. When probed for a deeper family history, he says that his mother and two cousins have had their thyroids removed. Which of the following conditions most likely accounts for the clinical scenario?

(A) Acromegaly
(B) ACTH-secreting pituitary adenoma
(C) Hyperparathyroidism
(D) Nonfunctioning pituitary adenoma
(E) Pheochromocytoma

12. Growth hormone is essential to normal human growth and development, and its secretion is tightly regulated via a feedback control system involving the hypothalamus, the pituitary gland, and the peripheral tissues. Which of the following is a stimulus for the secretion of growth hormone?

(A) Hypoglycemia
(B) Obesity
(C) Pregnancy
(D) Somatomedin excess
(E) Somatostatin therapy

13. The product of the cells shown in this image induces a rise in serum calcium levels. Which of the following types of cells are indicated by the arrows in this image?

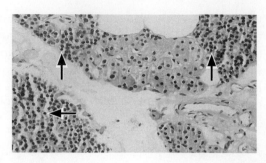

Image courtesy of Armed Forces Institute of Pathology.

(A) Adipocytes
(B) Parathyroid chief cells
(C) Parathyroid oxyphil cells
(D) Thyroid C cells
(E) Thyroid follicle cells

14. A 66-year-old man with chronic cough, dyspnea, and a 50-pack-year history of cigarette smoking comes to the clinic after noticing blood in his sputum. He says he feels lethargic and has lost 18 kg (40 lb) over the past 3 months with no changes in diet or exercise. Laboratory studies show a serum sodium level of 120 mEq/L. While awaiting CT, the patient suffers a seizure and is rushed to the emergency department. Which of the following is most likely to be elevated in this patient?

(A) ACTH
(B) ADH
(C) Parathyroid hormone
(D) Renin
(E) Tumor necrosis factor-α

15. A 65-year-old woman comes to her primary care physician complaining of progressive weakness and fatigue. On further questioning, she notes a recent weight gain and constipation as well as constant subjective chills. Physical examination shows a moderate nontender goiter. A biopsy shows a lymphocytic infiltrate. Which of the following best describes this patient's thyroid-stimulating hormone (TSH) and thyroid hormone levels relative to normal baseline values?

Choice	Thyroid-Stimulating Hormone	Total Thyroxine	Free Thyroxine
A	↑	↑	↑
B	↑	↓	↑
C	↑	↓	↓
D	↓	↓	↑
E	↓	↓	↓

(A) A
(B) B
(C) C
(D) D
(E) E

16. A 27-year-old woman presents to a new physician with muscle cramping and spasm. On physical examination, the physician notes shortened fourth and fifth metacarpals and metatarsals, short stature, a round face, and abnormal teeth. Her facial muscles twitched when her facial nerve was tapped, and her wrist twitched with the use of a blood pressure cuff. Laboratory studies show a decreased serum calcium level and a significantly elevated parathyroid hormone level. There is no evidence of renal disease, thus decreasing the likelihood of renal osteodystrophy. Which of the following is the most common mode of inheritance of this patient's disease?

(A) Autosomal dominant
(B) Autosomal recessive
(C) Mitochondrial
(D) X-linked dominant
(E) X-linked recessive

17. A 43-year-old woman presents with fatigue, a 4.5-kg (9.9-lb) weight gain over the past 3 months, cold intolerance, hair loss, and con-centration problems. Physical examination is significant for dry, coarse skin and bradycardia. She states that she had some slight swelling of her lower neck several months ago, which resolved without treatment. Results of antithyroglobulin antibody and antinuclear antibody tests are negative, but a thyroid peroxidase antibody test is positive. What other autoimmune diseases will this patient most likely have?

(A) Graves' disease and pernicious anemia
(B) Osteoarthritis and Addison's disease
(C) Rheumatoid arthritis and vitiligo
(D) Type 1 diabetes mellitus and celiac disease
(E) Whipple's disease and type 1 diabetes mellitus

18. A 45-year-old man comes to his primary care physician complaining of back pain. On questioning, the patient indicates a recent history of polyuria, polydipsia, hypertension, and weight gain. X-ray of the spine shows an L4-L5 compression fracture. Which of the following is most likely to be elevated in this patient?

(A) Cortisol
(B) Glucagon
(C) Growth hormone
(D) Insulin
(E) Thyroid hormones

19. A 60-year-old woman with a history of type 2 diabetes mellitus comes to the clinic for a follow-up examination after being placed on a new agent to help her achieve tighter glycemic control. She complains that she has suffered occasional abdominal cramps and diarrhea, adding that she has recently been experiencing increased flatulence, which has become an embarrassing nuisance. Which of the following agents best accounts for this patient's complaints?

(A) Acarbose
(B) Chlorpropamide
(C) Glipizide
(D) Metformin
(E) Orlistat
(F) Troglitazone

20. A 42-year-old man comes to the physician with loss of vision in the lateral periphery on both sides as well as decreased libido. On physical examination his features appear coarser and larger than in a photograph taken 1 year ago, and he states that his glove size and shoe size have changed over the past year as well. His MRI is shown in the image. Which of the following is the most likely diagnosis?

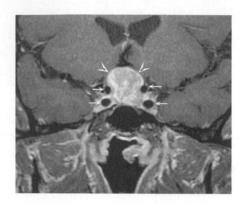

Reproduced, with permission, from Fauci AS, Braunwald E, Kasper DL, Hauser SL, Longo DL, Jameson JL, and Isselbacher KJ, eds. *Harrison's Principles of Internal Medicine*, 17th ed. New York: McGraw-Hill, 2008: Figure 333-4.

(A) ACTH-secreting pituitary adenoma
(B) Growth hormone-secreting pituitary adenoma
(C) Luteinizing hormone- and follicle-stimulating hormone-secreting pituitary adenoma
(D) Prolactin-secreting pituitary adenoma
(E) Thyroid-stimulating hormone-secreting pituitary adenoma

21. A 39-year-old woman is seen by a physician because of a lump in the front of her neck. Physical examination reveals a swollen thyroid gland. A biopsy of the enlarged but painless thyroid gland is found to contain psammoma bodies and thin projections of epithelium surrounding a fibrovascular core. The nuclei of many cells are optically clear. Which of the following risk factors is most commonly associated with her diagnosis?

(A) Chronic cigarette smoking
(B) Preexisting Graves' disease
(C) Presence of HLA-DR5 receptors
(D) Prior radiotherapy to the head or neck
(E) Recent pregnancy

22. Glucocorticoids are important in the treatment of inflammatory diseases; however, their use is associated with many adverse effects on multiple systems. The utility of glucocorticoids has to be weighed against the patient's ability to withstand the problems that are likely to arise. High-dosage glucocorticoid treatment can result in which ECG changes?

(A) Appearance of delta wave
(B) Appearance of U wave
(C) Peaked T wave
(D) PR segment elongation
(E) ST segment elevation

23. Surgery is planned to excise a hyperfunctioning adrenal adenoma from a patient with primary hyperaldosteronism. On CT scan of the abdomen, the adenoma is visible as a 4-cm mass just superior to the right kidney. In order to immediately relieve the patient's hyperaldosteronism, the surgeon must first ligate the primary venous drainage of the tumor. The primary venous drainage flows directly into which of the following structures?

(A) Abdominal aorta
(B) Inferior vena cava
(C) Portal vein
(D) Right gonadal vein
(E) Right renal vein

24. A 54-year-old man with a history of smoking and lung cancer develops hypercalcemia. He is enrolled in a research study to assess the efficacy of a new synthetic agent to treat this condition. After several days of treatment, he reports persistent numbness and tingling around his mouth. Physical examination is significant for facial spasm when the jaw is tapped and carpal spasm when the blood pressure cuff is inflated. Which of the following was most likely used to treat his hypercalcemia?

(A) Calcitonin
(B) Parathyroid hormone
(C) Parathyroid hormone-related peptide
(D) Thyroxine
(E) Vitamin D

25. A 34-year-old African-American woman presents to the physician with abdominal cramping that worsens during her menstrual period. The patient also says that her periods often last for more than 7 days. An ultrasound study shows multiple masses on the patient's uterus. Which of the following immunohistochemical stains would be the most appropriate for diagnosing this patient's condition?

(A) Cytokeratin
(B) Desmin
(C) Glial fibrillary acid proteins
(D) Neurofilament
(E) Vimentin

26. A 34-year-old woman goes to her primary care physician complaining of a recent feeling that "her heart was racing" and visual changes. During the interview, the physician notices that the patient is clearly anxious. During the review of systems, the patient reveals a recent unintentional 4-kg (8.8-lb) weight loss. On physical examination, the physician notes that the patient is tachycardic and has 2+ nonpitting edema in her lower extremities. Which of the following is the most likely etiology of this disease?

(A) Autoantibodies to the thyroid-stimulating hormone receptor
(B) Circulating antibodies to thyroid peroxidase and thyroglobulin
(C) Hyperfunctioning thyroid nodule
(D) Iodine deficiency
(E) Reaction to radiation

27. An 18-year-old woman is referred to a specialist because her periods have stopped. She reports occasional bouts of nausea, vomiting, and generalized weakness. Her blood pressure is 160/99 mm Hg; laboratory studies show a serum K+ level of 2.2 mEq/L. This patient suffers from a condition that affects the production of

two of the three adrenal hormones, leaving only one functioning hormone. In which area of the adrenal gland is this one hormone produced?

(A) Capsule
(B) Medulla
(C) Zona fasciculata
(D) Zona glomerulosa
(E) Zona reticularis

28. A 66-year-old man comes to the emergency department because of weight loss, hypotension, and hyperpigmented skin. Laboratory tests show decreased serum levels of sodium, chloride, and cortisol, but increased serum levels of potassium and ACTH. Additionally, the urinary level of 17-hydroxypregnenolone is decreased. Which of the following most likely explains this patient's symptoms and laboratory values?

(A) Autoimmune destruction of the adrenal glands
(B) Cortisol-secreting adrenal adenoma
(C) Ectopic ACTH production
(D) Hemochromatosis
(E) Pituitary corticotropin insufficiency

29. The predominant cells in this photomicrograph from the adrenal medulla secrete which of the following hormones into the bloodstream?

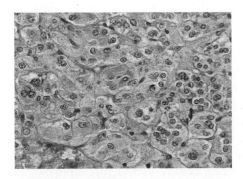

Image courtesy of Armed Forces Institute of Pathology.

(A) Aldosterone
(B) Androgens
(C) Cortisol
(D) Norepinephrine

30. A researcher investigating the action of thyroid hormones wants to develop an assay to analyze the activity of this hormone in various tissues. Which of the following strategies would be most effective in determining the level of activity of these hormones in a tissue sample?

    (A) Assessing cAMP levels
    (B) Assessing intracellular calcium levels
    (C) Assessing Na^+/K^+-ATPase mRNA levels
    (D) Assessing phospholipase C activity
    (E) Assessing phosphorylation of insulin receptor substrate 1

31. A 25-year-old woman presents to a primary care clinic complaining of galactorrhea, loss of libido, and vision changes. Further work-up reveals a mass in the sella turcica. Which of the following functions will most likely be preserved with normal functioning in this individual?

    (A) Free water resorption
    (B) Menstruation
    (C) Ovulation
    (D) Salt retention
    (E) Thyroid hormone production

32. A 24-year-old woman who has never been pregnant presents to her physician with galactorrhea. Her past medical history is significant for hypercalcemia and recurrent duodenal ulcers. Maternal family members have been diagnosed with a variety of tumors. Which of the following is the genetic inheritance pattern of this patient's disorder?

    (A) Autosomal dominant
    (B) Autosomal recessive
    (C) Mitochondrial
    (D) X-linked dominant
    (E) X-linked recessive

33. A 28-year-old man with a history of hypothyroidism comes to the physician because of a 3-day history of abdominal pain, diarrhea, palpitations, and fatigue. Physical examination is remarkable only for tachycardia. Which of the following medications most likely accounts for this patient's presentation?

    (A) Dobutamine
    (B) Iodide
    (C) Leuprolide
    (D) Levothyroxine
    (E) Propylthiouracil

34. A 22-year-old woman complains of recent-onset polydipsia and polyuria. She has no recent head trauma or known intracranial tumor. A recent blood test reveals that her plasma ADH levels are normal. Her plasma osmolarity is 290 mOsm/L, and her urine flow rate is 10 mL/min. If this patient has nephrogenic diabetes insipidus, which of the following urine osmolarity values most closely reflects her condition?

    (A) 100 mOsm/L
    (B) 290 mOsm/L
    (C) 350 mOsm/L
    (D) 425 mOsm/L
    (E) 1000 mOsm/L

35. An agitated and confused 44-year-old man is brought to the emergency department after collapsing at his office. The patient has a history of diabetes mellitus and was recently diagnosed with hypertension. He is conscious when the emergency medical team arrives and complains of fatigue and dizziness but denies any chest pain, palpitations, shortness of breath, sweating, fever, or chills. His diabetes has been poorly controlled with glyburide, and his most recent HbA1c was 8.5%. He is unable to recall the name of his antihypertensive drug. Which of the following agents is most likely responsible for this patient's condition?

    (A) Enalapril
    (B) Hydralazine
    (C) Hydrochlorothiazide
    (D) Propranolol
    (E) Triamterene

36. A 33-year-old woman with diabetes mellitus presents to the physician with loss of vision in both eyes. On physical examination, she is noted to be of tall stature with a lantern jaw, a prominent nose, and supraorbital ridges. She reports excessive sweating and a progressive in-

crease in her ring size. An MRI shows a mass at the base of the patient's brain; a biopsy is performed. Which of the following describes how this biopsied mass would most likely appear on staining?

(A) Acidophilic
(B) Basophilic
(C) Chromophobic
(D) Mixed acidophilic and basophilic
(E) Mixed basophilic and chromophobic

37. A patient undergoes successful thyroidectomy for Graves' disease and returns to a euthyroid state with the use of levothyroxine supplementation. In a follow-up examination, the patient reports resolution of all prior symptoms except for anxiety and irritability. She also reports frequent muscle spasms. On physical examination, tapping over the facial nerve elicits facial muscle spasm. An ECG shows QT prolongation. Which of the following most likely describes the current laboratory values of this patient?

Choice	Calcium	Phosphate	Parathyroid Hormone
A	↑	↓	↑
B	↑	↓	↓
C	↓	↑	↑
D	↓	↑	↓
E	Normal	Normal	Normal

(A) A
(B) B
(C) C
(D) D
(E) E

38. A 63-year-old patient using medication to control type 2 diabetes mellitus undergoes an arterial blood gas study that show the following results:

pH: 7.25
Po_2: 90 mm Hg
Pco_2: 28 mm Hg
HCO_3^-: 15 mEq/L
Anion gap: 20 mEq/L

Which of the following agents is the most likely cause of the abnormal blood gas findings?

(A) Acarbose
(B) Glipizide
(C) Metformin
(D) Pioglitazone
(E) Tolbutamide

39. A 65-year-old man comes to the physician because he awakens to urinate several times per night and has developed problems starting and stopping his stream of urine. A biopsy of the prostate shows enlargement and dilation of the prostatic glands but no dysplasia. Which of the following is the most appropriate pharmacological treatment for this patient?

(A) Finasteride
(B) Flutamide
(C) Ketoconazole
(D) Spironolactone
(E) Yohimbine

40. Steroid hormones are unique in that they enter the cell and act directly on the DNA to effect change, rather than acting only through intermediary proteins. Which of the following steps in the steroid hormone mechanism is the last step necessary before DNA binding within the nucleus?

(A) Hormone binding to a hormone-specific globulin in plasma
(B) Hormone binding to a membrane receptor
(C) Hormone binding to DNA enhancer element
(D) Hormone binding to intracellular receptor
(E) Transformation of the hormone-receptor complex

41. A white, 5-year-old, thin boy is brought to the physician complaining of recent weight loss accompanied by excessive hunger, thirst, and urination. His urine is positive for high levels of ketones and glucose. Which of following is the most likely mechanism and associated findings in this disease?

    (A) A deficiency of a brush border enzyme of the intestinal mucosal cells, causing an inability to break down all of the normally digested carbohydrates
    (B) An autoimmune process and an association with human leukocyte antigens DR3 and DR4
    (C) An autoimmune process associated with human leukocyte antigen B27
    (D) An increase in the body's resistance to insulin; association with obesity

42. A 56-year-old woman who has type 2 diabetes mellitus with recent onset hypertension comes to her physician because of a rash, changes in taste, and a mild cough. Physical examination shows patchy areas of edema throughout her body. Which of the following medications is the most likely cause of this patient's signs and symptoms?

    (A) Captopril
    (B) Hydrochlorothiazide
    (C) Losartan
    (D) Nifedipine
    (E) Propranolol

43. A 19-year-old female college student presents with rapid onset of malaise, myalgias, vomiting, photophobia, and a temperature of 39.8° C (103.6° F). Because she quickly develops leg pains along with a purpuric rash, she is transferred from university health services to a local hospital, where she is found to have a blood pressure of 82/49 mm Hg after receiving 2 L intravenous normal saline. Physical examination reveals positive Kernig's and Brudzinski's signs, a petechial rash on her lower extremity, and diffuse abdominal tenderness. Her arterial oxygen pressure is 58 mm Hg, platelet count is 81,000/mm³, International Normalized Ratio is 2.1, and D-dimer levels are elevated at 41,000 ng/mL. Cerebrospinal fluid shows 1300 WBCs/mm³ and 10 RBCs/mm³. Gram stain shows multiple gram-negative diplococci. Which aspect of this disease process most likely contributes to her hypotension, vomiting, and diffuse abdominal tenderness?

    (A) Bilateral adrenal hemorrhage
    (B) Disseminated intravascular coagulation
    (C) Hypoxemia
    (D) Meningitis
    (E) Viral gastroenteritis

44. A 65-year-old man with small cell lung cancer is receiving treatment for ectopic production of ADH. After beginning demeclocycline, he produces large volumes of dilute urine and drinks copious amounts of water. The patient is instructed to not drink any fluid for a 12-hour period. Despite the hold on fluids, the patient continues to produce dilute urine. ADH levels are increased, and serum hyperosmolarity and hypernatremia are noted. Which of the following is the most likely diagnosis?

    (A) Nephrogenic diabetes insipidus secondary to demeclocycline treatment
    (B) Neurogenic diabetes insipidus secondary to metastatic cancer
    (C) Primary hyperaldosteronism
    (D) Syndrome of inappropriate ADH secretion
    (E) Type 2 diabetes mellitus

45. A patient with osteodystrophy of chronic renal disease has abnormal activity of the large cell shown in the image. Which of the following hormones plays a key role in stimulating activity of this cell?

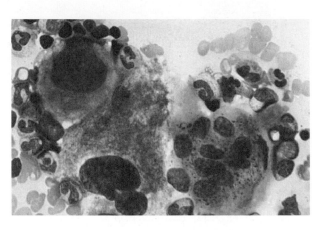

Reproduced, with permission, from Lichtman MA, Beutler E, Kipps TJ, Seligsohn U, Kaushansky K, Prchal JF. *Williams Hematology*, 7th ed. New York: McGraw-Hill, 2006: Plate XV-1.

(A) Angiotensin II
(B) Calcitonin
(C) Parathyroid hormone
(D) Renin
(E) Thyroid hormone

46. A 55-year-old woman presents to her doctor with feelings of fatigue, increased appetite, increased sweating, and palpitations. Physical examination is unremarkable except for exophthalmos. She receives pharmacologic treatment for her condition, but soon develops a fever and multiple infections in her throat and gastrointestinal tract. Her doctor quickly discontinues the medication. Which medication was she most likely prescribed?

(A) Folic acid
(B) Levothyroxine
(C) Propranolol
(D) Propylthiouracil
(E) Radioactive iodine

47. A 54-year-old woman presents to the physician with diabetes mellitus, osteoporosis, and hypertension. She has noted a recent weight gain and abdominal striae. Laboratory studies show a decreased ACTH level. A single mass is noted adjacent to the right kidney on abdominal CT scan. Neither low- nor high-dose dexamethasone suppresses the patient's cortisol production. Which of the following is the most likely explanation for these findings?

(A) Adrenal adenoma
(B) Bilateral adrenal hyperplasia
(C) Ectopic ACTH secretion
(D) Exogenous corticosteroid administration
(E) Pituitary adenoma

48. A 60-year-old woman with a 55-pack-year history of smoking presents to the emergency department with nausea and vomiting, headache, malaise, and diffuse aches. A CT scan shows a solitary nodule in the right upper lobe of the lung. Laboratory studies are significant for a serum calcium level of 14.2 mg/dL, a serum phosphate level of 1.5 mg/dL, and a serum alkaline phosphatase activity of 81 U/L. The factors that account for this patient's laboratory findings act primarily at which of the following locations?

(A) Adrenal cortex and intestines
(B) Adrenal cortex and renal tubules
(C) Intestines and bones
(D) Renal tubules and bones
(E) Renal tubules and pancreas

49. A researcher studying type 2 diabetes mellitus is inducing insulin resistance in normal mice. Inhibition of which of the following would produce this effect?

(A) Adenylate cyclase
(B) Guanylate cyclase
(C) Serine kinases
(D) Threonine kinases
(E) Tyrosine kinases

50. A 48-year-old man with a history of thyroid carcinoma for which he underwent thyroidectomy 5 years ago presents to his primary care physician complaining of a 6-week history of intermittent palpitations, diaphoresis, headaches, and anxiousness. His blood pressure is 180/90 mm Hg and heart rate is 135/min. After a complete workup, the patient is diagnosed with a pheochromocytoma, and his physician recommends surgery. Which of the following is the most appropriate preoperative management for this patient?

(A) α-Blockade followed by β-blockade
(B) β-Blockade followed by α-blockade
(C) Levothyroxine
(D) Prednisone
(E) Propylthiouracil

1. The correct answer is A. This patient presents as a classic case of Graves' disease. In Graves' disease, thyroid-stimulating IgG antibodies bind to TSH receptors and lead to thyroid hormone production. This causes glandular hyperplasia and enlargement characteristic of the goiter associated with Graves' disease. Graves' disease is the most common cause of thyrotoxicosis. Patients with this condition may have other autoimmune diseases, such as pernicious anemia or type 1 diabetes mellitus, and frequently present with anxiety, irritability, tremor, heat intolerance with sweaty skin, tachycardia and cardiac palpitations, weight loss, increased appetite, fine hair, diarrhea, and amenorrhea or oligomenorrhea. Signs include diffuse goiter, proptosis, periorbital edema, and thickened skin on the lower extremities. Laboratory values reveal increased thyroid hormone levels and decreased TSH levels.

Answer B is incorrect. Idiopathic replacement of thyroid and surrounding tissue with fibrous tissue is seen in Riedel's thyroiditis; patients may present with dysphagia, stridor, dyspnea, and hypothyroidism, although more than 50% of patients are euthyroid. The disease can mimic thyroid carcinoma, which is high on the list of differential diagnoses for a patient with Riedel's thyroiditis.

Answer C is incorrect. Most thyroid adenomas present as solitary nodules and are usually nonfunctional.

Answer D is incorrect. Thyroid hormone-producing ovarian teratomas are known as struma ovarii, a tumor consisting of thyroid tissue. These tumors can cause hyperthyroidism, but given the patient's history of autoimmune disease, Graves' disease is the better answer choice.

Answer E is incorrect. Viral infections such as mumps or coxsackievirus can lead to destruction of thyroid tissue and granulomatous inflammation, as seen in subacute granulomatous thyroiditis. Patients typically present with flu-like symptoms and thyroid tenderness and pain. The disease is typically self-limited and can include a transient hyperthyroid state.

2. The correct answer is D. Primary hyperaldosteronism is most commonly caused by an aldosterone-producing adenoma of the adrenal gland. It can also be found in patients with zona glomerulosa hyperplasia. The increased levels of aldosterone lead to hypertension, increased sodium and water retention, and the associated increase in excretion of potassium leading to hypokalemia. Increased blood pressure and aldosterone levels produce negative feedback to the kidneys, resulting in a decreased level of serum renin. Serum renin levels help differentiate between primary hyperaldosteronism, with increased aldosterone and decreased renin levels, and secondary hyperaldosteronism, with increased aldosterone levels and increased renin levels.

Answer A is incorrect. Addison's disease results from adrenal atrophy and causes hypofunction of the adrenal glands. Patients with Addison's disease display signs that are the opposite of those seen in hyperaldosteronism, including hypotension, hyponatremia, and hyperkalemia.

Answer B is incorrect. Patients with hyperthyroidism have heat intolerance, hyperactivity, weight loss, chest pain/palpitations, arrhythmias, diarrhea, hyperreflexia, fine hair, and warm, moist skin.

Answer C is incorrect. Patients with pheochromocytoma have increased levels of epinephrine and norepinephrine, which can lead to elevated blood pressure; however, sodium, potassium, and renin levels are not affected.

Answer E is incorrect. Lab values in secondary hyperaldosteronism would show hypernatremia and hypokalemia with an increase in renin levels. Secondary hyperaldosteronism occurs in settings in which the kidneys perceive low intravascular volume (renal artery stenosis, chronic renal failure, chronic heart failure, cirrhosis), resulting in an overactive renin-angiotensin system that acts as a stimulus for aldosterone secretion.

3. **The correct answer is B.** This patient has symptoms of a glucagonoma, a rare glucagon-secreting tumor that can cause hyperglycemia, diarrhea, and weight loss. The hyperglycemia seen in these patients will not respond to oral hypoglycemic agents because of the uncontrolled excess glucagon production that continues despite increased insulin levels. Glucagonomas are also associated with necrolytic migratory erythema, a skin rash consisting of painful, pruritic erythematous papules that blister, erode, and crust over.

Answer A is incorrect. Corticosteroid therapy can cause hyperglycemia; however, it is not the best answer choice for this question because it does not satisfactorily explain this patient's pancreatic mass and rash.

Answer C is incorrect. An insulinoma would cause hypoglycemia and not hyperglycemia.

Answer D is incorrect. It is unlikely that a 59-year-old man would present with type 1 diabetes mellitus. Furthermore, the pancreatic mass and rash cannot be explained by the diagnosis of diabetes mellitus.

Answer E is incorrect. Although VIPomas can cause diarrhea, hyperglycemia, and a pancreatic mass on CT scan, the rash cannot be explained by a diagnosis of VIPoma.

4. **The correct answer is A.** Usually, the thyroid gland develops beneath the tongue, descends along the thyroglossal duct, and eventually resides anterior to the trachea in the neck. Ectopic thyroid tissue may be found anywhere along the course of the duct, including its place of origin: beneath the tongue. This is a common congenital anomaly that does not affect thyroid function, and it should not be removed. Hypersecretion of thyroxine (T_4) from the ectopic gland can result in menstrual abnormalities, including amenorrhea and oligomenorrhea.

Answer B is incorrect. Cold intolerance is characteristic of hypothyroidism, which is a de-

creased secretion of T_4 from the thyroid gland. Hypersecretion of T_4 would cause heat intolerance, not cold.

Answer C is incorrect. Constipation is characteristic of hypothyroidism, which is a decreased secretion of T_4 from the thyroid gland. Hypersecretion of T_4 is not associated with constipation.

Answer D is incorrect. Hyperlipidemia is characteristic of hypothyroidism, which is a decreased secretion of T_4 from the thyroid gland. Hypersecretion of T_4 is not associated with hyperlipidemia.

Answer E is incorrect. Weight gain is characteristic of hypothyroidism, which is a decreased secretion of T_4 from the thyroid gland. Hypersecretion of T_4 is associated with hypermetabolism and weight loss, not weight gain.

5. **The correct answer is D.** The vignette is a classic case of a patient with type 2 diabetes mellitus: polydipsia, polyuria, and polyphagia in an individual >40 years old. This condition is due to increased resistance to insulin. The image shows nodular glomerulosclerosis, also known as Kimmelstiel-Wilson glomerulosclerosis. This represents the accumulation of nodules in the mesangial matrix, which is pathognomonic for diabetes mellitus. Kidneys of diabetic patients also show increased basement membrane thickness and diffuse mesangial matrix proliferation.

Answer A is incorrect. Bence-Jones proteins are not a histological feature. They are free immunoglobulin light chains found in the urine of patients with multiple myeloma. However, multiple myeloma can cause pathological change in the kidney through renal amyloidosis, in which eosinophilic amyloid deposits are found in the subendothelium and mesangium. The protein is best seen when stained with Congo red. Areas of positive staining are birefringent when viewed with polarized light.

Answer B is incorrect. Crescent formation results from a proliferation of Bowman's capsule epithelial cells, which appear to "crowd out" the glomerular tufts. It is classically seen in nephritic syndromes and suggests a poor prognosis.

Answer C is incorrect. Hyaline arteriolosclerosis is a homogeneous, eosinophilic thickening of arteriolar walls, producing a narrowed vessel lumen. It is a feature of benign nephrosclerosis seen in longstanding hypertension, which is a common cause of chronic renal failure. The image shown is of a glomerulus, not a renal arteriole.

Answer E is incorrect. The wire loop abnormality is characteristic of type 4 lupus nephropathy. It is caused by thickening of the glomerular basement membrane associated with immune complex deposition.

6. **The correct answer is B.** This patient is at risk for prednisone-induced Cushing's syndrome. Cushing's syndrome is associated with diabetes mellitus, which can be an adverse effect of chronic corticosteroid use owing to decreased glucose tolerance and the counterregulatory action of the hormone. Glucocorticoids increase the glucose production by the liver in part by stimulating gluconeogenesis, and also by stimulating proteolysis in the skeletal muscle and releasing glucogenic amino acids into the vasculature.

Answer A is incorrect. Diabetes mellitus, not diabetes insipidus, is an adverse effect of corticosteroids, owing to decreased glucose tolerance and the counterregulatory action of the hormone. Diabetes insipidus can develop due to either pituitary dysfunction (i.e., Sheehan's syndrome) or failure of kidneys to respond to circulating ADH (i.e., renal disease).

Answer C is incorrect. Hyperpigmentation of the skin may develop in a patient with Cushing's disease due to primary pituitary adenoma hypersecretion of ACTH. Elevated ACTH can result in skin hyperpigmentation because of its melanocyte properties. This patient is receiving exogenous corticosteroids; thus, his ACTH levels should be decreased from negative feedback inhibition, and skin hyperpigmentation should not occur.

Answer D is incorrect. Hypertension, not hypotension, is an adverse effect of corticosteroids.

This side effect is due to the mineralocorticoid properties of steroids, which lead to increased sodium retention and hence to hypertension.

Answer E is incorrect. Muscle wasting, not muscle hypertrophy, usually develops in Cushing's syndrome due to the catabolic effects of cortisol.

Answer F is incorrect. Sodium retention, not sodium wasting, can be an adverse effect of chronic corticosteroid treatment.

7. **The correct answer is D.** The sensory receptors responsible for transducing the sensation of vibration, pressure, and tension are the large, encapsulated pacinian corpuscles, which are located in the deeper layers of the skin, ligaments, and joint capsules. They can be distinguished histologically by their onionlike appearance on cross section. This patient is presenting with one of the complications of diabetes, neuropathy, and since pacinian corpuscles are responsible for transducing vibratory stimuli, it is these receptors that are involved in this patient's presentation.

Answer A is incorrect. Kraus end bulbs are sensory receptors found in the oropharynx and conjunctiva of the eye.

Answer B is incorrect. Meissner's corpuscles, which are responsible for conveying the sensation of light touch, are small encapsulated sensory receptors found just beneath the dermis of hairless skin, most prominently in the fingertips, soles of the feet, and lips. Meissner's corpuscles are involved in the reception of light discriminatory touch, not vibratory sensation, as is being tested in this case.

Answer C is incorrect. Merkel nerve endings are nonencapsulated and found in all skin types (both hairy and hairless) and, along with Meissner's corpuscles, are believed to be responsible for discriminatory touch.

Answer E is incorrect. Ruffini corpuscles are spindle-shaped, encapsulated mechanoreceptors that are found in the soles of the feet and are responsible for transducing pressure.

8. **The correct answer is E.** This patient had a disulfiramlike reaction after drinking alcohol at a cocktail party. Of the diabetes medications listed, only tolbutamide is associated with causing a disulfiramlike reaction after alcohol consumption. Tolbutamide is a sulfonylurea antidiabetic agent. Sulfonylureas lower blood glucose in patients with type 2 diabetes by directly stimulating the release of insulin from the pancreas. They do this by binding to the sulfonylurea receptor on the β islet cell, leading to the inhibition of potassium ion efflux, cell depolarization, subsequent opening of voltage-gated calcium channels, and calcium influx, which triggers the release of preformed insulin. Other drugs known to cause a disulfiramlike reaction include metronidazole, quinacrine, griseofulvin, and chloramphenicol, as well as some cephalosporins including cefamandole and cefoperazone.

Answer A is incorrect. Acarbose is an α-glucosidase inhibitor that may cause gastrointestinal disturbances. It does not cause disulfiramlike reactions. α-Glucosidases are attached to the intestinal brush border and acarbose will reduce the postprandial digestion and absorption of starch and disaccharides.

Answer B is incorrect. Glipizide and glyburide are second-generation sulfonylureas that may cause hypoglycemia, but they do not cause disulfiramlike reactions.

Answer C is incorrect. Glyburide and glipizide are second-generation sulfonylureas that may cause hypoglycemia, but they do not cause disulfiramlike reactions. Glyburide and glipizide are second-generation sulfonylureas that may cause hypoglycemia, but they do not cause disulfiramlike reactions. The mechanism of action of sulfonylureas is primarily to increase insulin release from the pancreas. However, two additional mechanisms of action have been proposed (1) a reduction of serum glucagon and (2) closure of potassium channels in extrapancreatic tissues.

Answer D is incorrect. A full explanation of the mechanism of action of metformin remains elusive. However the blood glucose-lowering action of metformin does not depend on the presence of functioning pancreatic β cells.

Answer F is incorrect. Troglitazone is a glitazone that may cause weight gain. It does not cause disulfiramlike reactions. Troglitazone is a glitazone or thiazolidinedione that may cause weight gain. It does not cause disulfiramlike reactions. As a drug class, thiazolidinediones are ligands of peroxisome proliferator-activated receptor-γ (PPAR-γ) that decrease insulin resistance. PPAR-γ receptors are nuclear receptors that modulate the expression of the genes involved in lipid and glucose metabolism.

9. **The correct answer is B.** The head of the pancreas and the duodenum share a dual blood supply from the gastroduodenal artery, a branch of the celiac trunk. This artery supplies the anterior and posterior superior pancreaticoduodenal arteries as well as the superior mesenteric artery, which supplies the anterior and posterior inferior pancreaticoduodenal arteries. Therefore, to resect any portion of the duodenum or the head of the pancreas, branches from both the gastroduodenal and superior mesenteric arteries must be ligated.

Answer A is incorrect. While the gastroduodenal artery is an important source of vascular supply to the head of the pancreas, the inferior mesenteric artery does not provide any vascular supply to this structure and thus provides no branches that would need to be ligated to remove the mass described in the question stem.

Answer C is incorrect. Neither the left gastric nor the inferior mesenteric arteries provide any significant arterial supply to the head of the pancreas; thus no branches from either of these vessels would need to be ligated to complete the resection.

Answer D is incorrect. While the superior mesenteric artery is an important source of vascular supply to the head of the pancreas, the left gastric artery does not provide any vascular supply to this structure and thus provides no branches that would need to be ligated to remove the mass.

Answer E is incorrect. Neither the proper hepatic nor the inferior mesenteric arteries provide any significant arterial supply to the head of the pancreas; thus no branches from either of these vessels would need to be ligated to complete the resection.

Answer F is incorrect. While the superior mesenteric artery is an important source of vascular supply to the head of the pancreas, the proper hepatic artery does not provide any vascular supply to this structure and therefore provides no branches that would need to be ligated to remove the mass.

10. **The correct answer is C.** This patient presents with acromegaly, the clinical syndrome that is a result of excessive growth hormone (GH) secretion in adults (after closure of the physes). Octreotide is a somatostatin analog that acts at the anterior pituitary to suppress GH secretion, and is used in the treatment of acromegaly. Surgical and radiotherapeutic approaches are also an option, depending on the etiology. Somatostatin is normally secreted by the hypothalamus to help regulate basal GH secretion.

Answer A is incorrect. Finasteride is a 5-α-reductase inhibitor that suppresses the conversion of testosterone to dihydrotestosterone and is used in the treatment of benign prostatic hypertrophy.

Answer B is incorrect. Leuprolide is a gonadotropin-releasing hormone analog that can exhibit both agonist and antagonist actions, depending on the timing of administration. It is used to treat infertility, prostate cancer, and uterine fibroids. Adverse effects include antiandrogen actions (e.g., gynecomastia, decreased libido), nausea, and vomiting.

Answer D is incorrect. Like somatrem, recombinant GH is useful in the treatment of GH deficiency, but would exacerbate the condition of a patient with acromegaly.

Answer E is incorrect. Somatrem is a somatotropin, or GH analog, that stimulates the release of somatomedin/insulin-like growth factor-1 from the liver and is useful in the treatment of GH deficiency. It would exacerbate the condition of a patient with acromegaly.

11. **The correct answer is E.** The headache, anxiety, and palpitations suggest an excess of catecholamines stimulating the sympathetic nervous system. A pheochromocytoma may be suspected, and since there appears to be familial involvement, the related multiple endocrine neoplasia (MEN) syndromes should also be considered. MEN type II (used to be called type 2a) consists of medullary thyroid carcinoma (MTC), pheochromocytoma, and tumors of the parathyroid. MEN type III (used to be type 2b) usually includes MTC, pheochromocytoma, and neuromas instead of parathyroid tumors. It is therefore likely that this patient's relatives had their thyroids removed due to MTC. One could further differentiate the two types by looking for neuromas on the lips, tongue, or eyelids or in the gastrointestinal tract causing constipation/diarrhea, or for hyperparathyroidism manifesting in bradycardia, hypotonia, fatigue, and bone pain.

Answer A is incorrect. Acromegaly can lead to headaches; however, it does not commonly cause palpitations and is not associated with multiple endocrine neoplasia. Clinical signs of acromegaly include coarse facies, enlarged tongue, and increased size of hands and feet.

Answer B is incorrect. An ACTH-secreting pituitary adenoma, which defines Cushing's disease, would cause hypercortisolemia secondary to ACTH stimulation from the anterior pituitary, with elevated serum ACTH levels. Clinical findings would include characteristic moon facies, striae, obesity, hypertension, weakness, and hirsutism.

Answer C is incorrect. Up to 80% of patients with hyperparathyroidism are asymptomatic at diagnosis, and their disease is caught by routine blood tests. Some have nonspecific symptoms such as fatigue, mild depression, and anorexia. If severe, metastatic calcification and osteoclastic bone lesions can occur.

Answer D is incorrect. A nonfunctioning pituitary adenoma could suppress ACTH in the serum and would generally be accompanied by hypocortisolemia. Clinical findings would include weight loss, hypotension, fatigue, nausea, abdominal pain, and muscle cramps.

12. **The correct answer is A.** In addition to being necessary to normal human growth and development, GH is critical in the stress response to starvation. GH is released in response to hypoglycemia and acts directly to decrease glucose uptake by cells and increase lipolysis, resulting in an increase in blood sugar levels.

Answer B is incorrect. GH secretion is not stimulated by obesity, but rather is reduced by this condition.

Answer C is incorrect. Pregnancy is not a stimulus for GH secretion. Rather, GH secretion decreases in pregnancy.

Answer D is incorrect. Somatomedins, or insulin-like growth factors, are secreted by the liver in response to GH and mediate the metabolic changes necessary for growth and development. These intermediaries also act on the hypothalamus and the anterior pituitary via a negative feedback mechanism to reduce GH secretion.

Answer E is incorrect. Somatostatin is not a stimulus for GH secretion but rather is a component of the negative feedback system that regulates GH secretion. Somatostatin is secreted by the hypothalamus in response to stimulation by insulin-like growth factors/somatomedins and acts on the anterior pituitary to reduce GH secretion. Somatostatin may be used clinically to control the diarrhea associated with carcinoid syndrome or VIPomas.

13. **The correct answer is B.** Parathyroid chief cells are small, pale cells with round central nuclei. These cells secrete parathyroid hormone, which raises serum calcium levels in three ways: (1) it acts directly on bone to increase osteoclastic resorption; (2) it acts directly on the kidney to increase resorption of calcium and inhibit resorption of phosphate; and (3) it promotes gastrointestinal absorption of calcium via increased levels of activated vitamin D.

Answer A is incorrect. Adipose tissue in the parathyroid gland increases with age but does not secrete hormones related to calcium regulation. The cells contain large vacuoles that appear white on hematoxylin and eosin stain.

Answer C is incorrect. Parathyroid oxyphil cells tend to occur in nodules and have abundant eosinophilic cytoplasm. They are larger than chief cells and do not secrete parathyroid hormone.

Answer D is incorrect. Thyroid C cells secrete calcitonin, which decreases bone resorption of calcium, leading to a decrease in serum calcium levels. C cells are distinguished by their extensive clear cytoplasm. Think "C" for "Clear Cytoplasm."

Answer E is incorrect. Thyroid follicular cells are simple cuboidal cells that line colloid follicles. They are responsible for the synthesis and secretion of triiodothyronine and thyroxine.

14. **The correct answer is B.** This vignette is most consistent with a syndrome of inappropriate secretion of ADH due to a lung neoplasm. ADH is secreted by the posterior pituitary and stimulates the expression of aquaporins in the renal collecting ducts, resulting in transport of water into the renal medulla from the ductal lumen and hence water retention in the kidneys. When levels of this hormone are inappropriately elevated, excessive water retention results in hyponatremia, which can lead to seizures. ADH can be produced ectopically in the setting of malignancy, classically by small cell lung cancer.

Answer A is incorrect. ACTH can be produced ectopically in the setting of malignancy, especially small cell lung cancer. However, excessive levels of ACTH would result in Cushing's syndrome, and the vignette provides no symptoms or signs that would be consistent with this condition.

Answer C is incorrect. Parathyroid hormone (PTH) can be produced ectopically in the setting of malignancy and is associated with a variety of neoplasia, including squamous cell lung cancer, breast cancer, and multiple myeloma. However, excessive levels of PTH would result in hypercalcemia, and the vignette does not provide any indication that would be most consistent with this condition. Note that these symptoms can also occur in the setting of malignancy due to production of PTH-related peptide by tumor cells.

Answer D is incorrect. Hyperreninemia does not typically occur as paraneoplastic syndrome and would generally cause hyperaldosteronism, resulting in hypernatremia and hypokalemia. While seizures can be a consequence of severe hypernatremia, the vignette does not mention any signs or symptoms of hypokalemia (nausea, vomiting, muscle weakness, cardiac dysrhythmias).

Answer E is incorrect. Tumor necrosis factor-α can be produced ectopically in the setting of malignancy and parallels parathyroid hormone both in causing secondary hypercalcemia and in the cancers with which excessive production is associated.

15. **The correct answer is C.** The vignette describes a classic history for hypothyroidism caused by Hashimoto's thyroiditis. This primary hypothyroidism is characterized by reduced secretion of thyroid hormone, resulting in decreased levels of free and total T_4 and increased levels of TSH due to the absence of negative feedback by T_4.

Answer A is incorrect. In the setting of a primary hypothyroidism, both total and free thyroxine levels should be decreased rather than increased. An elevated TSH in the setting of high total and free thyroxine levels could be seen in a TSH-secreting pituitary adenoma or, less commonly, in patients with thyroid hormone resistance syndrome.

Answer B is incorrect. Both total and free T_4 levels should be decreased rather than increased in setting of primary hypothyroidism. An elevated T_4 would otherwise result in decreased rather than increased TSH levels due to negative feedback. Furthermore, free and total T_4 levels should vary in the same direction in this setting, as there is no change in the binding capacity of the proteins in the blood.

Answer D is incorrect. Hashimoto's thyroiditis indicates that both total and free T_4 levels should be decreased rather than increased, while TSH levels should be increased rather than decreased. Furthermore, free and total thyroxine levels should vary in the same direction in this setting, as there is no change in the binding capacity of the proteins in the blood.

Answer E is incorrect. In a primary hypothyroidism such as Hashimoto's thyroiditis, the reduction of free and total thyroxine levels in the blood should eliminate feedback inhibition of TSH secretion, leading to increased rather than decreased TSH levels in the blood. A low TSH level in conjunction with low serum total and free thyroxine levels is rare, but can be seen with secondary hypothyroidism, in which the pituitary gland does not produce sufficient TSH.

16. **The correct answer is A.** This patient had pseudohypoparathyroidism. In all forms of pseudohypoparathyroidism, there is a defect in the peripheral organ response to PTH, leading to increased PTH levels. There are several types of pseudohypoparathyroidism, which vary in clinical presentation. This is an autosomal dominant disease, and penetrance is variable. Pseudohypothyroidism is caused by kidney unresponsiveness to PTH.

Answer B is incorrect. Pseudohypoparathyroidism is an autosomal dominant disease, and penetrance is variable.

Answer C is incorrect. Pseudohypoparathyroidism is an autosomal dominant disease, and penetrance is variable.

Answer D is incorrect. Pseudohypoparathyroidism is an autosomal dominant disease, and penetrance is variable.

Answer E is incorrect. Pseudohypoparathyroidism is an autosomal dominant disease, and penetrance is variable.

17. **The correct answer is D.** This patient has Hashimoto's thyroiditis, an autoimmune disorder in which patients have antibodies attacking thyroglobulin, thyroid peroxidase, or another part of the thyroid gland or thyroid hormone

synthesis pathway. Patients with Hashimoto's thyroiditis have a 20 times greater prevalence of celiac disease and type 1 diabetes mellitus than the general population.

Answer A is incorrect. This patient has Hashimoto's thyroiditis. She would not have Graves' disease as well.

Answer B is incorrect. Addison's disease does have a high prevalence in patients with Hashimoto's thyroiditis. However, osteoarthritis is not an autoimmune disease.

Answer C is incorrect. Rheumatoid arthritis and vitiligo are both autoimmune diseases, but they do not have as high of an association with Hashimoto's thyroiditis as do type 1 diabetes mellitus and celiac disease.

Answer E is incorrect. Whipple's disease is caused by *Tropheryma whippelii.*

18. **The correct answer is A.** This patient's recent history of hyperglycemic symptoms, hypertension, and weight gain are all consistent with a diagnosis of Cushing's syndrome, which is characterized by hypercortisolemia. This leads to exaggeration of the physiologic effects of cortisol, such as hyperglycemia and insulin resistance, immune suppression, and hypertension (a consequence of salt retention due to secondary elevation of aldosterone). One result of this syndrome is osteoporosis, which is caused by increased bone resorption in response to an elevated serum cortisol level. Vertebral compression fractures are common manifestations of osteoporosis.

Answer B is incorrect. Glucagon can account for hyperglycemia via its anti-insulin physiologic effects, but it has no known physiologic effects on bone metabolism.

Answer C is incorrect. GH can cause hyperglycemia and insulin resistance but cannot account for increased bone resorption resulting in osteoporosis. Rather, GH stimulates increased bone growth that results in linear growth; it is responsible for the pubertal growth spurt.

Answer D is incorrect. Insulin causes hypoglycemia rather than hyperglycemia and does not exert any physiologic effects on bone metabolism that may be exaggerated and thus manifested as pathology in the setting of insulin excess.

Answer E is incorrect. Thyroid hormones function primarily to increase basal metabolism by increasing the activity of the Na^+/K^+ ATPase but also cause hyperglycemia by stimulating increased glycogenolysis, gluconeogenesis, and lipolysis. However, thyroid hormones do not cause increased bone resorption, but rather stimulate bone growth.

19. **The correct answer is A.** Acarbose is an α-glucosidase inhibitor that decreases the hydrolysis and absorption of disaccharides and polysaccharides at the intestinal brush border, thereby reducing postprandial hyperglycemia. This drug can be used as monotherapy or in combination with oral hypoglycemic medications in the management of type 2 diabetes mellitus. Acarbose commonly causes gastrointestinal adverse effects that include abdominal cramps, diarrhea, and flatulence.

Answer B is incorrect. Chlorpropamide is a sulfonylurea that acts via stimulation of insulin secretion by the pancreas. Hypoglycemia is the most important adverse effect of this drug, but chlorpropamide can also cause disulfiram-like adverse effects. This agent is generally not known to cause significant gastrointestinal disturbances.

Answer C is incorrect. Glipizide is a sulfonylurea that acts via stimulation of insulin secretion by the pancreas. Hypoglycemia is the most important side effect of this drug. Glipizide is generally not known to cause significant gastrointestinal disturbances.

Answer D is incorrect. Metformin inhibits gluconeogenesis, thus reducing blood sugar levels. The most important side effect of this agent is lactic acidosis. Metformin can sometimes cause loose bowel movements but is generally not associated with increased flatulence.

Answer E is incorrect. Orlistat is an inhibitor of pancreatic lipases that, when ingested, decreases the absorption of triglycerides from the human diet. It is not used in the management of diabetes. This drug commonly causes gastrointestinal adverse effects that include abdominal cramps, diarrhea, and flatulence.

Answer F is incorrect. Troglitazone sensitizes the peripheral tissues to insulin action and is typically associated with weight gain and hepatotoxicity as adverse effects. Gastrointestinal disturbances are not characteristic of this agent or other agents in the same class.

20. **The correct answer is B.** Bitemporal hemianopsia (due to compression of the optic nerves at the chiasm) and diminished libido are common presenting symptoms of pituitary tumors in men. The MRI shows a pituitary adenoma. When these adenomas become large enough, they exert mass effect on the second cranial nerves at the chiasm. GH-secreting pituitary adenomas are slow-growing and often go undiagnosed for several years. GH hypersecretion is associated with acromegaly, resulting in bone overgrowth with increased hand and foot size, soft tissue swelling, oily skin, and proximal muscle weakness.

Answer A is incorrect. ACTH-secreting pituitary adenomas account for 70% of cases of Cushing's syndrome. Cortisol excess leads to thin skin, central obesity, hypertension, "moon facies," glucose intolerance, and osteoporosis. ACTH-secreting tumors are typically smaller than 5 mm, and half are undetectable on MRI, rendering the diagnosis a clinical one.

Answer C is incorrect. Gonadotropin-secreting tumors are typically nonfunctioning. These are as common as prolactinomas and are generally diagnosed late because there are few symptoms until mass effect occurs.

Answer D is incorrect. Causes of hyperprolactinemia in men include medications, primary hypothyroidism, and chest wall stimulation (from trauma or herpes zoster reactivation). The diagnosis of idiopathic hyperprolactinemia is made by exclusion of known causes. Forty percent of all pituitary tumors are prolactinomas.

Answer E is incorrect. Thyroid-stimulating hormone-secreting tumors are rare. Patients present with goiter and hyperthyroidism.

21. **The correct answer is D.** Papillary thyroid carcinoma is the most common type of thyroid cancer. It is always distinguished by its finger-like projections of epithelium surrounding a central fibrovascular core, calcified spheres (psammoma bodies), optically clear "Orphan Annie" nuclei, and molding of the nuclei. Patients often have a prior history of radiation to the head or neck. Papillary thyroid carcinoma carries a better prognosis than the other forms of thyroid cancer.

Answer A is incorrect. A 20-year history of cigarette smoking would certainly increase this patient's risk for many types of cancers, such as lung, oropharyngeal, esophageal, pancreatic, and bladder. However, smoking is not specifically a risk factor for developing thyroid carcinoma.

Answer B is incorrect. Graves' disease is an autoimmune disorder in which antibodies to the thyroid hormone-stimulating receptor stimulate increased release of thyroid hormone. Symptoms of Graves' disease include the clinical features of hyperthyroidism (restlessness, tremor, tachycardia, heat intolerance) as well as a tendency to develop exophthalmos and pretibial myxedema. Graves' disease is often seen in patients who have other autoimmune disorders, such as systemic lupus erythematosus, diabetes mellitus type I, and pernicious anemia. Patients with Graves' disease are not at a significantly increased risk of papillary thyroid carcinoma.

Answer C is incorrect. Individuals with HLA-DR5 receptors have an increased incidence of Hashimoto's thyroiditis, an autoimmune form of hypothyroidism. The biopsy of a patient with Hashimoto's thyroiditis would show substantial lymphocytic infiltration into the gland along with characteristic eosinophilic Hurthle cells. Like patients with Graves' disease, patients with Hashimoto's thyroiditis often have concurrent autoimmune conditions, but they are not at increased risk for papillary thyroid carcinoma.

Answer E is incorrect. Postpartum thyroiditis presents with a painless enlarged thyroid and symptoms of hyperthyroid function. The thyroid is often filled with a lymphocytic infiltrate. Women who experience one episode of postpartum thyroiditis are at increased risk of recurrence after another pregnancy. There is no association, however, between postpartum thyroiditis and an increased risk of thyroid carcinoma.

22. **The correct answer is B.** Acute high-dosage glucocorticoid treatment can cause a change in electrolyte levels by their cross-reactivity to the mineralocorticoid receptors, thus causing sodium retention and potassium depletion. Hypokalemia is manifested on ECG as a U wave, which is a small wave that follows the T wave.

Answer A is incorrect. Delta waves are the result of accessory conduction pathways, not hypokalemia. They are often seen in Wolff-Parkinson-White syndrome and look like sloped upstrokes in the QRS complex.

Answer C is incorrect. Peaked T waves on ECG are suggestive of hyperkalemia. In this case, the more likely result is hypokalemia instead of hyperkalemia; thus, T waves would not be expected to be peaked.

Answer D is incorrect. PR segment elongation is indicative of increased time for conduction between the atria and the ventricles. This is typically seen with first-degree heart block, which is not caused by glucocorticoid treatment.

Answer E is incorrect. ST segment elevation suggests transmural myocardial ischemia, which is not an adverse effect of glucocorticoids.

23. **The correct answer is B.** The right adrenal gland is drained via the right adrenal vein, which flows directly into the inferior vena cava

(IVC). Thus, a right-sided hyperfunctioning adrenal adenoma is drained via the right adrenal vein into the IVC. In contrast, the left adrenal gland is drained via the left adrenal vein into the left renal vein, which then flows into the IVC.

Answer A is incorrect. The abdominal aorta plays no role in the vascular drainage of any organ but rather provides arterial supply to the abdominal organs, including the kidneys and adrenals glands.

Answer C is incorrect. The portal vein is superior and anterior to the adrenal and renal vasculature and is not involved in the drainage of either of the adrenal glands. Instead, it drains most of the gastrointestinal tract down to the rectum into the liver.

Answer D is incorrect. The right gonadal vein drains the testes or ovaries directly into the inferior vena cava but does not drain the right adrenal gland in either sex.

Answer E is incorrect. Drainage of the right adrenal gland and hence a right-sided adrenal adenoma does not flow through the right renal vein, but instead the adrenal vein flows directly into the inferior vena cava.

24. **The correct answer is A.** This vignette describes a patient with classic symptoms and signs of hypocalcemia, including Chvostek's sign (facial spasm) and Trousseau's sign (carpal spasm). All of these findings can be attributed to the physiologic effects of calcitonin. Calcitonin is normally secreted in response to elevated levels of serum calcium and causes decreased bone resorption of calcium, resulting in lower calcium levels.

Answer B is incorrect. PTH acts to increase serum calcium and phosphate levels by increasing bone resorption and renal reabsorption of calcium. Additionally, PTH-related peptide (PTHrP) stimulates conversion of inactive 25-OH vitamin D to active 1,25-OH vitamin D, resulting in hypercalcemia rather than hypocalcemia.

Answer C is incorrect. PTHrP acts like PTH to increase serum calcium and phosphate levels by increasing bone resorption and renal re-absorption of calcium. Additionally, PTHrP stimulates conversion of inactive 25-OH vitamin D to active 1,25-OH vitamin D, resulting in hypercalcemia rather than hypocalcemia. Metastatic small cell lung cancer can plausibly account for a nodule palpable in the neck and is generally associated with paraneoplastichypercalcemia secondary to elaboration of PTHrP.

Answer D is incorrect. Thyroxine is generally not known to significantly affect serum calcium levels. Therefore, excess thyroxine would not be expected to cause hypocalcemia. The functions of thyroxine are summarized by the "4 B's": **B**rain maturation, **B**one growth, β-adrenergic effects, and increase **B**asal metabolic rate.

Answer E is incorrect. Vitamin D stimulates calcium and phosphate absorption from the intestines and increases bone resorption, resulting in increased serum calcium and phosphate levels. Hence, excess vitamin D would result in hypercalcemia rather than hypocalcemia, with nonspecific symptoms of hypercalcemia such as malaise, fatigue, depression, and diffuse aches and pains. Hypercalcemia and hyperophosphatemia are evident on laboratory evaluation.

25. **The correct answer is B.** This vignette describes leiomyomas, or fibroids, which are most often seen in African-American women. These tumors are benign and usually present with menstrual pain and menorrhagia (increased bleeding). They are estrogen-sensitive, increasing in size during pregnancy and decreasing with menopause. As their name suggests, leiomyomas are composed of muscle fibers; thus, the appropriate stain is desmin.

Answer A is incorrect. Cytokeratin staining would be most appropriate for epithelial cells.

Answer C is incorrect. Glial fibrillary acid protein staining would be most appropriate for neuroglia.

Answer D is incorrect. Neurofilament staining would be most appropriate for neurons.

Answer E is incorrect. Vimentin staining would be most appropriate for connective tissue.

26. **The correct answer is A.** This patient has Graves' disease, an autoimmune disorder resulting from IgG-type autoantibodies to the thyroid-stimulating hormone receptor. The three classic findings associated with Graves' disease are hyperthyroidism, ophthalmopathy, and dermopathy/pretibial myxedema.

Answer B is incorrect. Hashimoto's thyroiditis is an autoimmune disorder characterized by antibodies attacking thyroglobulin or thyroid peroxidase (the two most common autoantibodies in these patients) or antibodies against another part of the thyroid or thyroid hormone synthesis pathway. Although some cases of Hashimoto's thyroiditis may present as a transient hyperthyroidism (with symptoms including palpitations and increased metabolic rate) from an initial disruption of thyroid follicles, the majority of cases present with signs and symptoms of hypothyroidism, such as intolerance to cold weather, weight gain, and mental and physical slowness.

Answer C is incorrect. Plummer's disease is characterized by a nodular goiter that has a hyperfunctioning nodule, causing hyperthyroidism. As opposed to Graves' disease, Plummer's disease is not accompanied by ophthalmopathy or dermopathy/pretibial myxedema.

Answer D is incorrect. Iodine deficiency causes hypothyroidism, manifested with signs and symptoms that include intolerance to cold weather, weight gain, and mental and physical slowness.

Answer E is incorrect. Papillary carcinoma of the thyroid, the most common form of thyroid cancer, usually presents as an asymptomatic thyroid nodule with signs of obstruction from the tumor such as hoarseness, cough, dysphagia, or dyspnea or a cervical lymph node mass (as opposed to symptoms of hyper- or hypothyroidism). Radiation is a common cause of thyroid cancer.

27. **The correct answer is D.** 17-α-Hydroxylase deficiency, a form of congenital adrenal hyperplasia, is characterized by deficits in glucocorticoid and sex steroid synthesis. This is coupled with increased mineralocorticoid production due to the increased flow of precursors, such as pregnenolone and progesterone, through mineralocorticoid-yielding pathways. The resultant low serum cortisol and sex steroid levels with elevated mineralocorticoid levels manifest clinically with hypertension, hypokalemia, and a female phenotype with no sexual maturation. Aldosterone is produced in the zona glomerulosa. Aldosterone synthesis requires 21-β-hydroxylase but not 17-α-hydroxylase. Remember the mnemonic "Salt, Sugar, and Sex" for the layers of the adrenal cortex and their respective products.

Answer A is incorrect. The capsule does not produce any hormones.

Answer B is incorrect. The medulla produces catecholamines; neither 17-α-hydroxylase nor 21-β-hydroxylase is required for the synthesis of catecholamines.

Answer C is incorrect. Cortisol is produced in the zona fasciculata of the adrenal cortex. Cortisol synthesis requires 21-β-hydroxylase and 17-α-hydroxylase.

Answer E is incorrect. Sex hormones are produced in the zona reticularis. Synthesis of the sex hormones requires 17-α-hydroxylase but not 21-β-hydroxylase.

28. **The correct answer is A.** This patient's laboratory values are consistent with Addison's disease, a primary deficiency of aldosterone and cortisol due to adrenal hypofunction. This condition leads to hypotension and skin hyperpigmentation. Lack of aldosterone production results in the electrolyte imbalance seen in this patient's lab values: low aldosterone reduces renal sodium reabsorption and potassium secretion, resulting in low serum sodium and high serum potassium levels with hypotension. ACTH levels increase due to the loss of negative feedback from low cortisol levels. Adrenal atrophy can be due to a number of causes, including autoimmune destruction, infection, and adrenal hemorrhage. Importantly, adrenal

atrophy reduces the hydroxylation of pregnenolone by 17-α-hydroxylase present in the adrenals. This is the cause of reduced urinary 17-hydroxypregnenolone.

Answer B is incorrect. An adrenal adenoma producing cortisol would also lead to signs and symptoms consistent with Cushing's syndrome.

Answer C is incorrect. Ectopic ACTH production, as seen in the paraneoplastic syndrome associated with small cell lung cancer, would likely lead to increased, rather than decreased, levels of cortisol production. This would result in signs and symptoms consistent with Cushing's syndrome, including hypertension and weight gain.

Answer D is incorrect. Patients with hemochromatosis can also have changes in skin pigmentation due to deposition of hemosiderin in the skin. Hemochromatosis is associated with a triad of conditions consisting of micronodular pigment cirrhosis, bronze diabetes, and skin pigmentation, all of which are related to iron deposits and toxicity in associated organs. Hemochromatosis is not likely to cause the laboratory values seen in this patient. The mnemonic for hemochromatosis is "a tan man with diabetes."

Answer E is incorrect. Pituitary corticotropin insufficiency is an example of secondary adrenocortical insufficiency. Patients with pituitary insufficiency would likely have decreased cortisol and ACTH levels. Secondary insufficiency usually results in less mineralocorticoid malfunction and less, if any, change in skin pigmentation.

29. **The correct answer is D.** Chromaffin cells are neuroendocrine cells derived from the embryonic neural crest. They are found in the medulla of the adrenal gland and in sympathetic nervous system ganglia. Chromaffin cells of the adrenal medulla are innervated by the splanchnic nerve and secrete epinephrine, norepinephrine, and enkephalin into the bloodstream. They derive their name from their ability to be visualized by staining with chromium salts. These cells have large nuclei and are strongly basophilic, in contrast to the more eo-

sinophilic zona reticularis cells. They contain little endoplasmic reticulum and no stored lipid. Norepinephrine-secreting cells are distinguished from epinephrine-secreting cells by virtue of having dense core granules and a more strongly positive chromaffin reaction.

Answer A is incorrect. Aldosterone is secreted by zona glomerulosa cells, which are arranged in irregular ovoid clusters. These cells have round, strongly stained nuclei. The cytoplasm is acidophilic and contains abundant smooth endoplasmic reticulum and mitochondria. Glomerulosa cells contain less lipid and cytoplasm than cells of the zona fasciculata.

Answer B is incorrect. Androgens are secreted by cells in the zona reticularis, the innermost zone of the adrenal cortex. This zone is composed of an irregular network of branching cords and clusters of cells. There are few lipid droplets, and hematoxylin and eosin stains reveal the brown pigment lipofuscin.

Answer C is incorrect. Cortisol is secreted by cells of the zona fasciculata in the adrenal cortex. This zone is the middle and the broadest of the three cortical zones. It is identified histologically by radially arranged cords of single cell width. These cells have abundant, poorly staining cytoplasm and are rich in mitochondria and lipid droplets.

30. **The correct answer is C.** Thyroid hormones act via a nuclear hormone receptor. On binding with its ligand, the receptor translocates from the cytoplasm to the cell nucleus, and the ligand-receptor complex acts as a transcription factor. This results in gene transcription and new protein synthesis. This answer is the only one that involves assessment of gene transcription, and thus represents the only selection that refers to a nuclear hormone receptor mechanism. Furthermore, an important function of thyroid hormones is increasing basal metabolic rate, which is mediated by increasing Na^+/K^+-ATPase expression and activity. Other hormones that act through nuclear steroid hormone receptors include cortisol, aldosterone, vitamin D, testosterone, estrogen, and progesterone.

Answer A is incorrect. Adenylate cyclase and cAMP are critical in the mechanism of a number of different hormones, including glucagon, histamine, epinephrine, dopamine, and vasopressin. However, adenylate cyclase and cAMP are not important in the mechanism of thyroid hormones and other steroid hormones.

Answer B is incorrect. Increases in intracellular calcium levels are important in the mechanism of hormones such as norepinephrine, histamine, and vasopressin but are not important in the mechanism of thyroid hormones and other steroid hormones.

Answer D is incorrect. Activation of phospholipase C, resulting in the cleavage of phosphatidylinositol diphosphate into inositol triphosphate and diacylglycerol, is important in the mechanism of several hormones, including histamine and vasopressin, but is not important in the mechanism of thyroid hormones and other steroid hormones.

Answer E is incorrect. Phosphorylation of insulin receptor substrate 1 is important in the mechanism of intracellular insulin action via a tyrosine kinase cascade. Tyrosine kinases are not important in the mechanism of thyroid hormones and other steroid hormones.

31. **The correct answer is D.** Pituitary adenomas can lead to hypersecretion of hormones as demonstrated by this woman's galactorrhea suggesting high levels of prolactin. Due to their mass effect, an adenoma can also lead to deficiencies in other pituitary hormones and changes in vision. The key to answering this question is to realize which of the processes listed is not changed by a deficiency in a pituitary hormone. Salt retention is a primary action of aldosterone, which acts at the renal distal tubules to increase sodium and chloride reabsorption as well as increase potassium secretion. Aldosterone is produced in a multistep pathway from cholesterol, along with cortisol and the androgens, in response to ACTH stimulation. ACTH is secreted by the anterior pituitary and would likely be deficient due to impingement of an adenoma on this gland. However, ACTH deficiency does not cause salt

wasting, volume contraction, and hyperkalemia, because it does not result in clinically important deficiency of aldosterone.

Answer A is incorrect. Free water resorption is mediated by ADH that is secreted from the posterior pituitary. ADH secretion leads to insertion of water channels in the collecting duct of the nephron that resorb free water. In the absence of ADH, there would be a lack of water channels to resorb free water.

Answer B is incorrect. Luteinizing hormone secretion could be affected by a prolactinoma, which would, in turn, impact menstruation.

Answer C is incorrect. Ovulation is stimulated by the surge of luteinizing hormone (LH) just prior to the midpoint of the menstrual cycle. LH is secreted by the anterior pituitary and would likely be deficient due to impingement of an adenoma on the LH-secreting cells of this gland. Ovulation would likely be impaired in such a case.

Answer E is incorrect. Thyroid hormone is produced by the thyroid in response to TSH released by the anterior pituitary. Because TSH release occurs in the same place as the adenoma, its levels would be decreased, leading to lower levels of thyroid hormone.

32. **The correct answer is A.** The patient has tumors involving the "3 P's" of MEN type I, also known as Werner's syndrome. Her galactorrhea is likely due to a **P**rolactin-secreting pituitary tumor, and her hypercalcemia is likely due to a **P**arathyroid adenoma. Her recurrent duodenal ulcers are a manifestation of a gastrin-secreting tumor frequently located in the **P**ancreas, as seen in Zollinger-Ellison syndrome. The genetic inheritance of MEN I is autosomal dominant, as one would expect if multiple maternal family members are also affected by this disorder.

Answer B is incorrect. MEN type I is not inherited in an autosomal recessive pattern. Examples of autosomal recessive disorders include cystic fibrosis, Tay-Sachs disease, and phenylketonuria.

Answer C is incorrect. MEN type I is not inherited in a mitochondrial pattern. Diseases with a mitochondrial pattern of inheritance include mitochondrial myopathy and Leigh syndrome.

Answer D is incorrect. MEN type I is not inherited in an X-linked dominant pattern. An example of X-linked dominant disorders is Coffin-Lowry syndrome.

Answer E is incorrect. MEN type I is not inherited in an X-linked recessive pattern. Examples of X-linked recessive disorders include hemophilia A and B and Duchenne muscular dystrophy.

33. **The correct answer is D.** This patient presents with thyrotoxicosis, which can result due to excess endogenous or exogenous thyroid hormone. Levothyroxine is a synthetic form of thyroxine that is used in the treatment of hypothyroidism. Excessively high serum levels of levothyroxine result in symptoms of thyrotoxicosis, including those described in the vignette as well as heat intolerance, unexplained weight loss, agitation, and confusion.

Answer A is incorrect. Dobutamine is a β-adrenergic agonist that is useful in the acute treatment of congestive heart failure. While the effects of this drug can mimic the symptoms and signs of thyrotoxicosis, this agent cannot account for the gastrointestinal symptoms, the weight loss, and the heat intolerance that are characteristic symptoms of thyrotoxicosis.

Answer B is incorrect. Pharmacologic doses of iodide are used in the treatment of hyperthyroidism; they inhibit the synthesis of thyroid hormone and the release of preformed thyroid hormone. Iodide is administered orally, and adverse effects include sore mouth and throat, rashes, ulcerations of mucous membranes, and a metallic taste in the mouth, but not thyrotoxicosis.

Answer C is incorrect. Leuprolide is a gonadotropin-releasing hormone analog that can exhibit both agonist and antagonist actions, depending on the timing of administration. It is used to treat infertility, prostate cancer, and uterine fibroids. Adverse effects include antiandrogen actions (e.g., gynecomastia, decreased libido), nausea, and vomiting.

Answer E is incorrect. Propylthiouracil, which inhibits the synthesis of T_4 and the peripheral conversion of T_4 to triiodothyronine, is used in the treatment of hyperthyroidism. Rare toxicities due to this agent include agranulocytosis, rash, and edema.

34. **The correct answer is A.** Diabetes insipidus is characterized by an inability of the kidney to concentrate urine effectively. Concentration of urine is normally controlled by ADH, which regulates water pores in the renal collecting duct. Central diabetes insipidus results from decreased ADH levels, whereas nephrogenic diabetes insipidus results from a decrease in the kidney's ability to respond to ADH. In either condition, thirst and resulting polydipsia are caused by increased levels of plasma sodium and osmolarity. This change in osmolarity occurs due to loss of free water in the form of hypotonic urine. Since this patient's plasma osmolarity is 290 mOsm/L, only a urine osmolarity less than this value would indicate a hypotonic urine and diabetes insipidus. The correct answer from these choices is therefore 100 mOsm/L.

Answer B is incorrect. Because this patient's plasma osmolarity is 290 mOsm/L, only a urine osmolarity less than this value would indicate a hypotonic urine and diabetes insipidus.

Answer C is incorrect. Because this patient's plasma osmolarity is 290 mOsm/L, only a urine osmolarity less than this value would indicate a hypotonic urine and diabetes insipidus.

Answer D is incorrect. Because this patient's plasma osmolarity is 290 mOsm/L, only a urine osmolarity less than this value would indicate a hypotonic urine and diabetes insipidus.

Answer E is incorrect. Because this patient's plasma osmolarity is 290 mOsm/L, only a urine osmolarity less than this value would indicate a hypotonic urine and diabetes insipidus.

35. **The correct answer is D.** This patient is most likely hypoglycemic. Normally, hypoglycemia causes an increased sympathetic tone resulting in tachycardia, diaphoresis, tremor, and anxiety. Diabetic patients who are on β blockers may be unable to produce this sympathetic response, which makes it difficult to recognize the onset of hypoglycemia. Sulfonylureas, such as glyburide and glipizide, are known for causing hypoglycemia—more than other agents, such as metformin.

Answer A is incorrect. Enalapril is an angiotensin converting enzyme inhibitor that may lead to cough, hypotension, and edema. Adverse events include dizziness and possible syncope, but not agitation or confusion.

Answer B is incorrect. Hydralazine is used to treat severe hypertension and may cause tachycardia and fluid retention.

Answer C is incorrect. Hydrochlorothiazide toxicity includes hyperglycemia, hyperlipidemia, hyperuricemia, and hypercalcemia.

Answer E is incorrect. Triamterene is a potassium-sparing diuretic that may lead to hyperkalemia, which presents with cardiac manifestations.

36. **The correct answer is A.** The patient is showing signs and symptoms of acromegaly. On further testing, the bilateral vision loss is likely to be a bitemporal hemianopsia from the GH-secreting adenoma compressing the optic chiasm. GH-secreting tumors cause gigantism if the epiphyses have not closed, as in children, and cause acromegaly in adults. Other characteristics of acromegaly include coarse features such as enlarged jaw, face, hands, and feet. Osteoporosis, hyperglycemia, and hypertension may also be associated with excess GH secretion. This second most common pituitary tumor is composed of acidophilic-staining cells.

Answer B is incorrect. Basophilic-staining cells of the pituitary gland can be remembered by the mnemonic "B-FLAT Major": Basophilic = FSH, LH, ACTH, TSH, MSH.

Answer C is incorrect. Chromophobic-staining cells of the pituitary gland include prolactin-producing cells.

Answer D is incorrect. A growth hormone-secreting adenoma would not be expected to consist of mixed acidophilic and basophilic components.

Answer E is incorrect. A growth hormone-secreting adenoma would not be expected to consist of mixed basophilic and chromophobic components.

37. **The correct answer is D.** Causes of hypoparathyroidism include thyroidectomy, metastatic cancer, and DiGeorge's syndrome. Signs and symptoms of hypoparathyroidism include anxiety and irritability, neuromuscular excitability, tetany, intracranial calcifications, dental abnormalities, and cardiac conduction abnormalities. Laboratory values reflect a state of hypocalcemia and hyperphosphatemia with low parathyroid hormone levels.

Answer A is incorrect. These laboratory values are seen in primary hyperparathyroidism.

Answer B is incorrect. The patient would be hypoparathyroid; however, hypoparathyroidism causes hypocalcemia and hyperphosphatemia, not hypercalcemia and hypophosphatemia as indicated in this answer choice.

Answer C is incorrect. These laboratory values are seen in secondary hyperparathyroidism.

Answer E is incorrect. This patient's history of radioactive iodine therapy and signs and symptoms of irritability, neuromuscular excitability, positive Chvostek's sign, and QT prolongation all point to a diagnosis of hypocalcemia secondary to hypoparathyroidism. It is unlikely that his calcium, phosphate, and parathyroid hormone levels are normal.

38. **The correct answer is C.** The mechanism of action of metformin is not entirely understood. It may inhibit gluconeogenesis and increase glycolysis, leading to a decrease in serum glucose levels. Metformin is used as an oral hypoglycemic agent and can be used in patients without islet cell function. Lactic acidosis, one possible cause of an anion-gap metabolic acidosis, is the most serious adverse effect of metformin.

Answer A is incorrect. Acarbose is an intestinal brush border α-glucosidase inhibitor that delays hydrolysis of sugars and absorption of glucose, helping to decrease postprandial hyperglycemia. Because sugars remain in the intestine undigested, patients often experience osmotic diarrhea, which limits the utility of this drug.

Answer B is incorrect. Glipizide is a second-generation sulfonylurea that closes potassium channels in the β cell membrane, stimulating cell depolarization, an increase in calcium influx, and the release of endogenous insulin in patients with type 2 diabetes mellitus. This oral hypoglycemic agent requires some residual islet cell function in order to be effective. Common adverse effects include hypoglycemia.

Answer D is incorrect. Pioglitazone can be used as a monotherapy for type 2 diabetes mellitus or in combination with other agents. Pioglitazone enhances target cell response to insulin. Weight gain is a side effect of the drug and results from increased responsiveness to insulin, a growth factor.

Answer E is incorrect. Tolbutamide is a first-generation sulfonylurea that works via the same mechanism as glipizide. First-generation sulfonylureas are less likely to cause hypoglycemia than second-generation drugs but are more likely to cause a disulfiram-like effect.

39. **The correct answer is A.** Benign prostatic hyperplasia (BPH) is a common entity in men older than age 50. Pathophysiologically, estradiol levels increase with age and they are thought to sensitize the prostate to the effects of dihydrotestosterone (DHT), causing the prostatic cells to grow. Common symptoms of BPH include increased frequency of urination, noc-

turia, problems with initiating and stopping urination, and pain on urination. Finasteride is a 5α-reductase inhibitor that inhibits conversion of testosterone to DHT, therefore preventing further growth of the prostate, as well as promoting hair growth.

Answer B is incorrect. Flutamide is a competitive inhibitor of testosterone and its receptor and is used in the treatment of prostatic carcinoma, not benign prostatic hypertrophy.

Answer C is incorrect. Ketoconazole is a commonly used antifungal that also has antiandrogen effects. In the latter capacity, it is used in the treatment of polycystic ovarian syndrome to prevent hirsutism.

Answer D is incorrect. Spironolactone is a K+-sparing diuretic that also has antiandrogenic effects. In addition to use in the treatment of hyperaldosteronism, hypokalemia, and congestive heart failure, it can be used in preventing hirsutism in polycystic ovarian syndrome.

Answer E is incorrect. Yohimbine is an α-2-selective inhibitor with questionable usage in the treatment of impotence.

40. **The correct answer is E.** The steroid hormone circulates in the plasma bound to a hormone-specific binding globulin. At the target organ, it enters a cell at the cell membrane due to its lipophilic properties and binds to an intracellular receptor either in the cytoplasm or within the nucleus. The hormone-receptor complex must transform in order to reveal the hormone's DNA binding domain; without this step, it is unable to carry out its action. Once the binding domain is revealed, the hormone binds the DNA enhancer element and generates gene transcription.

Answer A is incorrect. Binding a hormone-specific globulin in the plasma helps the hormone reach its target cell population but does not directly affect its DNA binding capacity.

Answer B is incorrect. Steroid hormones do not act through transmembrane receptors and second messengers like protein hormones do.

Answer C is incorrect. Binding to the DNA enhancer element is the desired action of the hormone, but this is not possible without first binding to an intracellular receptor.

Answer D is incorrect. Binding to the intracellular receptor alone does not enable DNA binding.

41. **The correct answer is B.** This patient most likely has diabetes mellitus type 1. The symptoms are due to a lack of insulin production by pancreatic β cells, which is believed to be caused by autoimmune/immune-related injury to the pancreas. The genetic predisposition to type 1 diabetes is not as strong as that for type 2 diabetes, but type 1 is associated with human leukocyte antigens (HLA)-DR3 and -DR4. Among whites with type 1 diabetes, 95% have HLA-DR3, HLA-DR4, or both.

Answer A is incorrect. These characteristics are commonly used to describe lactase deficiency, which causes an inability to properly digest the disaccharide lactose into glucose and galactose. The development of some cases is associated with viral or bacterial enteric infections. Note that other brush border enzymes include trehalase, which breaks down the disaccharide trehalose into glucose, and sucrase, which breaks down the disaccharide sucrose into glucose and fructose.

Answer C is incorrect. Crohn's disease, a type of inflammatory bowel disease, is associated with HLA-B27. Crohn's disease is often characterized by "skip lesions," referring to the occurrence of multiple diseased gastrointestinal segments adjacent to normal-appearing uninvolved bowel.

Answer D is incorrect. These are concepts used to describe type 2 diabetes mellitus, which is characterized by erratic insulin secretion (levels may be low, normal, or high) and insulin resistance; the insulin that is secreted from the pancreas does not function properly. About 80% of patients with type 2 diabetes are obese.

42. **The correct answer is A.** Captopril is the prototypical angiotensin-converting enzyme (ACE) inhibitor. Common adverse effects are cough, angioedema, taste changes, and rash. Although ACE inhibitors are not indicated as first-line treatment for new-onset hypertension in the general population (lifestyle modification should be tried first), those with diabetes should be placed on an ACE inhibitor at the first sign of hypertension to preserve renal function.

    Answer B is incorrect. Hydrochlorothiazide (HCTZ) is a sulfa-derived diuretic used as a first-line treatment for hypertension, but it is not associated with angioedema. Adverse effects of HCTZ include dehydration, metabolic alkalosis, hypokalemia, hypomagnesemia, hypercalcemia, rash (sulfa allergy), hyperglycemia, and hypercholesterolemia/hypertriglyceridemia.

    Answer C is incorrect. Losartan is an angiotensin II receptor inhibitor and is indicated for patients who experience the adverse effects of angiotensin-converting enzyme inhibitors. Its adverse effect profile is very similar to that of captopril, but the incidence of angioedema and cough are far less frequent.

    Answer D is incorrect. Nifedipine is a dihydropyridine calcium channel blocker (CCB) and it is not known to cause a dry cough or angioedema. Because it primarily acts on peripheral vasculature and minimally affects atrioventricular nodal conduction, it is far less likely than nondihydropyridine CCBs (such as diltiazam or verapamil) to cause heart block.

    Answer E is incorrect. β-Blockers such as propranolol do not cause angioedema. Common adverse effects include asthma exacerbation, sedation, bradycardia, and atrioventricular block, Sudden withdrawal of the drug can cause tachycardia due to receptor upregulation.

43. **The correct answer is A.** This patient has disseminated meningococcal infection, characterized by meningitis (cerebrospinal fluid [CSF] pleocytosis and positive examination findings), hypoxemia, disseminated intravascular coagulation (DIC), and acute onset adrenal insufficiency. Acute onset adrenal insufficiency in the context of disseminated meningococcemia is termed Waterhouse-Friderichsen syndrome and is caused by bilateral adrenal hemorrhage. It is important to recognize that the clinical presentation of adrenal insufficiency is often nonspecific, and may include fever, nausea, vomiting, diffuse abdominal tenderness, and hypotension that is mainly refractory to large amounts of intravenous hydration.

    Answer B is incorrect. Although this patient indeed has DIC (thrombocytopenia, coagulopathy, elevated D-dimer, and a petechial rash), these findings are not likely contributing to her abdominal tenderness.

    Answer C is incorrect. This patient's hypoxemia is likely due to sepsis secondary to meningococcal bacteremia. Hypoxemia may cause cyanosis and dyspnea, but it does not cause hypotension and diffuse abdominal tenderness.

    Answer D is incorrect. This patient also has meningitis, characterized by photophobia, fevers, positive Kernig's and Brudzinski's signs, and CSF pleocytosis with positive Gram stains. However, meningitis alone does not cause diffuse abdominal tenderness.

    Answer E is incorrect. Viral gastroenteritis is a common cause of hypotension, vomiting, and diffuse abdominal tenderness. However, in this case of Waterhouse-Friderichsen syndrome (which is due to disseminated meningococcemia), a concomitant viral gastroenteritis is unlikely.

44. **The correct answer is A.** Demeclocycline, like lithium, can inhibit the kidneys' response to ADH, resulting in diabetes insipidus (DI). Symptoms of DI include polydipsia, polyuria, hypotonic urine, serum hyperosmolarity, and hypernatremia. In nephrogenic DI, the problem is with the renal response to ADH, so the administration of exogenous ADH has no effect because the kidney is unable to respond the ADH. In an attempt to enhance this response, the posterior pituitary increases ADH production, and consequently ADH plasma

levels are also elevated. In contrast, central DI is a defect in the central production of ADH by the hypothalamic-pituitary axis. ADH is produced by the hypothalamic fibers that descend into the posterior pituitary (neurohypophysis). Mass effect due to compressive tumors in the diencephalon, for example, can cause depression of ADH release from the hypothalamus, resulting in neurogenic DI. In these patients, the serum ADH level will be low. Moreover, the resulting DI can be resolved with exogenous ADH administration.

Answer B is incorrect. In neurogenic DI, unlike nephrogenic DI, exogenous ADH is beneficial because the disease is a result of lack of central ADH production; ADH plasma levels are thus reduced.

Answer C is incorrect. Primary hyperaldosteronism would also cause hypernatremia and hypokalemia. Dilute urine, however, would not be expected.

Answer D is incorrect. ADH levels are frequently elevated in patients with the syndrome of inappropriate ADH secretion; however, these patients produce hypertonic urine and have serum hypoosmolarity and hyponatremia.

Answer E is incorrect. Although polydipsia and polyuria are also seen in uncontrolled type 2 diabetes mellitus, hypernatremia would not be expected.

45. **The correct answer is C.** The large cell shown in the image is an osteoclast, which is responsible for bone resorption. Osteoclasts can be identified by their multiple nuclei, ruffled cytoplasmic border adjacent to the surface of bone tissue, and vacuoles and lysosomes within the cytoplasm. Patients with chronic renal disease usually have increased serum phosphorus levels, a tendency towards decreased serum calcium levels, and a compensatory increase in PTH levels. The increase in PTH levels leads to an increase in osteoclast bone resorption and thus an increase in serum calcium and alkaline phosphatase.

Answer A is incorrect. Angiotensin II, which is converted from angiotensin I in the lung capil-laries by ACE, is a product of the renin-angiotensin system and thus can be affected in patients with chronic renal disease; however, angiotensin II does not stimulate activity of osteoclasts.

Answer B is incorrect. Calcitonin inhibits osteoclast activity and thus decreases bone resorption, which would not be the expected physiologic response to hypocalcemia.

Answer D is incorrect. Although renin levels can be affected in patients with chronic renal disease, renin does not stimulate activity of osteoclasts.

Answer E is incorrect. Thyroid hormone does not stimulate activity of osteoclasts.

46. **The correct answer is D.** The patient most likely has Graves' disease-induced hyperthyroidism, the most prominent feature being the exophthalmos seen in the image. In addition, her fatigue, sweating, palpitations, and increased appetite are also symptoms of hyperthyroidism. She could be treated with an agent such as propylthiouracil at this point, which would help with the symptoms, although it will not reverse the eye changes. Unfortunately, it can have the adverse effect of agranulocytosis, and thus blood work needs to be done when first prescribing this agent to a patient. Agranulocytosis can lead to infection and may be life threatening.

Answer A is incorrect. Folic acid is not used in the treatment of hyperthyroidism. It also does not cause agranulocytosis. It is often given to patients who are anemic. It is important that pregnant women receive adequate amounts of folic acid to reduce the incidence of neural tube defects.

Answer B is incorrect. Levothyroxine is used to treat hypothyroidism and would be contraindicated in this patient as it would worsen her current symptoms.

Answer C is incorrect. Propranolol is also used to treat hyperthyroidism. However, it is not associated with agranulocytosis. Its most common adverse effect is fatigue.

Answer E is incorrect. Radioactive iodine is used to treat hyperthyroidism. The treatment is permanent and often results in hypothyroidism. It does not cause agranulocytosis.

47. **The correct answer is A.** The patient has signs and symptoms suggestive of hypercortisolism, also known as Cushing's syndrome. Etiologies of hypercortisolism include a cortisol-producing adrenal adenoma, an ACTH-producing pituitary adenoma, paraneoplastic ectopic production of ACTH, and exogenous cortisol or ACTH administration. The dexamethasone suppression test can help distinguish between possible etiologies of hypercorticism. In normal individuals, low doses of dexamethasone suppress cortisol production. In patients with ACTH-producing pituitary adenomas, high doses of dexamethasone are needed to suppress cortisol production. In patients with adrenal adenomas or ectopic sources of ACTH, both low and high doses of dexamethasone fail to suppress cortisol production. Unlike patients with ectopic ACTH production, patients with an adrenal adenoma are expected to have low levels of ACTH due to negative feedback inhibition from the increased cortisol levels, as noted in this patient.

Answer B is incorrect. Bilateral adrenal hyperplasia suggests increased stimulation of the adrenal glands due to increased ACTH production from either a pituitary adenoma or an ectopic ACTH source.

Answer C is incorrect. Ectopic ACTH production is seen in paraneoplastic syndromes associated with bronchogenic cancer, pancreatic cancer, and thymomas. Bilateral adrenal hyperplasia and failed dexamethasone suppression are characteristics of ectopic ACTH production. A single mass noted on abdominal CT scan adjacent to a kidney is more suggestive of an adrenal adenoma than bilateral adrenal hyperplasia.

Answer D is incorrect. Although exogenous corticosteroid administration, like adrenal adenomas, results in decreased levels of ACTH, a mass on abdominal CT scan would be unlikely in a patient with exogenous corticosteroid administration.

Answer E is incorrect. An ACTH-secreting pituitary adenoma would cause bilateral adrenal hyperplasia and elevated ACTH levels, which are usually suppressed with high-dose dexamethasone.

48. **The correct answer is D.** This vignette describes a patient suffering from hypercalcemia secondary to malignancy. The laboratory data show hypercalcemia coupled with hypophosphatemia in the setting of an elevated serum alkaline phosphatase activity. This is consistent with hypercalcemia due to the action of PTHrP, which produces physiologic effects that mimic those of PTH: increased bone resorption and increased renal absorption of calcium, resulting in elevated levels of these electrolytes in the serum.

Answer A is incorrect. PTH and PTHrP do not act at the adrenal cortex or the intestines. The adrenal cortex is the primary site of action for ACTH and ACTH-like peptide; the intestines are the primary site of action for 1,25-dihydroxycholecalciferol.

Answer B is incorrect. PTH and PTHrP have no action at the adrenal cortex. ACTH and ACTH-like peptide (both of which can be elaborated by neoplastic cells, resulting in Cushing's syndrome) act primarily at the adrenal cortex.

Answer C is incorrect. The intestines and bones are primary sites of action for 1,25-dihydroxycholecalciferol (vitamin D). While PTH and PTHrP stimulate production of 1,25-dihydroxycholecalciferol, producing secondary effects at the intestines, these hormones do not act primarily on the intestines.

Answer E is incorrect. PTH and PTHrP act primarily at the renal tubules and bones to increase serum calcium levels. These hormones do not influence the pancreas, although pancreatic tumors have been shown to occasionally secrete PTHrP.

49. **The correct answer is E.** The actions of insulin are mediated at the cellular level by binding of the insulin to its receptor followed by autophosphorylation of tyrosine residues on the insulin receptor; this generates a tyrosine kinase that participates in an intracellular signaling cascade. Inhibition of tyrosine kinase function would preclude downstream signaling and block the physiologic changes associated with insulin action, regardless of the amount of insulin present in the blood.

Answer A is incorrect. Adenylate cyclase and its product, cAMP, are involved in numerous important intracellular signaling systems, including the systems that mediate autonomic sympathetic nervous stimulation, ADH action, renal calcium and phosphate transport, and glucagon action. However, adenylate cyclase and cAMP are not involved in the system that mediates insulin action.

Answer B is incorrect. Guanylate cyclase and its product, cGMP, are involved in many intracellular signaling systems, including those that mediate the transduction of visual stimuli into electrical signals in the nervous system and the relaxation of vascular smooth muscle throughout the body. However, guanylate cyclase and cGMP are not involved in the system that mediates insulin action.

Answer C is incorrect. Serine kinases are involved in a number of intracellular signaling cascades, but they are not involved in the signaling cascade that mediates insulin action.

Answer D is incorrect. Threonine kinases are involved in a number of intracellular signaling cascades, but they are not involved in the signaling cascade that mediates insulin action.

50. **The correct answer is A.** This patient has a pheochromocytoma, a chromaffin cell tumor of the adrenal medulla that secretes excess epinephrine and norepinephrine. Signs and symptoms of pheochromocytoma include episodic hypertension, headache, sweating, tachycardia, palpitations, and pallor. Pheochromo-

cytomas may occur sporadically or as part of the MEN syndromes, which are a group of autosomal dominant syndromes in which more than one endocrine organ is dysfunctional. Given his history of thyroid carcinoma requiring a thryoidectomy, this patient most likely has MEN type II, which is characterized by the combination of medullary carcinoma of the thyroid, pheochromocytoma, and parathyroid hyperplasia. Pheochromocytomas are treated surgically, but must first be managed preoperatively with both a nonselective α-antagonist (usually phenoxybenzamine) to normalize blood pressure, followed by a β-blocker (e.g., propranolol) to control tachycardia. The β-blocker should never be started prior to α-blockade because it would result in unopposed α-receptor stimulation, leading to a further elevation in blood pressure.

Answer B is incorrect. Pheochromocytomas are treated surgically, but must first be managed preoperatively with both a nonselective β-antagonist (usually phenoxybenzamine) to normalize blood pressure, followed by a β-blocker (e.g., propranolol) to control tachycardia. The β-blocker should never be started prior to α-blockade because it would result in unopposed α-receptor stimulation, leading to a further elevation in blood pressure.

Answer C is incorrect. Levothyroxine is thyroid hormone replacement that is used to treat hypothyroidism and myxedema. It is not indicated in the treatment of pheochromocytoma.

Answer D is incorrect. Prednisone is a glucocorticoid that is used to treat many inflammatory, allergic, and immunologic disorders, but is not indicated in the treatment of pheochromocytoma.

Answer E is incorrect. Propylthiouracil is used to treat hyperthyroidism. It acts by inhibiting the organification and coupling of thyroid hormone synthesis, and by decreasing the peripheral conversion of thyroxine to triiodothyronine. It is not indicated in the treatment of pheochromocytoma.

CHAPTER 10

Gastrointestinal

1. A 35-year-old woman who is HIV-positive presents to the physician with jaundice and right upper quadrant abdominal pain. The patient reports having had multiple episodes of jaundice over the past 10 years. A hepatitis panel is positive for HBsAg and anti-HBc IgM, but negative for HBsAb and anti-HAV IgM. Which of the following would most likely be lower than normal in this patient?

(A) Albumin
(B) Alkaline phosphatase
(C) Bilirubin
(D) Prothrombin time
(E) Transaminases

2. A 1-year-old boy presents to the emergency department with bilious vomiting, bloody stools, and abdominal distention. The new intern orders an abdominal radiograph and abdominal ultrasound. The abdominal radiograph is shown in the image. The abdominal ultrasound shows the superior mesenteric artery and vein twisting in a clockwise fashion. Which of the following conditions is the most likely cause of this patient's symptoms?

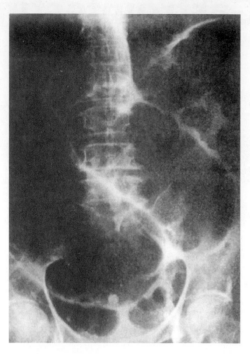

Reproduced, with permission, from Tintinalli JE, Kelen GD, Stapczynski JS, Ma OJ, Cline DM. *Tintinalli's Emergency Medicine: A Comprehensive Study Guide*, 6th ed. New York: McGraw-Hill, 2004: Figure 79-1.

(A) Colorectal carcinoma
(B) Duodenal atresia
(C) Esophageal atresia
(D) Intussusception
(E) Volvulus

3. A 35-year-old woman that is pregnant with her fourth child comes to the physician because of painful gastrointestinal bleeding for the past month. The pain and bleeding are worse when she defecates. Which of the following is the most likely diagnosis?

(A) Colorectal carcinoma
(B) External hemorrhoids
(C) Internal hemorrhoids
(D) Perianal abscess
(E) Squamous cell carcinoma

4. A 45-year-old woman presents to her physician with a 2-day history of right upper quadrant pain, nausea, gas, and vomiting. She reports that her symptoms are worse after she eats a fatty meal. Which of the following substances inhibits the hormone causing her right upper quadrant pain?

   (A) Cholecystokinin
   (B) Gastrin
   (C) Pepsin
   (D) Secretin
   (E) Somatostatin

5. A healthy 25-year-old man comes to the physician for a routine examination. His laboratory tests show a serum bilirubin level of 4 mg/dL and a direct bilirubin level of 0.3 mg/dL. The patient's liver function tests are normal. Which of the following best explains this patient's serum and indirect bilirubin levels?

   (A) Extrahepatic biliary obstruction
   (B) Glucuronosyltransferase deficiency
   (C) Heme oxygenase deficiency
   (D) Intrahepatic biliary obstruction
   (E) Liver cell damage

6. A 39-year-old white woman who suffers from polycythemia vera presents to the clinic complaining of severe and constant right upper quadrant pain over the past 2 days. Physical examination reveals an enlarged liver. What other finding would most likely be seen at presentation?

   (A) Ascites
   (B) Asterixis
   (C) Esophageal varices
   (D) Hyperpigmented skin
   (E) Spider angiomata

7. A 30-year-old woman presents to her physician complaining of chest pain and difficulty swallowing. Results of ECG and x-ray of the chest were normal, but the following image was seen during a barium swallow study. Which of the following actions is most likely absent in this patient?

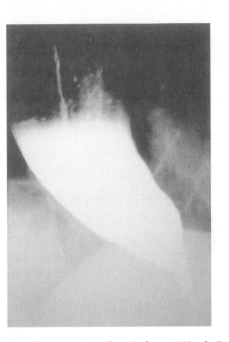

Reproduced, with permission, from Lalwani AK, ed. *Current Diagnosis & Treatment in Otolaryngology—Head & Neck Surgery*, 2nd ed. New York: McGraw-Hill, 2008: Figure 35-3A.

   (A) Contraction of the lower esophageal sphincter
   (B) Contraction of the upper esophageal sphincter
   (C) Initiation of swallowing in the oropharynx
   (D) Relaxation of the lower esophageal sphincter
   (E) Relaxation of the upper esophageal sphincter

8. An unconscious 57-year-old man is brought to the emergency department by ambulance with massive, bright red emesis. On arrival, his blood pressure is 80/40 mm Hg and his heart rate is 124/min. He appears jaundiced with multiple spider angiomas on his chest and arms. He has an enlarged abdomen that is dull to percussion and positive for a fluid wave. He has spleno-megaly and muscle wasting in his extremities. Which of the following vessel anastomoses is responsible for the patient's bleeding?

(A) Left gastric artery and left gastric vein
(B) Left gastric vein and azygos vein
(C) Paraumbilical vein and inferior epigastric vein
(D) Portal vein and inferior vena cava
(E) Splenic vein and left renal vein

9. A 43-year-old man with a 20-year history of ul-cerative colitis presents to the physician with complaints of worsening bloody diarrhea, pro-gressive fatigue, pruritus, visual disturbances, and arthralgias. On physical examination, he is found to have icteric sclera, finger clubbing, and several small ulcerations with necrotic edges on both legs. Endoscopic retrograde cho-langiopancreatography (ERCP) shows alternat-ing strictures and dilations of the bile ducts. Which of the following conditions is consistent with these ERCP findings?

(A) Cholelithiasis
(B) Pancreatic carcinoma
(C) Primary biliary cirrhosis
(D) Primary hemochromatosis
(E) Primary sclerosing cholangitis

10. A 17-year-old girl who is being treated with an-tibiotics for recurrent sinus tract infections presents to the physician with intractable wa-tery diarrhea and cramps. Which of the follow-ing is most often associated with this patient's condition?

(A) *Clostridium difficile*
(B) *Clostridium perfringens*
(C) *Escherichia coli*
(D) *Staphylococcus aureus*
(E) *Vibrio cholerae*
(F) *Yersinia enterocolitica*

11. A 65-year-old white woman presents to the emergency department with persistent right upper quadrant pain with nausea and vomit-ing. Abdominal CT scan reveals a polypoid mass of the gallbladder protruding into the lu-men, diffuse thickening of the gallbladder wall, and enlarged lymph nodes. This patient most likely has a history of which of the following?

(A) *Ascaris lumbricoides*
(B) Cigarette smoking
(C) Gallstones
(D) *Schistosoma haematobium*
(E) Tuberculosis

12. Which of the following types of hepatocellular injury is commonly seen after acetaminophen overdose?

(A) Acute hepatitis
(B) Centrilobular necrosis
(C) Fibrosis
(D) Granuloma formation
(E) Microvesicular fatty change

13. A 46-year-old woman comes to the physician because of voluminous, malodorous, bulky stools. The diarrhea usually abates on fasting. Fecal analysis shows an increased stool osmo-lality and fat content (fecal fat excretion 32 g/day [normal: <7 g/day]). Laboratory tests show a sodium level of 149 mEq/L, potassium of 3.5 mEq/L, chloride of 110 mEq/L, and bicarbon-ate of 18 mEq/L. Which of the following is the pathologic mechanism most likely responsible for the patient's presentation?

(A) Exudative diarrhea
(B) Malabsorption
(C) Motility derangement
(D) Osmotic diarrhea
(E) Secretory diarrhea

14. A 62-year-old woman has had persistent nausea for 5 years with occasional vomiting. Gastroin-testinal endoscopy reveals a small area of gastric mucosa in the fundus without rugal folds, and a biopsy demonstrates well-differentiated adeno-carcinoma confined to the mucosa. Upper gas-trointestinal endoscopy performed 5 years ago showed a pattern of gastritis. Microscopy at that

time showed chronic inflammation with the presence of *Helicobacter pylori*. Which of the following best characterizes this patient's neoplasm?

(A) Favorable prognosis
(B) Highest incidence in the United States
(C) Linitis plastica
(D) Metastases limited to regional lymph nodes
(E) On light microscopy, a signet ring cell pattern

15. A 23-year-old man presents to the physician with abdominal distention and tenderness with no vomiting or diarrhea. Physical examination shows hepatosplenomegaly. Bowel sounds are normal. On questioning, the patient says that he traveled to eastern South America 1 year ago. Several weeks after returning from his trip, he remembers having fever, diarrhea, weight loss, and "funny looking stools." Ultrasonography shows ascites and hepatic periportal fibrosis. Which of the following is most likely responsible for this patient's present symptoms?

(A) Appendicitis
(B) Bowel obstruction
(C) Enterocolitis
(D) Portal hypertension
(E) Ruptured viscus

16. A 62-year-old woman with rheumatoid arthritis and no other past medical history comes to the emergency department complaining of severe epigastric pain, nausea, and vomiting. She says that she vomited blood earlier in the day. A gross image of the gastric mucosa is shown. Which of the following is the most likely cause of this patient's symptoms?

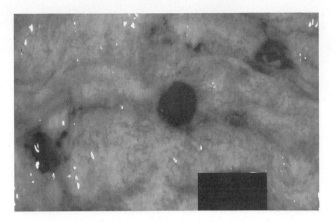

Reproduced, with permission, from PEIR Digital Library (http://peir.net).

(A) Amyloidosis
(B) Infection with *Helicobacter pylori*
(C) Nonsteroidal anti-inflammatory drugs
(D) Prednisone
(E) Uremia

17. A 20-year-old man with Crohn's disease refractory to treatment with high-dose methylprednisolone is started on therapy with infliximab, a chimeric monoclonal antibody with anti-inflammatory effects. This drug is administered intravenously every 2 months and produces substantial improvement in the patient's symptoms between doses. Which of the following best describes infliximab's mechanism of action?

(A) Acting as a partial agonist at some estrogen receptors and as an antagonist at others
(B) Binding a growth factor receptor to target a cell for killing
(C) Binding to and neutralizing a secreted cytokine
(D) Inhibiting a fusion protein with tyrosine kinase activity
(E) Irreversibly inhibiting the enzyme cyclooxygenase

18. A 2-month-old boy is brought to his pediatrician for a regular check-up. His parents report that he has a poor appetite and is very constipated. He has small bowel movements once a week, which his parents believe are very painful. Although he was at the 75th percentile for both height and weight at birth, he is currently at the 25th percentile for height and is below the 5th percentile for weight. His abdomen is distended, but his bowel sounds are normal and his abdomen does not appear to be tender. Barium enema shows a narrow rectosigmoid with a dilation of the segment above the narrowing, and a rectosigmoid biopsy shows a conspicuous absence of acetylcholinesterase-positive ganglion cells. Which of the following genetic conditions is most commonly associated with this patient's disease?

(A) Cystic fibrosis
(B) Down's syndrome
(C) Sickle cell disease
(D) Tay-Sachs disease
(E) Turner's syndrome

19. An 8-year-old boy presents to the emergency department with a 2-hour history of vomiting after eating dinner at a seafood buffet. Arterial blood gas analysis reveals a pH of 7.50, an bicarbonate level of 34 mEq/L, and partial carbon dioxide pressure of 40 mm Hg. Which of the following best describes the acid-base disturbance occurring in this patient?

(A) Metabolic acidosis
(B) Metabolic acidosis/respiratory acidosis
(C) Metabolic acidosis/respiratory alkalosis
(D) Metabolic acidosis/respiratory compensation
(E) Metabolic alkalosis
(F) Metabolic alkalosis/respiratory compensation

20. A 37-year-old woman is found by police in a confused state and is brought to the emergency department for evaluation. The patient is unable to answer any of the physician's questions. Physical examination reveals jaundice. Despite aggressive therapy the patient dies. An autopsy is performed and a microscopic view of the patient's liver is shown in the image. Which of

the following conditions is most consistent with these findings?

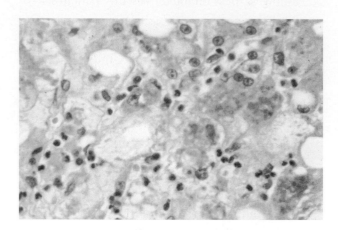

Reproduced, with permission, from PEIR Digital Library (http://peir.net).

(A) α_1-Antitrypsin deficiency
(B) Acute viral hepatitis
(C) Alcoholic hepatitis
(D) Fatty liver of pregnancy
(E) Neonatal hepatitis

21. A 24-year-old man presents to the physician with diarrhea and abdominal cramps. A fecal occult blood test is positive. On questioning, it is learned that the patient went swimming in a lake during a camping trip 2 days ago. A stool sample is sent for laboratory evaluation. This patient is most likely infected with which of the following?

(A) *Cryptosporidium*
(B) *Entamoeba histolytica*
(C) *Giardia lamblia*
(D) *Leishmania donovani*
(E) *Naegleria fowleri*
(F) *Toxoplasma gondii*

22. A 27-year-old man goes to the doctor for an annual physical examination. On rectal examination, masses are palpated. The patient is referred for a colonoscopy, which reveals adenomatous polyps located diffusely throughout the colon. When asked about his family history, the patient states that his father passed away from colon cancer. A diagnosis of familial adenomatous polyposis is suspected, and the patient asks how he got this. Which of the following is the inheritance pattern of this condition?

(A) Autosomal dominant
(B) Autosomal recessive
(C) Autosomal trisomy
(D) Sex chromosome abnormality
(E) X-linked recessive

23. A 10-year-old girl living in New Jersey is brought to the physician because she has had a fever and headache accompanied by abdominal pain and bloody diarrhea. Her stool smear shows leukocytes. A stool culture incubated at 42° C (107.6° F) in a microaerophilic environment shows many comma-shaped organisms each with a single polar flagellum. She has no history of recent travel or sick contacts. She has a pet puppy, which the mother says has had diarrhea for the past week. Based on the above information, the physician suspects bacterial gastroenteritis. The organism responsible for this patient's sickness is thought to be associated with the possible later development of which of the following symptoms?

(A) Acute renal failure and thrombocytopenia with hemolytic anemia
(B) Fever, migratory polyarthritis, and carditis
(C) Fever, new murmur, small erythematous lesions on the palms, and splinter hemorrhages on the nail bed
(D) Petechial rash and bilateral hemorrhage into the adrenal glands
(E) Symmetric ascending muscle weakness beginning in the distal lower extremities

24. A 2-year-old girl who has recently been adopted from an impoverished family is brought to the clinic by her adopted parents. They are concerned because the child seems to be having trouble with her vision at in low-light conditions. The vitamin most likely deficient in this child is absorbed by the gastrointestinal system using what mechanism?

(A) Apoferritin-mediated transport
(B) Intrinsic factor-mediated transport
(C) Micelle-mediated transport
(D) Sodium-dependent cotransport
(E) Vitamin D-dependent binding protein-mediated transport

25. A 46-year-old white woman with rheumatoid arthritis presents with severe pruritus. She denies any history of alcohol or drug use. On physical examination, she is found to have icteric sclera, palpebral xanthomas, and hepatomegaly. She tests positive for antimitochondrial antibody and increased alkaline phosphatase activity. Which of the following is most likely responsible for this patient's presentation?

(A) Destruction of intrahepatic bile ducts
(B) Hepatic parenchymal destruction
(C) Obstruction of extrahepatic bile ducts
(D) Portal vein thrombosis
(E) Stenosis of extrahepatic and intrahepatic bile ducts

26. A 10-year-old boy presents to the pediatrician with weight loss and multiple purpuric lesions all over his body. The patient has bulky, greasy yellow stools associated with abdominal pain and flatulence that most often occurs after meals. Which of the following will most likely be seen on bowel biopsy?

(A) Benign mucosa
(B) Continuous linear mucosal lesions
(C) Diffuse severe atrophy and blunting of the villi
(D) Foamy macrophages in the lamina propria
(E) Skip lesions with crypt abscesses and granulomas

27. A 26-year-old man with hepatitis C is being medically treated while he awaits liver transplantation. One of the drugs he is taking causes him to have periodic fevers and chills and a sense of depression that he did not have prior to treatment. Which of the following is most likely responsible for this patient's adverse effects?

(A) Intravenous immunoglobulin
(B) Lamivudine
(C) Pegylated interferon
(D) Ribavirin
(E) Tumor necrosis factor-α

28. A 19-year-old man presents to the emergency department with a new onset of right lower quadrant abdominal pain. On physical examination, the patient has a temperature of 38.5° C (101.3° F) and a WBC count of 13,000/mm³. Flexion at his hip elicits pain. Release of manual pressure on the abdomen causes more pain than deep palpation. Which of the following is also most likely present in this patient?

(A) Abdominal distention
(B) Dyspnea
(C) Hunger
(D) Nausea and vomiting
(E) Profuse watery diarrhea

29. A 4-year-old child is brought to the pediatrician because of abdominal pain, vomiting, and diarrhea containing mucus and blood. The child has a fever of 39.4° C (103° F). On stool culture, the causative organism is shown to be a non-lactose-fermenting and non-hydrogen sulfide-producing bacterium. Which of the following is most likely responsible for the child's illness?

(A) Enteroinvasive *Escherichia coli*
(B) Enterotoxigenic *Escherichia coli*
(C) *Salmonella* spp.
(D) *Shigella* species
(E) *Vibrio cholerae*

30. A 42-year-old man visits his primary care physician to discuss possible cholesterol-lowering agents. His last blood test showed that he had elevated LDL cholesterol and triglyceride levels. The physician decides to prescribe gemfibrozil and schedules the man for a follow-up visit in 1 month. Which of the following results are likely to be seen on this patient's next blood test?

(A) A decrease in LDL cholesterol and a slight increase in triglycerides
(B) A decrease in LDL cholesterol with little to no effect on HDL or triglycerides
(C) A large decrease in LDL cholesterol, an increase in HDL cholesterol, and a slight decrease in triglycerides

(D) A large decrease in triglycerides, a slight decrease in LDL cholesterol, and a slight increase in HDL cholesterol
(E) An increase in LDL cholesterol, a slight decrease in HDL cholesterol, and a decrease in triglycerides

31. A 76-year-old man with chronic obstructive pulmonary disease presents at his annual clinic visit with complaints of black stools and epigastric pain relieved by meals. He reports a 4.5-kg (10-lb) weight gain over the past 4 months. He has no other medical problems and takes no medications. Physical examination is unremarkable. His plasma calcium and phosphate levels are within the normal ranges. Endoscopy reveals mucosal ulceration in the duodenal bulb. Which of the following is the most likely risk factor for this patient's duodenal ulcer?

(A) Alcohol use
(B) Chronic nonsteroidal anti-inflammatory use
(C) Excessive salt intake
(D) Primary hyperparathyroidism
(E) Tobacco use

32. An 8-year-old boy returns from a camping trip complaining of abdominal cramping, diarrhea, and excessive gas. A duodenal aspirate reveals the organism shown in the image. What is the most likely explanation for his symptoms?

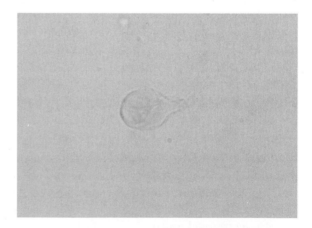

Reproduced, with permission, from the Centers for Disease Control and Prevention's Public Health Image Library; content provider Dr. Mae Melvin.

(A) Activation of enteral adenylate cyclase
(B) Deficiency of an enzyme
(C) Invasion of the lining of the intestine
(D) Small bowel inflammation and villous atrophy
(E) Viral infection of the cells of the small intestinal villi

33. A 20-year-old man presents to his physician with a 2-day history of fever, vomiting, and diarrhea. His laboratory studies are unremarkable except for a serum albumin level of 7.5 g/dL. Which of the following conditions would most likely cause this patient's laboratory abnormality?

(A) Acute infection
(B) Chronic liver disease
(C) Dehydration
(D) Nephrotic syndrome
(E) Poor nutritional status

34. A 33-year-old man with active gastroesophageal reflux disease returns to his physician for the second time in 2 weeks complaining of a worsening sore throat. The patient was previously diagnosed with penicillin-sensitive *Streptococcus pyogenes* on throat culture and, because he is allergic to penicillin, was given ciprofloxacin. Suspicious of an interaction, the physician asks the patient if he has been taking any other medications. Which of the following medications is this patient most likely taking?

(A) Aspirin
(B) Calcium carbonate
(C) Cimetidine
(D) Misoprostol
(E) Omeprazole

35. A 50-year-old alcoholic man presents with intermittent "stomach" pain that also seems to be present "between his shoulder blades." The pain is often associated with nausea and vomiting. He also states that every once in a while he has a few days of bulky, foul-smelling stools.

He also says he has been admitted to the hospital several times over the past few years for the same reason. Which of the following is the most likely finding associated with this patient's illness?

(A) Abdominal air-fluid levels on x-ray
(B) Abdominal free air under the right hemidiaphragm on x-ray
(C) Pancreatic calcifications on computed tomography
(D) Pancreatic cysts
(E) Pancreatic granuloma formation

36. A 51-year-old man with a long history of medication-dependent reflux esophagitis sees his physician for an annual physical, which reveals a blood gastrin level three times the upper limit of normal. His physician is concerned that the patient might develop atrophic gastritis. Which of the following medications is this patient most likely taking?

(A) Aluminum hydroxide
(B) Bismuth
(C) Cimetidine
(D) Misoprostol
(E) Omeprazole

37. A 22-year-old man presents to the physician with a 1-year history of chronic recurrent right lower quadrant abdominal pain and diarrhea. The patient also has had low-grade fevers and a 6.7-kg (15-lb) weight loss during this period. Colonoscopy reveals multiple lesions of the terminal ileum and colon. Biopsies of these lesions reveal full-thickness inflammation and ulceration of the involved mucosa. Which of the following is the most likely diagnosis?

(A) Celiac sprue
(B) Collagenous colitis
(C) Crohn's disease
(D) Irritable bowel syndrome
(E) Ulcerative colitis

38. A 57-year-old woman comes to the physician 6 weeks after returning from a trip to Greece. She has had a fever of 38.8° C (101.8° F) that rises during the day and decreases at night. She says that she feels tired and has lost weight. She mentions she enjoyed her vacation and trying the local specialties, including fresh goat cheese. Her physical examination is notable for hepatosplenomegaly and generalized lymphadenopathy. Which of the following organisms is most likely responsible for this patient's symptoms?

(A) *Bartonella henselae*
(B) *Brucella melitensis*
(C) *Pasteurella multocida*
(D) *Plasmodium malariae*

39. A 53-year-old man with a history of drinking 1–2 bottles of vodka a day for the past 25 years presents to the emergency department with massive hematemesis. He takes antacids for mild acid reflux but has no other known medical problems or medications. His temperature is 36.7° C (98.1° F), pulse is 110/min, respiratory rate is 23/min, and blood pressure is 80/40 mm Hg. Physical examination reveals a regular rate and rhythm with no murmurs and his lungs are clear to auscultation. There is no abdominal tenderness or distension and bowel sounds are present. His stool is negative for blood. Which of the following is the most likely diagnosis?

(A) Esophageal laceration (Mallory-Weiss syndrome)
(B) Esophageal metaplasia (Barrett's esophagus)
(C) Esophageal squamous cell carcinoma
(D) Esophageal stricture
(E) Hiatal hernia

40. A 32-year-old woman presents to the physician with alternating bouts of diarrhea and constipation. She also has chronic abdominal pain relieved by frequent bowel movements. Her symptoms are exacerbated by stress. The patient denies fever or weight loss. She has a negative hemoccult test. Colonoscopy and endoscopy reveal no abnormalities. The most probable diagnosis in this patient is commonly associated with which of the following?

(A) Leukocytosis
(B) Normal biopsy
(C) Primary sclerosing cholangitis
(D) Strictures in the small bowel
(E) Villous flattening in the small intestine

41. A 55-year-old female farmer from Venezuela with a past medical history significant for smoking and alcoholism presents to her primary care physician's office with concerns regarding recent episodes of intermittent hemoptysis and chest pain. On questioning the patient describes symptoms of a chronic cough and dyspnea. She denies any fever, night sweats, weight loss, or anorexia. On physical examination the physician notes dullness to percussion on the right base of the lung and bronchial breathing on auscultation. Results of laboratory tests, including serum electrolytes, complete blood cell count, and liver function tests, are within normal limits. X-ray of the chest is shown in the image. What potentially life-threatening complication is most likely to result from this patient's disease?

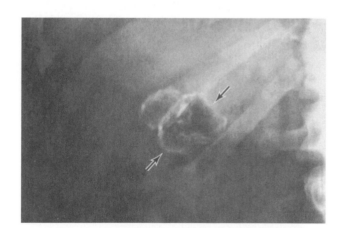

Reproduced, with permission, from Tanagho EA, McAnnich JW. *Smith's Geneal Urology.* 17th ed. New York: McGraw-Hill, 2008: Figure 14-5.

(A) Anaphylactic shock
(B) Disseminated intravascular coagulation
(C) Hepatitis
(D) Metastatic spread
(E) Myocardial infarction

42. A healthy 55-year-old woman presents to the physician with a 1-year history of an unchanging, palpable mass in her left cheek. A parotid gland biopsy reveals groups of well-differentiated epithelial cells in a chondromyxoid stroma surrounded by a fibrous capsule; multiple cell types are visible on light microscopy. The pathologic description of the mass is most consistent with which of the following conditions?

(A) Adenoid cystic carcinoma
(B) Mucoepidermoid carcinoma
(C) Pleomorphic adenoma
(D) Sialic duct stone
(E) Warthin's tumor

43. A 45-year-old woman who was diagnosed with scleroderma 5 years ago presents to her physician with increasing difficulty swallowing. Which of the following abnormalities of esophageal muscle function is the most likely cause of these symptoms?

(A) Atrophy of smooth muscle in the lower two thirds of the esophagus
(B) Atrophy of smooth muscle in the upper two thirds of the esophagus
(C) Atrophy of striated muscle in the lower two thirds of the esophagus
(D) Atrophy of striated muscle in the middle one third of the esophagus
(E) Atrophy of striated muscle in the upper two thirds of the esophagus

44. A previously healthy 70-year-old man presents to the emergency department with lower abdominal pain, fever, and an elevated WBC count. Which of the following is the most likely etiology of this patient's condition?

(A) Embolic arterial occlusion of the superior mesenteric artery leading to bowel infarction
(B) Idiopathic transmural inflammation of the distal colon
(C) Increased intraluminal pressure leading to perforation of a bowel outpouching
(D) Malignant cells invading one of the vessels supplying the colon
(E) Twisting of the sigmoid colon about its mesenteric base

45. A 26-year-old man presents to the clinic with bradykinesia, rigidity, and resting tremor. Serum aminotransferase levels are mildly elevated. A liver biopsy is shown in the image. What is the chance that this patient's sister will have the same condition?

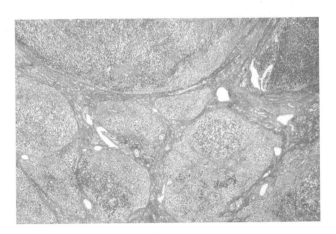

Reproduced, with permission, from PEIR Digital Library (http://peir.net).

(A) 0%
(B) 25%
(C) 50%
(D) 66.6%
(E) 100%

46. A woman comes to the physician because of profuse vomiting and watery, nonbloody diarrhea that developed 5 hours after she had eaten tuna salad. She is diagnosed with food poisoning. Which of the following is a characteristic of the most likely cause of her symptoms?

(A) Microscopic examination of the patient's stool will demonstrate gram-positive, catalase-positive, and coagulase-negative bacteria
(B) One would expect to observe a positive quellung reaction from a culture of the tuna salad
(C) Thayer-Martin media could be used to culture the pathologic organism from this patient's stool
(D) The contaminated canned fish was the source of the pathologic organism
(E) The enterotoxin is preformed in food; therefore there is a short incubation time for the development of the disease

47. A newborn presents to the pediatrician with kernicterus, jaundice, and elevation of serum unconjugated bilirubin; the patient dies soon after her first birthday. This patient most likely had a deficiency in which of the following enzymes?

(A) Aldolase B
(B) Galactose-1-phosphate uridyltransferase
(C) Glucose 6-phosphatase
(D) Uridine diphosphate-glucuronosyltransferase
(E) Uroporphyrinogen decarboxylase

48. A 45-year-old man presents with severe anal pain. He is noted to have a fluctuant red and tender mass consistent with a perianal abscess. The patient has had cyclical fevers. He has a temperature of 38.2° C (100.8° F), a heart rate of 89/min, a blood pressure of 129/85 mm Hg, and a respiratory rate of 18/min. The abscess is drained and a specimen of the pus is examined under a microscope. The specimen is shown to contain a predominance of neutrophils. Which of the following factors is most abundant in the pus specimen?

(A) Leukotriene B_4
(B) Prostaglandin I_2
(C) Thromboxane A_2
(D) Vascular endothelial growth factor
(E) von Willebrand factor

49. A 40-year-old white man presents to the emergency department complaining of burning retrosternal chest pain after meals. His pain is relieved by antacids. The patient's ECG is normal, and his x-ray of the chest is remarkable for an 8-cm hiatal hernia. This patient is at risk for developing which of the following types of cancer?

(A) Adenocarcinoma of the esophagus
(B) Krukenberg's tumor
(C) Non-small cell adenocarcinoma of the lung
(D) Squamous cell carcinoma of the esophagus
(E) Stomach carcinoma

50. A 50-year-old man presents to his physician because of a 6.8-kg (15-lb) weight loss over the past month, epigastric pain radiating to the back, and jaundice. Laboratory studies show an amylase level of 500 U/L, a lipase level of 300 U/L, and an alkaline phosphatase level of 500 U/L. Levels of CA 19-9 and carcinoembryonic antigen are also elevated. Which of the following is most likely responsible for this patient's symptoms?

(A) Acute cholecystitis
(B) Acute pancreatitis
(C) Carcinoid tumor
(D) Colon cancer
(E) Pancreatic adenocarcinoma

1. **The correct answer is A.** This patient has a flare-up of her chronic hepatitis B infection, as evidenced by the presence of HBsAg and anti-HBc IgM and lack of HBsAb. Hepatitis B typically presents with jaundice and right upper quadrant pain and can be transmitted via parenteral, sexual, and maternal-fetal routes. Chronic hepatitis B is marked by the presence of HBsAg for >6 months. While most patients will develop HBsAb and eliminate HBsAg from the blood, chronically infected patients do not. A patient with HIV may have a history of risky sexual behavior and would be at risk for hepatitis B infection; in fact, chronic HBV infection affects about 10% of HIV-infected patients worldwide. This patient's chronic liver disease would lead to a decrease in albumin, as it is typically produced by the liver.

Answer B is incorrect. A patient with chronic liver disease would have an elevation in alkaline phosphatase activity due to decreased function of the biliary tree.

Answer C is incorrect. A patient with chronic liver disease would have an elevation of serum bilirubin, due to difficulty with release into the bile.

Answer D is incorrect. A patient with chronic liver disease would have an increase in prothrombin time, as the liver is the site of production of all major coagulation factors, except factor VIII.

Answer E is incorrect. A patient with chronic liver disease would have an elevation of transaminases, as these indicate hepatocellular damage.

2. **The correct answer is E.** This is an example of volvulus, a twisting of the bowel that results in compression of portions of the intestine by other loops of bowel. In adults, volvulus occurs with equal frequency in both the small and large intestines. In children, volvulus almost always occurs in the small intestine and is often the result of intestinal malrotation that occurred during development of the embryonic gut. This patient has symptoms of advanced volvulus: bilious vomiting, abdominal distention, and bloody stools. On the abdominal radiograph, he exhibits the nonspecific "double-bubble," which is a sign of intestinal obstruction. In the image, the white arrow points to the smaller bubble representing the proximal duodenum, while the black arrow points to the stomach. The twisting of the superior mesenteric artery and vein on abdominal ultrasound are more specific for a diagnosis of volvulus as a result of malrotation.

Answer A is incorrect. Colorectal carcinoma may be papillary or polypoid. A 1-year-old patient is unlikely to have colorectal carcinoma that would be large enough to cause clinical and radiologic signs of bowel obstruction.

Answer B is incorrect. Duodenal atresia is the failure of the duodenum to recanalize normally during embryonic development. Duodenal atresia is usually diagnosed prior to birth (usually with a fetal ultrasound showing polyhydramnios) or early in the postpartum period (when the infant displays bilious vomiting or absent bowel movements). About 30% of patients with duodenal atresia have Down's syndrome. Infants with duodenal atresia do exhibit the "double bubble" sign on abdominal radiograph, but do not have twisting of the superior mesenteric artery and vein in a clockwise fashion.

Answer C is incorrect. Esophageal atresia is a developmental defect causing a blind-ended pouch of the esophagus. As a result there is an interruption in the connection between the proximal and distal ends of the esophagus. Patients with esophageal atresia are diagnosed shortly after birth, when they exhibit coughing or turning blue with feedings, excessive drooling, or immediate regurgitation after feeding. In addition, patients do not exhibit bilious vomiting because the defect is at a more proximal location of the alimentary canal. Additionally, patients do not have the "double bubble" sign on radiographs, nor do they have a clockwise twisting of the superior mesenteric artery and vein.

Answer D is incorrect. Intussusception occurs when one segment of the small intestine telescopes into the immediately distal segment of the bowel. Although intussusception can cause vomiting and is common in children, the radiologic findings make volvulus, and not intussusception, the more accurate answer.

3. **The correct answer is B.** This patient has external hemorrhoids. External hemorrhoids are thromboses (blood clots) in the veins of the external rectal venous plexus. Since they originate below the pectinate line, external hemorrhoids receive somatic innervation and are therefore painful. Rectal bleeding is also a common symptom with hemorrhoids. Some of the predisposing factors for hemorrhoids include, but are not limited to, pregnancy, constipation, heavy weight lifting, or any other cause that results in increased intra-abdominal pressure.

Answer A is incorrect. The peak incidence of colorectal carcinoma is between the ages of 60 and 80 years. When it is found in a younger person, ulcerative colitis, familial adenomatous polyposis, or another preexisting precancerous syndrome must be suspected. The clinical features of colorectal carcinoma include fatigue, weakness, iron deficiency anemia, constipation, painless rectal bleeding, and abdominal pain. This patient's painful rectal bleeding and lack of other clinical evidence of a malignant lesion make this option unlikely.

Answer C is incorrect. Internal hemorrhoids are prolapses of rectal mucosa containing the normally dilated veins of the internal venous plexus. In contrast to external hemorrhoids, internal hemorrhoids originate above the pectinate line, have an autonomic nerve supply, and usually present with painless rectal bleeding.

Answer D is incorrect. Abscesses are localized collections of purulent inflammatory tissue. Perianal abscess may follow infection of anal fissures or rectal trauma. In this patient, the lack of evidence or history of infection does not support a diagnosis of abscess.

Answer E is incorrect. Squamous cell carcinomas can occur in the lower anal canal and are commonly associated with human papillomavirus infection. They can also present with pain on defecation, bleeding, and obstruction. However, this patient's lack of weight loss, intermittent course, and association of symptoms with pregnancy make this diagnosis highly unlikely.

4. **The correct answer is E.** This patient's symptoms are classic for gallstone cholecystitis. Somatostatin is released by D cells of the pancreas and gastrointestinal mucosa. It inhibits gastric acid, pepsinogen, insulin, glucagon, pancreatic and small intestine fluid secretion, and (as in this patient) gallbladder contraction.

Answer A is incorrect. Cholecystokinin is released by I cells of the duodenum and jejunum and is responsible for gallbladder contraction, pancreatic enzyme secretion, and sphincter of Oddi relaxation.

Answer B is incorrect. Gastrin is released by G cells in the antrum and duodenum and stimulates secretion of gastric acid, intrinsic factor, and pepsinogen.

Answer C is incorrect. Pepsin is secreted by chief cells of the stomach and facilitates protein digestion.

Answer D is incorrect. Secretin is secreted by S cells of the duodenum; it inhibits gastric acid secretion and stimulates bicarbonate secretion from the pancreas. It also increases bile secretion, which would act to potentiate the patient's pain.

5. **The correct answer is B.** This patient has an indirect bilirubinemia with a high total serum bilirubin but a normal direct bilirubin. In a healthy 25-year-old individual, this is most likely due to a deficiency in functional glucuronosyltransferase (GST), otherwise known as Gilbert's disease. Crigler-Najjar syndrome also results from a deficiency in this enzyme. Type I Crigler-Najjar syndrome (complete absence of GST) is always fatal, while type II (partial defect) is generally mild with occasional kernicterus. Mild GST deficiency causes an indirect hyperbilirubinemia only, while the other an-

swer choices cause an elevation in both direct and indirect bilirubin levels.

Answer A is incorrect. Extrahepatic biliary obstruction due to a tumor, stone, or stricture causes an elevation of both indirect and direct bilirubin levels.

Answer C is incorrect. The first step in the breakdown of heme into bilirubin is the formation of biliverdin by heme oxygenase. A deficiency in this enzyme would not elevate indirect bilirubin specifically.

Answer D is incorrect. Intrahepatic biliary obstruction causes a defect in excretion and results in an increase in both direct and indirect bilirubin levels.

Answer E is incorrect. Liver cell damage such as that seen in chronic hepatitis causes an elevation of both direct and indirect bilirubin due to impairments in uptake, conjugation, and excretion of bilirubin.

6. **The correct answer is A.** This is an acute presentation of Budd-Chiari syndrome, or thrombosis of two or more hepatic veins. This condition is associated with hypercoagulable states such as myeloproliferative disorders, inherited coagulation disorders, intra-abdominal cancers, oral contraceptive use, and pregnancy. The increased intrahepatic pressure leading to ascites is present in 90% of patients with Budd-Chiari syndrome. The disease can also present in a subacute manner or in a chronic manner, and diagnosing this condition may then be more challenging because the classic triad of abdominal pain, hepatomegaly, and ascites may not be present.

Answer B is incorrect. Asterixis is associated with hepatic encephalopathy in the setting of liver failure. The underlying mechanisms linking liver failure to asterixis are not completely understood.

Answer C is incorrect. Esophageal varices are associated with portal hypertension, in which portosystemic shunts occur to bypass the hepatic circulation and return blood to the heart.

Answer D is incorrect. Skin hyperpigmentation can occur in several settings, such as hemochromatosis or Addison's disease (adrenal atrophy), but none of these diseases fit the present clinical picture.

Answer E is incorrect. Spider angiomata are usually associated with cirrhosis; their pathogenesis is not completely understood but they are believed to occur in the setting of defects in the metabolism of sex hormones. They can also be present in pregnant women and malnourished patients.

7. **The correct answer is D.** The barium swallow study shows esophageal dilatation and a "bird's beak" sign of the distal esophagus, which are characteristic of achalasia. This disease presents with difficulty swallowing, abnormal contractions of esophageal muscles, absence of peristalsis, and absence of relaxation of the lower esophageal sphincter on swallowing.

Answer A is incorrect. In achalasia, the lower esophageal sphincter fails to relax. If the lower esophageal sphincter fails to close completely, a patient may experience symptoms of gastroesophageal reflux and not achalasia.

Answer B is incorrect. In achalasia, the lower esophageal sphincter is affected, not the upper esophageal sphincter.

Answer C is incorrect. There is no difficulty with initiation of swallowing in achalasia.

Answer E is incorrect. In achalasia, the lower esophageal sphincter is affected, not the upper esophageal sphincter.

8. **The correct answer is B.** The patient's presentation is consistent with ruptured esophageal varices. Portal systemic shunting of blood occurs when the liver becomes so fibrotic that there is an increase in resistance in blood flow from the portal vein and portal hypertension develops. When the pressure in the portal system is greater than the venous pressure in the systemic system, blood will find alternate routes to return to the heart. One of those alternate routes is from the left gastric vein into the azygos vein. The veins around the

esophagus and upper stomach that carry this blood may become enlarged and rupture, as in this case. Mortality from ruptured esophageal varices approaches 50%, so it is important to look for symptoms of liver disease and portal hypertension in anyone with massive hematemesis. It is also important to screen cirrhotic patients with serial endoscopies to look for varices that can be treated before they rupture.

Answer A is incorrect. The portal system is a system of veins that drain the gastrointestinal tract and deliver the blood to the liver. The left gastric artery is upstream of the portal system, and an anastomosis between the left gastric artery and vein would bypass the portal system altogether and would not contribute to the formation of esophageal varices.

Answer C is incorrect. Anastomoses between these two vessels leads to the formation of caput medusae, the spokes-of-a-wheel veins radiating from the umbilicus in patients with portal hypertension.

Answer D is incorrect. There is no route for blood to flow from the portal vein to the inferior vena cava. If there were, however, this would relieve the pressure in the portal system and would reduce the risk of bleeding from varices. In fact, creating a portacaval shunt (TIPS, or transjugular intrahepatic portosystemic shunt) is a current treatment for portal hypertension with massive ascites.

Answer E is incorrect. Anastomoses between the splenic vein and the left renal vein are retroperitoneal vessels that are not near the esophagus.

9. **The correct answer is E.** This patient presents with a number of classic extraintestinal manifestations of ulcerative colitis. Progressive fatigue, pruritus, and icteric sclera are clinical manifestations of primary sclerosing cholangitis, an irreversible condition characterized by inflammation, obliterative fibrosis, and segmental constriction of intrahepatic and extrahepatic bile ducts seen in patients with ulcerative colitis. On endoscopic retrograde cholangiopancreatography (a radiographic visualization of the pancreatic duct and biliary tree), these bile duct

changes are visualized as alternating strictures and dilations, or "beading."

Answer A is incorrect. Cholelithiasis, also known as gallstones, is not associated with ulcerative colitis. Endoscopic retrograde cholangiopancreatography may be used to visualize a ductal stone but is not a modality of choice for gallstone detection.

Answer B is incorrect. Pancreatic carcinoma is not associated with ulcerative colitis. On endoscopic retrograde cholangiopancreatography, it is characterized by a double-duct sign that results from tumor obstruction of both the common bile duct and the main pancreatic duct, not beading.

Answer C is incorrect. Primary biliary cirrhosis is a nonsuppurative, granulomatous destruction of medium-sized intrahepatic bile ducts. It is not associated with ulcerative colitis. Endoscopic retrograde cholangiopancreatography findings in this condition are nonspecific.

Answer D is incorrect. Primary hemochromatosis is a familial defect in control of iron absorption with massive accumulation of hemosiderin in hepatic and pancreatic parenchymal cells. This condition is not associated with ulcerative colitis and has no specific endoscopic retrograde cholangiopancreatography findings.

10. **The correct answer is A.** Pseudomembranous or antibiotic-associated colitis is an acute colitis characterized by the formation of adherent inflammatory exudates (pseudomembranes) on the injured mucosa. It is usually caused by the two protein exotoxins (A and B) of *Clostridium difficile*, a bacterium normally found in the gut. This disease commonly occurs in patients after a course of broad-spectrum antibiotic therapy (especially clindamycin). Alteration of the normal colonic flora allows these toxin-producing strains to thrive. Patients usually present with severe bouts of watery diarrhea, which can be life threatening. The first step in treating these patients is to immediately discontinue the offending antibiotic.

Answer B is incorrect. *Clostridium perfringens* is not associated with pseudomembranous colitis. Intestinal infection by this organism causes watery diarrhea, with some strains producing a severe necrotizing enterocolitis with perforation.

Answer C is incorrect. *Escherichia coli* is not associated with the development of pseudomembranous colitis. However, clinical features such as fever and diarrhea are common to both *E. coli and Clostridium difficile* infections.

Answer D is incorrect. Although *Staphylococcus aureus* has been implicated in pseudomembranous colitis the incidence of *S. aureus* pseudomembranous colitis is rare relative to *Clostridium difficile* colitis.

Answer E is incorrect. *Vibrio cholerae* is not implicated in pseudomembranous colitis. It usually causes massive secretory diarrhea.

Answer F is incorrect. *Yersinia enterocolitica* is not associated with pseudomembranous colitis. However, this organism can also cause fever and diarrhea secondary to intestinal epithelial invasion.

11. **The correct answer is C.** The patient's clinical presentation is consistent with adenocarcinoma of the gallbladder. Gallbladder adenocarcinoma is associated with chronic gallbladder inflammation, typically from a history of gallstones, which can be seen with the thickening of the gallbladder wall on CT. Gallbladder polyps, the polypoid lesion, are also associated with an increased risk of gallbladder adenocarcinoma. The enlarged lymph nodes point to local invasion and spread, which is unfortunately common on initial presentation. Gallbladder cancer is a disease of the elderly and is more common in women than men. Most (90%) patients with gallbladder cancer have concomitant stones. In general, the treatment for adenocarcinoma of the gallbladder is surgical excision but prognosis is generally poor if not found incidentally.

Answer A is incorrect. *Ascaris lumbricoides* is associated with gastrointestinal irritation, cough, and eosinophilia.

Answer B is incorrect. Cigarette smoking is associated with many malignancies, particularly of the lung, pancreas, and esophagus; it has not been linked to adenocarcinoma of the gallbladder.

Answer D is incorrect. *Schistosoma haematobium* infection is associated with the development of squamous cell carcinoma of the bladder.

Answer E is incorrect. Tuberculosis is associated with hemoptysis, cough, and weight loss.

12. **The correct answer is B.** Acetaminophen is known to cause centrilobular necrosis. This type of necrosis occurs immediately around the terminal hepatic vein. In addition to acetaminophen, centrilobular necrosis can be caused by carbon tetrachloride, bromobenzene, halothane, and rifampin. Diffuse hepatic necrosis has also been reported with acetaminophen toxicity.

Answer A is incorrect. Drugs causing acute hepatitis include methyldopa, isoniazid, nitrofurantoin, and phenytoin. Acetaminophen is not associated with acute hepatitis.

Answer C is incorrect. Hepatic fibrosis is commonly associated with drugs that cause chronic hepatitis and/or hepatocellular injury. Some of the culprits include ethanol, methotrexate, and amiodarone. Acetaminophen is not associated with fibrotic liver changes.

Answer D is incorrect. Granuloma formation does not occur with acetaminophen overdose. Some of the drugs associated with granuloma formation include sulfonamides, methyldopa, quinidine, hydralazine, and allopurinol.

Answer E is incorrect. Microvesicular fatty change does not occur with acetaminophen overdose. It is usually seen with tetracycline, salicylates, and ethanol use.

13. **The correct answer is B.** The patient's symptoms, characterized by voluminous, malodorous bulky stools that improve with fasting, combined with increased stool osmolality and

72-hour fecal fat, are suggestive of malabsorption. Malabsorption can result from multiple causes, including defective intraluminal digestion (e.g., pancreatitis), primary mucosal cell abnormalities (e.g., celiac sprue, tropical sprue), reduced small intestinal surface area (e.g., small bowel resection), lymphatic obstruction (e.g., Whipple's disease), and impaired mucosal cell absorption secondary to an infectious agent (e.g., *Giardia lamblia*). One of the easier ways to test for malabsorption is to perform a 72-hour fecal fat collection. This involves putting a patient on a 100-g fat diet for 3 days followed by fecal fat measurement in the stool.

Answer A is incorrect. Exudative diseases are characterized by mucosal destruction that leads to purulent and bloody stools. Exudative diarrhea persists with fasting.

Answer C is incorrect. Motility derangement such as that which occurs with diabetic neuropathy or hyperthyroidism results from failure of gut neuromuscular function. This type of diarrhea would not improve with fasting. Furthermore, stool osmolality would be expected to be normal.

Answer D is incorrect. Osmotic diarrhea is characterized by abundant stool output per day that is relieved with fasting. This type of diarrhea has an osmotic gap ($290 - 2$ [$Na_{in\ stool}$ + $K_{in\ stool}$])>50 mOsm, similar to that of malabsorptive diarrhea. However, osmotic diarrhea would not normally increase fecal fat.

Answer E is incorrect. In secretory diarrhea, net intestinal fluid secretion also leads to significantly increased amounts of stool output. Unlike diarrhea secondary to malabsorption, however, secretory diarrhea will be isotonic with respect to plasma and will not abate with fasting.

14. **The correct answer is A.** This patient has early gastric cancer, defined as adenocarcinoma limited to the gastric mucosa and submucosa. It begins in glandular epithelium, but if allowed to advance may invade muscularis propia. The prognosis for early gastric carcinoma is quite good.

Answer B is incorrect. The incidence of gastric cancer is highest in Japan. Its incidence dropped in the US with the advent of refrigeration, purportedly due to an increase in the consumption of uncontaminated, fresh foodstuffs.

Answer C is incorrect. Linitis plastica or "leather bottle" stomach is a poor prognostic factor in late-stage gastric carcinoma. It occurs when the neoplasm extends into the muscular layer of the stomach, causing stiffening and narrowing of the organ.

Answer D is incorrect. Metastasis occurs in more advanced adenocarcinoma. Cancer can spread to nearby structures such as the liver and pancreas, or to more distant locations, including lungs. As endoscopy suggested signs of gastritis only 5 years ago, the cancer likely has not developed to the point of metastasis.

Answer E is incorrect. Signet cells appear in poorly differentiated, late-stage gastric adenocarcinoma. Mucus released by tumor cells builds up inside individual cells, pushing the nucleus to the periphery. This gives the appearance of a ring.

15. **The correct answer is D.** Schistosomiasis is a helminthic disease with hepatic involvement. *Schistosoma mansoni* cercaria, which are commonly found in fresh waters of South America, penetrate the host's skin, invade the peripheral vasculature, and eventually settle in the portal or pelvic venous vasculature. Several weeks following infection, patients may develop symptoms similar to the ones described, such as fever, diarrhea, and weight loss; the "funny looking stools" likely represent *S. mansoni* eggs. Chronic infection may eventually lead to portal hypertension and hepatosplenomegaly, leading in turn to ascites and eventually cirrhosis. In addition, the hepatosplenomegaly leads to esophageal varices, producing bleeding that can often be the first clinical sign.

Answer A is incorrect. Appendicitis commonly presents with right lower quadrant abdominal pain, fever, nausea, vomiting, and leukocytosis.

The ascites seen in this patient is not a typical finding with appendicitis.

Answer B is incorrect. Bowel obstruction generally presents with nausea, vomiting, and decreased or absent bowel sounds. This patient has none of these signs or symptoms.

Answer C is incorrect. Enterocolitis would not present with signs and symptoms of ascites. It usually manifests with diarrhea.

Answer E is incorrect. Ruptured viscus may present with signs of peritonitis such as rebound tenderness. It may result from ischemic bowel disease or obstruction. This patient's history, physical examination, and imaging studies are inconsistent with this etiology.

16. **The correct answer is C.** The symptoms of upper gastrointestinal bleeding associated with epigastric pain in a patient with rheumatoid arthritis are most consistent with acute erosive hemorrhagic gastritis. The image shows diffusely hyperemic gastric mucosa, a typical finding in acute gastritis. Given this patient's history of rheumatoid arthritis, the most likely cause of her presentation is nonsteroidal anti-inflammatory drug use. As many as 25% of patients who take daily aspirin for rheumatoid arthritis eventually develop acute gastritis.

Answer A is incorrect. Amyloidosis is associated with chronic gastritis, not acute gastritis.

Answer B is incorrect. *Helicobacter pylori* infection is associated with chronic gastritis and not acute erosive hemorrhagic gastritis. *H. pylori* infection can be associated with a mild acute gastritis, but the patient's history of rheumatoid arthritis should prompt the consideration of nonsteroidal anti-inflammatory drug use.

Answer D is incorrect. Steroid treatment is not a known risk factor for acute gastritis.

Answer E is incorrect. Although uremia is a risk factor for developing acute gastritis, this patient has no evidence of kidney failure or symptoms to suggest uremia.

17. **The correct answer is C.** Recent studies have demonstrated the benefit of infliximab for the treatment of Crohn's disease that is refractory to steroid treatment. It is also approved for use in a variety of other autoimmune diseases such as ulcerative colitis, ankylosing spondylitis, psoriasis, and psoriatic arthritis. Infliximab is a monoclonal chimeric antibody that binds soluble TNF-α, and as a result blocks its effects. TNF-α is a proinflammatory cytokine secreted by macrophages that is found in high concentrations in the stool of Crohn's patients. The chimeric antibody is 75% human and 25% murine. A single infusion produces a clinical response in 65% of patients. Common side effects are increased susceptibility to upper respiratory infections, headache, and gastrointestinal distress.

Answer A is incorrect. This answer choice describes selective estrogen receptor modulators (SERMs), such as tamoxifen and raloxifene. These drugs have the ability to serve as estrogen antagonists in some tissues (such as the breast), while acting as a partial agonist in others (such as the bone). SERMs can be used to treat estrogen receptor-positive breast cancers or can be given as prophylaxis in patients with a strong family history of breast cancer. They can also be used to prevent the progression of osteoporosis in postmenopausal women. A complication of tamoxifen therapy is an increased risk of developing endometrial cancer (raloxifene does not carry this risk because unlike tamoxifen, it serves as an estrogen antagonist on endometrial cells).

Answer B is incorrect. This answer choice describes the drug trastuzumab (Herceptin), which is a monoclonal antibody specific for c-erbB2 (Her-2/neu), the epidermal growth factor receptor. Hyperexpression of this cell marker is a poor prognostic factor for carcinoma of the breast.

Answer D is incorrect. This answer choice describes the drug imatinib (Gleevec), which is an inhibitor of the bcr-abl fusion protein that results from the 9:22 translocation producing what is called the Philadelphia chromosome. This translocation is commonly seen in chronic myelogenous leukemia and can also be found in gastrointestinal stromal tumors. It results in an overly active abl tyrosine kinase that has oncogenic effects.

Answer E is incorrect. This answer choice describes aspirin, which nonselectively and irreversibly inhibits cyclo-oxygenase 1 and 2. Aspirin produces anti-inflammatory effects by preventing the synthesis of prostaglandins. However, these effects would not be strong enough for the treatment of refractory Crohn's disease.

18. **The correct answer is B.** This patient suffers from Hirschsprung's disease, which develops when neural crest cells fail to migrate to the distal colon. Consequently, enteric neurons do not form in a segment of the rectosigmoid; these neurons are normally responsible for relaxation of the rectum to allow defecation. Ten percent of cases of Hirschsprung's disease occur in children with Down's syndrome, caused by trisomy 21. Children with Down's syndrome also have an increased risk of duodenal atresia, congenital heart disease, and acute lymphoblastic leukemia.

Answer A is incorrect. Cystic fibrosis (CF) is caused by recessive mutations in the *CFTR* gene on chromosome 7. Infants with CF have an increased risk of meconium ileus, and also show a variable spectrum of pancreatic insufficiency. Later in life, patients with CF develop characteristic bronchiectasis with chronic lung infections with *Pseudomonas* species.

Answer C is incorrect. Sickle cell disease is caused by homozygous G12V mutations in the β-globin gene. Neonates with sickle cell disease are often asymptomatic, as fetal hemoglobin persists.

Answer D is incorrect. Tay-Sachs disease is caused by deficiency in hexosaminidase A, leading to accumulation of GM2 ganglioside. Infants with Tay-Sachs disease show progressive neurodegeneration, cherry-red spots, and developmental delay. There is no known association between Tay-Sachs disease and Hirschsprung's disease.

Answer E is incorrect. Infants with Turner's syndrome (XO) commonly show coarctation of

the aorta, but there is no association between Turner's syndrome and Hirschsprung's disease.

19. **The correct answer is E.** Vomiting typically induces a metabolic alkalosis due to a loss of hydrogen ions from the stomach, leading to an increase in pH. This leaves an increased bicarbonate concentration (generally >24 mEq/L) in the bloodstream. In this case, the partial carbon dioxide pressure is still normal; thus, no respiratory compensation has occurred, and the patient has uncompensated metabolic alkalosis.

Answer A is incorrect. This patient is presenting with a metabolic alkalosis (pH >7.4), not an acidosis.

Answer B is incorrect. This patient has an alkalosis, as evidenced by the pH. The partial carbon dioxide pressure is normal, indicating that there is no respiratory acidosis. Sometimes patients will present with more than one condition causing acid-base imbalance. These are known as complicated or mixed conditions, but this is not true of the patient in the above vignette.

Answer C is incorrect. There is no metabolic acidosis, because the bicarbonate concentration is actually increased. There has been no respiratory change, either, because the partial carbon dioxide pressure is normal.

Answer D is incorrect. This patient does not have an acidosis.

Answer F is incorrect. The patient does have metabolic alkalosis, but because partial carbon dioxide pressure is normal, there has been no respiratory compensation. In respiratory compensation, the partial carbon dioxide pressure would be increased to create more free H^+ in the bloodstream. This could be accomplished by hypoventilation.

20. **The correct answer is C.** The image shows fatty change, Mallory bodies, and a neutrophilic infiltrate. These histopathologic findings, as well as the patient's jaundice, are consistent with hepatitis seen in severe exposure to alcohol. Intracytoplasmic hyaline inclusions derived from cytokeratin intermediate fila-

ments are called Mallory bodies, which are also seen in primary biliary cirrhosis, Wilson's disease, chronic cholestatic syndromes, and hepatocellular tumors. Prolonged alcohol abuse may result in alcoholic cirrhosis, an irreversible condition characterized by nodular fibrosis of the liver parenchyma.

Answer A is incorrect. α_1-Antitrypsin deficiency is an autosomal recessive disorder that may result in both liver failure and emphysema. Histologically, this condition is characterized by the presence of cytoplasmic globular inclusions in hepatocytes. These inclusions are strongly periodic acid-Schiff positive on staining, a specific feature for this disease.

Answer B is incorrect. In acute viral hepatitis, hepatocyte injury takes the form of diffuse swelling (ballooning degeneration). Fatty change is unusual, with the exception of hepatitis C virus. In contrast to alcoholic hepatitis, Mallory bodies are not seen.

Answer D is incorrect. Fatty liver of pregnancy is an acute hepatic failure during the third trimester of pregnancy associated with microvesicular liver change. Pathologically, this condition is not characterized by Mallory body formation and neutrophilic infiltrates.

Answer E is incorrect. Neonatal hepatitis commonly results in jaundice during the first few weeks of life. Liver biopsy in neonatal hepatitis may reveal panlobular multinucleated giant cells among other morphologic manifestations. Mallory bodies and neutrophilic infiltrates are not typically seen in this condition.

21. **The correct answer is B.** *Entamoeba histolytica* infection presents with bloody diarrhea (dysentery), abdominal cramps with tenesmus, and pus in the stool. It can also cause right upper quadrant pain and liver abscesses. *E. histolytica* is transmitted via cysts in water (fecal-oral transmission). On microscopy, one observes amebas with ingested RBCs. Treatment for *E. histolytica* infection includes metronidazole and iodoquinol.

Answer A is incorrect. *Cryptosporidium* species infection presents with severe diarrhea in HIV-positive patients and with mild watery diarrhea in HIV-negative patients. *Cryptosporidium* is transmitted via cysts in water (fecal-oral transmission). Microscopically, acid-fast staining cysts are found. Unfortunately, there is no treatment available for *Cryptosporidium* species infection. In healthy patients, however, cryptosporidiosis is self-resolving.

Answer C is incorrect. *Giardia lamblia* infection presents with bloating, flatulence, foul-smelling diarrhea, and light-colored fatty stools. *G. lamblia* is transmitted via cysts in water (fecal-oral transmission). On microscopy, one observes teardrop-shaped trophozoites with a ventral sucking disc or cysts. Metronidazole is used to treat *G. lamblia* infection.

Answer D is incorrect. *Leishmania donovani* presents with hepatomegaly and splenomegaly, malaise, anemia, and weight loss. *L. donovani* is transmitted via the sandfly. Microscopically, macrophages containing amastigotes are observed. Sodium stibogluconate is used to treat *L. donovani* infection.

Answer E is incorrect. *Naegleria fowleri* presents with headache, fever, nausea, vomiting, and meningismus with progression to third, fourth, and sixth cranial nerve palsies as well as seizures and coma. It is transmitted through inhalation of contaminated dust or water. Prognosis is poor; the only survivors have been treated with amphotericin B and rifampin.

Answer F is incorrect. *Toxoplasma gondii* infection presents with brain abscesses in HIV-positive patients and with birth defects if infection occurs during pregnancy (toxoplasmosis is one of the ToRCHeS organisms). *Toxoplasma gondii* is transmitted via cysts in raw meat or cat feces. The definitive stage (sexual stage) occurs in cats. Microscopically, acid-fast staining cysts are found. Sulfadiazine and pyrimethamine are used to treat toxoplasmosis.

22. **The correct answer is A.** Familial adenomatous polyposis (FAP) is an autosomal dominant condition characterized by a germline mutation on chromosome 5, specifically at the adenomatous polypsis coli (APC) locus. The *APC*

gene is thought to have tumor suppressive effects, and its loss is associated with more than colonic cancers. Patients with FAP are at increased risk for developing duodenal, gastric, liver, thyroid, and central nervous system neoplasms.

Answer B is incorrect. Examples of autosomal recessive conditions include cystic fibrosis, sickle cell anemia, and hemochromatosis.

Answer C is incorrect. Examples of autosomal trisomy conditions include Down's syndrome (trisomy 21), Edwards' syndrome (trisomy 18), and Patau's syndrome (trisomy 13).

Answer D is incorrect. Examples of conditions related to sex chromosome abnormalities include Klinefelter's syndrome (XXY), Turner's syndrome (XO), and double-Y males (XYY).

Answer E is incorrect. Examples of X-linked recessive conditions include fragile X syndrome, hemophilia A and B, glucose-6-phosphate dehydrogenase deficiency, and Lesch-Nyhan syndrome.

23. **The correct answer is E.** Guillain-Barré syndrome is characterized by rapidly progressing ascending paralysis. It is an autoimmune-mediated illness that can occur following a variety of infectious diseases, such as cytomegalovirus, Epstein-Barr virus, HIV, mycoplasma pneumonia, and gastroenteritis caused by *Campylobacter jejuni*. *C. jejuni* gastroenteritis is characterized by bloody diarrhea together with the finding of comma-shaped organisms with a single polar flagellum when cultured at 42° C (107.6° F) in a microaerophilic environment. Other enteric pathogens with this morphology include bacteria of the Vibrio genus (*V. cholera* and *V. parahaemolyticus*). These species, however, are not endemic to the United States, and would not be expected in a patient without a recent travel history. Domestic animals serve as a source of *C. jejuni*, which are then transmitted to humans via the fecal-oral route.

Answer A is incorrect. Hemolytic-uremic syndrome (HUS) is characterized by acute renal failure and thrombocytopenia with hemolytic anemia. HUS can be a complication of infection caused by *Escherichia coli* O157:H7 and not *Campylobacter jejuni*. Like *C. jejuni*, *E. coli* O157:H7 is a gram-negative rod that can cause enteritis. *E. coli*, however, are characterized by numerous flagella and aerobic metabolism.

Answer B is incorrect. Rheumatic fever is characterized by fever, migratory polyarthritis, and carditis. It may follow group A *streptococcal pharyngitis*.

Answer C is incorrect. Fever, a new murmur, Janeway lesions, and nail-bed hemorrhages are all signs of bacterial endocarditis. Acute endocarditis is caused by *Staphylococcus aureus* and subacute infection can be caused by *Streptococcus viridans*.

Answer D is incorrect. Waterhouse-Friderichsen syndrome is characterized by high fever, shock, purpura, and adrenal insufficiency. It is classically associated with *Neisseria meningitides* septicemia.

24. **The correct answer is C.** This patient has vitamin A deficiency, which is characterized by early symptoms of night blindness, dry conjunctivae, and gray plaques, or late symptoms of corneal ulceration and necrosis leading to perforation and blindness. This deficiency is typically seen in children and pregnant women whose diets are deficient in vitamin A, especially those from Southeast Asia. Vitamin A deficiency can also result from malabsorption following intestinal surgery, especially of the ileum. Vitamins A, D, E, and K (the fat-soluble vitamins) are absorbed in the small intestine and absorption requires micelles formed with bile salts.

Answer A is incorrect. Fe^{2+} is absorbed in the small intestine and absorption requires apoferritin binding.

Answer B is incorrect. Vitamin B_{12} is absorbed in the terminal ileum and absorption requires intrinsic factor.

Answer D is incorrect. Water-soluble vitamins are absorbed in the small intestine and absorption requires sodium contransport.

Answer E is incorrect. Calcium is absorbed in the small intestine and absorption requires a vitamin D-dependent calcium binding protein.

25. **The correct answer is A.** The triad of jaundice (icteric sclera), hypercholesterolemia (palpebral xanthomas), and pruritus with positive antimitochondrial antibody titers and elevated alkaline phosphatase activity is classic for primary biliary cirrhosis. Primary biliary cirrhosis is a cholestatic disease with chronic, progressive, and often fatal liver injury characterized by the destruction of medium-sized intrahepatic bile ducts with eventual liver failure. Liver transplantation is the definitive treatment.

Answer B is incorrect. Hepatic parenchymal destruction occurs only as a late sequela of primary biliary cirrhosis secondary to intrahepatic bile duct compromise. This patient's acute presentation suggests early disease.

Answer C is incorrect. Obstruction of extrahepatic bile ducts is seen with secondary biliary cirrhosis resulting from obstructive conditions such as cholelithiasis, neoplasms, surgical procedures, biliary atresia, and cystic fibrosis. Primary biliary cirrhosis is not characterized by extrahepatic bile duct obstruction.

Answer D is incorrect. Portal vein thrombosis is not a mechanism responsible for this patient's presentation. Portal vein thrombosis has multiple etiologies, including hypercoagulable states, inflammatory diseases (e.g., ulcerative colitis), iatrogenic causes, infections, and liver disease. Unlike primary biliary cirrhosis, it commonly presents with variceal hemorrhage and/or melena.

Answer E is incorrect. Stenosis of extrahepatic and intrahepatic bile ducts is seen with primary sclerosing cholangitis and not with primary biliary cirrhosis. Primary sclerosing cholangitis often presents with jaundice, right upper quadrant pain, and fever.

26. **The correct answer is C.** This patient's clinical presentation is consistent with celiac disease. The physical exam would most likely reveal an anorexic-appearing child with temporal wast-ing and multiple nonblanching purpuric lesions located on the upper and lower extremities, called dermatitis herpetiformis. Celiac disease (gluten-sensitive enteropathy) is characterized by blunting and atrophy of the small bowel villi and lymphocytic infiltrates resulting in malabsorption of most nutrients, accounting for the symptoms and physical findings present in this patient. The gliadin fraction in wheat is responsible for disease activation. Thus, introduction of cereals into the diet is responsible for most patients' presentations. Discontinuation of gliadin-containing foods such as cereals usually results in complete remission.

Answer A is incorrect. Benign mucosa would be expected if the patient were lactose intolerant. While lactose intolerance would account for the patient's nausea and vomiting, it would fail to account for the steatorrhea and pruritic lesions.

Answer B is incorrect. Continuous linear mucosal lesions are the hallmark of ulcerative colitis, which presents with a relapsing bloody diarrhea and mucus, abdominal pain, and cramps. Because the lesions are continuous from the colon, there is often little or no malabsorption of nutrients. Stress is often an inducer of the attacks, and treatment is initially medical with sulfasalazine, with surgery reserved for prolonged and severe cases.

Answer D is incorrect. Foamy macrophages strongly point to Whipple's disease, a diagnosis confirmed by rod-shaped bacilli on electron microscopy. *Tropheryma whippelii* is the causative organism and resides in macrophages, distending them and leading to lymphatic blockage and lipid deposition, all characteristically without neutrophil inflammation. Patients are typically in their 30s to 40s, men, and exposed to rural regions, and they present with arthropathy, diarrhea, and weight loss.

Answer E is incorrect. Skip mucosal lesions (referred to as "cobblestoning") and granulomas are characteristic of Crohn's disease. These patients present with mild, typically nonbloody diarrhea, fever, and abdominal pain along with migratory polyarthritis and other extraintestinal manifestations. Mild disease can be treated medically with sulfasalazine. However, stricture and fistula formations are common and often necessitate surgical intervention, usually within 10 years of diagnosis.

27. **The correct answer is C.** Pegylated interferon is a cytokine derivative that improves the body's antiviral response. It is used in the treatment of hepatitis B and C. Adverse effects of interferon therapy include a flu-like reaction that manifests as episodic fevers and chills, as well as occasional profound depression. As a result, interferon is contraindicated in severely depressed or suicidal patients. Although interferon is not a cure for hepatitis, it is recommended to slow the progression of cirrhotic liver disease in some patients. Pegylated interferon is a longer-acting form of interferon.

    Answer A is incorrect. Intravenous immunoglobulin is an engineered antibody that is used to clear the serum of protein products. It is often used in treatment of autoimmune diseases such as Guillain-Barré syndrome. Adverse effects include flu-like reaction and anaphylactoid reaction.

    Answer B is incorrect. Lamivudine is a nucleotide reverse transcriptase inhibitor used in the treatment of HIV and hepatitis B. Its principal adverse effect is hepatotoxicity.

    Answer D is incorrect. Ribavirin is an antiviral drug used in the treatment of hepatitis C, respiratory syncytial virus, and, occasionally, other viral illnesses. It is not associated with depression or a flu-like reaction.

    Answer E is incorrect. Tumor necrosis factor-α is a cytokine involved in the antiviral and antitumor response. It is not currently used as a treatment for hepatitis C.

28. **The correct answer is D.** New onset of right lower quadrant abdominal pain in a young patient with a fever and an elevated WBC count is suggestive of appendicitis. Patients with appendicitis typically present with periumbilical or right lower quadrant abdominal pain. Fifty to sixty percent will also present with nausea

and vomiting. They may also exhibit a psoas sign (pain on hip flexion) and rebound tenderness.

Answer A is incorrect. Distention is rare in a patient with appendicitis unless diffuse peritonitis has developed.

Answer B is incorrect. Dyspnea is uncommon in acute appendicitis. Shortness of breath is more often associated with primary cardiopulmonary disease, anemia, exercise, and environmental irritants.

Answer C is incorrect. Patients with appendicitis typically present with anorexia. Hunger in a patient with appendicitis should make one reconsider the diagnosis.

Answer E is incorrect. While diarrhea can occur in a patient with appendicitis, profuse watery diarrhea is more suggestive of acute gastroenteritis than appendicitis.

29. **The correct answer is D.** *Shigella* species produce gastroenteritis characterized by abdominal pain, bloody diarrhea, and nausea and/or vomiting. Additionally, since *Shigella* species invade intestinal epithelial cells, the illness is accompanied by fever. *Shigella* is a nonlactose fermenter, and it does not produce gas or hydrogen sulfide. *Shigella* infection usually affects preschool-age children and populations in nursing homes. Transmission occurs by the fecal-to-oral route via fecally contaminated water and hand-to-hand contact.

Answer A is incorrect. *Escherichia coli* can also cause a bloody diarrhea, and the enteroinvasive species can cause fever. Unlike *Shigella*, however, *E. coli* is a lactose fermenter. *E. coli* is a common cause of traveler's diarrhea.

Answer B is incorrect. Enterotoxigenic *Escherichia coli* infection causes gastroenteritis characterized by watery diarrhea. *E. coli* is a lactose fermenter.

Answer C is incorrect. Like infection with *Shigella*, *Salmonella* infection can also lead to fever, abdominal pain, and bloody stools. *Salmonella* is capable of invading the mucosal epithelium, causing salmonellosis. It is a non-lactose fermenter but, unlike *Shigella*, produces gas and hydrogen sulfide. *Salmonella* infection results from fecal-oral transmission and lives in the gastrointestinal tract of animals. It infects humans when there is contamination of food or water by animal feces.

Answer E is incorrect. *Vibrio cholerae* produces a gastroenteritis characterized by high-volume, watery diarrhea. This microorganism infects travelers and children in endemic areas.

30. **The correct answer is D.** Gemfibrozil functions mainly to reduce the circulating level of triglycerides. It is a fibric acid derivative that acts on peroxisome proliferator-activated receptor-α protein to increase the activity of lipoprotein lipase and facilitate enhanced clearance of triglycerides. There is also a slight reduction in cholesterol synthesis.

Answer A is incorrect. Bile acid resins such as cholestyramine and colestipol bind to bile acids and steroids in the small intestine, preventing their absorption. They cause a reduction in LDL cholesterol and a slight increase in triglycerides.

Answer B is incorrect. Ezetimibe blocks cholesterol and phytosterol (a plant sterol) absorption in the small intestine, resulting in a decrease in LDL cholesterol with little to no effect on HDL cholesterol or triglyceride levels.

Answer C is incorrect. 5-Hydroxy-3-methylglutaryl-coenzyme A reductase inhibitors (statins) act to reduce cholesterol biosynthesis in the liver by preventing the formation of the cholesterol precursor mevalonate. They produce a large decrease in LDL cholesterol, an increase in HDL cholesterol, and a slight decrease in triglycerides.

Answer E is incorrect. This option describes a drug that would increase LDL cholesterol levels. This is not caused by any of the cholesterol-lowering drugs.

31. **The correct answer is E.** Given this patient's history of chronic obstructive pulmonary dis-

ease, the most likely factor contributing to the development of his duodenal ulcer is tobacco use. The incidence of peptic ulcers in smokers is twice as great as in nonsmokers.

Answer A is incorrect. Unlike acute gastritis, alcohol use is not a known risk factor for peptic ulcer development.

Answer B is incorrect. Chronic use of nonsteroidal anti-inflammatory drugs is a known risk factor for peptic ulcer disease. However, in this patient, there is no reason to suspect long-term use of these medications.

Answer C is incorrect. Excessive salt intake is not a risk factor for peptic ulcer disease.

Answer D is incorrect. Primary hyperparathyroidism is associated with peptic ulcer disease. This condition is a possibility in this patient given his increased risk for bronchogenic squamous cell carcinoma; however, his recent weight gain and normal calcium and phosphate plasma levels argue against primary hyperparathyroidism.

32. **The correct answer is D.** Colonization of the gut by *Giardia* trophozoites results in inflammation and villous atrophy, reducing the gut's absorptive capability. The image shows these pear-shaped trophozoites from a duodenal aspirate. Duodenal aspiration can be used to diagnose infection with *Giardia*. Trophozoites have four pairs of flagella and two nuclei. They attach to epithelial cells in duodenal and jejunal crypts through a sucking disk on their ventral surface. They absorb nutrients from the host and cause inflammation and malabsorption, but they do not invade the intestinal wall.

Answer A is incorrect. Some strains of the bacteria *Escherichia coli* possess heat-labile enterotoxin, which increases cyclic adenosine monophosphate by activating adenylate cyclase through the GTP-dependent ADP ribosylation of specific membrane proteins. This gives rise to secretory diarrhea. The heat-labile toxin is closely related in structure and function to the enterotoxin expressed by *Vibrio cholerae*.

Answer B is incorrect. Deficiency of the enzyme lactase (called lactose intolerance) allows undigested lactose to pass into the colon, which causes an osmotic diarrhea. Colonic bacteria can further ferment the sugar (lactose) to hydrogen gas and organic acids, producing bowel distention, bloating, cramping, and abdominal pain.

Answer C is incorrect. Several organisms have the ability to invade the lining of the intestine when they infect humans. Cryptosporidiosis, caused by infection with the protozoan *Cryptosporidium*, is one example. It causes non-bloody, mucousy diarrhea; flatulence and bloating; and a low-grade fever. Amebiasis, an infection caused by the protozoal organism *Entamoeba histolytica*, is another invasive organism. Patients with amebic colitis typically present with a history of several weeks of abdominal pain, diarrhea, and bloody stools. A characteristic finding of *E. histolytica* trophozoites is that they often have ingested RBCs in their cytoplasm, whereas the cystic forms have a distinctive "ring and dot" nucleus and chromatoid bodies.

Answer E is incorrect. Viral enteritis is caused by viral infection of the epithelial cells of the small intestinal villi, especially those near the tips of the villi. Because the villi are important for the digestion of carbohydrates and absorption of fluid and electrolytes, enteric viruses can lead to malabsorption by decreased hydrolysis of carbohydrates and excess fluid loss from the intestine. On microscopy, there is often only an inflammatory infiltrate and intestinal villus blunting. With extensive damage, one may see fusion of adjacent villi resulting in significantly decreased absorptive surface area.

33. **The correct answer is C.** Hyperalbuminemia is only significant when it may indicate dehydration. A patient with a 2-day history of vomiting and diarrhea is most likely dehydrated due to loss of volume.

Answer A is incorrect. Acute infection typically causes hypoalbuminemia due to decreased protein synthesis.

Answer B is incorrect. Chronic liver disease causes hypoalbuminemia as albumin is typically produced in the liver.

Answer D is incorrect. Nephrotic syndrome causes hypoalbuminemia due to excessive protein loss.

Answer E is incorrect. Poor nutritional status causes hypoalbuminemia due to poor protein intake.

34. **The correct answer is B.** The oral absorption of ciprofloxacin is impaired by divalent cations, including those in antacids such as calcium carbonate, which this patient takes for gastroesophageal reflux disease. Ciprofloxacin belongs to the family of fluroquinolones, whose mechanism of action is to block bacterial DNA synthesis by inhibiting bacterial topoisomerase II (DNA gyrase) and topoisomerase IV. Inhibition of DNA gyrase prevents the relaxation of positively supercoiled DNA that is required for normal transcription and replication.

Answer A is incorrect. Unlike the other drugs listed, aspirin is not used as a pharmacotherapeutic agent for gastroesophageal reflux disease and in fact is strongly associated with gastric ulcers. Although many patients take aspirin for its antiplatelet effect, this patient has no indication for using aspirin and drug interactions are not expected between aspirin and ciprofloxacin.

Answer C is incorrect. Cimetidine, an H_2 antagonist, is associated with inhibition of the cytochrome P-450 system. However, it does not significantly affect the metabolism or pharmacokinetics of ciprofloxacin.

Answer D is incorrect. Misoprostol is a prostaglandin E_1 analog that can be used to prevent nonsteroidal anti-inflammatory drug-induced peptic ulcers. It is also used as a medical abortifacient in many countries and is therefore strictly contraindicated in pregnant women. Misoprostol would not decrease the absorption nor increase the metabolism of ciprofloxacin.

Answer E is incorrect. Omeprazole is a proton pump inhibitor considered first-line therapy for gastroesophageal reflux disease. Omeprazole will decrease intragastric acidity but will not affect the intestinal absorption, metabolism, or excretion of ciprofloxacin.

35. **The correct answer is C.** Chronic pancreatitis is a disease characterized by recurrent episodes of pancreatic inflammation with associated loss of pancreatic parenchyma. It is commonly associated with alcoholism. Chronic pancreatitis is a disabling disease. Chronic malabsorption may develop secondary to exocrine insufficiency. Diabetes mellitus is also a common manifestation of chronic pancreatitis. A relatively specific finding in chronic pancreatitis is visualization of pancreatic calcifications on CT scan.

Answer A is incorrect. An abdominal x-ray finding of air-fluid levels in the small intestine is suggestive of bowel obstruction. This feature is not common with chronic pancreatitis, but may occur with acute pancreatitis.

Answer B is incorrect. Free air under the right hemidiaphragm on x-ray of the chest suggests a ruptured abdominal viscus. This feature is not common with chronic pancreatitis, but may occur with acute pancreatitis.

Answer D is incorrect. Chronic pancreatitis may be characterized by pseudocysts, but not cystic lesions. Pseudocysts are collections of fluid, usually pancreatic secretions, that form after inflammation of the pancreas. Unlike pancreatic cysts, they lack true epithelial lining.

Answer E is incorrect. Pancreatic granuloma formation is not commonly seen in chronic pancreatitis. Pancreatic granuloma is a rare condition that may be seen with extrapulmonary tuberculosis and, uncommonly, with sarcoidosis. It is not commonly associated with chronic pancreatitis.

36. **The correct answer is E.** Omeprazole is a proton pump inhibitor (PPI) that exerts its action by covalently binding and irreversibly inactivating the hydrogen/potassium ATPase on the luminal surface of the gastric parietal cell. Gastrin levels are regulated by a feedback loop in which intragastric acidity stimulates D-cells in the gastric antrum to release somatostatin, which works in a paracrine fashion, binding G-cells in the gastric antrum and inhibiting gastrin release. PPIs will effectively raise the intragastric pH so that gastrin levels rise two- to four-fold. Omeprazole is associated with atrophic gastritis due to hypergastrinemia. It may also be associated with carcinoid tumors.

Answer A is incorrect. Aluminum hydroxide is an antacid and is associated with constipation and hypophosphatemia.

Answer B is incorrect. Bismuth binds to ulcers, allowing a physical protective barrier, and has no known significant adverse effects.

Answer C is incorrect. Cimetidine is an H_2-antagonist and is associated with inhibition of the cytochrome P-450 system. Inhibition of the proton pumps by omeprazole has a greater effect on the intragastric acidity that regulates the gastrin feedback loop than antagonizing the H_2-receptors by cimetidine.

Answer D is incorrect. Misoprostol is a prostaglandin E_1 analog that can be used to prevent nonsteroidal anti-inflammatory drug-induced peptic ulcers. It is also used as a medical abortifacient in many countries and is therefore strictly contraindicated in pregnant women.

37. **The correct answer is C.** A history of recurrent right lower quadrant abdominal pain with diarrhea, fevers, and weight loss is characteristic of an inflammatory bowel disease. Crohn's disease typically presents in adolescent patients with fever, weight loss, and abdominal pain with frequent, sometimes bloody diarrhea. These symptoms result from chronic transmural inflammation of the bowel, which usually occurs in the terminal ileum, but may involve any intestinal tissue between the mouth and the anus. Treatment consists of anti-inflammatory agents and/or immunosuppressants.

Answer A is incorrect. Celiac sprue is a gluten-sensitive enteropathy that commonly results in intestinal malabsorption. However, it would not present with fevers and mucosal erosions. Instead, endoscopy with biopsy of the small intestine would demonstrate villous flattening.

Answer B is incorrect. Patients with collagenous colitis, which is the lymphocytic infiltration of the colonic mucosa and thickening of the submucosal collagen layer, usually have normal endoscopic findings.

Answer D is incorrect. Irritable bowel syndrome, characterized by abdominal pain, constipation, and/or diarrhea, is a functional disorder and does not present with abnormalities on colonoscopy.

Answer E is incorrect. Ulcerative colitis shares many features with Crohn's disease. However, the contiguous, superficial ulcerative lesions of ulcerative colitis are usually limited to the colon.

38. **The correct answer is B.** This patient is exhibiting signs and symptoms of undulant fever, caused by infection by *Brucella* species. *B. melitensis* enters the body after the ingestion of contaminated milk products or direct contact with contaminated livestock. It is an intracellular bacterium that causes undulating fever, weakness, and loss of appetite.

    Answer A is incorrect. *Bartonella henselae* is the causative agent of cat scratch disease and may also lead to bacillary angiomatosis. Like Brucella, Bartonella infection can lead to lymphadenopathy and fever, but exposure to unpasteurized milk in this case strongly points to Brucella as the etiologic agent.

    Answer C is incorrect. *Pasteurella* infection commonly results from dog or cat bite wounds and typically causes a cellulitis. High fever, hepatosplenomegaly, and exposure to unpasteurized milk products are not generally associated with infection.

    Answer D is incorrect. *Plasmodium malariae* is a protozoan that causes malaria. This disease is characterized by episodes of fever and chills every 72 hours. It is spread through the bite of the *Anopheles* mosquito. While splenomegaly is often present, lymphadenopathy is not.

39. **The correct answer is A.** This patient has Mallory-Weiss syndrome. Repeated bouts of

prolonged vomiting can cause longitudinal lacerations in the distal esophagus, normally at the esophagogastric junction or in the proximal gastric mucosa, with extension to submucosal arteries that can bleed massively. Untreated, this bleeding can be fatal. Mallory-Weiss syndrome generally presents with hematemesis following a bout of retching or vomiting; however, new research suggests that this classic history may be obtained in only about 50% of patients. Bleeding from esophageal varices should also be suspected in a patient with a significant drinking history like this patient has.

Answer B is incorrect. Metaplasia of esophageal mucosa is associated with chronic reflux causing inflammation, sometimes leading to ulceration. This can cause bleeding, but it is usually not massive as in this patient. Barrett's esophagus is of concern primarily because of its association with adenocarcinoma.

Answer C is incorrect. Esophageal squamous cell carcinoma would cause ulceration of the esophageal mucosa, but massive bleeding is uncommon.

Answer D is incorrect. Esophageal stricture is typically caused by scaring, from reflux, toxic ingestions, or scleroderma. It is a chronic problem most commonly manifesting as dysphagia, not hematemesis.

Answer E is incorrect. Hiatal hernia is usually an incidental finding, most commonly causing nausea and substernal pain. Bleeding is very uncommon and is rarely massive.

40. **The correct answer is B.** Any biopsy would likely show normal structures. Irritable bowel syndrome is a functional gastrointestinal disorder characterized by abdominal pain and altered bowel habits in the absence of demonstrable organic pathology. It is a diagnosis of exclusion based on clinical features such as the ones presented. Most commonly patients have alternating diarrhea and constipation, chronic abdominal pain that improves with stools, a change in stool frequency and consistency, and onset after emotional and/or stressful life events. These symptoms occur in the absence

of fevers, lower gastrointestinal bleeding, leukocytosis, and weight loss.

Answer A is incorrect. Pseudomembranous colitis usually follows broad-spectrum antibiotic therapy and is characterized by bloody diarrhea, fever, and leukocytosis. Absence of these manifestations in the patient argues against this diagnosis.

Answer C is incorrect. Primary sclerosing cholangitis is an extraintestinal manifestation of ulcerative colitis. On colonoscopy mucosa shows continuous superficial ulceration with inflammatory "pseudopolyps."

Answer D is incorrect. Crohn's disease has a highly variable presentation; however, "skip lesions," fissures, and/or strictures are generally evident on colonoscopy, endoscopy, and/or radiography.

Answer E is incorrect. Celiac sprue is a disease of malabsorption characterized by bulky, fatty stools following meals. Endoscopic findings reveal villous flattening in the small intestine.

41. **The correct answer is A.** This patient has major environmental risk factors for hydatid disease caused by infection with the tapeworm *Echinococcus granulosus*. Hydatid disease or echinococcosis remains one of the most intractable and lethal helminthic diseases. The parasitic life cycle of *E. granulosus* is fairly complex, requiring both definitive hosts (usually carnivores such as dogs) and intermediate hosts (usually herbivores such as sheep and cattle). Humans can also function as intermediate hosts. Infection with *E. granulosus* typically results in the formation of hydatid cysts in the liver, lungs, kidney, and spleen in the intermediate host. Although laboratory values are generally unrevealing, imaging often shows well-demarcated cystic masses in involved organs. Patients can present with a wide range of symptoms, including being asymptomatic to experiencing sudden death from anaphylactic shock after spontaneous rupture of cysts. Anaphylaxis usually occurs secondary to biopsy or surgical intervention when the diagnosis is overlooked. This hypersensitivity reaction is related to the release of antigenic material within cysts and secondary immunologic reactions. Lung cysts tend to develop thin pericyst capsules, which can rapidly become larger and are more prone to spontaneous rupture.

Answer B is incorrect. Disseminated intravascular coagulation is not associated with hydatid disease, and the major risk factor associated with cyst rupture is systemic anaphylaxis.

Answer C is incorrect. Although this patient has both liver and lung involvement, hepatitis is not a common manifestation or complication of hydatid disease. Cysts can commonly rupture into the biliary tree and produce biliary colic, obstructive jaundice, cholangitis, or pancreatitis. Hepatic abscess formation is also common.

Answer D is incorrect. Although this patient's past history of smoking and symptoms of hemoptysis are concerning for malignancy, the radiographic findings of multiple circular, well-circumscribed, and homogenous shadows are not consistent with malignancy. Hydatid disease is a much more probable cause of this patient's symptoms given her occupational history and the results of imaging.

Answer E is incorrect. Myocardial infarction is not a common outcome of hydatid disease. Rarely, infection of the heart itself can result in mechanical rupture with widespread dissemination or pericardial tamponade.

42. **The correct answer is C.** The most common tumor of the parotid gland is the pleomorphic adenoma or the mixed tumor, which constitute 50% of salivary tumors. The pleomorphic adenoma is a benign, well-differentiated, well-circumscribed mass that grows slowly over the course of months to years. On histopathology, it is characterized by the presence of multiple cell types, classically epithelial cells in a chondromyxoid stroma.

Answer A is incorrect. Adenoid cystic carcinoma is an invasive, poorly differentiated cancer characterized by gland-forming tissue and a cystic, fluid-filled cavity. It tends to infiltrate perineurial spaces and cause pain. This type of tumors constitutes 5% of tumors and is malignant.

Answer B is incorrect. Mucoepidermoid carcinoma is an invasive, poorly differentiated cancer composed of mucosal and epidermal cell types. This type constitutes 15% of salivary gland tumors and is malignant.

Answer D is incorrect. A sialic duct stone is an inorganic precipitate mechanically obstructing the opening of the sialic duct, resulting in an erythematous and inflamed oral mass.

Answer E is incorrect. Warthin's tumor is a benign mass of lymphoid cells. A well-circumscribed mass of lymphoid cells in a salivary gland is virtually pathognomonic for a Warthin's tumor, which make up an additional 5%–10% of salivary tumors.

43. **The correct answer is A.** The upper one third of the esophagus is made up of striated muscle. The middle one third of the esophagus is made up of both striated and smooth muscle. The lower one third of the esophagus is made up of smooth muscle. Patients with scleroderma develop dysphagia (usually to solids) secondary to atrophy of smooth muscle of the lower two thirds of the esophagus and incompetence of the lower esophageal sphincter. The wall of the esophagus becomes thin and atrophic and can have regions of fibrosis.

Answer B is incorrect. Patients with scleroderma develop dysphagia secondary to atrophy of smooth (not striated) muscle in the lower (not upper) two thirds of the esophagus and incompetence of the lower esophageal sphincter.

Answer C is incorrect. Patients with scleroderma develop dysphagia secondary to atrophy of smooth (not striated) muscle contractions in the lower two thirds of the esophagus and incompetence of the lower esophageal sphincter.

Answer D is incorrect. Patients with scleroderma develop dysphagia secondary to atrophy of smooth (not striated) muscle contractions in the lower (not middle) two thirds of the esophagus and incompetence of the lower esophageal sphincter.

Answer E is incorrect. Patients with scleroderma develop dysphagia secondary to atrophy of smooth (not striated) muscle contractions in the lower (not upper) two thirds of the esophagus and incompetence of the lower esophageal sphincter.

44. **The correct answer is C.** A diverticulum is an outpouching of the mucosa, usually occurring in weaker areas of the bowel, such as where vessels penetrate the muscle wall. Diverticulosis is a common condition in Western countries due to the typical low-fiber and high-fat diet, which leads to low bulk stools and increased straining of the bowel during peristalsis and defecation. Inflammation and microperforation of one of these diverticula leads to diverticulitis, in which the patient would present with lower abdominal pain, anorexia, and systemic symptoms of inflammation, such as fever and leukocytosis. Diverticular bleeding, which is seen in approximately 5% of patients with diverticulosis, is uncommon in the setting of acute diverticulitis.

Answer A is incorrect. Bowel infarction would lead to the acute onset of abdominal pain, bloody diarrhea, and nausea. However, this condition is uncommon in healthy individuals; it is mostly seen in patients with a past cardiac or vascular condition.

Answer B is incorrect. Patients with ulcerative colitis have bloody stools; in addition, they tend to present at a younger age and other extraintestinal symptoms may be evident.

Answer D is incorrect. An older patient presenting with abdominal complaints should always raise the suspicion for cancer. However, gastrointestinal bleeding is often seen in this setting, and this patient's pain and signs of an inflammatory response such as fever would not likely be present.

Answer E is incorrect. Volvulus would lead to intestinal obstruction, with constipation and possibly obstipation. Fever and leukocytosis would be unlikely to occur in this setting.

45. The correct answer is B. This is a presentation of Wilson's disease. The patient has parkinsonian symptoms due to the death of neurons in the basal ganglia (particularly in the putamen and globus pallidus). Wilson's disease is an autosomal recessive disease in which there is a mutation in *ATP7B*, a gene in chromosome 13 that encodes for a copper-transporting ATPase. Copper accumulates in the liver, basal ganglia, bones, joints, kidneys, and Descemet's membrane in the cornea (Kayser-Fleischer rings). Because Wilson's disease follows an autosomal recessive pattern of inheritance, the patient's sister has a 25% chance of also having the disease.

The correct answer is A. The patient's sister would have nearly 0% chance of getting the disease if this condition followed an X-linked pattern of inheritance. Examples of X-linked disorders include Duchenne's muscular dystrophy and Lesch-Nyhan syndrome.

Answer C is incorrect. Fifty percent would be the answer in the case of an autosomal dominant disorder such as hereditary spherocytosis, familial adenomatous polyposis, and adult polycystic kidney disease.

Answer D is incorrect. If the sister were healthy, she would have a 66.6% chance of being a carrier of the mutated gene.

Answer E is incorrect. A 100% chance of getting a disease is not common, unless one is referring to the likelihood a child has of inheriting a disease with a mitochondrial pattern of inheritance from a mother with the condition. Examples of diseases with this inheritance pattern include mitochondrial myopathies and Leber's hereditary optic neuropathy.

46. The correct answer is E. *Staphylococcus aureus* food poisoning is characterized by more vomiting than diarrhea. Since the enterotoxin is preformed in food, the incubation time is short (1–8 hours). Contaminated mayonnaise has been shown to be a frequent source of S. *aureus* food poisoning.

Answer A is incorrect. *Staphylococcus aureus* is a gram-positive, catalase-positive, and coagulase-positive bacterium. Gram-positive, catalase-positive, and coagulase-negative bacteria include *Staphylococcus epidermidis* and S. *saprophyticus*, common pathogens in indwelling devices and urinary tract infections, respectively Regardless, the organism would not likely be present in the stool as this is a toxin-mediated reaction.

Answer B is incorrect. A positive quellung reaction is seen with encapsulated bacteria only, such as *Streptococcus pneumoniae* or *Neisseria meningitidis*. *Staphylococcus aureus* is not an encapsulated bacterium.

Answer C is incorrect. *Neisseria gonorrhoeae* is cultured on Thayer-Martin media.

Answer D is incorrect. Contaminated seafood is a common source of *Vibrio parahaemolyticus* and V. *vulnificus*. *Staphylococcus aureus* is commonly found in the mayonnaise portion of the tuna salad.

47. The correct answer is D. This constellation of symptoms is suggestive of Crigler-Najjar syndrome type I, a hereditary hyperbilirubinemia that is fatal within 18 months of life secondary to kernicterus (bilirubin deposition in brain tissue). Multiple genetic defects in the allele for the bilirubin uridine diphosphate-glucuronosyltransferase (UGT1) may give rise to this disorder. This enzyme is responsible for conjugating bilirubin with one or two molecules of glucuronic acid. The liver is morphologically normal by light and electron microscopy.

Answer A is incorrect. Aldolase B is responsible for conversion of fructose-1-phosphate to dihydroxyacetone phosphate and glyceraldehyde. The deficiency of this enzyme leads to jaundice, cirrhosis, and hypoglycemia, not kernicterus, as seen in Crigler-Najjar syndrome type I.

Answer B is incorrect. Deficiency in galactose-1-phosphate uridyltransferase (responsible for synthesis of glucose-1-phosphate from galctose-1-phosphate) causes cataracts, hepatosplenomegaly, and mental retardation and not the presentation seen in Crigler-Najjar syndrome type I.

Answer C is incorrect. Glucose 6-phosphatase is an enzyme that catalyzes the dephosphorylation of glucose 6-phosphate to glucose. Its deficiency results in severe fasting hypoglycemia and increased glycogen deposition in the liver (von Gierke's disease). Presentation of this disease is drastically different from Crigler-Najjar syndrome type I.

Answer E is incorrect. A deficiency of uroporphyrinogen decarboxylase (involved in heme synthesis) leads to porphyria cutanea tarda, the most commonly diagnosed porphyria. In some instances this disorder can result in secondary hemochromatosis, but not in the presentation of Crigler-Najjar syndrome type I.

48. **The correct answer is A.** Leukotriene (LT) B_4 is a neutrophil chemotactic agent and will be abundant during an acute inflammatory process. LTB_4 is produced via the 5-lipoxygenase pathway primarily by neutrophils and macrophages and is one of the most effective chemoattractant mediators known. It is found in elevated concentrations in a number of inflammatory and allergic conditions, such as asthma, psoriasis, rheumatoid arthritis, and inflammatory bowel disease, and has been implicated in the pathogenesis of these diseases.

Answer B is incorrect. Prostaglandin I_2 is synthesized by vascular endothelium and smooth muscle. Its effects include inhibition of platelet aggregation, relaxation of smooth muscle, reduction of systemic and pulmonary vascular resistance by direct vasodilation, and natriuresis in kidney. It is produced via the cyclooxygenase pathway.

Answer C is incorrect. Thromboxane A_2 is a potent inducer of platelet aggregation and vasoconstriction.

Answer D is incorrect. Vascular endothelial growth factor is a substance made by cells that stimulates new blood vessel formation and is a mitogen for endothelial (vessel lining) cells.

Answer E is incorrect. von Willebrand factor (vWF) is made by the cell lining in the walls of blood vessels (veins and arteries). It binds plate-let glycoprotein-1b and facilitates platelet adhesion at the site of injury. vWF is also a carrier of factor VIII.

49. **The correct answer is A.** The quality and location of this patient's pain, combined with alleviation with medication and the radiographic findings, are suggestive of gastroesophageal reflux disease. This disorder increases the risk of developing esophageal mucosal metaplasia, called Barrett's esophagus. In turn, patients with Barrett's esophagus are at increased risk for developing adenocarcinoma of the esophagus.

Answer B is incorrect. Krukenberg's tumor is bilateral involvement of the ovaries by metastatic carcinoma of the stomach. This neoplasm bears no relation to gastroesophageal reflux disease.

Answer C is incorrect. Non-small cell adenocarcinoma of the lung is commonly caused by cigarette smoking but is not associated with gastroesophageal reflux disease.

Answer D is incorrect. Squamous cell carcinoma is not known to correlate with gastroesophageal reflux disease. Squamous cell carcinoma is thought to be associated with tobacco and alcohol use.

Answer E is incorrect. Stomach cell carcinoma is not associated with gastroesophageal reflux disease. Risk factors for stomach adenocarcinoma include *Helicobacter pylori* infection, nitrosamine exposure, excessive salt intake, and low intake of fresh fruit and vegetables. This type of carcinoma is predisposed by achlorhydria and chronic gastritis.

50. **The correct answer is E.** Patients with pancreatic adenocarcinoma often present with jaundice, epigastric pain radiating to the back, and weight loss. Laboratory studies show an increased amylase, lipase, alkaline phosphatase, CA 19-9, and carcinoembryonic antigen (CEA). Pancreatic cancers are more common in patients with a history of smoking, diabetes mellitus, and chronic pancreatitis. Treatment for pancreatic adenocarcinoma is surgical re-

moval, yet for most patients this is impossible, as the cancer has already metastasized prior to its discovery. If possible, pancreaticoduodenectomy or distal pancreatectomy is preferred to a total pancreatectomy to preserve some of the pancreatic function.

Answer A is incorrect. Patients with acute cholecystitis will present with pain in the right upper quadrant and vomiting. Patients rarely present with jaundice and do not present with weight loss.

Answer B is incorrect. Patients with acute pancreatitis often present with epigastric abdominal pain radiating to the back as well as with nausea and vomiting. Patients do not often present with jaundice or weight loss. Amylase and lipase will also be elevated, but the tumor markers CA 19-9 and CEA will not be elevated in a patient with acute pancreatitis.

Answer C is incorrect. Patients with carcinoid tumor will present with weight loss and symptoms of carcinoid syndrome, including flushing, diarrhea, and valvular heart disease. The laboratory values that are elevated in this patient most likely would not be elevated in a patient with a carcinoid tumor.

Answer D is incorrect. Patients with colon cancer will present with weight loss and may or may not have a change in bowel function, based on the location of the tumor. CEA levels will be elevated in these patients.

CHAPTER 11

Hematology-Oncology

1. A 23-year-old woman presents to her physician with a nevus on her arm that is asymmetrical with irregular borders. She has noticed a change in the color of this nevus in recent weeks. The nevus is removed and sent to the pathologist. On examination of the specimen, the pathologist determines that it is a melanoma. Which of the following features of this lesion is the greatest indicator of a poor prognosis for this patient?

(A) Depth within the dermis of >2 mm
(B) Growth location on her arm
(C) Lateral spread within the epidermis of >5 mm
(D) Previous basal cell carcinoma lesions
(E) Very large average size of neoplastic cells

2. A 57-year-old smoker presents to her primary care physician with a lump in the upper outer quadrant of her right breast. Mammography confirms a 2.5-cm lesion and core needle biopsy yields invasive ductal carcinoma. The patient undergoes lumpectomy with axillary lymph node dissection, and is referred to an oncologist to begin chemotherapy. Which of the following should be coadministered with the chemotherapy that this patient will most likely receive?

(A) Leucovorin
(B) Mesna
(C) Thymidine
(D) Vitamin B_{12}
(E) Vitamin B_6

3. A 43-year-old man comes to the physician because of increasing epigastric pain, heartburn, and weight loss over the past 4 months. When asked about bowel habits, the patient recalls a few occasions on which he had black, tarry stools. On physical examination, the physician notes that the patient is thin and pale and has diffuse tenderness over the epigastric area. Serum levels of which of the following substances are likely to be elevated in this patient?

(A) Cholecystokinin
(B) Gastrin

(C) Intrinsic factor
(D) Secretin
(E) Somatostatin

4. A 65-year-old man presents with a 2-month history of a cough. He also complains of a droopy right eyelid and dry facial skin. On a head and neck examination, the physician finds the right pupil is more constricted than the left one. CT scan reveals a 3-cm nodule in one lung. Based on these symptoms, which of the following is the most likely location of the tumor found on CT scan?

(A) Apex of left upper lobe
(B) Apex of right upper lobe
(C) Hilum
(D) Right lower lobe
(E) Right middle lobe

5. A 58-year-old woman presented to her physician after discovering a lump in her left breast. The physician examines the lump and finds it to be hard, nontender, and moveable. Which of the following increases this woman's risk of breast cancer?

(A) Drinking 4 cups of coffee every day
(B) Having a history of a cyst that drained straw-colored fluid
(C) Having a history of fibroadenoma of the left breast
(D) Having gone through menopause 2 years ago
(E) Taking St. John's wort every day

6. Low-molecular-weight heparins (LMWH) are distinct from unfractionated heparin in several ways. Which of the following is the primary target of LMWH?

(A) Antithrombin III
(B) Factor IIa
(C) Factor VII
(D) Factor Xa
(E) Factors II, IX, and X

7. A 4-year-old girl is brought to the emergency department with an 8-hour history of projectile

vomiting and headache. Her parents say that the patient was well until 2 months ago, when they noted that she was becoming increasingly clumsy. Physical examination shows nystagmus in all directions of gaze, as well as truncal ataxia. Laboratory studies of blood show a WBC count of 7200/mm³, a hemoglobin level of 12.3 g/dL, and a platelet count of 225,000/mm³. A CT scan shows a lesion in the cerebellar vermis with associated dilation of the third and lateral ventricles. Which of the following is most likely to be evident on histopathologic examination of the lesion?

(A) Deeply staining nuclei with scant cytoplasm arranged in pseudorosettes
(B) Pleomorphic anaplastic cells with foci of necrosis in a palisading pattern
(C) Regular round cells aligned smoothly with spherical nuclei surrounded by clear cytoplasm and finely granular chromatin associated with calcifications
(D) Stratified squamous epithelial cells embedded in spongy reticular stroma with prominent peripheral gliosis
(E) Whorls of meningothelial cells with oval-shaped nuclei with indistinct cytoplasm and psammoma bodies

8. A 17-year-old boy presents to the emergency department with severe abdominal pain. Laboratory tests show a deficit in uroporphyrinogen I synthetase and excess δ-aminolevulinate and porphobilinogen in the urine. Which of the following symptoms would most likely also be present in this patient?

(A) Chest pain
(B) Hypotension
(C) Neuropsychiatric disturbances
(D) Polyphagia
(E) Stiff neck

9. A 35-year-old woman visits her primary care physician after feeling a hard lump in her neck. Her physician notes that she has a single, hard, nontender nodule in the left lobe of her thyroid that moves when she swallows. There is no cervical lymphadenopathy. The patient denies any changes in her recent health. The patient does not have tremor, restlessness, heat intolerance, or an increased level of anxiety. Blood tests show normal thyroid hormone and calcitonin levels. A scintiscan shows a cold nodule in the left lobe of her thyroid. Tissue is obtained and a histological section is shown in the image. This patient most likely has which of the following?

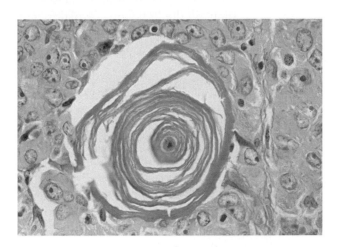

Image courtesy of Armed Forces Institute of Pathology.

(A) Follicular carcinoma
(B) Medullary carcinoma
(C) Multinodular goiter
(D) Papillary carcinoma
(E) Thyroglossal duct cyst

10. A 7-year-old African-American boy is brought to see his pediatrician. His father says he has noticed that the boy has been complaining of right knee pain for the past week. On physical exam, multiple ecchymoses are noted on both upper and lower extremities. His father claims that the boy has always bruised easily, and he has recently learned how to ride a bicycle. Which of the following elements of the coagulation cascade is most likely to be missing in this child?

(A) Antithrombin III
(B) Factor VII
(C) Factor VIII
(D) Factor IX
(E) Protein C

11. A 16-year-old boy is brought to the emergency department because of the acute onset of fever, chills, and a productive cough. X-ray of the chest shows an infiltrate restricted to the left lower lobe. Samples taken of the sputum show α-hemolytic gram-positive cocci in pairs. The patient says that he has had similar infections over the past year. A peripheral blood smear is done, and results show several sickle-shaped RBCs. Which of the following explains why this patient is susceptible to this particular type of infection?

(A) Bone marrow infiltration resulting in neutropenia and compromised immune function
(B) Large vessel occlusions in the cerebral vasculature resulting in neurologic events and aspiration pneumonia
(C) Microvascular infarcts resulting in pulmonary failure
(D) Microvascular infarcts resulting in splenic dysfunction
(E) Vaso-occlusion in the renal medulla

12. A 55-year-old man presents to his physician with easy bruising, splenomegaly, and fatigue. A peripheral blood smear is shown in the image. Which of the following is the most likely diagnosis?

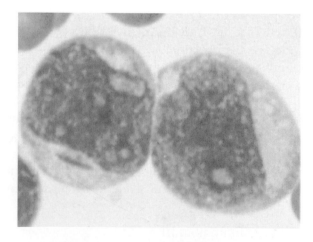

Reproduced, with permission, from Lichtman MA, Beutler E, Kipps TJ, Seligsohn U, Kaushansky K, Prchal JF. *Williams Hematology*, 7th ed. New York: McGraw-Hill, 2006: Color Plate XVI-2.

(A) Acute myeloid leukemia
(B) Chronic idiopathic myelofibrosis
(C) Chronic lymphocytic leukemia
(D) Chronic myelogenous leukemia
(E) Hairy cell leukemia

13. During autopsy of a 65-year-old woman, the liver is examined, revealing multiple tumors of various sizes throughout both lobes. This pattern, along with the fact that most tumors found in the liver are metastases, leads the pathologist to suspect that a primary tumor exists in another organ. Which of the following is the most likely location of the primary tumor?

(A) Breast
(B) Colon
(C) Kidney
(D) Lung
(E) Thyroid

14. A child is brought to the pediatrician because her parents are concerned about lead poisoning since their house is known to contain lead-based paint. A complete blood cell count reveals anemia. Lead poisoning causes anemia because it does which of the following?

(A) Disrupts heme synthesis by causing decreased iron absorption from the gut
(B) Disrupts heme synthesis by increasing the activity of aminolevulinate dehydratase
(C) Disrupts heme synthesis by inhibiting ferrochelatase
(D) Disrupts hemoglobin function by binding to hemoglobin with high affinity, preventing oxygen binding
(E) Disrupts RBC DNA synthesis, causing megaloblastic changes in RBCs

15. A 10-year-old boy with jaundice, splenomegaly, and chronic normocytic, normochromic anemia with an abnormal osmotic fragility test and increased mean corpuscular hemoglobin concentration presents to the clinic for a consult. He has had these symptoms for most of his life, and his parents are requesting a definitive cure. Which of the following confers a definitive cure for this patient's disease?

(A) Blood transfusions
(B) Bone marrow transplant
(C) Folate therapy
(D) Iron therapy
(E) Splenectomy

16. A 60-year-old woman presents to her physician with findings of decreased proprioception in her lower extremities and gait instability consistent with subacute combined degeneration secondary to cobalamin deficiency. However, blood tests show normal hematocrit and near-normal mean cell volume. The physician orders additional tests. Which of the following laboratory results would support a diagnosis of cobalamin deficiency?

(A) Decreased level of lactate dehydrogenase
(B) Elevated methylmalonic acid
(C) Elevated WBC count
(D) Increased cobalamin levels
(E) Microcytosis
(F) Negative anti-intrinsic factor antibody
(G) Negative Schilling test

17. A 73-year-old woman is brought to the emergency department after passing out on the subway. The patient has a 3-month history of burning epigastric pain that is worse after eating, along with dark stool. Physical examination shows a blood pressure of 95/52 mm Hg, a pulse of 97/min, epigastric tenderness, and guaiac-positive stool. Laboratory tests show a hemoglobin level of 9.5 g/dL, a hematocrit of 28%, and a mean corpuscular volume of 75 μm^3. Which of the following is the most likely diagnosis?

(A) Anemia of chronic disease secondary to peptic ulcer disease
(B) Iron deficiency anemia secondary to blood loss
(C) Iron deficiency anemia secondary to pernicious anemia
(D) Megaloblastic anemia secondary to blood loss
(E) Megaloblastic anemia secondary to pernicious anemia

18. Breast cancer is the leading cause of cancer in women in the United States and the second leading cause of cancer deaths in women. Age, a family history of breast cancer, and mutations in the *BRCA1* and *BRCA2* genes are important risk factors for the development of breast cancer. Which of the following drugs is used as prophylaxis in women at high risk for developing breast cancer?

(A) Abciximab and aspirin
(B) Flutamide and leuprolide
(C) Tamoxifen and raloxifene
(D) Testosterone and prednisone
(E) Vincristine and vinblastine

19. A 47-year-old woman from the Middle East presents to the clinic with fever, general malaise, and weight loss. Physical examination reveals hepatomegaly and massive splenomegaly, along with edema. Laboratory tests show moderate anemia and a peripheral WBC count <4000/mm³. Macrophages containing amastigotes are seen on histologic analysis. Which of the following parasites does the woman most likely harbor?

(A) *Babesia* species
(B) *Entamoeba histolytica*
(C) *Giardia lamblia*
(D) *Leishmania donovani*
(E) *Plasmodium ovale*

20. A type of lymphoma is characterized by onset in middle age and by neoplastic cells that resemble normal germinal center B lymphocytes. Additionally, it is the most common type of non-Hodgkin's lymphoma in the United States. What is the characteristic chromosomal translocation and protein that is produced by this translocation?

(A) t(8:14), c-myc
(B) t(9:22), bcr-abl
(C) t(11:22), EWS-FL-1
(D) t(14:18), bcl-2
(E) t(15:17), PML-RAR-α

21. A 52-year-old heart transplant patient on chronic immunosuppressive therapy that includes cyclosporine develops bacterial sinusitis. The patient's physician decides to start him on antibiotic therapy but is having difficulty choosing between amoxicillin and erythromycin to treat the infection. Concurrent use of erythromycin and cyclosporine would most likely lead to which of the following serum drug levels?

    (A) Decreased cyclosporine serum concentrations
    (B) First decreased, then increased serum cyclosporine concentrations
    (C) First increased, then decreased serum cyclosporine concentrations
    (D) Increased cyclosporine serum concentrations
    (E) Unchanged cyclosporine serum concentrations

22. A 56-year-old man is diagnosed with transitional cell carcinoma and treated with excision and chemotherapy. Which of the following risk factors most likely led to this patient's cancer?

    (A) Alcohol use
    (B) Exposure to aniline dyes
    (C) Exposure to asbestos
    (D) Hypertension
    (E) Previous pyelonephritis

23. A 70-year-old man with no prior surgical history presents with a tingling sensation of the extremities, weakness, and an enlarged tongue that is sore and smooth. Preliminary laboratory studies are negative for antinuclear antibodies and antimitochondrial antibodies, and peripheral blood smear reveals a macrocytic megaloblastic anemia. When the patient is given an oral dose of radiolabeled cyanocobalamin, none of that compound is detected in his urine. What is the function of the protein that is most likely deficient and/or affected in this disease process?

    (A) Binds free vitamin B_{12} in ileal cells for transport through the bloodstream
    (B) Binds free vitamin B_{12} in the stomach
    (C) Complex with free vitamin B_{12} in the small intestine and then binds to receptors on the wall of the ileum
    (D) Splits R-protein/vitamin B_{12} complexes in the duodenum
    (E) Splits vitamin B_{12} from its exogenous ingested protein-bound form

24. A 2-year-old boy is brought to a clinic because his mother noticed a large, unilateral, painless abdominal mass while she was bathing him. While performing an ultrasound-guided biopsy, the technician notes that the kidney calyces are highly distorted by the mass. Which of the following is most likely the origin of this lesion?

    (A) An autosomal dominant gene that also leads to cystic masses in the liver
    (B) Embryonic renal cells from the embryonic kidney
    (C) Malignant transformation of renal tubular cells
    (D) Malignant transformation of uroepethilial cells
    (E) Primitive neural crest cells

25. An 8-year-old boy is brought to the pediatrician after his parents noticed very dark urine in the toilet earlier that morning. Initial laboratory studies show intravascular hemolysis; further testing shows that his RBCs are susceptible to complement-mediated lysis. This patient most likely has which of the following conditions?

    (A) Autoimmune hemolytic anemia
    (B) Common bile duct stricture
    (C) Hereditary spherocytosis
    (D) Paroxysmal nocturnal hemoglobinuria
    (E) Thrombotic thrombocytopenic purpura

26. A 58-year-old man has a past medical history significant for chronic renal insufficiency. He was recently diagnosed with transitional cell carcinoma of the bladder and will be started on chemotherapy. Which of the following chemotherapeutic agents should be avoided in this patient?

    (A) Bleomycin
    (B) Cisplatin
    (C) Cytarabine

(D) Doxorubicin

(E) Tamoxifen

27. A 3-year-old girl was in her usual state of good health 1 month ago when she developed an acute viral upper respiratory infection. She now presents to the emergency department with nonblanching purple skin lesions. The rest of her physical examination is unremarkable. The complete blood count demonstrates a low platelet count, while the peripheral blood smear is notable only for large platelets. Which of the following laboratory findings would most likely be present in this patient?

(A) Antiplatelet antibodies

(B) Decreased megakaryocytes on bone marrow biopsy

(C) IgA deficiency

(D) Increased fibrin split products

(E) Vitamin K deficiency

28. A 57-year-old woman is diagnosed with small-cell lung carcinoma. She has gained weight, and she says that her face has recently "ballooned." Which of the following symptoms is this patient likely to be experiencing in addition to the ones mentioned?

(A) Cold intolerance and hair loss

(B) Galactorrhea and amenorrhea

(C) Insatiable thirst and polyuria

(D) Poor wound healing and hirsutism

(E) Restlessness and tremor

29. A 45-year-old woman arrives in the emergency department complaining of intense pain in her upper abdomen for the past 4 hours. She had a similar episode in the past, but it went away within an hour. Her history is significant for a recent flu-like infection and a prolonged feel-ing of fatigue and general exhaustion. Physical examination reveals that her sclerae are icteric, her palate is abnormally pigmented, and her skin has a yellow hue. Ultrasound shows radiopaque gallstones. A Coombs' test is negative. A peripheral blood smear shows small RBCs, several of which have no central pallor. Which of the following is the most likely cause of this patient's condition?

(A) A mutation in the gene encoding ankyrin

(B) A mutation in the glucose 6-phosphate dehydrogenase gene

(C) Circulating antibodies targeted against erythrocytes

(D) Iron deficiency anemia

(E) RBC hemolysis because of a mechanical heart valve

30. A research group is studying sickle cell disease in a small community of 6000 people in central Africa and performs a genetic analysis on every community member. At the beginning of the year, it is determined that 10% are homozygous for hemoglobin S and therefore have sickle cell disease. Thirty percent of the community is heterozygous for the mutant allele. Over the course of the year, 100 infants are born, six of whom are diagnosed with sickle cell disease. Of the 80 people who die during the year, three had sickle cell disease. Which of the following describes the current prevalence of homozygous sickle cell disease in this population?

(A) 3/6020

(B) 6/100

(C) 6/6020

(D) 603/6020

(E) 606/6100

31. A 65-year-old man comes to a local clinic complaining of back pain. After ruling out the most common causes of back pain, the treating physician becomes suspicious of a malignant process. He sends the patient for a bone marrow biopsy, with the results shown in the image. Which of the following is the most likely diagnosis?

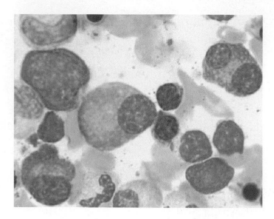

Reproduced, with permission, from Lichtman MA, Beutler E, Kipps TJ, Seligsohn U, Kaushansky K, Prchal JF. *Williams Hematology*, 7th ed. New York: McGraw-Hill, 2006: Color Plate XXI-2.

(A) Bone marrow suppression
(B) Lymphoma
(C) Metastatic prostate cancer
(D) Multiple myeloma
(E) Normal bone marrow

32. A 23-year-old woman presents to the emergency department following a motor vehicle crash. Her injuries are minor, and she states that she feels a bit dizzy and tired but has felt this way recently anyway. The physician notices that her laboratory results are consistent with megaloblastic anemia. Upon further questioning, she reports that she has been taking antibiotics off and on over the last several months for frequent urinary tract infections. Which of the following medications is this patient most likely taking?

(A) Chloramphenicol
(B) Clindamycin
(C) Erythromycin

(D) Gatifloxacin
(E) Trimethoprim

33. A 60-year-old woman presents to the physician because of red-brown streaks of blood in her stool. She reports no pain with bowel movements. Initial laboratory tests show:

Hematocrit: 33%
Hemoglobin: 11 g/dL
Mean corpuscular volume: 73 µm³
WBC count: 8000/mm³
Platelet count: 200,000/mm³

Which of the following is the most important next step in management?

(A) Abdominal plain films
(B) Colonoscopy
(C) CT scan of the abdomen
(D) Esophagoduodenoscopy
(E) Pelvic ultrasound

34. A patient with relapsing Hodgkin's disease presents with weight gain, foot ulcers, vision problems, elevated blood sugar, oral candidiasis, and new onset of wildly swinging mood changes. What is the most likely etiology of this patient's psychiatric symptoms?

(A) Adverse effects of bleomycin
(B) Adverse effects of prednisone
(C) Adverse effects of vincristine
(D) Normal psychiatric response to having cancer
(E) Progression of disease

35. A 41-year-old pregnant woman sees her obstetrician because of new-onset vaginal bleeding. Although she is only 4 months pregnant, her doctor notes that her uterus is the size usually seen at 6 months of gestation. Maternal blood works shows a β-human chorionic gonadotropin (β-hCG) level >5 times the upper limit of normal. If left untreated, what is a possible consequence of the patient's condition?

(A) Choriocarcinoma
(B) Coma
(C) Fetal neural tube defects
(D) Ovarian cancer
(E) Uterine bleeding and exsanguination

36. Hydrops fetalis occurs in the setting of a certain type of thalassemia. What is the underlying mechanism leading to this event?

    (A) Excess α-globin chains binding tighter to oxygen
    (B) Excess α-globin chains binding weaker to oxygen
    (C) Excess β-globin chains binding tighter to oxygen
    (D) Excess β-globin chains binding weaker to oxygen
    (E) Excess gamma-globin chains binding tighter to oxygen
    (F) Excess gamma-globin chains binding weaker to oxygen

37. A 56-year-old man who is a health care worker presents to his physician with vague abdominal discomfort. A physical examination reveals a tender liver, palpable to 6 cm below the costal margin and scleral icterus. His laboratory studies are significant for an aspartate aminotransferase activity of 200 U/L and an alanine aminotransferase activity of 450 U/L. A CT scan of the abdomen shows a dominant solid nodule in the liver. The marker most likely to be elevated in this patient is also a good indicator of which of the following malignancies?

    (A) Choriocarcinoma
    (B) Colorectal carcinoma
    (C) Melanoma
    (D) Neuroblastoma
    (E) Prostatic carcinoma
    (F) Yolk sac carcinoma

38. A 57-year-old man presents to his physician with a 4-month history of worsening fatigue and generalized weakness. Further questioning reveals that his clothes fit him more loosely now than they had in the past. Physical examination reveals generalized lymphadenopathy and hepatosplenomegaly. Lymph node biopsy specimens are sent to the pathologist with the presumptive diagnosis of lymphoma. Which of the following types of neoplastic cell is most common in non-Hodgkin's lymphoma?

    (A) B lymphocyte
    (B) Myeloblast

(C) Plasma cell
(D) Reed-Sternberg cell
(E) T lymphocyte

39. A 29-year-old man presents to his primary care physician with a painless testicular mass. Laboratory studies show an elevated serum human chorionic gonadotropin level. Which of the following is the most likely site of nodal metastasis in this tumor?

    (A) Deep inguinal lymph nodes
    (B) External iliac lymph nodes
    (C) Gluteal lymph nodes
    (D) Para-aortic lymph nodes
    (E) Superficial inguinal lymph nodes

40. A 28-year-old woman comes to the physician concerned about an excessive amount of bleeding from her gums when she brushes her teeth. Her laboratory results show an increased partial thromboplastin time and an increased bleeding time, but are otherwise unremarkable. Which of the following treatments will most likely alleviate this patient's symptoms?

    (A) Cryoprecipitate
    (B) Factor VIII concentrate
    (C) Fresh frozen plasma
    (D) Low-molecular-weight heparin
    (E) Protamine sulfate

41. A 29-year-old woman, who is 32 weeks' pregnant and has been in the hospital for 3 days because of pyelonephritis, starts oozing blood from her intravenous lines and bleeding from her gums. Petechiae are also noted in her skin. Laboratory tests show a platelet count of 98,000/mm³, hematocrit of 38%, WBC count of 8000/mm³, and a prolonged prothrombin time. What other laboratory anomaly would also be expected?

    (A) Elevated D-dimer levels
    (B) Elevated factor VII levels
    (C) Elevated fibrinogen levels
    (D) Elevated protein C levels
    (E) Elevated protein S levels

42. A 62-year-old woman presents to the clinic complaining of frequent bleeding while brushing her teeth and easy bruising. She reports she recently had pneumonia and was treated with a broad-spectrum antibiotic. Laboratory tests show:

Prothrombin time: 18 seconds
Partial thromboplastin time: 37 seconds
Platelet count: 231,000/mm³
Hematocrit: 37%
WBC count: 4800/mm³

The cofactor that is deficient in this patient is needed for the carboxylation of glutamate residues of which of the following?

(A) Factors II, VII, VIII, and X
(B) Factors VII, VIII, IX, and XII
(C) Proteins C and S and factors IX, X, XI, and XII
(D) Proteins C and S and factors XII, IX, and X
(E) Proteins C and S, prothrombin, and factors VII, IX, and X

43. A 20-year-old African-American man develops anemia after being treated for a urinary tract infection. A peripheral blood smear shows RBC lysis and precipitates of hemoglobin within the RBCs. Which of the following drug classes most likely caused his hemolytic anemia?

(A) Aminoglycosides
(B) Fluoroquinolones
(C) Macrolides
(D) Sulfonamides
(E) Tetracyclines

44. Several drugs are used to prevent myocardial infarction in patients with acute coronary syndrome. One class of drugs binds to the glycoprotein receptor IIb/IIIa on activated platelets, thereby interfering with platelet aggregation. This prevents renewed formation of clots that could block the lumen of the cardiac vessels. Which of the following is an example of this class of drug?

(A) Abciximab
(B) Clopidogrel
(C) Leuprolide

(D) Selegiline
(E) Ticlopidine

45. A 49-year-old man presents to the emergency department complaining that "my skin has turned yellow." Physical examination reveals the man is significantly jaundiced. He has no abdominal pain and has a negative Murphy's sign. The physician is concerned that he can feel the patient's gallbladder and orders a CT scan. What is the most likely cause of this patient's jaundice?

(A) Acute hepatitis
(B) Choledocholithiasis
(C) Cholelithiasis
(D) Hemolytic anemia
(E) Pancreatic cancer

46. A 34-year-old man comes to the emergency department complaining of the sudden onset of vomiting and epigastric abdominal pain radiating to the back. On physical examination, the patient is afebrile and has abdominal tenderness; decreased bowel sounds are noted, as is diffuse bruising that he describes as having appeared suddenly. He also reports continuous epistaxis. Laboratory tests show a slightly elevated WBC count, thrombocytopenia, increased amylase and lipase activity, increased prothrombin time (PT) and partial thromboplastin time (PTT), and the presence of fibrin split products. An abdominal ultrasound performed at the bedside shows a dilated common bile duct. Which of the following is the most likely etiology of this patient's abnormal coagulation profile?

(A) Acute hepatitis
(B) Acute pancreatitis
(C) Appendicitis
(D) Perforated gastric ulcer
(E) von Willebrand's disease

47. A 70-year-old man comes to his physician for a routine physical examination. Although he is asymptomatic, a blood test shows an abnormal level of immunoglobulin. After further testing, he is diagnosed with monoclonal gammopathy of undetermined significance. Which of the

following is the current treatment for monoclonal gammopathy of undetermined significance?

(A) Alendronate
(B) Anticoagulation
(C) High-dose steroids
(D) No treatment
(E) Vinca alkaloids

48. An 8-year-old boy has a chronic history of severe hemolytic anemia, hepatosplenomegaly, and maxillary overgrowth. He has received blood transfusions since early infancy but has not received a transfusion in over 4 months. A hemoglobin electrophoresis shows marked elevation of HbF, increased HbA_2, and absence of HbA_1. Which of the following diagnoses is most consistent with this patient's electrophoresis?

(A) α-Thalassemia minor
(B) β-Thalassemia major
(C) β-Thalassemia minor
(D) Glucose 6-phosphate dehydrogenase deficiency
(E) HbH disease
(F) RBCs containing hemoglobin Barts

49. A 69-year-old man has a tumor removed from the cerebellopontine angle because a CT scan shows a 2-cm sharply circumscribed mass adjacent to the right pons extending into the right cerebellar hemisphere. He reports a 3-month history of dizziness and a 4-year history of progressive hearing loss. Grossly, the tumor specimen appears as a single irregular fragment of tan-pink soft tissue that measures slightly less than 2 cm. A microscopic pathology report indicates that the specimen consists of compact areas of spindle cells with pink cytoplasm that form whirls and palisades. Which of the following types of tumors would most likely result in these findings?

(A) Medulloblastoma
(B) Meningioma
(C) Neurofibroma
(D) Oligodendroglioma
(E) Schwannoma

50. A 22-year-old man is diagnosed with medullary thyroid carcinoma, and his blood tests are significant for hypercalcemia and increased plasma catecholamine levels. He reports that his mother also had medullary thyroid carcinoma in her twenties and that she recently had surgery to remove her parathyroid glands. These findings suggest a possible mutation in which of the following genes?

(A) erb-B2
(B) MEN I
(C) ras
(D) Rb
(E) ret

1. **The correct answer is A.** In the vertical growth phase of melanoma, neoplastic cells grow deeply into the dermis. Considering that invasion of lymphatics or blood vessels (deep structures) is necessary for distant metastasis of any cancer, it can easily be understood why the depth of invasion is so important in highly labile melanoma. The depth of invasion into the dermis is an established prognostic factor for the patient, since most melanoma patients die due to complications of metastatic melanoma involvement of other organs (lung or brain). Patients with a tumor depth <1.7 mm have a more favorable prognosis. Remember the **AB-CDE's** of melanoma: **A**symmetry, **B**orders (irregular), **C**olor variation, **D**iameter >6 mm, and **E**levation/**E**volution.

Answer B is incorrect. Location of the lesion on an extremity, rather than the central body, indicates a more favorable prognosis.

Answer C is incorrect. Lateral spread within the epidermis is not as important as depth in determining metastatic potential.

Answer D is incorrect. Previous lesions do not have an impact on the likelihood of this nevus to metastasize.

Answer E is incorrect. Size of neoplastic cells is not a factor in determining prognosis.

2. **The correct answer is B.** The patient has invasive ductal carcinoma, which must be resected and then treated with chemotherapy. There are many chemotherapy combinations used to treat breast cancer, two of the most common being (1) cyclophosphamide, methotrexate, and 5-fluorouracil (5-FU) and (2) cyclophosphamide, doxorubicin, and 5-FU. Almost all of the regimens use the drug cyclophosphamide, an alkylating agent, which is commonly also used to treat non-Hodgkin's lymphoma and ovarian cancer. The most important toxicity of this drug is hemorrhagic cystitis, which can lead to transitional cell carcinoma. Hemorrhagic cystitis is prevented by coadministration of mesna. This is especially important in this patient because she is a smoker, which is independently a significant risk factor for transitional cell carcinoma.

Answer A is incorrect. Leucovorin can be used to reverse the myelosuppression that may occur with the use of methotrexate. Although methotrexate is likely one of the drugs that the patient will receive, there is no need to reverse its action until there is clear evidence of problematic immunosuppression. Conversely, administering mesna from the start is appropriate and makes sense, as it is protective of the bladder.

Answer C is incorrect. Thymidine can be used to reverse the myelosuppression that may occur with the use of 5-FU. Although 5-FU is likely one of the drugs that the patient will receive, there is no need to reverse its action until there is clear evidence of problematic immunosuppression. Conversely, administering mesna from the start is appropriate and makes sense, as it is protective of the bladder.

Answer D is incorrect. Coadministration of vitamin B_{12} would not be helpful for this patient. However, administration of vitamin B_{12} is necessary for a vitamin B_{12} deficiency caused by malabsorption, pernicious anemia, or a diseased terminal ileum.

Answer E is incorrect. Coadministration of vitamin B_6 would not be helpful for this patient. However, coadministration of vitamin B_6 can prevent neurotoxicity in a patient taking isoniazid for tuberculosis.

3. **The correct answer is B.** The question stem describes a case of a pancreatic gastrinoma leading to Zollinger-Ellison syndrome. This syndrome results from hypergastrinemia. Gastrin is normally produced by the G cells of the antrum and duodenum. For example, ectopic and unregulated production of gastrin by malignant pancreatic islet cells stimulates excess secretion of acid by parietal cells of the stomach. Gastrin also promotes hypertrophy of the stomach. Increased stomach acid leads to

symptoms of gastroesophageal reflux disease and to ulceration and gastric bleeding, as evidenced by the patient's pallor and melena. Elevated serum gastrin would be diagnostic of gastrinoma.

Answer A is incorrect. Cholecystokinin (CCK) is produced by the I cells of the duodenum and jejunum. CCK stimulates gallbladder contraction and pancreatic enzyme secretion. CCK inhibits gastric acid secretion.

Answer C is incorrect. Intrinsic factor is also released by the parietal cells of the stomach; its function is to bind vitamin B_{12} to enable its absorption. High intrinsic factor levels would be unlikely to produce the symptoms of elevated gastrin secretion in this case.

Answer D is incorrect. Secretin is produced normally by the S cells of the duodenum and promotes pancreatic bicarbonate secretion while inhibiting gastric acid secretion.

Answer E is incorrect. Somatostatin is produced by the pancreatic islets and gastrointestinal mucosa. Unlike gastrin, somatostatin inhibits gastric acid and pepsinogen secretion in addition to counteracting the actions of CCK and secretin. Somatostatin also inhibits the release of insulin and glucagons.

4. **The correct answer is B.** The question stem describes a case of Pancoast's tumor, in which a lung neoplasm of any type located in the apex impinges on the cervical sympathetic plexus. This impingement results in Horner's syndrome of ptosis, miosis, and anhidrosis, as described in this patient. The symptoms are ipsilateral to the damaged plexus, so the tumor must be located in the apex of the right upper lobe.

Answer A is incorrect. The symptoms are ipsilateral to the injured plexus, so a tumor in the left apex would have presented with Horner's syndrome on the left side, not the right.

Answer C is incorrect. Squamous cell carcinoma of the lung usually appears at the hilum, but such a tumor mass would not cause Horner's syndrome.

Answer D is incorrect. A tumor in the right lower lobe would not manifest in these symptoms.

Answer E is incorrect. A tumor located in the right middle lobe could not result in these symptoms because it would not be located near the cervical sympathetic plexus.

5. **The correct answer is D.** Late menopause (>50 years old) is associated with an increased risk of breast cancer. Other risk factors include being female, older age, early first menarche (<12 years old), delayed first pregnancy (>30 years old), and family history of a first-degree relative with breast cancer at a young age.

Answer A is incorrect. Breast cancer risk is not increased by caffeine intake.

Answer B is incorrect. Breast cancer risk is not increased by nonhyperplastic cysts. Had the cyst drained bloody fluid, it would have been more worrisome for a malignant process.

Answer C is incorrect. Breast cancer risk is not increased by fibroadenoma.

Answer E is incorrect. Breast cancer risk is not increased by use of St. John's wort.

6. **The correct answer is D.** LMWHs act predominantly on Xa, whereas unfractionated heparin targets both Xa and IIa. A major advantage of using LMWHs over unfractionated heparin is that there is no need for monitoring of APTT.

Answer A is incorrect. Heparin targets both antithrombin III and Xa.

Answer B is incorrect. Factor IIa, or thrombin, is the enzyme that catalyzes the final step of the clotting cascade, the formation of fibrin. Thrombin is a vitamin K-dependent factor that is not influenced by low-molecular-weight heparin.

Answer C is incorrect. Factor VII is part of the extrinsic pathway and is one of the vitamin K-dependent factors.

Answer E is incorrect. Warfarin blocks the activation of vitamin K-dependent factors II, VII, IX, and X.

7. **The correct answer is A.** The diagnosis is medulloblastoma, which occurs predominantly in children and is found exclusively in the cerebellum, accounting for 20% of brain tumors in children. On microscopic examination the tumor is very cellular with sheets of anaplastic cells. Each tumor cell is small with little cytoplasm and crescent-shaped, deeply staining nuclei (due to high mitotic activity) arranged in pseudorosettes. These tumors are frequently radiosensitive.

Answer B is incorrect. This micropathologic description is characteristic of glioblastoma multiforme, which is the most common primary brain tumor of adults and occurs in the cerebral hemispheres. It carries a particularly grave prognosis, with a survival rate at 5 years of almost zero. Most patients live less than 1 year after diagnosis. This is seldom a tumor of childhood and typically presents with severe headache and symptoms consistent with increased intracranial pressure.

Answer C is incorrect. This description is consistent with a diagnosis of oligodendroglioma, which is a relatively rare, slow-growing, benign tumor that is most often found in the frontal lobes. The clinical features are nonspecific and vary based on the location and extent of disease. General symptoms include headaches, seizures, and changes in cognition, while focal lesions can present with localized weakness, sensory loss, or aphasia. The micropathologic appearance is classically described as consisting of "fried egg" cells that have round nuclei with clear cytoplasm and are often calcified.

Answer D is incorrect. This histopathology describes a craniopharyngioma, the most common supratentorial tumor in children. It is embryologically derived from remnants of Rathke's pouch. The clinical presentation typically involves severe headaches, visual changes, and pituitary dysfunction (growth failure in children). It has a bimodal distribution of affected ages, with a second peak in the fifth decade of life.

Answer E is incorrect. This is a description of a meningioma, a nonmalignant primary intracranial neoplasm arising from arachnoid granulations. Clinically these tumors often present with seizures or a neurological deficit that gradually worsens over time. Focal symptoms vary by location. These tumors are slow growing and expand locally rather than by infiltration.

8. **The correct answer is C.** This patient suffers from acute intermittent porphyria (AIP), an autosomal dominant disorder caused by a lack of uroporphyrinogen I synthetase. The buildup of toxic levels of δ-aminolevulinate (ALA) and porphobilinogen lead to the associated symptoms of abdominal pain (more than 90% of cases), neuropathy, high sympathetic tone, and neuropsychiatric disturbances, including anxiety, depression, seizures, and paranoia. AIP almost never presents before puberty, and it can be hard to diagnose because of its acute nature. Untreated, it can lead to paralysis and death.

Answer A is incorrect. The differential diagnosis for chest pain is long and includes cardiac, pulmonary, gastrointestinal, and musculoskeletal etiologies. However, attacks of acute intermittent porphyria are not associated with chest pain.

Answer B is incorrect. Due to the high sympathetic tone caused by the pain of the crisis, hypertension may be associated with acute intermittent porphyria, but not hypotension.

Answer D is incorrect. Polyphagia, or greatly increased hunger, is one of the cardinal symptoms associated with diabetes mellitus, not acute intermittent porphyria.

Answer E is incorrect. A stiff neck may be associated with meningeal irritation and can be found in meningitis or with musculoskeletal problems, but it is not found in acute intermittent porphyria.

9. **The correct answer is D.** This patient has papillary carcinoma, the most common form of thyroid cancer. Patients are frequently in their 20s–40s and many have a history of exposure to ionizing radiation. Most papillary carcinomas are cold masses on scintiscan. On histologic exam, papillary carcinomas show branching papillae with a fibrovascular stalk. These

papillae are lined by epithelial cells with empty-looking, ground-glass nuclei often called "Orphan Annie eye" nuclei. Also characteristic of papillary carcinoma is the concentrically calcified psammoma bodies shown in the image above. Psammoma bodies are almost never seen in follicular or medullary carcinomas. The prognosis of papillary carcinoma is excellent. The overall 10-year survival rate is about 98%, especially in patients without lymph node metastases.

Answer A is incorrect. Follicular carcinoma is the second most common form of thyroid cancer and generally presents in women in their 40s and 50s. Follicular carcinomas may present as well-circumscribed nodules or infiltrative lesions. Like papillary carcinomas, they show up as cold lesions on scintigrams; however, their histology is different. Microscopically, follicular carcinomas present as uniform cells surrounding colloid-filled follicles with Hurthle cells (cells with abundant granular eosinophilic cytoplasm). There are no psammoma bodies seen in follicular carcinoma. The prognosis is excellent, with 10-year survival rates >92%.

Answer B is incorrect. Medullary carcinoma is a neoplasm of the parafollicular or C cells of the thyroid. These cells secrete calcitonin, which causes increased serum calcitonin levels. Medullary carcinoma can be sporadic, in which case it tends to be unilateral. Medullary carcinoma may also be associated with multiple endocrine neoplasia types IIA and IIB, in which case it tends to affect both the right and left lobes of the thyroid. On histologic exam, sheets of spindle-shaped cells are seen in amyloid stroma.

Answer C is incorrect. Multinodular goiters are asymmetrically enlarged thyroid glands that may be toxic or nontoxic, meaning that they may or may not overproduce thyroid hormone. Multinodular goiter may cause dysphagia due to compression of the esophagus. It may also cause compression of the large vessels in the neck. The presentation of multinodular goiter does not correlate with the clinical picture presented in this case.

Answer E is incorrect. A thyroglossal cyst is a congenital abnormality caused by the persistence of the diverticulum formed during the migration of the thyroid gland from the foramen cecum to the tracheal cartilage. These lesions are found in the midline and do not localize to one lobe.

10. **The correct answer is C.** This patient has hemophilia A, an X-linked disorder caused by factor VIII deficiency. Bleeding frequently occurs in joints and the retroperitoneal space. It is the most common inherited coagulopathy, as 1:10,000 males has a deficiency or dysfunction of factor VIII.

Answer A is incorrect. Mutations leading to antithrombin III deficiency result in a rare cause of inherited hypercoagulability. The history of multiple ecchymoses on both upper and lower extremities and easy bruising argues against a hypercoaguable disorder.

Answer B is incorrect. Factors II, VII, IX, and X are vitamin K-dependent clotting factors. None of them is deficient in patients with hemophilia A, and deficiencies of these factors are exceedingly rare.

Answer D is incorrect. Factor IX deficiency is the cause of hemophilia B, another X-linked disorder. The incidence of hemophilia B (also called Christmas disease) is 1:100,000 in males.

Answer E is incorrect. Protein C or protein S deficiency is another uncommon inherited cause of hypercoagulability.

11. **The correct answer is D.** This patient has sickle cell disease, as evidenced by the erythrocyte sickling in the peripheral blood smear. Patients with this disease are prone to microvascular infarcts in several vascular beds in the body. Over time, multiple micro-infarcts in the spleen result in functional asplenia, making patients particularly susceptible to infections with encapsulated organisms. This patient presents with pneumonia caused by *Streptococcus pneumoniae*. This is an encapsulated bacterium, which can be confirmed by a positive quellung reaction.

Answer A is incorrect. Sickle cell patients are at risk of having an aplastic crisis, often associated with parvovirus B19 infection, during which time bone marrow activity is suppressed. Some patients may subsequently develop bone marrow necrosis. Although these patients are at risk of developing a host of infections, this particular complication is not specifically associated with susceptibility to infections with encapsulated organisms.

Answer B is incorrect. Strokes in sickle cell patients due to large vessel occlusion can be a serious cause of morbidity. Aspiration pneumonia could be a complication of these neurologic events, but this does not explain increased susceptibility to infection with encapsulated bacteria.

Answer C is incorrect. Although microinfarcts in the pulmonary vasculature are a chronic complication of sickle cell disease and constitute a leading cause of death for these patients, they are not responsible for the patient's susceptibility to infections with encapsulated organisms.

Answer E is incorrect. The renal medulla is particularly prone to vaso-occlusive complications in sickle cell patients; renal failure and uremia could be possible complications. This can result in isothenuria, in which the kidney is not fully able to concentrate the urine.

12. **The correct answer is A.** The cytoplasmic inclusions seen in the myelocytic precursors in the image are fused lysosomal granules known as Auer rods. Release of these fused granules may cause acute disseminated intravascular coagulation (DIC) and fatal hemorrhage. Auer rods define a cell as being of myelocytic lineage as opposed to lymphocytic and are seen in acute myeloid leukemia (AML), especially in the subgroup of acute promyelocytic leukemia, also known as M3 in the French American British system (FAB). AML is the most common form of leukemia in adults and constitutes approximately one-fifth of acute leukemia cases in children. Symptoms of AML are related to complications of pancytopenia (i.e., anemia, neutropenia, and thrombocytopenia)

and include weakness and easy fatigue, infections, and hemorrhagic findings such as gingival bleeding, ecchymoses, epistaxis, or menorrhagia. The prognosis for patients with AML is poor; many patients die within a few years of diagnosis.

Answer B is incorrect. Chronic idiopathic myelofibrosis also can present with splenomegaly and fatigue; however, peripheral blood smear would show teardrop-shaped RBCs, nucleated red cell precursors, and granulocytic precursor cells without the presence of Auer rods.

Answer C is incorrect. Chronic lymphocytic leukemia is more common in patients >60 years old. The disease has an insidious onset, with patients presenting early on with fatigue and weight loss and later with lymphadenopathy and hepatosplenomegaly. The peripheral blood smear reflects a marked lymphocytosis, with a typically normocytic, normochromic anemia. As the disease progresses, the platelet count may drop. Auer rods are not a feature of lymphocytic lymphomas or leukemias.

Answer D is incorrect. Characteristics of chronic myelogenous leukemia include lymphadenopathy, splenomegaly, marked leukocytosis, mature myeloid precursor cells, and minimal blasts and promyelocytes. Auer rods are not typically seen on peripheral blood smear.

Answer E is incorrect. Although hairy cell leukemia affects middle-aged men who tend to present with massive splenomegaly and fatigue, Auer rods are not present in leukemic cells of this disease. Hairy cell leukemia derives its name from the hairlike filamentous projections characteristic of affected leukemic cells.

13. **The correct answer is B.** The liver and lung are the most common sites of metastasis (after lymph nodes) due to the high blood flow through these organs. Therefore, primary tumors in any of the locations listed may metastasize to the liver. However, given that the blood vessels from the gastrointestinal tract drain into the hepatic circulation, the most likely primary tumor that metastasizes to the liver would be from a gastrointestinal source such as the colon.

Answer A is incorrect. Breast tumors may also metastasize to the liver, but with less frequency than gastrointestinal cancers. Breast metastases are more often found in brain and bone.

Answer C is incorrect. Tumors of the kidney, such as renal cell carcinoma, metastasize to the brain and bone, and less so to the liver.

Answer D is incorrect. Lung tumors often metastasize to brain and bone, and less often to the liver.

Answer E is incorrect. Thyroid cancer often leads to bone metastases.

14. **The correct answer is C.** Lead inhibits δ-aminolevulinate (ALA) dehydratase and ferrochelatase, preventing both porphobilinogen formation and the incorporation of iron into protoporphyrin IX, the final step in heme synthesis. Inhibition of both of these steps results in ineffective heme synthesis and subsequent microcytic (hemoglobin-poor) anemia.

Answer A is incorrect. Lead poisoning does not affect iron absorption from the gut.

Answer B is incorrect. Lead inhibits ALA dehydratase, preventing porphyrin synthesis beyond the formation of ALA; it does not increase its actions. This causes ALA to accumulate in the urine.

Answer D is incorrect. Lead does not have a high affinity for hemoglobin. This type of pathology is seen in carbon monoxide (CO) poisoning. CO binds to hemoglobin with much higher affinity than oxygen, resulting in decreased oxygen-carrying capacity.

Answer E is incorrect. Lead does not interrupt RBC DNA synthesis. Folate and/or vitamin B_{12} deficiencies disrupt DNA synthesis, specifically thiamine synthesis, resulting in megaloblastic changes in RBCs.

15. **The correct answer is E.** The patient is exhibiting symptoms of a hemolytic anemia because he is anemic and has jaundice, which results from the breakdown of RBCs leading to the formation of excess bilirubin. Moreover, his anemia is normochromic and normocytic with an abnormal osmotic fragility test and increased mean corpuscular hemoglobin concentration (MCHC). These are all characteristics of hereditary spherocytosis, an intrinsic, extravascular hemolysis due to spectrin or ankyrin defect. RBCs are small and round with no central pallor. The osmotic fragility test detects hemolysis by measuring the fraction of hemoglobin released from RBCs at progressively more dilute salt concentrations. It detects hemolysis in spherocytes at salt concentrations that do not affect normal RBCs. The MCHC measures the concentration of hemoglobin in a given volume of packed RBCs and is elevated only in hereditary spherocytosis. The definitive treatment of hereditary spherocytosis is splenectomy because the spleen is responsible for the breakdown of the defective RBCs in this disease. Once eliminated, the spleen no longer hemolyzes the RBCs, and thus, the anemia improves.

Answer A is incorrect. Blood transfusions are indicated in hereditary spherocytosis for severe anemia, but are only temporary and not definitive treatment.

Answer B is incorrect. Bone marrow transplant is not indicated for hereditary spherocytosis. Splenectomy is curative and poses significantly less risks than bone marrow transplant.

Answer C is incorrect. Folate therapy is indicated for hereditary spherocytosis, but is not a definitive treatment. It is only a supportive treatment that does not eliminate the problem.

Answer D is incorrect. Iron therapy is not indicated in hereditary spherocytosis.

16. **The correct answer is B.** In a minority of patients with cobalamin (vitamin B_{12}) deficiency, hematocrit and mean corpuscular volume can be normal. In these cases, laboratory testing for elevated homocysteine and methylmalonic acid can be used to make the diagnosis.

Answer A is incorrect. Lactate dehydrogenase would be increased in vitamin B_{12} deficiency due to failed hematopoiesis.

Answer C is incorrect. Neutropenia with hypersegmented neutrophils is typically seen in vitamin B_{12} deficiency.

Answer D is incorrect. Decreased cobalamin levels would support a diagnosis of vitamin B_{12} deficiency.

Answer E is incorrect. Vitamin B_{12} deficiency presents as a macrocytic anemia. Peripheral blood smear typically shows macro-ovalocytosis of RBCs.

Answer F is incorrect. A positive anti-intrinsic factor antibody would suggest autoimmune destruction of parietal cells in the stomach leading to decreased intrinsic factor and vitamin B_{12} absorption.

Answer G is incorrect. In the Schilling test, radioactive cobalamin is given orally with a non-radioactive parenteral load. Radioactivity measured in the urine can be used to estimate oral cobalamin absorption. A positive Schilling test would suggest a defect in absorption.

17. **The correct answer is B.** This patient is suffering from iron deficiency anemia secondary to blood loss from the gastrointestinal tract. Since the body possesses a limited ability to absorb iron from the gut (which occurs mainly in the duodenum), occult blood loss can quickly lead to a depletion of existing iron stores and hence to an iron deficiency anemia. The burning epigastric pain that worsens after eating is consistent with a gastric ulcer. The black stool is melena, which occurs with blood loss in the upper gastrointestinal tract (bleeding in the lower gastrointestinal tract causes visibly bloody red stools). Iron deficiency anemia is shown by the low hematocrit level and mean corpuscular volume. The most common cause of iron deficiency anemia in postmenopausal women is occult blood loss, often from a gastrointestinal source.

Answer A is incorrect. Anemia of chronic disease is typically a normocytic anemia due to a chronic inflammatory, infectious, malignant, or autoimmune disease. This patient's anemia is microcytic and is likely due to a condition involving blood loss.

Answer C is incorrect. Although this patient's lab values are consistent with iron deficiency anemia, pernicious anemia results instead in megaloblastic anemia.

Answer D is incorrect. The low mean corpuscular volume is not consistent with megaloblastic anemia, which is normally caused by a deficiency of folate or vitamin B_{12}, not blood loss.

Answer E is incorrect. Pernicious anemia is caused by B_{12} deficiency and presents with a macrocytic, megaloblastic anemia. The low mean corpuscular volume is not consistent with megaloblastic anemia.

18. **The correct answer is C.** Use of tamoxifen and raloxifene as prophylaxis in women at high risk for breast cancer has been shown to reduce the incidence of breast cancer by 50%–80% in this population. It is thought that selective estrogen receptor modulators have a selective benefit in reducing the incidence of estrogen receptor-positive cancers for *BRCA2*-positive women. The decision to begin tamoxifen and raloxifene, however, is not one that should be taken lightly. These drugs have many adverse effects that impact quality of life, such as hot sweats and amenorrhea associated with early menopause and increased risk of stroke and pulmonary embolism. Women who have previously been diagnosed with breast cancer are also often put on tamoxifen as prophylaxis against a second cancer.

Answer A is incorrect. Abciximab is an antiplatelet drug used to treat acute coronary syndromes. Aspirin is an irreversible inhibitor of cyclooxygenase often used in the treatment and secondary prevention of acute coronary syndromes.

Answer B is incorrect. Flutamide is a nonsteroidal antiandrogen that competitively inhibits androgens at the testosterone receptor. Gonadotropin-releasing hormone analogs such as leuprolide are used in continuous dosing regimens in the treatment of prostate cancer.

Answer D is incorrect. Testosterone is an androgen that is approved by the Food and Drug Administration for palliation therapy in metastatic breast cancer. Adverse effects of testosterone treatment include virilization, edema, and jaundice. Prednisone is a systemic corticosteroid that is used in various anticancer treatment regimens. The combination of testosterone and prednisone is not used as prophylaxis treatment for women at high risk for breast cancer.

Answer E is incorrect. Vincristine and vinblastine are microtubule inhibitors used to treat testicular carcinoma as well as Hodgkin's and non-Hodgkin's lymphomas.

19. **The correct answer is D.** *Leishmania donovani* infection presents with hepatomegaly and splenomegaly, malaise, anemia, leukopenia, and weight loss. *L. donovani* is transmitted via the sandfly. Microscopically, macrophages containing amastigotes are observed. Sodium stibogluconate is used to treat *L. donovani* infection.

Answer A is incorrect. *Babesia* species infection presents with a malaria-like syndrome. Babesiosis is transmitted by the *Ixodes* tick and is found in the same regions as Lyme disease. On microscopic examination, one observes no red blood cell pigment and the Maltese cross-appearing parasite. Quinine is used to treat babesiosis.

Answer B is incorrect. *Entamoeba histolytica* infection presents with intestinal amebiasis (bloody diarrhea and abdominal pain) and less commonly liver abscesses. Patients are infected by ingestion of amebic cysts, usually from contaminated food or water. These cysts pass through the small intestine and form trophozoites, which can invade the mucosa of the colon. Microscopy will demonstrate cysts or trophozoites in the stool. Symptomatic patients should be treated with metronidazole.

Answer C is incorrect. *Giardia lamblia* infection presents with bloating, flatulence, foul-smelling diarrhea, and light-colored fatty stools. Abdominal pain, nausea, and vomiting may also be present, although in endemic regions two-thirds of infected individuals are asymptomatic. *G. lamblia* is transmitted via cysts in water (fecal-oral transmission) and is common in all areas of the world, but more prevalent in developing countries (although one should consider *Giardia* infection in patients who present with symptoms after camping trips). Domestic cats and dogs, along with beavers and other mammals, have recently been shown to have a high prevalence of the disease and may be reservoirs for humans. On microscopy, one observes teardrop-shaped trophozoites with a ventral sucking disc or cysts with "falling leaf" motility. Metronidazole is used to treat *G. lamblia* infection.

Answer E is incorrect. *Plasmodium ovale* is a form of malaria carried by the *Anopheles* mosquito that causes a 48-hour cyclic fever. Like other forms of malaria, it presents as a febrile illness with fevers accompanied by headaches, sweats, malaise, and anemia (due to lysed RBCs). A feature unique to both *P. ovale* and *P. vivax* is that they can form hypnozoites that can remain dormant in the liver for long periods, only to resurface later. Thus after the systemic infection is cleared, these forms must be treated with primaquine to kill any organisms remaining in the liver. *P. ovale* infection can be treated with chloroquine.

20. **The correct answer is D.** The question stem describes follicular lymphoma, the most common type of non-Hodgkin's lymphoma in the United States. The characteristic chromosomal translocation is t(14:18), which juxtaposes the IgH locus on chromosome 14 next to the BCL2 locus on chromosome 18. This causes overproduction of the bcl-2 protein, an anti-apoptotic factor, facilitating the survival of the cancer. An important simplifying fact to help remember the different chromosomal translocations is that those involving the immunoglobulin loci on chromosome 14 tend to be cells that normally produce antibodies (e.g., B lymphocytes). Thus, these translocations are common in B-lymphocyte lymphomas.

Answer A is incorrect. The t(8:14) rearrangement is most commonly found in Burkitt's lymphoma as well as in some cases of acute lymphocytic leukemia. Translocation of the c-myc gene next to the immunoglobulin heavy chain locus results in constitutive overproduction of the c-myc oncogene, promoting neoplastic proliferation.

Answer B is incorrect. The t(9:22) translocation results in the Philadelphia chromosome, which is most commonly found in chronic myelogenous leukemia as well as in other chronic myeloproliferative disorders and acute lymphocytic leukemia, where it confers a poor prognosis. The translocation results in a bcr-abl fusion protein that functions as a constitutively active tyrosine kinase to promote leukemia growth.

Answer C is incorrect. The t(11:22) chromosomal translocation is associated with Ewing's sarcoma. (Note that it does not involve the immunoglobulin locus.) It overproduces a chimeric transcription factor that activates the c-myc promoter and produces excessive amounts of the EWS-FL-1 protein. Ewing's sarcoma is a small round cell tumor of the bone usually found in the long bones of teenagers. X-ray will show a lytic tumor with reactive bone deposited around it in an onion-skin fashion.

Answer E is incorrect. The t(15:17) translocation denotes the acute promyelocytic leukemia (APL) subtype of acute myelogenous leukemia. The characteristic fusion of the promyelocytic leukemia (PML) gene with the retinoic acid receptor-α (RAR-α) gene blocks differentiation of immature myeloid blasts, most likely by blocking activity of other retinoic acid receptors. Treatment with all-*trans*-retinoic acid (termed differentiation therapy) overwhelms the blockade of the other retinoic acid receptors, restores differentiation, and can induce temporary remission. Combination differentiation treatment together with conventional chemotherapy can result in long-term survival rates of 70%–80%, unique among the acute leukemias. APL patients also typically present with dysfunctional coagulopathies, predisposing them to excess bleeding, a major source of mortality.

21. **The correct answer is D.** Cyclosporine is an immunosuppressant that binds to cyclophilins, thereby blocking the differentiation and activation of T lymphocytes by inhibiting the production of interleukin-2 (IL-2). Erythromycin is a macrolide antibiotic that binds to the 50S ribosomal subunit and inhibits protein synthesis. Amoxicillin is a β-lactam antibiotic that inhibits bacterial cell wall synthesis. Studies have shown

similar results with amoxicillin and erythromycin in the treatment of bacterial sinusitis. Concurrent use of erythromycin and cyclosporine could lead to elevated cyclosporine serum concentrations because erythromycin inhibits the cytochrome P-450 enzyme system in the liver. The cytochrome P-450 enzyme superfamily is a major site of drug metabolism and is responsible for the oxidation, reduction, and hydrolysis of drug compounds, including cyclosporine.

Answer A is incorrect. Erythromycin will increase, not decrease, cyclosporine concentrations.

Answer B is incorrect. Erythromycin will increase cyclosporine concentrations both initially and over time.

Answer C is incorrect. Erythromycin will increase cyclosporine concentrations both initially and over time.

Answer E is incorrect. Erythromycin will increase cyclosporine concentrations.

22. **The correct answer is B.** Transitional cell carcinoma (TCC) is a malignant tumor that arises from the transitional epithelium of the renal pelvis. It can spread to adjacent tissues and often recurs after removal. It is the most common tumor of the urinary tract system. While it can occur in renal calyces, the renal pelvis, and the ureters, the most common site for TCC is in the bladder. There is significant association of TCC with phenacetin (a common painkiller), smoking, aniline dyes, and cyclophosphamide (a chemotherapeutic drug); remember the mnemonic "associated problems in your **Pee SAC.**" Painless hematuria is the most common presenting sign of TCC. The presence of otherwise unexplained hematuria denotes cancer in the urinary tract in individuals over the age of 40 years until proven otherwise. Commonly, TCC is treated surgically. Other treatment modalities include radiation and chemotherapy as either adjuvant or primary treatment, depending on the case.

Answer A is incorrect. Alcohol use is not a risk factor associated with transitional cell carcinoma, but is associated with many other cancers, including esophageal and liver cancers.

Answer C is incorrect. Exposure to asbestos is not a risk factor associated with transitional cell carcinoma, but is associated with an increased risk for developing mesothelioma.

Answer D is incorrect. Hypertension is not a risk factor associated with transitional cell carcinoma.

Answer E is incorrect. Previous pyelonephritis is not a risk factor associated with transitional cell carcinoma.

23. **The correct answer is C.** The clinical and laboratory findings are consistent with pernicious anemia. This chronic progressive anemia is caused by a deficiency of intrinsic factor, a protein produced by gastric parietal cells. Once vitamin B_{12} is released from food, it binds R-proteins upon which it travels to the duodenum. In the duodenum, vitamin B_{12} is released from R-proteins and then complexes with intrinsic factor. The intrinsic factor-B_{12} complex binds to receptors in the ileum, where it is endocytosed by enterocytes. Pernicious anemia is believed to be caused by immune-mediated destruction of gastric mucosa, leading to a loss of parietal cells. A Schilling test (as described in the stem) will reveal whether the labeled vitamin B_{12} is being absorbed and eliminated in the urine (as in normal individuals), or whether a lack of intrinsic factor or malabsorption is preventing the radiolabeled compound from appearing in the urine.

Answer A is incorrect. Transcobalamin II, a plasma protein, binds free vitamin B_{12} in ileal cells for transport through the bloodstream.

Answer B is incorrect. R proteins are vitamin B_{12}-binding proteins produced by the salivary gland that bind vitamin B_{12} once it has been split from its exogenous protein-bound form by pepsin in the stomach.

Answer D is incorrect. Pancreatic proteases are secreted into the duodenum, which split the R-protein/vitamin B_{12} complexes, producing vitamin B_{12} that is free to bind intrinsic

factor to form intrinsic factor/vitamin B_{12} complexes.

Answer E is incorrect. Pepsin, which is active in creating the acidic pH of the stomach, splits vitamin B_{12} from its exogenous protein-bound form, leaving it free to bind R proteins produced by the salivary gland.

24. **The correct answer is B.** Wilms' tumor arises from neoplastic embryonal renal cells of the metanephros. Wilms' tumor is the most common solid tumor of childhood (most commonly occurring between the ages of 2 and 4 years) and is rarely seen in adults. It commonly presents with a huge palpable flank mass and is seen with hemihypertrophy (abnormal enlargement of one side of the body). It is associated with the deletion of tumor suppressor gene *WT1* on chromosome 11. Since it arises from the kidney parenchyma, it distorts the kidney calyces as it grows.

Answer A is incorrect. Adult polycystic disease is an autosomal dominant genetic disorder that presents with bilateral cystic enlargement of the kidneys. Individuals with this disorder also suffer from cystic enlargement of the liver, berry aneurysms, and mitral valve prolapse.

Answer C is incorrect. Clear cell carcinoma of the kidney is a malignancy derived from the renal tubular cells. It is common for patients to present with an abdominal mass, but patients with clear cell carcinoma are commonly men 50–70 years old, with an increased incidence found in smokers. Patients with renal cell carcinoma present with a range of symptoms, such as hematuria, a palpable mass, polycythemia, flank pain, and fever.

Answer D is incorrect. TCC is a malignant tumor that arises from the uroepithelial cells of the urinary tract. TCC is the most common tumor of the urinary tract (as it can occur in the renal calyx, renal pelvis, ureters, and bladder). Painless hematuria and urinary outflow obstruction are the most common presenting signs of TCC.

Answer E is incorrect. Malignancy that is derived from the primitive neural crest cells as an abdominal mass in a young child is neuroblastoma. The tumor does not arise in the kidney; instead, it forms from the adrenal medulla and paraspinal sympathetic ganglia. Therefore, it does not distort the kidney architecture.

25. **The correct answer is D.** This patient suffers from paroxysmal nocturnal hemoglobinuria, an acquired disease caused by RBC susceptibility to complement-mediated cell lysis. This is due to insufficient synthesis of GPI anchors, which anchor proteins that protect RBCs from this process. Clinical manifestations include intravascular hemolysis with hemoglobin release into the blood and subsequent hemoglobinuria, thrombotic complications (such as Budd-Chiari syndrome), and aplastic anemia.

Answer A is incorrect. Autoimmune hemolytic anemia is caused by IgG antibodies that are targeted against RBC antigens. This patient's symptoms are all due to acute intravascular hemolysis. In this condition the hemolysis is extravascular and antibody-mediated and is not due to complement-mediated lysis.

Answer B is incorrect. Although common bile duct stricture may cause darker urine due to elevated bilirubin in the blood, it would not cause intravascular hemolysis or complement-mediated lysis. Common bile duct strictures caused by carcinomas of the pancreatic head are the most common causes of painless jaundice.

Answer C is incorrect. Hereditary spherocytosis is caused by mutations that result in an unstable erythrocyte cytoskeleton. When those erythrocytes pass through the spleen, the reticuloendothelial cells remove pieces of the membrane, causing spherocyte formation. This results in extravascular hemolysis and is not due to complement-mediated lysis.

Answer E is incorrect. The normal von Willebrand factor (vWF) protease is absent in patients with thrombotic thrombocytopenic purpura (TTP), resulting in high levels of large vWF multimers and causing excessive platelet adhesion and clearance. Because of diffuse thrombus formation in the microvasculature, evidence of intravascular hemolysis is found due to microangiopathy. The classic pentad of TTP consists of fever, thrombocytopenia, microangiopathic hemolysis, neurologic symptoms, and renal insufficiency. RBC lysis is caused by shear trauma in the vessels and is not secondary to complement-mediated lysis.

26. **The correct answer is B.** Cisplatin has been shown to cause nephrotoxicity and acoustic nerve damage. Use of cisplatin requires that the patient be vigorously hydrated in order to prevent kidney damage. In patients with documented kidney dysfunction, cisplatin should be avoided altogether due to these patients' greater susceptibility to dose-related nephrotoxicity.

Answer A is incorrect. Bleomycin toxicity includes pulmonary fibrosis, hypertrophic skin changes, and minimal myelosuppression. It is not associated with nephrotoxicity.

Answer C is incorrect. Cytarabine causes leukopenia, thrombocytopenia, and megaloblastic anemia. It is not associated with nephrotoxicity.

Answer D is incorrect. Toxic effects of doxorubicin include cardiotoxicity, myelosuppression, and alopecia. It is not associated with nephrotoxicity.

Answer E is incorrect. Tamoxifen has been noted to cause hot flashes, nausea/vomiting, skin rash, and vaginal bleeding. It is not associated with nephrotoxicity.

27. **The correct answer is A.** This patient presents with clinical features of idiopathic thrombocytopenic purpura (ITP), the most common cause of thrombocytopenia in childhood. ITP is an autoimmune disease and is most commonly instigated by a viral illness. Bleeding disorders due to platelet defects or deficiencies will present with microhemorrhage of the mucous membranes and of the skin, like the nonblanching purple skin lesions (purpura) seen in this patient. ITP is a diagnosis of exclusion but classically presents with thrombocytopenia, antiplatelet antibodies, as well as signs of a compensatory increase in platelet production,

including large platelets on peripheral blood smear and increased megakaryocytes on bone marrow biopsy. As ITP only affects platelets, patients will have normal prothrombin time and normal partial thromboplastin time.

Answer B is incorrect. Decreased megakaryocytes on bone marrow biopsy suggest a defect in platelet production which can result from malignancy, infection, or drug reactions.

Answer C is incorrect. Patients with IgA deficiency present with frequent respiratory, urinary, and gastrointestinal infections and would not present with isolated thrombocytopenia.

Answer D is incorrect. Increased fibrin split products are a sign of activation of the coagulation cascade and may be associated with thrombocytopenia in the case of DIC. DIC is caused by a systemic activation of the clotting cascade leading to global depletion of clotting factors in addition to depletion of platelets. DIC leads to complications from both the systemic microthrombi and the increased risk of bleeding from clotting factor and platelet depletion. While patients with DIC will present with thrombocytopenia, they will also have an increased prothrombin time and partial thromboplastic time and schistocytes on their peripheral blood smears. In addition to the microhemorrhage of the skin and mucous membranes due to the platelet deficiency, patients with DIC can also develop macrohemorrhage in joints and internal organs as a result of the clotting factor deficiencies.

Answer E is incorrect. Vitamin K deficiency leads to a deficiency in the Vitamin K-dependent clotting factors, II, VII, IX, and X, causing an elevated prothrombin time and increasing the risk of macrohemorrhage. Vitamin K deficiency, however, should not lead to thrombocytopenia seen in this patient.

28. **The correct answer is D.** Although her symptoms may be somewhat nonspecific, the fact that this patient has small-cell lung carcinoma (SCLC) should be a clue that her symptoms may be part of a paraneoplastic syndrome. SCLC is notorious for production of ACTH and ADH. In this case, excessive ACTH pro-

duction has lead to increased glucocorticoids. Weight gain and redistribution of body fat (in contrast to the cachexia typical of cancers alone) and moon facies are classic signs of Cushing's syndrome. Poor wound healing (due to inhibition of collagen synthesis by glucocorticoids) and hirsutism (stimulation of androgen production by ACTH) are also part of Cushing's syndrome.

Answer A is incorrect. Cold intolerance and hair loss are symptoms of hypothyroidism.

Answer B is incorrect. Galactorrhea and amenorrhea are symptoms of hyperprolactinemia, as may occur in cases of anterior pituitary tumors.

Answer C is incorrect. Insatiable thirst and polyuria are symptoms of ADH deficiency or diabetes insipidus.

Answer E is incorrect. Restlessness and tremor are symptoms of hyperthyroidism.

29. **The correct answer is A.** This woman suffers from hereditary spherocytosis (HS), typically caused by mutations in the genes that code for either ankyrin or spectrin. Both of these proteins contribute to the erythrocyte cytoskeleton. When the erythrocytes with abnormal membranes pass through the spleen, the reticuloendothelial cells remove pieces of the membrane, causing a decreased membrane-to-cytoplasm ratio. This results in spherocyte formation. HS is often associated with hemolytic crisis resulting in jaundice and pigmented gallstones.

Answer B is incorrect. Glucose 6-phosphate dehydrogenase (G6PD) deficiency is due to an X-linked mutation and therefore typically occurs only in males. Although hemolysis in the setting of G6PD could be secondary to infection, Heinz bodies and bite cells will be found in the peripheral blood smear, not spherocytes.

Answer C is incorrect. Autoimmune hemolytic anemia is due to antibodies against erythrocytes. This will cause a positive Coombs' test and therefore is unlikely in this setting.

Answer D is incorrect. Iron deficiency anemia causes a microcytic anemia. This does not fit the hemolytic picture and is not associated with spherocytes.

Answer E is incorrect. Hemolysis because of a mechanical valve is caused by mechanical trauma as the erythrocytes flow across the foreign surface. This results in schistocytes in a peripheral blood smear. This diagnosis is unlikely given the absence of a unique heart sound on examination and an absence of schistocytes in the smear.

30. **The correct answer is D.** Prevalence is the total number of cases in a population divided by the total population; that is, the proportion of the total population with the disease. The total number of cases at the beginning of the study can be calculated by multiplying the initial population (6000) by the initial prevalence (10%), yielding 600 cases. Over the course of the year, there was a net gain of 3 patients with sickle cell disease (6 births – 3 deaths), bringing the new total to 603. Likewise, the new total population is 6020, a net gain of 20 people. Therefore, the current prevalence of sickle cell disease is 603/6020.

Answer A is incorrect. Prevalence is the total number of cases in a population divided by the total population. The value in this answer choice describes the net gain in the number of cases divided by the population, and therefore is incorrect.

Answer B is incorrect. Prevalence is commonly confused with incidence, which is the number of new cases in a unit of time divided by the number of susceptible people. This answer choice represents the incidence of sickle cell disease during the year, not the prevalence. Because the genotype of all community members is already known, only newborn infants are truly at risk for the disease. Therefore, of the 100 people at risk for sickle cell disease, 6 were diagnosed, yielding an incidence of 6/100.

Answer C is incorrect. This value would represent the incidence of the disease if the entire population were at risk. However, because the genotypes of all preexisting members of the community are already known, only newborn infants are truly at risk for sickle cell disease, and thus the denominator in the calculation of incidence would be 100, not 6020.

Answer E is incorrect. This answer fails to take into account the deaths that occurred during the year, which would affect both the total number of current cases and the current population.

31. **The correct answer is D.** This bone marrow biopsy is consistent with multiple myeloma. Plasma cells can be clearly seen throughout this image, recognized by their off-center nuclei and clock-face chromatin distribution. Also commonly seen on a blood smear are stacked RBCs, in what is known as a rouleaux formation.

Answer A is incorrect. Bone marrow suppression appears as a paucity of cells on histology. This image has too many plasma cells to represent bone marrow suppression.

Answer B is incorrect. Lymphoma is a neoplastic disorder of the lymphoid tissue. There are many different types of lymphoma, two of the most distinctive histologic types being Burkitt's lymphoma and Hodgkin's lymphoma. Burkitt's lymphoma shows a "starry sky" pattern on histology. This pattern is created by macrophage ingestion of tumor cells. Hodgkin's lymphoma is distinguished by its Reed-Sternberg cells. The Reed-Sternberg cells are binucleate and display prominent nucleoli.

Answer C is incorrect. Prostate cancer is typically adenocarcinoma. It commonly metastasizes to the axial skeleton and can cause back pain and spinal cord compression. It causes osteoblastic lesions in bone.

Answer E is incorrect. This image shows too many plasma cells to represent normal bone marrow.

32. **The correct answer is E.** Trimethoprim is associated with megaloblastic anemia, leukopenia, and granulocytopenia. These effects may be reduced with a folic acid supplement.

Answer A is incorrect. Chloramphenicol is a broad-spectrum antibiotic that is particularly effective against bacterial meningitis and is associated with aplastic anemia and gray baby syndrome.

Answer B is incorrect. Clindamycin is associated with pseudomembranous colitis due to *Clostridium difficile* overgrowth.

Answer C is incorrect. Erythromycin is a macrolide and is associated with cholestatic hepatitis.

Answer D is incorrect. Gatifloxacin is a fluoroquinolone and is associated with tendinitis.

33. **The correct answer is B.** Rectal bleeding or anemia in anyone age 50 years or older is considered colorectal cancer until proven otherwise. The gold standard for diagnosis of colorectal cancer is colonoscopy with possible tissue biopsy of suspicious lesions. Current cancer screening recommendations suggest colonoscopy or double-contrast barium enema every 10 years, sigmoidoscopy every 5 years, and/or fecal occult blood testing in people ≥50 years old.

Answer A is incorrect. Abdominal plain films are best used to visualize radiopaque renal lithiasis, free air, or fluid.

Answer C is incorrect. Abdominal CT scans can visualize many abdominal pathologies; however, colonoscopy is a more sensitive test for colorectal cancer screening.

Answer D is incorrect. Esophagoduodenoscopy is best used to evaluate for lesions of the upper gastrointestinal tract.

Answer E is incorrect. Pelvic ultrasound is best used to evaluate abnormalities of the ovaries, uterus, and vagina.

34. **The correct answer is B.** This patient is presenting with some of the classic adverse effects of steroid therapy, which is often part of treatment for Hodgkin's disease. These include the physical signs of Cushing's syndrome (weight gain, moon facies, thin skin, muscle weakness, and brittle bones), along with cataracts, hypertension, increased appetite, elevated blood sugar, indigestion, insomnia, nervousness, restlessness, and immunosuppression. However, in addition, prednisone is known to produce profound mood changes known as glucocorticoid psychosis.

Answer A is incorrect. The typical adverse effects of bleomycin are pulmonary fibrosis, skin changes, and myelosuppression. Bleomycin is part of the **ABVD** cancer chemotherapy regimen against Hodgkin's: **A**driamycin (doxorubicin), **B**leomycin, **V**inblastine, and **D**acarbazine.

Answer C is incorrect. Common adverse effects of vincristine are areflexia and peripheral neuritis. Vincristine is part of the **MOPP** cancer chemotherapy regimen used against Hodgkin's disease: **M**echlorethamine, vincristine (**O**ncovin), **P**rocarbazine, and **P**rednisone.

Answer D is incorrect. Wildly swinging mood is suggestive of cyclothymic disorders, which are common in patients with chronic medical illness. However, given that this disorder requires 2 years of symptoms before a definitive diagnosis can be made, the most likely cause is glucocorticoid psychosis.

Answer E is incorrect. The progression of Hodgkin's disease typically does not involve profound psychiatric symptoms.

35. **The correct answer is A.** The patient has a hydatidiform mole. Hydatidiform moles are cystic swellings of the chorionic villi. They usually present in the fourth and fifth months of pregnancy with vaginal bleeding. On exam the uterus is larger than expected for gestational age and the serum β-hCG level is much higher than normal. Moles can be either partial or complete and are caused by either fertilization of an egg that has lost its chromosomes or fertilization of a normal egg with two sperm. Partial moles may contain some fetal tissue but no viable fetus, and a complete mole contains no fetal tissue. Hydatidiform moles must be surgically removed because the chorionic villi may embolize to distant sites and because moles may lead to choriocarcinoma, an aggressive

neoplasm that metastasizes early but is very responsive to chemotherapy.

Answer B is incorrect. Coma is a possible outcome of eclampsia, not of a hydatidiform mole. Preeclampsia is the triad of hypertension, proteinuria, and edema. Eclampsia occurs when seizures accompany the symptoms of preeclampsia. This patient does not have any of these symptoms.

Answer C is incorrect. Neural tube defects are usually detected in utero by increased α-fetoprotein levels in amniotic fluid and maternal serum; β-hCG levels are normal in these patients.

Answer D is incorrect. Ovarian cancers are often accompanied by an increase in blood cancer antigen 125 levels, not β-hCG levels. This patient has a hydatidiform mole, not ovarian cancer. Hydatidiform moles do not predispose patients to ovarian cancer.

Answer E is incorrect. If undetected, tubal pregnancies may rupture, causing unilateral lower quadrant pain and uterine bleeding. Because the patient may exsanguinate, ruptured ectopic pregnancy is a surgical emergency. This patient does not have the symptoms of a tubal pregnancy. Also, because of the small size of the fallopian tubes, tubal pregnancies present long before 4 months of gestation.

36. **The correct answer is E.** When the α-globin genes are missing (as in the most severe type of α-thalassemia), excess gamma-globin chains accumulate, leading to the formation of tetramers known as hemoglobin Barts. These tetramers bind so strongly to oxygen that the fetal tissues are not oxygenated properly. This severe tissue anoxia leads to hydrops fetalis, an abnormal fluid accumulation in at least 2 fetal compartments.

Answer A is incorrect. α-Thalassemia occurs when one or more α-globin genes is deleted, leading to accumulation of other globin chains. For this reason, one would not expect to see accumulation of α-globin chains in α-thalassemia. Excess α-globin chains would be expected in β-thalassemia minor or major. β-Thalassemia

usually does not have negative effects on the fetus because β-chains are not expressed until after birth.

Answer B is incorrect. There is no excess of α-chains in α-thalassemia

Answer C is incorrect. Excess β-globin chains would be seen in the case of hemoglobin H (HbH) disease (another type of α-thalassemia), in which three α-globin chains have been deleted. Here, β-globin chains make tetramers known as HbH. HbH does have a higher affinity for oxygen, and there is usually tissue hypoxia associated with this disease. However, hydrops fetalis is not associated with this condition because the hypoxia occurs in the adult when β-chains are expressed.

Answer D is incorrect. Excess β-globin chains leading to hemoglobin H actually bind more strongly to oxygen.

Answer F is incorrect. In hemoglobin Barts, the hemoglobin binds more strongly to oxygen, not more weakly.

37. **The correct answer is F.** This vignette suggests a malignancy of the liver. Hepatomas are highly associated with chronic hepatitis B and C infections, which are often found in health care workers due to needle stick injuries. Other risk factors for hepatomas include Wilson's disease, hemochromatosis, alcoholic cirrhosis, α-1-antitrypsin deficiency, and carcinogens. α-Fetoprotein is a marker for hepatomas but can also be elevated in patients with germ cell tumors, such as yolk sac tumors. Tumor markers should not be used for primary diagnoses, but for confirmation and to monitor therapy.

Answer A is incorrect. The marker for choriocarcinoma is β-human chorionic gonadotropin. This marker is also elevated with hydatidiform moles and gestational trophoblastic tumors. The presence of a hepatoma has no effect on this marker.

Answer B is incorrect. The marker for colorectal carcinoma is carcinoembryonic antigen. This marker is nonspecific and is also produced by pancreatic, gastric, and breast carcinomas. The presence of a hepatoma has no effect on this marker.

Answer C is incorrect. The marker for melanoma is S-100. This marker also is elevated with neural tumors and astrocytomas. The presence of a hepatoma has no effect on this marker.

Answer D is incorrect. The marker for neuroblastoma is bombesin. This marker also is elevated with lung and gastric cancers. The presence of a hepatoma has no effect on this marker.

Answer E is incorrect. The marker for prostatic carcinoma is prostate-specific antigen. The presence of a hepatoma has no effect on this marker.

38. **The correct answer is A.** Neoplastic B lymphocytes are the cells of origin in most non-Hodgkin's lymphomas (90% of cases), with the notable exception of lymphoblastic lymphoma, which is typically dominated by T lymphocytes.

Answer B is incorrect. Myeloblasts are the neoplastic cells in acute myelogenous leukemia.

Answer C is incorrect. Plasma cells are the neoplastic cells in multiple myeloma. Multiple myeloma also affects patients in their 50s and 60s. However, at presentation patients with multiple myeloma usually have pathologic fracture caused by lytic lesions, hypercalcemia because of bone resorption, and repeated infection because of decreased production of normal immunoglobulins. Urine analysis in patients with multiple myeloma shows Bence Jones proteinuria with a monoclonal spike on electrophoresis.

Answer D is incorrect. Reed-Sternberg cells are the neoplastic cells in Hodgkin's disease. Under light microscopy, Reed-Sternberg cells appear as large binucleate cells with abundant cytoplasm and large "owl-eye" nucleoli.

Answer E is incorrect. T-lymphocyte lymphomas are less common and include lymphoblastic lymphomas and a minority of diffuse large cell lymphomas.

39. **The correct answer is D.** The testes begin life high in the abdomen and descend to their final resting place in the scrotum. The lymphatic drainage from the testes, therefore, is to the para-aortic lymph nodes in the lumbar region just inferior to the renal arteries.

Answer A is incorrect. The deep inguinal nodes drain the vessels in the spongy urethra and may become enlarged in some sexually transmitted diseases or other causes of urethritis.

Answer B is incorrect. External iliac nodes drain the bladder.

Answer C is incorrect. Gluteal lymph nodes drain the deep tissue of the buttocks.

Answer E is incorrect. Tumors of the scrotum itself, but not of the testes, may spread to the superficial inguinal lymph nodes. The scrotum is an outpouching of abdominal skin, and drainage of this skin is to the superficial inguinal nodes. The testes, however, which lie inside the scrotum, begin life in the abdomen, and lymph drainage follows embryologic origins.

40. **The correct answer is A.** This woman suffers from von Willebrand's disease, the most common inherited bleeding disorder; it results from a defective form or overall deficiency of vWF. vWF has two functions: it serves as the ligand for platelet adhesion to a damaged vessel wall, and it also is the plasma carrier of factor VIII. Due to platelet dysfunction and lack of a carrier for factor VIII, the unique lab finding in this disease consists of an increased bleeding time and an increased partial thromboplastin time. Cryoprecipitate is the precipitate that remains when fresh frozen plasma is thawed. It contains sufficient normal vWF to correct the bleeding dyscrasia. In addition to prolonged bleeding from mucosal surfaces as in this patient, other symptoms include easy bleeding and skin bleeding.

Answer B is incorrect. Factor VIII concentrate is used to treat individuals with hemophilia A, an inherited condition that results in factor VIII deficiency.

Answer C is incorrect. Fresh frozen plasma (FFP) is used to treat several factor deficiencies, including V, VII, X, and XI. FFP administration will replace several factor deficiencies, although factor concentrations in FFP tend to vary. Unlike cryoprecipitate, FFP does not contain von Willebrand factor or fibrinogen. FFP may be needed for inherited factor XI deficiency or as a source of factor V in severe cases of disseminated intravascular coagulation when platelet concentrates and cryoprecipitate do not correct the factor V, VIII, and fibrinogen consumption defects.

Answer D is incorrect. LMWH is an anticoagulant that acts predominantly on factor Xa. This patient is in need of a procoagulant rather than an anticoagulant. LMWH can be administered subcutaneously. One advantage of LMWH over heparin is that the partial thromboplastin time does not need to be routinely monitored with this drug.

Answer E is incorrect. Protamine sulfate is used for reversal of heparinization. It is a positively charged molecule that acts by binding to heparin, a negatively charged molecule. Protamine would have no therapeutic benefit for this patient.

41. **The correct answer is A.** DIC can occur in the setting of obstetric complications, sepsis, malignancy, and other conditions. It is described as a thrombohemorrhagic process because there are microthrombi throughout the body, and coagulation factors and platelets are consumed actively. The active conversion of fibrinogen to fibrin as part of the convergence of both clotting cascades leads to decreased levels of fibrinogen. At the same time, anticoagulation factors such as plasmin and protein C are being activated, leading to fibrinolysis and increased levels of D-dimers in the circulation.

Answer B is incorrect. DIC leads to consumption of coagulation factors; therefore, a drop in factor VII levels would be expected.

Answer C is incorrect. Fibrinogen is actively converted to fibrin in the setting of DIC; there-

fore, a decrease in the levels of fibrinogen would be expected.

Answer D is incorrect. Because the anticoagulation factors are also being activated and consumed during DIC, protein C levels would decrease.

Answer E is incorrect. Because anticoagulation factors are being consumed during DIC, protein S levels would decrease.

42. **The correct answer is E.** The patient has a prolonged prothrombin time, likely indicating a deficiency in one of the factors involved with the extrinsic pathway. Vitamin K is a fat-soluble vitamin that is a cofactor for the γ-carboxylation of glutamate residues of prothrombin; factors VII, IX, and X; and proteins C and S. Vitamin K deficiency is uncommon; however, it can occur in the setting of oral broad-spectrum antibiotics, which suppress the flora of the bowel and interfere with the absorption and synthesis of this vitamin. It can also be associated with other conditions related to fat malabsorption and diffuse liver disease, or in the neonatal period when the intestinal flora have not developed and the liver reserves of vitamin K are small. Vitamin K deficiency usually presents with bleeding diathesis, hematuria, melena, bleeding gums, and ecchymoses.

Answer A is incorrect. The activity of factor VIII does not depend on vitamin K.

Answer B is incorrect. The activities of factors VIII and XII do not depend on vitamin K.

Answer C is incorrect. The activities of factors IX and XII do not depend on vitamin K.

Answer D is incorrect. The activity of factor XII does not depend on vitamin K.

43. **The correct answer is D.** This patient likely has glucose 6-phosphate dehydrogenase deficiency, which is common in African-Americans, and demonstrates characteristic Heinz bodies (precipitates of hemoglobin) within RBCs. Hemolysis can be precipitated by certain drugs, such as sulfonamides, isoniazid, aspirin, ibuprofen, primaquine, and nitrofurantoin.

Answer A is incorrect. Aminoglycosides are commonly associated with nephro- and ototoxicity.

Answer B is incorrect. Fluoroquinolones may cause some gastrointestinal upset, damage to cartilage in children, and tendonitis and tendon rupture in adults.

Answer C is incorrect. Macrolide toxicity includes gastrointestinal discomfort, acute cholestatic hepatitis, eosinophilia, and skin rashes.

Answer E is incorrect. Tetracycline toxicity includes gastrointestinal distress, tooth discoloration and inhibition of bone growth in children, and photosensitivity reactions.

44. **The correct answer is A.** Abciximab functions by binding to the glycoprotein receptor IIb/IIIa on activated platelets, preventing fibrinogen from binding and interfering with platelet aggregation. It is used in acute coronary syndrome and angioplasty.

Answer B is incorrect. Both clopidogrel and ticlopidine function by inhibiting the ADP pathway involved in the binding of fibrinogen to platelets during platelet aggregation.

Answer C is incorrect. Leuprolide is a gonadotropin-releasing hormone analog that acts as an agonist when administered in a pulsatile fashion and as an antagonist when administered in a continuous fashion. It is used to treat infertility (when administered as an agonist), prostate cancer (when administered as an antagonist), and uterine fibroids.

Answer D is incorrect. Selegiline is a selective monoamine oxidase B inhibitor that causes an increase in the availability of dopamine. It is used with levodopa in the treatment of Parkinson's disease.

Answer E is incorrect. Both clopidogrel and ticlopidine function by inhibiting the ADP pathway involved in the binding of fibrinogen to platelets during platelet aggregation.

45. **The correct answer is E.** This patient's physical exam demonstrates Courvoisier's sign: jaundice and a palpable, enlarged, nontender gallbladder. This sign is often found in patients with cancer in the head of the pancreas, which is obstructing the gallbladder from emptying.

Answer A is incorrect. Acute hepatitis is associated with tenderness in the right upper quadrant, and it should not produce an enlarged gallbladder.

Answer B is incorrect. Choledocholithiasis is the presence of a stone in the common bile duct. It is a common cause of cholecystitis, which is associated with tenderness in the right upper quadrant.

Answer C is incorrect. Cholelithiasis simply refers to stones within the gallbladder. It is generally painless, and does not cause jaundice or an enlarged gallbladder.

Answer D is incorrect. Hemolytic anemia is a cause of painless jaundice, however, it is not associated with an enlarged gallbladder.

46. **The correct answer is B.** This patient has DIC secondary to an acute case of pancreatitis. Common causes of DIC are gram-negative sepsis, malignancy, acute pancreatitis, trauma, transfusion reactions, and obstetric complications. During DIC, there is a massive activation of the coagulation cascade that results in thrombus formation throughout the microvasculature. Rapid consumption of both platelets and coagulation factors follows, with subsequent easy bleeding and bruising. Concurrent with this consumptive coagulopathy is activation of the fibrinolytic system. In this patient, thrombocytopenia, elevated prothrombin time/partial thromboplastin time, and the presence of fibrin split products all suggest DIC. Pancreatitis as the cause is supported by the clinical presentation of epigastric pain that may radiate to the back, nausea, vomiting, and increased amylase and lipase levels. The presence of a dilated common bile duct suggests that gallstones may have been the cause of the pancreatitis episode. Dilation of the common bile duct can be seen proximal to an area of current or past obstruction. An obstruction in the ampulla of Vater or simply

the passing of a gallstone through the ampulla can block the flow of pancreatic exocrine enzymes from the pancreatic duct, and the backflow of these enzymes into the pancreas leads to autodigestion of the pancreatic parenchyma. This autodigestion leads increased blood levels of the pancreatic enzymes amylase and lipase.

Answer A is incorrect. Acute hepatitis is an inflammatory process leading to liver cell death, likely caused by viral agents, drugs, or poisons. Signs and symptoms of acute hepatitis vary greatly among patients but can range from asymptomatic to fatal. Patients may present with nausea and vomiting. Easy bruising and bleeding secondary to decreased hepatic product of clotting factors may occur, with subsequent prolongation to PT and PTT. Thrombocytopenia may occur secondary to decreased hepatic production of thrombopoietin, with subsequent prolongation of bleeding time. Gallstones, as suggested by a dilated common bile duct, could cause obstruction of the biliary tree and damage the liver. However, unlike the presentation in this patient, pain associated with acute hepatitis is likely to develop in the right upper abdominal quadrant. Fever may also be present, especially with viral etiologies. While aspartate aminotransferase, alanine aminotransferase, and alkaline phosphatase levels are commonly elevated in acute hepatitis, amylase and lipase levels are not. Fibrin split products are unlikely to be present.

Answer C is incorrect. Acute cholecystitis is defined as inflammation of the gallbladder generally associated with cholelithiasis. Pathogenesis typically involves obstruction of the cystic duct by gallstones. Acute cholecystitis may present with elevated WBC counts, nausea, and vomiting. However, unlike in this patient, the pain is more likely to be located in the right upper quadrant and may radiate to the scapula or shoulder. A low-grade fever is common. Because the obstruction by gallstones is generally restricted to the cystic duct and not to the hepatic duct or biliary tree, liver damage is not common. In fact, total bilirubin and alkaline phosphatase levels are elevated in only a minority of cases, and hepatic produc-

tion of clotting factors and thrombopoietin is not often impaired. This, combined with the low likelihood of disseminated intravascular coagulation in acute cholecystitis, means that PT, PTT, and platelet counts should be normal, and there should be no signs of easy bleeding or bruising. Also, amylase and lipase levels should be normal in acute cholecystitis. Ultrasounds would likely show cholelithiasis, but cholecystitis is not necessarily associated with dilation of the common bile duct since the obstruction usually occurs in the cystic duct.

Answer D is incorrect. Gastric ulcers may present clinically as epigastric pain radiating to the back and may be associated with increased amylase activity, especially if perforation has occurred. However, ulcers are not typical causes of disseminated intravascular coagulation or subsequent findings of thrombocytopenia, increased PT and PTT, and fibrin split products. Furthermore, gastric ulcers will not cause increased amylase and lipase levels and are not generally related to common bile duct dilation.

Answer E is incorrect. von Willebrand's disease is characterized by defect or deficiency of vWF. During clot formation in hemostasis, vWF functions to link platelets to collagen in exposed endothelium and serves as a carrier for factor VIII. Symptoms include easy bruising and bleeding. Like this patient, people with von Willebrand's disease are likely afebrile. Bleeding time would be prolonged due to decreased platelet adhesion, and PTT would be increased due to decreased available VIII (a component of the intrinsic pathway). However, the sudden onset of disease as an adult makes this hereditary disease a less likely cause of this patient's symptoms. Furthermore, abdominal pain, fever, increased WBC counts, thrombocytopenia, increased PT, fibrin split products, and common bile duct dilation would not be likely findings in von Willebrand's disease.

47. **The correct answer is D.** Monoclonal gammopathy of undetermined significance (MGUS) is characterized as a plasma cell dyscrasia, de-

fined by the presence of a monoclonal immunoglobulin, also called an M protein, in the serum or urine of persons without evidence of multiple myeloma, Waldenström's macroglobulinemia, amyloidosis, or other lymphoproliferative disorders. MGUS is a preneoplastic condition. There is no accepted treatment for this disorder because one cannot predict which patients will progress to develop multiple myeloma.

Answer A is incorrect. Bisphosphonates such as alendronate and risedronate are used to treat multiple myeloma, which is known to cause bone destruction due to increased osteoclast activity. Bisphosphonates have been shown to decrease pain and fractures in multiple myeloma by reducing the number and activity of osteoclasts.

Answer B is incorrect. Anticoagulation is not the recommended treatment for MGUS.

Answer C is incorrect. High-dose steroids are not a current treatment modality for MGUS.

Answer E is incorrect. Vinca alkaloids such as vincristine and vinblastine are microtubule inhibitors used in the treatment of some cancers. However, vinca alkaloids are not currently the recommended treatment for MGUS.

48. **The correct answer is B.** Thalassemias are genetic diseases involving decreased synthesis or complete absence of either the α-globin chain or the β-globin chain. This patient has classic symptoms of thalassemia: hemolytic anemia, hepatosplenomegaly, and "chipmunk facies," cased by extramedullary hematopoeisis in the bones of the face. The requirement for blood transfusions since birth should raise the suspicion for β-thalassemia major in this patient, but the hemoglobin electrophoresis results alone can be used to arrive at this conclusion. This patient shows increased HbF (α-2 γ-2) and HbA2 (α-2 δ-2); thus, synthesis of the α chain is intact. Absence of HbA_1 (α-2 β-2) supports an absence of β-chain synthesis and, therefore, a diagnosis of β-thalassemia major. Death in these individuals is often caused by cardiac failure secondary to hemochromatosis.

Answer A is incorrect. α-Thalassemia minor is associated with a two-gene deletion of α globin (two gene regions are intact). Deletion of only a single α gene results in an asymptomatic carrier with no hematologic manifestations, as there are four α globin genes and two will still function properly. Results of electrophoresis should rule out α-thalassemia minor.

Answer C is incorrect. β-Thalassemia minor (the heterozygous defect) would show decreased but not absent HbA_1. This is a less severe form of the disease.

Answer D is incorrect. Glucose 6-phosphate dehydrogenase deficiency would not present with abnormal hemoglobin electrophoresis.

Answer E is incorrect. HbH is less severe than Hb Barts and is associated with three-gene deletion of α globin. The abnormal hemoglobin molecule (HbH) contains four β chains. The β-thalassemias are more prevalent in Mediterranean populations and the α-thalassemias are more prevalent in Asian and African populations.

Answer F is incorrect. Hb Barts is the most severe of the genotypes involving deletion of α globin genes; it is associated with complete absence of all α-globin chains. This results in the absence of all hemoglobins that require this chain, and in the formation of tetramers of the γ chain (normally a component of HbF). This condition leads to hydrops fetalis and intrauterine fetal death.

49. **The correct answer is E.** This patient had an acoustic schwannoma removed from the cerebellopontine angle. Schwann cell tumors are the third most common primary intracranial tumor, are often localized to cranial nerve VIII (acoustic neuroma), and are commonly seen at the cerebellopontine angle. The most common signs and symptoms of schwannomas include hearing loss, tinnitus, vertigo, hydrocephalus, and increased intracranial pressure. Most are benign, slow-growing tumors that can be resected. Histologically, two patterns are found: (1) Antoni A, or spindle cells palisading and forming a whirl appearance; and (2) An-

toni B, or loosely arranged tissue after degeneration in the tumor. The histopathologic description of this patient's tumor is consistent with Antoni A.

Answer A is incorrect. Medulloblastomas are highly malignant radiosensitive tumors that are typically found in the posterior fossa. These tumors are of neuroectodermal origin, and histopathologic examination shows a rosette or perivascular pseudorosette pattern. Peak incidence occurs in childhood.

Answer B is incorrect. Meningiomas are slow-growing tumors that most often occur in the hemispheric convexities and parasagittal regions. Rarely they can appear in the cerebellopontine angle. However, the histology would classically show psammoma bodies, or areas of calcification.

Answer C is incorrect. Neurofibromas are tumors of peripheral origin. This patient's tumor is intra-axial, as shown on the CT scan. Histologically, these cells appear as loosely arranged spindle cells with intervening collagen.

Answer D is incorrect. Oligodendrogliomas are relatively uncommon, slow-growing tumors that occur most often in the frontal lobes. The tumor comprises homogeneous sheets of cells with uniformly rounded nuclei and an associated network of finely branching blood vessels.

50. **The correct answer is E.** The characteristics described in the question are found in patients with the most common hyperplasias/tumors associated with multiple endocrine neoplasia (MEN) type IIA, also known as Sipple's syndrome. MEN IIA is associated with parathyroid hyperplasia or tumor leading to hypercalcemia, medullary carcinoma of the thyroid, and pheochromocytoma, which commonly causes elevated plasma catecholamine levels. The MEN syndromes follow an autosomal dominant pattern of inheritance and both MEN IIA and MEN IIB (MEN III) are linked to distinct mutations in the *ret* oncogene.

Answer A is incorrect. The *erb*-B2 oncogene is associated with breast, ovarian, and gastric carcinomas.

Answer B is incorrect. Mutations in the *MEN I* gene are found in patients with multiple endocrine neoplasia I, also known as Wermer's syndrome, which is characterized by hyperplasia or tumor of the "**3 P's**": **P**ituitary, **P**arathyroid, and **P**ancreas.

Answer C is incorrect. The *ras* oncogene mutation is associated with carcinoma of the colon.

Answer D is incorrect. The *Rb* gene is a tumor suppressor gene located on chromosome 13q. Mutation of the gene is associated with retinoblastoma and osteosarcoma.

CHAPTER 12

Musculoskeletal and Connective Tissue

1. A recent immigrant from Central America presents to the dermatologist with the cutaneous hypopigmented lesions shown in the image. The lesions are concentrated in the extremities and buttocks. The patient reports recent loss of eyebrows along with several episodes of epistaxis. Past medical history is significant for childhood asthma and atopic dermatitis. The dermatologist performs both a sensory neurologic examination and a biopsy of the cutaneous nodules. Which of the following cytokines, when administered locally, would most likely improve this patient's condition?

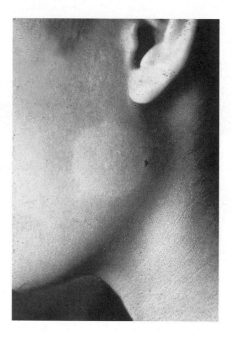

Reproduced, with permission, from Wolff K, Johnson RA, Suurmond D. *Fitzpatrick's Color Atlas & Synopsis of Clinical Dermatology*, 5th ed. New York: McGraw-Hill, 2005: Figure 73-10.

(A) Interferon-γ
(B) Interleukin-4
(C) Interleukin-5
(D) Interleukin-10
(E) Transforming growth factor-β

2. A 19-year-old woman is admitted to a Colorado hospital immediately after returning from an extended hiking trip in the mountains. She presents with malaise and a diffuse red rash over most of her body except the palms of her hands and the soles of her feet. Physical examination is remarkable for fever, tachycardia, elevated respiratory rate, and orthostatic hypotension. No obvious signs of infection are found. The patient reports that this is the fourth day of her menstrual cycle. When questioned, she reports that she has only changed her tampon once during this period due to the circumstances of being outdoors. She denies alcohol use, drug use, or recent exposure to febrile individuals. The patient is immediately started on intravenous antibiotics and gradually improves. Which of the following is the most likely causative agent in this patient's condition?

(A) *Clostridium perfringens* enterotoxin
(B) Disseminated *Staphylococcus aureus* infection
(C) *Rickettsia rickettsii*
(D) *Staphylococcus aureus* exotoxin
(E) *Treponema pallidum*

3. A 76-year-old man is scheduled to undergo repair of an abdominal hernia that is easily reduced by pushing the abdominal contents back through the external ring. During repair, the surgeon sees that the hernial sac protrudes from the abdominal wall superior to the inguinal ligament and medial to the inferior epigastric vessels. Which of the following types of hernia does this patient have?

(A) Diaphragmatic hernia
(B) Direct inguinal hernia
(C) Femoral hernia
(D) Hiatal hernia
(E) Indirect inguinal hernia

4. A 22-year-old college student presents to the school health service complaining of worsening weakness in his arms and legs. He says that over the past day he has also begun to feel weakness in his chest and back. He mentions that he thinks he had food poisoning earlier in

the week, which caused stomach pain and bloody diarrhea. Physical examination reveals that the deep tendon reflexes in his lower extremities are absent. His physician sends his stool to be cultured. The results show infection with *Campylobacter jejuni*. Which one of the following statements is most consistent with the disease process connecting the patient's gastrointestinal infection and his neurological symptoms?

(A) An excessive immune response to a gastrointestinal *Campylobacter jejuni* infection led to an autoimmune inflammation of peripheral nerves

(B) Dissemination of *Campylobacter* jejuni gastrointestinal infection led to infiltration of peripheral nerves with *C. jejuni*

(C) Dissemination of *Campylobacter jejuni* gastrointestinal infection led to infiltration of peripheral muscle cells with *C. jejuni*

(D) Toxins secreted by *Campylobacter jejuni* infiltrated into peripheral nerves, causing their destruction

(E) Toxins secreted by *Campylobacter jejuni* infiltrated into peripheral muscle cells

5. An 81-year-old man complains of back pain that is dull and constant, regardless of his activity level. Laboratory tests reveal an elevated serum alkaline phosphatase level. The patient dies, and a sample of his vertebra at autopsy is shown in the image. What was the most likely cause of this patient's pain?

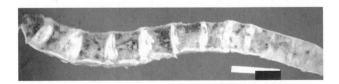

Reproduced, with permission, from PEIR Digital Library (http://peir.net).

(A) Chondrosarcoma
(B) Ewing's sarcoma
(C) Metastatic carcinoma
(D) Osteosarcoma
(E) Paget's disease of bone

6. An otherwise healthy infant boy born via vaginal delivery has an abnormal appearance of his right upper limb. His arm hangs by his side, pronated and medially rotated. Which of the following muscles is still functioning in this patient?

(A) Biceps
(B) Deltoid
(C) Infraspinatus
(D) Supraspinatus
(E) Triceps

7. A 19-year-old man comes to the physician after returning from a vacation in Tennessee with a fever of 39.5° C (103.1° F). He also has a severe headache and red conjunctivae. A couple of hours after the onset of these symptoms, a rash appears on his palms and soles. Which of the following statements regarding his illness is correct?

(A) Cold antibody agglutination is a classic finding for rickettsial infections
(B) He should promptly be treated with doxycycline
(C) The causative agent is a virus
(D) The causative bacterium is a facultative intracellular parasite
(E) The causative bacterium is spread by the tsetse fly

8. A 16-year-old gymnast presents to the emergency department after landing awkwardly on her ankle. She is diagnosed with a sprained ankle. Which of the following ligaments is most commonly injured in an ankle sprain?

(A) Anterior talofibular ligament
(B) Calcaneofibular ligament
(C) Talonavicular ligament
(D) Tibiocalcaneal ligament
(E) Tibiotalar ligament

9. A 13-month-old boy is admitted to the hospital with a broken tibia. This is the fourth broken bone the patient has sustained. On physical examination, the patient is found to have multiple poorly healing superficial wounds on his arms and legs; he also has a blue tint to his sclerae. The patient is subsequently diagnosed with the most common form of this disease. Which of the following would most likely be affected in this patient?

(A) Blood vessels, skin, uterus
(B) Bone, interstitial tissue, cartilage
(C) Bone, tendons, skin
(D) Cartilage, blood vessels, vitreous humor
(E) Skin, cellular basement membrane, blood vessels

10. A 17-year-old girl comes to the physician complaining of a painful, swollen left elbow and fever. She notes that in the previous few days her right knee was also swollen and slightly painful. Upon physical examination, the physician notices an edematous and tender left elbow. He also notices that the patient's cheeks are slightly red but do not appear tender to the touch. Laboratory tests are negative for anti-double-stranded DNA antibodies but positive for antibodies against Smith nuclear antigen and antinuclear antibodies. Also, results of Venereal Disease Research Laboratory testing are positive. The patient is shocked when informed of her positive result for syphilis, stating that she has no past sexual history. Which of the following is the most likely diagnosis?

(A) Polyarteritis nodosa
(B) Rheumatoid arthritis
(C) Secondary syphilis
(D) Systemic lupus erythematosus
(E) Tertiary syphilis

11. A 14-year-old boy presents to his family physician with complaints of muscle weakness affecting his ability to play on his soccer team. Physical examination reveals pseudohypertrophy of his calf muscles. The boy's family history is positive for similar symptoms in a maternal uncle, whose condition progressed to a wheelchair-bound state by the age of 30 years.

Which of the following is the etiology of this disorder?

(A) Autosomal dominant
(B) Autosomal recessive
(C) Mitochondrial inheritance
(D) Somatic mutation
(E) X-linked dominant
(F) X-linked recessive

12. A biopsy of one of several red, tender, subcutaneous nodules from the anterior lower legs of a 27-year-old man is obtained by a dermatologist. On histopathology, she sees a panniculitis (inflammation of subcutaneous fat) with widening of tissue septa from edema, increased neutrophils, and fibrin exudation. Which of the following diseases is often present in someone with these nodules?

(A) Acne vulgaris
(B) Crohn's disease
(C) Eczema
(D) Pancreatitis
(E) Psoriasis

13. A 23-year-old man comes to the clinic complaining of a severe headache that started 2 hours ago. He describes the headache as being "the worst in his life." His blood pressure is 138/95 mm Hg, and his heart rate is 56/min. On examination, the physician notes hyperextensible joints and increased skin elasticity, with hyperpigmentation over bony prominences. The examination is otherwise unremarkable. The patient states that he has not had any medical problems in the past. A CT scan of the head reveals blood in the sulci indicative of a subarachnoid hemorrhage. What is the most likely defect associated with this patient's disease?

(A) Antibodies to U1RNP
(B) Deficient hydroxylation of propyl and lysyl residues
(C) Keratin gene mutation
(D) Type III collagen gene mutation
(E) Type IV collagen gene mutation

14. A 64-year-old man with no prior medical history has had increasing back pain and right hip

pain for the past decade. The pain is worse at the end of the day. On physical examination, he has bony enlargement of the distal interphalangeal joints (see image). Which of the following diseases is most likely the cause of this patient's symptoms?

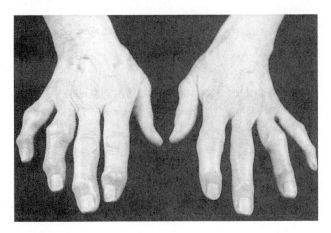

Reproduced, with permission, from Fauci AS, Braunwald E, Kasper DL, Hauser SL, Longo DL, Jameson JL, and Loscalzo J, eds. *Harrison's Principles of Internal Medicine*, 17th ed. New York: McGraw-Hill, 2008: Figure 326-2.

(A) Gout
(B) Osteoarthritis
(C) Osteomyelitis
(D) Pseudogout
(E) Rheumatoid arthritis

15. A 31-year-old man comes to the clinic complaining of red and itchy eyes for the past 8 hours. The patient has had pain on urination and diffuse joint pain for 1 month, but tested negative for gonorrhea and chlamydia on a previous visit 3 weeks ago. He has also tested negative for rheumatoid factor, and his human leukocyte antigen (HLA) status is HLA-B27. When asked about any recent illnesses, all the patient can recall is going to the emergency department 2 months ago for a bad case of diarrhea. Which of the following is the most likely diagnosis?

(A) Lyme arthritis
(B) Psoriatic arthritis
(C) Reiter's syndrome

(D) Rheumatoid arthritis
(E) Systemic lupus erythematosus

16. A 50-year-old slightly obese man comes to the emergency department with his wife at 3 am complaining of severe pain in his left great toe. He said the pain began 5 hours ago while he was walking home after dinner, which consisted of steak and a few beers. His serum studies are unremarkable except for negative blood cultures and an elevated uric acid level. When asked about allergies, the patient states that he is allergic to nonsteroidal anti-inflammatory drugs. An aspiration of the toe reveals negatively birefringent crystals. Which of the following is the best acute treatment for this condition?

(A) Allopurinol
(B) Ceftriaxone
(C) Colchicine
(D) Hydrochlorothiazide
(E) Ibuprofen
(F) Indomethacin
(G) Naproxen

17. A 20-year-old woman presents to the emergency department with several deep lacerations on the medial side of her wrist after a suicide attempt. She receives prompt psychiatric evaluation. The function of which of the following muscles might be affected by these injuries?

(A) Abductor pollicis brevis
(B) Adductor pollicis
(C) Flexor pollicis brevis
(D) Lumbricals (1 and 2)
(E) Opponens pollicis

18. A 50-year-old man presents to the emergency department because of severe pain with even slight abduction of his arm following a skiing accident. He is diagnosed with a rotator cuff tear. Which of the following is most commonly injured in a rotator cuff tear?

(A) Infraspinatus tendon
(B) Subacromial bursa
(C) Subscapularis tendon
(D) Supraspinatus tendon
(E) Teres minor tendon

19. A 58-year-old man comes to the doctor complaining of arthralgias in his hands and knees and mild fever. Physical examination reveals hepatomegaly, but there is no rash or neurologic findings. Laboratory studies show no hematologic abnormalities or renal disease. The patient is positive for antinuclear antibody and negative for anti-DNA antibodies. The patient mentions that he started a new medication a few months ago. Which of the following medications is most likely be responsible for this patient's symptoms?

(A) Bleomycin
(B) Enalapril
(C) Haloperidol
(D) Hydralazine
(E) Rifampin

20. A 34-year-old man injures his lateral pterygoid muscle. Which of the following activities will be adversely affected by this injury?

(A) Closing the jaw
(B) Smiling
(C) Swallowing
(D) Whistling
(E) Yawning

21. A 33-year-old woman develops an erythematous, finely punctate, blanchable rash. The rash first develops on her trunk and neck. Within a day, it progresses to her extremities but spares the face. The rash is worse in the creases of her axillae and groin. On physical examination, the physician notes an erythematous oropharynx and paleness around the mouth. Which of the following is the most likely diagnosis?

(A) Bacterial meningitis
(B) Rubella
(C) Scarlet fever
(D) Streptococcal pharyngitis
(E) Toxic shock syndrome

22. A 12-year-old African-American girl is brought to the physician with complaints of fever, malaise, and pain in her left forearm for the past 4 days. Her mother reports no history of trauma or fracture, but recounts an upper respiratory infection a few days ago. The patient has been hospitalized three times for abdominal pain, for which she takes hydroxyurea. Her temperature is 39.8° C (103.6° F) and the rest of her vital signs are stable. On examination the left forearm is erythematous, warm, and tender to palpation. Blood samples for culture are drawn. Which of the following is most likely to be isolated from this patient's blood?

(A) *Escherichia coli*
(B) *Pseudomonas aeruginosa*
(C) *Salmonella* species
(D) *Staphylococcus aureus*
(E) *Streptococcus pyogenes*

23. The skeletal system develops via a process known as ossification, in which bones are created from preexisting mesoderm. By which of the following processes do the long bones ossify?

(A) Chondrocytes deposit minerals directly from the mesoderm
(B) Osteoblasts deposit minerals directly from the mesoderm
(C) Osteoblasts deposit minerals over a hyaline cartilage mold
(D) Osteoclasts deposit minerals over a hyaline cartilage mold

24. A couple brings their 3-year-old son to the emergency department, reporting that he fell down the stairs and broke his arm. The boy has a tearful face and gingerly holds his right arm by the elbow, but refuses to look the physician in the eye or to answer any questions. X-ray of the boy's arm is performed. Which of the following types of fracture is most likely to suggest an etiology of child abuse?

(A) Bowing fracture
(B) Buckle fracture
(C) Greenstick fracture
(D) Spiral fracture

25. A 42-year-old woman comes to the clinic complaining of blurry vision. She states that for the past 3 weeks her eyes have been very dry and itchy, and she is unable to make tears. She also states that she has had a very dry mouth despite

drinking adequate fluids. Physical examination reveals bilateral dry, ulcerated corneas and fissures on the sides of her lips. In addition, both of her knees are erythematous and swollen. When asked about her knees, she says, "Yes, my knees and wrists tend to be swollen and stiff in the morning, but my mom had arthritis." Testing for several autoantibodies reveals she is rheumatoid factor-positive and antibody-SS-B (La)-positive. Which of the following is the most likely diagnosis?

(A) CREST syndrome
(B) Cystic fibrosis
(C) Sicca syndrome
(D) Sjögren-Larsson syndrome
(E) Sjögren's syndrome

26. A 14-year-old football player is side tackled during a high school football game. When he tries to stand up, his right leg buckles. He is taken to the emergency department, where physical examination reveals that the patient's tibia is easily moved anterior in relation to the femur. An MRI of the patient's knee is shown in the image. Which injured structure is responsible for the findings in the patient's physical examination?

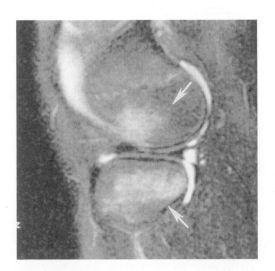

Reproduced, with permission, from Chen MYM, Pope TL, Ott DJ. *Basic Radiology.* New York: McGraw-Hill, 2004: Figure 7-21.

(A) Anterior cruciate ligament
(B) Lateral collateral ligament
(C) Medial collateral ligament
(D) Posterior cruciate ligament
(E) Ulnar collateral ligament

27. A 25-year-old man comes to the emergency department because of rapidly spreading cellulitis on his right hand. He tells the physician that he was bitten by a cat the previous day. Which of the following organisms is most likely responsible for this patient's infection?

(A) *Francisella tularensis*
(B) *Pasteurella multocida*
(C) Rabies virus
(D) *Sporothrix schenckii*
(E) *Staphylococcus aureus*

28. A 1-year-old adopted, darkly pigmented boy is brought to the pediatrician for his first well-child check-up. The adoptive parents do not know any of the infant's past medical history or family history. Physical examination reveals an unusual widening of the child's wrists and ankles and marked enlargement of the child's costochondral junctions. What is a characteristic laboratory finding used to support the most likely diagnosis?

(A) Increased intact parathyroid hormone level
(B) Increased serum calcium level
(C) Increased serum 1,25-dihydroxycholecalciferol level
(D) Increased serum 25-hydroxycholecalciferol level
(E) Increased serum phosphorus level

29. A 21-year-old man presents to the emergency department following an injury to his shoulder that he sustained while playing football. His shoulder appears flattened, and he is not able to abduct his arm. He is found to have a fracture at the surgical neck of his humerus. The muscle that is most likely injured in this patient receives innervation from which of the following nerve roots?

(A) C3-5
(B) C5-6
(C) C6-7
(D) C7-8
(E) C8-T1

30. A 42-year-old woman has had increasing pain and swelling of the joints of her hands and feet for several months. It is becoming very difficult for her to perform common household tasks. A microscopic image of the synovium of a proximal interphalangeal joint in her hand is shown. Which of the following laboratory serologic findings would most likely be positive in this patient?

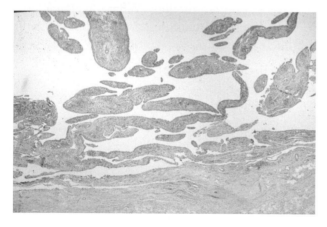

Reproduced, with permission, from PEIR Digital Library (http://peir.net).

(A) Anti-centromere antibody
(B) Anti-nuclear antibody
(C) Borrelia burgdorferi antibody
(D) HLA-B27
(E) IgM anti-IgG

31. A 60-year-old man presents to the physician with a limp that he has had since childhood. When he walks, the patient takes a step with his right leg, then leans all the way over to his right so that he can swing his left leg to take a step. He reports one major illness as a child, after which he developed this limp. Which of the following nerve(s) is most likely injured in this patient?

(A) Inferior gluteal nerve
(B) L5 and S1
(C) Obturator nerve
(D) S1 and S2
(E) Superior gluteal nerve

32. A 45-year-old computer programmer notices atrophy and weakness of his thumb. Laboratory tests reveal an increased erythrocyte sedimentation rate and leukocyte count. Sensation to which of the following cutaneous areas is most likely to be decreased?

(A) Dorsal aspect of fifth digit
(B) Dorsal aspect of fourth digit
(C) Palmar aspect of second digit
(D) Volar aspect of lateral wrist
(E) Volar aspect of medial wrist

33. A 61-year-old man presents to the physician with frequent headaches and increasing deafness. The patient notes that his winter hat fits more snugly than usual. Laboratory values show a marked increase in alkaline phosphatase activity. A diagnosis of Paget's disease is made. Dysfunction of the cell type shown in the image is associated with Paget's disease. Which of the following is the embryologic origin of this dysfunctional cell?

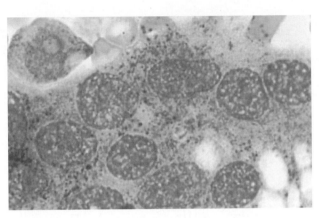

Reproduced, with permission, from Lichtman MA, Beutler E, Kipps TJ, Seligsohn U, Kaushansky K, Prchal JF. *Williams Hematology*, 7th ed. New York: McGraw-Hill, 2006: Color Plate VI-2.

(A) Endoderm
(B) Mesoderm
(C) Neural crest cells
(D) Neuroectoderm
(E) Surface ectoderm

34. A 22-year-old woman who is a professional tennis player presents to the physician with pain on the lateral aspect of her elbow radiating down her forearm. Repetitive use of which of the following muscles most likely lead to this patient's condition?

(A) Biceps
(B) Extensor carpi radialis
(C) Extensor carpi ulnaris
(D) Flexor carpi ulnaris
(E) Pronator teres

35. A 50-year-old man who recently returned from a trip to Southeast Asia comes to the physician with exquisitely tender and enlarged lymph nodes. He also complains of fever, chills, and general weakness. On physical examination, the physician notes a painful ulcer surrounded by dark, hemorrhagic purpura on the right arm in the area where, according to the patient, a flea had bitten him 5 days ago. Which of the following organisms is most likely responsible for this patient's symptoms?

(A) *Babesia microti*
(B) *Bacillus anthracis*
(C) *Leishmania donovani*
(D) *Trichinella spiralis*
(E) *Yersinia pestis*

36. An 8-year-old boy is brought to his pediatrician by his parents with complaints of swelling and pain over his right femur for the past 2–3 weeks. The child and parents deny any history of trauma to the region. The patient reports that the pain is often worse at night, and his mother states that he has been having low-grade fevers of 37.8°–38.1° C (100.0°–100.6° F). On physical examination there is no erythema of the region, but a firm immobile tender mass is palpable. Fine needle aspiration cytology reveals anaplastic small blue cells. Genetic evaluation of this patient is most likely to reveal which of the following?

(A) t(9,22) chromosomal translocation
(B) t(11,22) chromosomal translocation
(C) Trisomy 18
(D) Trisomy 21
(E) XXY

37. A 38-year-old man comes to the clinic with a swollen, sausage-like left middle finger along with diffuse joint swelling of his left hand and right foot over the past 3 days. The patient also has scaly plaques with well-defined borders along the skin just distal to both elbows. His uric acid level is within normal limits. Which of the following is most likely to be seen in this patient?

(A) Antigliadin antibodies
(B) Elevated erythrocyte sedimentation rate
(C) Negatively bifringent crystals in joint fluid
(D) Positive rheumatoid factor
(E) Weakly positively bifringent crystals in joint fluid

38. A 20-year-old man presents to the physician with a nontender indurated mass over his mandible. He has had this mass for 4 months and decided to come to the physician because the mass started to ooze a thick yellow exudate. Yellow granules are seen on microscopic examination of the discharge. Which of the following organisms is most likely responsible for this man's lesion?

    (A) *Actinomyces israelii*
    (B) *Nocardia asteroides*
    (C) *Prevotella melaninogenica*
    (D) *Staphylococcus aureus*
    (E) *Trichinella spiralis*

39. A 29-year-old man develops a flu-like illness 10 days after a trip to upstate New York. On physical examination, he has lymphadenopathy and a circular, nonpruritic, erythematous, macular rash on his left arm. One red spot is particularly big and has a clear area in the center. Which of the following statements is correct?

    (A) A diagnosis of late stage Lyme disease is best made based on clinical presentation
    (B) Erythema multiforme is the characteristic rash of Lyme disease
    (C) Lyme disease is best treated with a fluoroquinolone
    (D) The late stage, stage 3, of Lyme disease is characterized by acute, aseptic meningitis
    (E) The reservoir of *Borrelia burgdorferi* is the white-footed mouse

40. The diagram shows a cross-section of normal human skin. Patients with pemphigus vulgaris suffer from production of autoantibodies against which of the following labeled layers in this image?

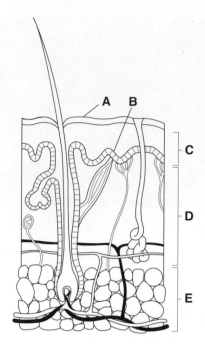

Reproduced, with permission, from USMLERx.com.

    (A) A
    (B) B
    (C) C
    (D) D
    (E) E

41. A 25-year-old man develops acute onset of fever, malaise, muscle pain, hypertension, abdominal pain, bloody stool, and prerenal failure 6 months after recovering from an acute hepatitis B infection. Which of the following disease processes is most likely responsible for the patient's findings?

    (A) Buerger's disease
    (B) Giant cell (temporal) arteritis
    (C) Kawasaki's syndrome
    (D) Polyarteritis nodosa
    (E) Takayasu's arteritis

42. A 36-year-old woman presents to the clinic with a new complaint of fatigue of several months' duration. She also reports stiffness in both hands that is worse in the morning and decreases after soaking them in her warm morning bath each day. Physical examination reveals a low-grade fever. Subcutaneous nodules are palpated along her forearm bilaterally. What type of hypersensitivity reaction is causing this patient's arthritis?

(A) Arthus reaction
(B) Delayed cell-mediated hypersensitivity reaction
(C) Immune complex hypersensitivity reaction
(D) Type I hypersensitivity reaction
(E) Type II hypersensitivity reaction

43. A 27-year-old man comes to the physician's office with a 6-month history of low back pain and stiffness that wakes him up during the night and is worst in the morning. The patient was diagnosed with bilateral sacroiliitis 4 months ago because of his tenderness to percussion of the sacroiliac joints and pain on springing the pelvis up. He has severe limitation of motion of his lumbar spine. Laboratory test results arc negative for antinuclear antibody and rheumatoid factor, and show the patient's human leukocyte antigen status is B27-positive. Which of the following is the most likely diagnosis?

(A) Ankylosing spondylitis
(B) Osteoarthritis
(C) Psoriatic arthritis
(D) Reiter's syndrome
(E) Rheumatoid arthritis
(F) Vertebral compression fracture

44. A 15-year-old boy is brought to the emergency department because he has pain in his hand following a fist fight. The physician tells the patient that he has broken his hand. Which of the following is the most likely site of this patient's fracture?

(A) Distal radius
(B) Hamate
(C) Metacarpals
(D) Phalanges
(E) Scaphoid

45. A 5-year-old boy comes to the emergency department with fever, malaise, nausea, decreased urine output (despite normal fluid intake), and smoky brown urine that began 10 days after he had recovered from a sore throat. Which of the following are the most likely pathologic findings on biopsy of the kidney?

(A) Enlarged hypercellular glomeruli on light microscopy; dense humps found on the epithelial side of the glomerular basement membrane on electron microscopy
(B) Linear deposition of antibodies against glomerular basement membrane found on immunofluorescence
(C) Mesangial proliferation on light microscopy; mesangial deposition of IgA on immunofluorescence
(D) Normal-appearing glomeruli on light microscopy; effacement of the foot processes of the visceral epithclial cells on electron microscopy
(E) Widespread and pronounced thickening and splitting of the glomerular basement membrane on electron microscopy

HIGH-YIELD SYSTEMS

Musculoskeletal

1. **The correct answer is A.** This clinical example demonstrates the importance of CD4+ T-helper (Th) cell differentiation into a Th_1 or Th_2 phenotype. Th_1 cells drive a cell-mediated immune response that includes activation of macrophages and cytotoxic T lymphocytes. Th_2 cells orchestrate an antibody-mediated response. As an intracellular pathogen that infects macrophages, *Mycobacterium leprae* is most effectively controlled by Th_1 cells. The patient described presents with severe lepromatous disease, which results when the CD4+ Th cells differentiate into Th_2 instead of Th_1 effectors. Indeed, a biopsy would most likely show widespread acid-fast bacilli inside of macrophages. Individuals that mount a Th_1 response to the mycobacteria can better control the disease (their clinical condition is named tuberculous leprosy), and their macrophages can contain the bacilli within granulomas. Interferon-γ is secreted by Th_1 cells, and one important role of this cytokine is to activate macrophages. Therefore, local administration of this cytokine will alleviate the cutaneous lesions.

Answer B is incorrect. Interleukin-4 is a Th_2 cytokine important in antibody class switching.

Answer C is incorrect. Interleukin-5 is a Th_2 cytokine important in antibody class switching.

Answer D is incorrect. Interleukin-10 is a Th_2 cytokine important in antibody class switching.

Answer E is incorrect. Transforming growth factor-β has immunosuppressive effects.

2. **The correct answer is D.** The question stem describes a classic clinical vignette associated staphylococcal toxic shock syndrome (a menstruating female who did not change a tampon for an extended period of time). The *Staphylococcus aureus* exotoxin "toxic shock syndrome toxin 1" (TSST-1) is an example of a superantigen. Bacterial/viral superantigens are proteins that nonspecifically cross-link MHC class II molecules with certain T-cell receptor (TCR) subsets, leading to the inappropriate activation of these T-cells. Depending on the superanti-

gen, anywhere from 2%–20% of all T lymphocytes can be activated. The massive T-lymphocyte activation leads to supraphysiologic production of cytokines, including interleukin (IL)-1, tumor necrosis factor-α, IL-6, IL-12, and interferon-γ. It is these cytokines that are most responsible for the clinical symptoms of toxic shock syndrome. Thus, the most likely cause of the patient's symptoms is a toxin released from S. *aureus* TSST-1 and not the bacterium itself.

Answer A is incorrect. *Clostridium perfringens* is the causative agent of gas gangrene. While *Clostridium perfringens* enterotoxin is also a superantigen, physical examination revealed no signs of cutaneous infections, and thus this pathogen is less likely to be the causative agent.

Answer B is incorrect. The clinical vignette is most likely indicative of toxic shock syndrome, a result of a circulating staphylococcal toxin and not the bacterium itself. In fact, blood cultures are most often negative. In this patient's case, vaginal cultures may be positive for S. *aureus* and may have been taken.

Answer C is in correct. *Rickettsia rickettsii* is the causative agent of Rocky Mountain spotted fever. While rash is often a presenting symptom, it classically includes the palms and soles. The setting of this clinical scenario in Colorado is purely a distracter. The name *Rocky Mountain Spotted Fever* is actually a misnomer, as it is much more common in the Southeastern United States.

Answer E is incorrect. In secondary syphilis, rash is often a presenting symptom, but it often includes the palms and soles. Nothing else in the patient's presentation or history is consistent with syphilis.

3. **The correct answer is B.** Direct inguinal hernias protrude directly through the abdominal wall in Hesselbach's triangle, which is bordered by the inguinal ligament, rectus abdominis muscle, and inferior epigastric vessels. Remem-

ber that the issue of direct versus indirect has nothing to do with whether or not the hernia enters the scrotum through the external ring, as both direct and indirect hernias can do this. Direct versus indirect distinguishes where the hernia enters the inguinal canal, either through the internal ring (indirect) or straight through the abdominal wall (for direct hernias, think **directly** through the wall). In this case, the abdominal contents pierced through the abdominal wall and through the external inguinal ring. Direct hernias are often discovered in older patients, as the hernia is a result of pressure and tension exerted over time that eventually leads the abdominal wall to give way. Direct hernias are less common and have less risk of strangulation than indirect hernias.

Answer A is incorrect. Diaphragmatic hernias are serious birth defects that are lethal unless repaired soon after birth. A defective development of the diaphragm leads to herniation of abdominal contents into the thorax, displacing the lung. Even after repair of such lesions, children may have poor pulmonary function due to poor lung development in utero.

Answer C is incorrect. Femoral hernias protrude inferior to the inguinal ligament and do not go through the external inguinal ring.

Answer D is incorrect. Hiatal hernias are hernias of the stomach protruding superiorly through the diaphragm.

Answer E is incorrect. Indirect inguinal hernias occur when abdominal contents enter the internal inguinal ring through a patent processus vaginalis, exit the inguinal canal through the external ring, and often enter the scrotum of male patients. The examiner's finger would go through the external ring and would pass posterior to the epigastric vessels and through the internal ring. These hernias are the most common type found in both men and women, and the recommendation is that they be repaired when they are discovered to avoid the complication of strangulation and bowel infarction.

4. **The correct answer is A.** This patient has Guillain-Barré as a result of his gastroenteritis.

The important message here is that Guillain-Barré syndrome is thought to be primarily an autoimmune disorder against peripheral nerves and the cells that myelinate them (Schwann cells). Thus, it makes sense that an excessive immune response to an infection (such as from a pathogen like *Campylobacter jejuni*) can lead to an autoimmune process. Histologically, this disease is characterized by perivenular and endoneurial infiltration with lymphocytes, macrophages, and plasma cells.

Answer B is incorrect. The mechanism suggested in this answer choice is not thought to be the primary disease process in Guillain-Barré syndrome.

Answer C is incorrect. Guillain-Barré syndrome is a disease that primarily attacks peripheral nerves and Schwann cells. The ascending paralysis and muscle weakness that occur as a consequence are secondary to the neuropathy.

Answer D is incorrect. While *Campylobacter jejuni* does produce an enterotoxin, the mechanism described in this answer choice is not the major hypothesized pathogenesis of Guillain-Barré syndrome.

Answer E is incorrect. Guillain-Barré syndrome is a disease that primarily attacks peripheral nerves and Schwann cells. The ascending paralysis and muscle weakness that occur as a consequence are secondary to the neuropathy.

5. **The correct answer is C.** This image shows several nodular, tan lesions, indicative of metastases. Metastatic neoplasia should be strongly considered in older adults with elevated alkaline phosphatase levels, particularly older men with back pain, often a sign of bone lesions due to prostate cancer. Metastases to bone are far more common than primary bone tumors. The most common cancers that metastasize to bone are breast, lung, thyroid, testes, kidney, and prostate.

Answer A is incorrect. Chondrosarcoma is a malignant cartilaginous tumor. It is most common in men 30–60 years old. Chondrosarcoma is rarely seen in the spine.

Answer B is incorrect. Ewing's sarcoma is an anaplastic blue cell malignant tumor most common in boys under 15 years of age. It is typically aggressive but highly responsive to chemotherapy.

Answer D is incorrect. Osteosarcoma is the most common malignant tumor of bone, with a peak incidence in teenage males (10–20 years old). It is most commonly found in the metaphysis of long bones, most commonly in the lower extremities. It commonly presents with systemic symptoms and a palpable soft tissue mass.

Answer E is incorrect. Paget's disease of bone is characterized by accelerated bone turnover leading to increased bone formation and resorption, resulting in its characteristic "mosaic" pattern. It presents most commonly with pain, skeletal deformities, and fractures. It is associated with secondary osteosarcoma and fibrosarcoma. It does not cause nodular lesions like those shown here.

6. **The correct answer is E.** This infant has Erb-Duchenne palsy, a condition seen following trauma during delivery, due to traction/tear of the C5-C6 roots in the brachial plexus (superior trunk). This condition results in paralysis of abductors, lateral rotators, and biceps. Of the muscles listed above, only the triceps is not involved in these actions; it functions to extend the elbow and adduct the arm. It is innervated by the radial nerve, which is supplied by C6-C8.

Answer A is incorrect. The biceps muscle functions to supinate and flex the arm. It is innervated by the musculocutaneous nerve, which comes from the superior trunk of the brachial plexus.

Answer B is incorrect. The deltoid is supplied by the axillary nerve, which comes from the superior trunk of the brachial plexus. It functions to abduct the arm.

Answer C is incorrect. The infraspinatus muscle helps laterally rotate the arm and is supplied by the suprascapular nerve from the superior trunk of the brachial plexus.

Answer D is incorrect. The supraspinatus muscle helps abduct the arm and is supplied by the suprascapular nerve from the superior trunk of the brachial plexus.

7. **The correct answer is B.** The patient presents with signs and symptoms of Rocky Mountain spotted fever and should promptly be treated (even before confirmatory lab results are available) with a tetracycline (such as doxycycline) or chloramphenicol, as delay in antibiotic therapy can lead to death.

Answer A is incorrect. Cold antibody agglutination is used to detect *Mycoplasma* infection. The Weil-Felix reaction can detect a rickettsial infection due to cross-reacting antigens from *Proteus vulgaris*.

Answer C is incorrect. Although many viral infections can cause rash in a young patient (i.e., measles), a rash that begins on the palms and soles suggests Rocky Mountain spotted fever.

Answer D is incorrect. *Rickettsia rickettsii* is an obligate intracellular parasite that replicates freely in the cytoplasm and is depended on host nicotinamide adenine dinucleotide and coacetyl A.

Answer E is incorrect. *Rickettsia rickettsii*, the causative bacterium of Rocky Mountain spotted fever, has two arthropod vectors, the ticks *Dermacentor andersoni* and *D. variabilis*. The tsetse fly spreads African sleeping sickness.

8. **The correct answer is A.** The lateral ligaments are more commonly injured than the medial ligaments, since they are weaker. The anterior talofibular ligament is the most common of the lateral ligaments to be injured.

Answer B is incorrect. The calcaneofibular ligament is a lateral ligament that is injured frequently, but less frequently than the anterior talofibular ligament.

Answer C is incorrect. The lateral ligaments are more commonly injured than the medial ligaments, since they are weaker. The talonavicular ligament is a medial ligament so it is much less likely to be injured.

Answer D is incorrect. The lateral ligaments are more commonly injured than the medial ligaments, since they are weaker. The tibiocalcaneal ligament is a medial ligament so it is much less likely to be injured.

Answer E is incorrect. The lateral ligaments are more commonly injured than the medial ligaments, since they are weaker. The tibiotalar ligament is a medial ligament so it is much less likely to be injured.

9. **The correct answer is C.** The most likely diagnosis is osteogenesis imperfecta (OI). OI is characterized by multiple spontaneous bone fractures, retarded wound healing, and characteristically blue sclerae. This disease is caused by a variety of gene defects leading to abnormal collagen synthesis. The most common form of OI is an autosomal dominant defect in type I collagen synthesis. Type I collagen has high tensile strength and is found in skin, bone, tendons, eyes, ears, and teeth. Other symptoms of type I OI include hearing impairment and joint laxity. Thinning of the sclerae from reduced type I collagen causes the characteristic blue tint noted in the whites of these patient's eyes.

Answer A is incorrect. Type III cartilage is characterized by thin, pliable fibrils found in blood vessels, skin, and the uterus. This collagen is not abnormal in type I OI.

Answer B is incorrect. Interstitial tissue is composed of types V and VI collagen. Cartilage contains type II and IX collagen. Of these tissues only bone contains type I cartilage, the type of cartilage affected by type I OI.

Answer D is incorrect. Type II collagen is primarily found in cartilage and vitreous humor. Blood vessels contain collagen types III and V, thus none of these tissues are affected in type I OI.

Answer E is incorrect. Skin contains type I collagen and type VII collagen at the dermal-epidermal junction. Cellular basement membrane is composed of type IV collagen. Blood vessels contain types III and V cartilage. Of

these three structures, only skin contains the collagen affected most commonly in OI.

10. **The correct answer is D.** This patient has systemic lupus erythematosus (SLE), which is diagnosed by the presence of 4 of the following 11 findings designated by the American Rheumatism Association, and summarized by the mnemonic "**BRAIN SOAP, MD**": **B**lood dyscrasias (such as hemolytic anemia or thrombocytopenia), **R**enal disorder, **A**rthritis (in two or more peripheral joints), **I**mmunologic disorder (such as anti-DNA antibody and anti-Smith antibody), **N**eurologic disorder, **S**erositis (such as pleuritis or pericarditis), **O**ral ulcers, **A**ntinuclear antibody (elevated titers in the absence of drugs associated with drug-induced lupus syndrome), **P**hotosensitivity, **M**alar rash, and **D**iscoid rash. Many patients with SLE have antiphospholipid antibodies, which are actually believed to be antibodies against proteins that complex to phospholipids. Since these antibodies also bind to the cardiolipin antigen used in syphilis serology, patients with SLE may test false-positive for syphilis.

Answer A is incorrect. Polyarteritis nodosa, a necrotizing immune complex vasculitis that usually affects small or medium-sized muscular arteries, commonly presents with fever, malaise, myalgias, and hypertension. Findings may include pericarditis, myocarditis, palpable purpura, and cotton-wool spots (white opacities in the retina).

Answer B is incorrect. The American Rheumatism Association diagnostic criteria for rheumatoid arthritis requires four out of the following seven findings: (1) Morning stiffness for more than 6 weeks; (2) Arthritis of hand joints for more than 6 weeks; (3) Arthritis involving three or more joint areas for more than 6 weeks; (4) Symmetric arthritis for more than 6 weeks; (5) Rheumatoid nodules (small lumps of tissue most commonly found over bony prominences, that are histologically characterized by a center of fibrinoid necrosis surrounded by histiocytes, numerous lymphocytes, and plasma cells); (6) Positive serum rheumatoid factor; and (7) Radiologic changes (such as bony erosion in or near the area of symptomatic joints).

Answer C is incorrect. Secondary syphilis often develops 6 weeks after an untreated primary chancre of syphilis has healed and is characterized by fever, lymphadenopathy, skin rashes (widespread small, flat lesions that particularly involve the palms, soles, and oral mucosa), and condylomata lata (painless wartlike lesions that present in the vulva, the scrotum, or other warm, moist areas of the body).

Answer E is incorrect. Tertiary syphilis may develop 6–40 years after primary syphilis and may present with gummas (noninfectious granulomatous lesions, often found in skin and bone), tabes dorsalis (inflammatory damage to the posterior columns and dorsal roots of the spinal cord), aneurysm of the ascending aorta or aortic arch, and Argyll Robertson pupils (pupils that constrict during accommodation but do not react to light).

11. **The correct answer is F.** X-linked recessive inheritance shows affected male individuals inheriting a defective copy of the X chromosome from heterozygous (asymptomatic) mothers. There is no male-to-male transmission. Heterozygous females may be affected, but usually not as severely as males. Becker's muscular dystrophy is a milder, slower-developing form of dystrophinopathy with manifestations similar to those of Duchenne's muscular dystrophy.

Answer A is incorrect. Autosomal dominant inheritance shows disease in many generations, with both males and females affected. It is possible for a male or a female to transmit the defective gene to their offspring. Becker's muscular dystrophy is not inherited in this manner.

Answer B is incorrect. In autosomal recessive inheritance, a defective gene from each carrier parent is transmitted to the offspring. Disease is often seen in only one generation. Males and females are equally likely to be affected. Becker's muscular dystrophy is not inherited in this manner.

Answer C is incorrect. In mitochondrial inheritance, all children (male and female) of an affected mother exhibit the disease. The disease is not transmitted from fathers to any of their children (only maternal transmission). Becker's muscular dystrophy is not inherited in this manner.

Answer D is incorrect. Somatic mutations occur in the somatic (non-germ) tissues; they are unable to be transmitted to offspring and often occur in isolated individuals within a family. Males and females are equally susceptible to somatic mutations. Becker's muscular dystrophy is not inherited in this manner.

Answer E is incorrect. X-linked dominant inheritance shows disease in any offspring who inherit the affected X chromosome. It is transmitted from fathers to all their daughters but none of their sons, and from mothers to sons or daughters. Becker's muscular dystrophy is not inherited in this manner.

12. **The correct answer is B.** This patient has erythema nodosum, an inflammation of subcutaneous fat that is often accompanied by fever and malaise that is described clinically and pathologically in the question stem. The exact mechanism is unknown, but it often occurs together with inflammatory bowel disease (Crohn's disease or ulcerative colitis), sarcoidosis, certain drugs (such as oral contraceptives and sulfonamides), certain malignant neoplasms, and certain infections (such as tuberculosis, β-hemolytic streptococci, coccidioidomycosis, histoplasmosis, and leprosy).

Answer A is incorrect. Acne vulgaris is a disorder of the epidermis that has both inflammatory and noninflammatory variants. It is associated with the bacterium *Propionibacterium acnes*.

Answer C is incorrect. Eczema is an inflammatory skin disorder that is associated with contact allergies, asthma, ultraviolet light exposure, repeated physical skin rubbing, and certain drugs. It is not associated with erythema nodosum.

Answer D is incorrect. Pancreatitis, which is associated with many cases of biliary tract disease and alcoholism, is not associated with erythema nodosum.

Answer E is incorrect. Psoriasis is a nonpruritic inflammatory skin disorder associated with arthritis, enteropathy, spondylitic disease, and certain HLA types, including HLA-B27, HLA-13, and HLA-17.

13. **The correct answer is D.** Ehlers-Danlos syndrome (EDS) is a heterogeneous group of inherited connective tissue disorders characterized by joint hypermobility, cutaneous fragility, and hyperextensibility. There are 11 different types of EDS identified. This presentation is most consistent with type IV EDS, which also is characterized by vascular problems including arterial or uterine rupture. Although confusing, Type IV EDS is characterized by a decreased amount of type III collagen, which is a structural protein in blood vessels. It is a rare, but severe form and patients often have a shortened lifespan because of the spontaneous rupture of a large artery.

Answer A is incorrect. Antibodies to U1RNP are common in mixed connective tissue disease, which is also characterized by Raynaud's phenomenon, arthralgias, myalgias, fatigue, and esophageal hypomotility.

Answer B is incorrect. Vitamin C deficiency results in an inability to hydroxylate the propyl and lysyl residues between tropocollagen molecules necessary for the production of collagen. This deficiency may lead to scurvy, a disease that is characterized by hypertrophic, bleeding gums and poor wound healing but not intracranial arterial rupture.

Answer C is incorrect. Mutations in keratin genes lead to a group of blistering disorders including epidermolysis bullosa, in which skin and related epithelial tissues break and blister as the result of minor trauma. These disorders are not associated with berry aneurysms nor subarachnoid hemorrhage.

Answer E is incorrect. Mutations in type IV collagen are found in patients with Alport's syndrome. Alport's syndrome is an X-linked disorder characterized by nephritis, sensorineural deafness, and ocular disorders. It is not associated with berry aneurysms nor subarachnoid hemorrhage.

14. **The correct answer is B.** Osteoarthritis is a disease of wear and tear leading to destruction of articular cartilage, subchondral bone formation, osteophytes, sclerosis, and other degenerative changes. It is common and progressive, and becomes more so with age. It classically presents in weight-bearing joints as pain after use, improving with rest. It commonly affects the distal interphalangeal joints as well. Common imaging findings include narrowing of the joint space, sclerosis, and the presence of osteophytes.

Answer A is incorrect. Gout is a painful swelling of a joint, most commonly the metatarsophalangeal joint, caused by precipitation of monosodium urate crystals. It is diagnosed by viewing the crystals in the joint's synovial fluid, which are negatively birefringent. It is not associated with osteophytes or sclerosis with narrowing.

Answer C is incorrect. Osteomyelitis is an infection in the bone. It presents most commonly with tenderness, warmth, swelling, and more acute pain, rather than joint narrowing. The pain typically is present with and without movement.

Answer D is incorrect. Pseudogout causes symptoms that mimic those of gout, but is caused by the precipitation of calcium pyrophosphate crystals within the joint space. These crystals are positively birefringent. This disease classically affects large joints, most commonly the knee, in men over 50 years old. It is not associated with osteophytes or sclerosis with narrowing.

Answer E is incorrect. Rheumatoid arthritis is an autoimmune arthritis caused by inflammatory destruction of synovial joints. It is associated with pain that is worst in the morning, improving with use, and classically affects the proximal interphalangeal joints. It is not associated with osteophytes or sclerosis with narrowing.

15. **The correct answer is C.** Reiter's syndrome is diagnosed by conjunctivitis in a patient who has had both urethritis (or cervicitis) and arthritis for at least 1 month. Most patients are in their 20s or 30s, and 80% are positive for HLA-B27. It is thought to be caused by an autoimmune reaction within several weeks of a gastrointestinal or genitourinary infection.

Answer A is incorrect. Lyme arthritis, usually caused by a bite from a tick harboring the spirochete *Borrelia burgdorferi*, presents as an initial local skin infection followed by monarticular/polyarticular arthritis. Its late sequelae include myocardial, pericardial, and neurologic changes.

Answer B is incorrect. Patients with psoriatic arthritis can have joint pain, conjunctivitis, and human leukocyte antigen-B27, but the diagnosis requires the presence of psoriasis, which is characterized by nonpruritic scaly/silvery erythematous plaques with well-defined borders.

Answer D is incorrect. While rheumatoid factor is not necessary to diagnose rheumatoid arthritis, the patient's human leukocyte antigen status, urethritis, and conjunctivitis make it a less likely diagnosis.

Answer E is incorrect. Systemic lupus erythematosus is diagnosed by the presence of 4 of the 11 symptoms summarized by the mnemonic "**BRAIN SOAP, MD**": **B**lood dyscrasias (such as hemolytic anemia or thrombocytopenia), **R**enal disorder, **A**rthritis, **I**mmunologic disorder (such as anti-DNA antibody and anti-Smith antibody), **N**eurologic disorder, **S**erositis (such as pleuritis or pericarditis), **O**ral ulcers, **A**ntinuclear antibody (elevated titers in the absence of drugs associated with drug-induced lupus syndrome), **P**hotosensitivity, **M**alar rash, and **D**iscoid rash.

16. **The correct answer is C.** Gout is characterized by a raised blood uric acid level that leads to uric acid deposition in tissues, particularly the joints. In some patients, gout is precipitated by eating foods rich in purine, such as meats (especially organ meats, like kidneys). The first-line therapy in the treatment of gout consists of non-steroidal anti-inflammatory drugs (NSAIDs) such as ibuprofen, naproxen, and indomethacin. However, since the patient is allergic to NSAIDs, colchicine is the next best therapy for an acute gouty attack. It is considered an alternate drug because adverse effects include diarrhea, gastrointestinal upset, and (in patients with renal or hepatic insufficiency) bone marrow suppression, myopathy, and neuropathy. Colchicine works by inhibiting microtubule polymerization by binding to tubulin, one of the main constituents of microtubules. This inhibits immune cell motility and activity, thus promoting an anti-inflammatory result.

Answer A is incorrect. Allopurinol is used in the chronic treatment of gout but has no beneficial effect in an acute gouty attack; in fact, it may initially precipitate an attack or make an existing attack worse.

Answer B is incorrect. Ceftriaxone would be given for gonococcal arthritis, which most frequently involves the knee. Early stages yield positive blood cultures for gonococci and later stages may yield positive joint cultures and/or purulent synovial fluid.

Answer D is incorrect. Hydrochlorothiazide is a diuretic and is not indicated for gout. In fact, people who take hydrochlorothiazide may develop gout because it increases the renal tubular reabsorption of uric acid.

Answer E is incorrect. The patient is allergic to NSAIDs, so ibuprofen is not a good choice.

Answer F is incorrect. The patient is allergic to NSAIDs, so indomethacin is not a good choice.

Answer G is incorrect. The patient is allergic to NSAIDs, so naproxen is not a good choice.

17. **The correct answer is B.** Wrist slashing on the medial aspect of the arm may injure the ulnar artery and ulnar nerve. The adductor pollicis is innervated by a branch of the ulnar nerve and adducts the thumb. Other muscles innervated by the ulnar nerve include the hypothenar muscles, lumbricals (3 and 4), dorsal interossei, and palmar interossei.

Answer A is incorrect. The abductor pollicis brevis is innervated by a branch of the median nerve and functions in abduction and opposition of the thumb.

Answer C is incorrect. The flexor pollicis brevis is innervated by a branch of the median nerve and flexes the thumb.

Answer D is incorrect. The first and second lumbricals are innervated by the median nerve.

Answer E is incorrect. The opponens pollicis is innervated by a branch of the median nerve and functions in opposition of the thumb.

18. **The correct answer is D.** The supraspinatus tendon is most commonly injured in a rotator cuff tear. This muscle aids the deltoid in abduction of the arm, especially in the first 15 degrees. Rotator cuff tear is very uncommon in the young but often occur in older individuals when an abducted arm receives an indirect force.

Answer A is incorrect. The infraspinatus muscle is less commonly injured in rotator cuff tears. It functions to laterally rotate the arm.

Answer B is incorrect. The subacromial bursa separates the supraspinatus tendon from the coracoacromial ligament, acromion, and deltoid. Injury to this bursa causes severe pain with abduction from 50 to 130 degrees, not slight abduction.

Answer C is incorrect. The subscapularis muscle is less commonly injured in rotator cuff tears. It functions to medially rotate and adduct the arm.

Answer E is incorrect. The teres minor muscle is less commonly injured in rotator cuff tears. It functions to laterally rotate and adduct the arm.

19. **The correct answer is D.** This is the clinical picture of drug-induced lupus, which affects males and females equally (as opposed to systemic lupus erythematosus, which has a higher incidence in females). Although anti-nuclear antibodies are identified in this patient's serum, he does not have hypocomplementemia or anti-DNA antibodies, which are normally present in systemic lupus erythematous. Hydralazine is the only drug among those listed that is associated with this syndrome. Other drugs known to cause lupus are procainamide, isoniazid, chlorpromazine, penicillamine, sulfasalazine, methyldopa, and quinidine.

Answer A is incorrect. Bleomycin is most commonly associated with pulmonary fibrosis.

Answer B is incorrect. Enalapril, an angiotensin-converting enzyme inhibitor, is most often associated with a dry cough.

Answer C is incorrect. Haloperidol can lead to hepatomegaly but would not cause a clinical picture suggestive of drug-induced lupus.

Answer E is incorrect. Isoniazid, not rifampin, is associated with drug-induced lupus.

20. **The correct answer is E.** The muscles involved in jaw movement are fourfold: lateral pterygoid, masseter, temporalis, and medial pterygoid. The lateral pterygoid opens the jaw while the other three close the jaw. All four are innervated by the trigeminal nerve (V3). One can remember this with the mnemonic "M's Munch" and "Lateral Lowers." Yawning would be impaired with a lateral pterygoid injury.

Answer A is incorrect. Closing the mouth is performed by the masseter, temporalis, and medial pterygoid.

Answer B is incorrect. Smiling requires the function of many facial muscles, including the zygomaticus major.

Answer C is incorrect. Swallowing is mediated by the pharynx and the tongue.

Answer D is incorrect. Whistling is mediated by the tongue and facial muscles, such as the buccinator and orbicularis oris.

21. **The correct answer is C.** Scarlet fever is caused by *Streptococcus pyogenes* and is characterized by a typical sandpaper rash, strawberry tongue, beefy-red pharynx, and circu-

moral pallor. As the rash heals, the skin peels off in fine scales.

Answer A is incorrect. The signs of meningitis are fever, headache, photophobia, nuchal rigidity, and possibly seizures. This patient does not have these symptoms.

Answer B is incorrect. Rubella presents with a prodrome of malaise and suboccipital lymphadenopathy. A maculopapular rash develops first on the face and then generalizes and resolves in 3–5 days. The patient's rash is not consistent with a diagnosis of rubella.

Answer D is incorrect. Inflammation, exudates, fever, and tender cervical lymph nodes characterize pharyngitis. While scarlet fever may sometimes complicate cases of primary *Streptococcus pyogenes* pharyngitis, pharyngitis does not appear to be a prominent feature of this particular presentation.

Answer E is incorrect. *Staphylococcus aureus* and *Streptococcus pyogenes* toxic shock syndromes are characterized by abrupt onset of local or diffuse pain, fever, confusion, and signs of soft tissue infection. The former is sometimes (but not exclusively) associated with women using hyperabsorbable tampons during menses. A diffuse erythema that subsequently desquamates as the patient recovers may be present in 10% of patients. It does not involve the symptoms described in the question.

22. **The correct answer is C.** This patient has acute osteomyelitis and a history of sickle cell disease as evidenced by her multiple hospitalizations (likely for episodes of painful crises) and medication (hydroxyurea reduces the incidence of painful crises in sickle cell disease by increasing the amount of fetal hemoglobin). Osteomyelitis is an infection of the bone tissue. It is common in young children and usually results from the hematogenous spread of organisms from another site of infection (upper respiratory infection in this case). *Salmonella* species are the most common organisms responsible for osteomyelitis in patients with sickle cell disease.

Answer A is incorrect. *Escherichia coli* causes osteomyelitis in infants, but *Salmonella* species are the most common organisms responsible for osteomyelitis in patients with sickle cell disease.

Answer B is incorrect. *Pseudomonas aeruginosa* typically causes infections in immunocompromised hosts and patients with cystic fibrosis.

Answer D is incorrect. *Staphylococcus aureus* is the most common cause of osteomyelitis in the general population, but not in patients with sickle cell disease.

Answer E is incorrect. *Streptococcus pyogenes* causes osteomyelitis in children, but *Salmonella* species are the most common organisms responsible for osteomyelitis in patients with sickle cell disease.

23. **The correct answer is C.** The long bones of the limbs form via endochondral ossification. In this process, mesoderm is first converted to a cartilaginous model by hypertrophic chondrocytes. Bone then forms at the primary ossification center at the diaphysis as cells differentiate into osteoblasts. Besides the long bones, other bones that form via endochondral ossification include the sphenoid, ethmoid, incus, stapes, malleus, limb girdles, vertebrae, sternum, and ribs.

Answer A is incorrect. Chondrocytes are important in endochondral (not intramembranous) ossification. They do not deposit minerals.

Answer B is incorrect. In the process of intramembranous ossification, bone forms directly from mesoderm without an intermediate cartilaginous mold. The long bones do not undergo this process, but rather form via endochondral ossification with a cartilaginous intermediate. Bones that form via intramembranous ossification include the frontal, parietal, maxilla, zygomatic, palatine, and mandible.

Answer D is incorrect. Osteoclasts are important for growth, remodeling, and mineral homeostasis throughout the development of the long bones. They do not, however, deposit minerals; rather, they are responsible for breaking bone down.

24. **The correct answer is D.** A spiral fracture is one that is caused by a twisting, rotational force to the bone. While child abuse may manifest with any kind of fracture, a spiral fracture should raise increased suspicion of intentionally inflicted injury. Spiral fractures in child abuse are usually caused by the twisting of the bone by an angry adult.

Answer A is incorrect. A bowing fracture, also known as a bending fracture, is one in which the cortex of the diaphysis is deformed, but without injury to the periosteum. The pediatric bone structure has greater compliance and porousness than adult bone, resulting in injuries that deform or bend the bone rather than causing a line fracture. Bowing fractures are common pediatric fractures. While a bowing fracture could be caused by child abuse, it is not the most likely of the listed choices to suggest that etiology.

Answer B is incorrect. A buckle fracture, also known as a torus fracture, is caused by compression, resulting in a bulging or buckling of the periosteum, rather than a complete fracture line. Buckle fractures are one of the more common pediatric fractures and are frequently caused by accidents. While a buckle fracture could be caused by child abuse, it is not the most likely of the listed choices to suggest that etiology.

Answer C is incorrect. A greenstick fracture is an incomplete cortical fracture in which cortical disruption and periosteal tearing occurs on the convex aspect of the bone, but the concave aspect has an intact periosteum. Greenstick fractures are one of the more common pediatric fractures and are frequently caused by accidents. While a greenstick fracture could by caused by child abuse, it is not the most likely of the listed choices to suggest that etiology.

25. **The correct answer is E.** This patient has Sjögren's syndrome. The vast majority of patients with this syndrome are women between the ages of 35 and 45 years, and the disease is characterized by dry eyes (keratoconjunctivitis sicca), dry mouth (xerostomia), and one other connective tissue or autoimmune disease (such as rheumatoid arthritis). The eye and mouth dryness is from autoimmune destruction of the lacrimal and salivary glands.

Answer A is incorrect. CREST syndrome is a variant of scleroderma (progressive systemic sclerosis), which is a disease characterized by extensive fibrosis throughout the body (most notably of the skin). **CREST** stands for Calcinosis, **R**aynaud's phenomenon, **E**sophageal dysfunction, **S**clerodactyly, and **T**elangiectasia.

Answer B is incorrect. Cystic fibrosis also causes dysfunction of the exocrine glands (such as the lacrimal and salivary glands), but it is due to a mutation in the cystic fibrosis transmembrane conductance regulator gene on chromosome 7. Individuals with cystic fibrosis also tend to have pulmonary and pancreatic dysfunction.

Answer C is incorrect. When only the first two criteria are present (dry eyes and dry mouth) it is called sicca syndrome.

Answer D is incorrect. Sjögren-Larsson syndrome is an autosomal recessive syndrome that is characterized by congenital ichthyosis (dry and scaly fishlike skin) and associated with mental retardation and spastic paraplegia; it is caused by a mutation in the fatty aldehyde dehydrogenase gene on chromosome 17p.

26. **The correct answer is A.** The MRI shows torn fibers of the anterior cruciate ligament (ACL). The ACL is one of four major ligaments of the knee and bridges the femur and tibia. Part of the "unhappy triad" (ACL, medial collateral ligament, and medial meniscus) of structures involved in common knee injuries, the ACL resists anterior movement of the tibia in relation to the femur and limits anterolateral rotation at the knee. Thus, to test its integrity, one can check for the so-called anterior drawer sign: With the patient's knees in a flexed position, stand in front of the patient and place your hands behind the calf muscles. The sign

is positive if, as you pull toward yourself, there is significant anterior dislocation.

Answer B is incorrect. The lateral collateral ligament is one of four major ligaments of the knee and bridges the femur and the fibula. It prevents excessive lateral movement of the knee.

Answer C is incorrect. The medial collateral ligament is one of four major ligaments of the knee and bridges the femur and the tibia. Part of the "unhappy triad" (anterior cruciate ligament, medial collateral ligament, and medial meniscus) of structures involved in common knee injuries, it prevents excessive medial movement of the knee.

Answer D is incorrect. The posterior cruciate ligament is one of four major ligaments of the knee and bridges the femur and tibia. It acts to limit posterior anterior movement of the tibia in relation to the femur.

Answer E is incorrect. The ulnar collateral ligament is in the upper extremity at the elbow. It forms connections between the ulna and the humerus.

27. **The correct answer is B.** *Pasteurella multocida* is associated with cat and dog bites. Cellulitis appears around the bite site and can sometimes lead to osteomyelitis.

Answer A is incorrect. *Francisella tularensis* is transmitted by wild animals, including rabbits, deer, and ticks, and causes tularemia. Tularemia can vary clinically from the sudden onset of an influenza-like syndrome to a prolonged course of fever and adenopathy.

Answer C is incorrect. Rabies virus causes rabies. The signs of this disease include a prodrome of fever and anorexia followed by confusion, lethargy, and increased salivation.

Answer D is incorrect. *Sporothrix schenckii* is a fungus that typically causes necrotizing, granulomatous lymphocutaneous skin infections in the distribution of draining lymph nodes following trauma by tainted vegetation. Its association with recent outdoor activity, particularly gardening, accounts for its nickname, "rose gardener's disease."

Answer E is incorrect. *Staphylococcus aureus* is one of the major causes of cellulitis but is not particularly associated with an animal bite.

28. **The correct answer is A.** This patient has symptoms and signs consistent with vitamin D-deficient rickets, which results from the decreased or absent mineralization of osteoid (bone matrix) secondary to decreased serum calcium and/or phosphorous levels. Vitamin D normally promotes absorption of calcium and phosphorous from the gastrointestinal tract. In vitamin D-deficient patients, areas of bone growth (e.g., wrists, ankles, costochondral junctions) contain patches of unmineralized, soft osteoid that give rise to the classically reported signs, including widened wrists and/or ankles and enlarged costochondral junctions (rachitic rosary). In cases of severe vitamin D deficiency, laboratory studies typically demonstrate decreased serum calcium, decreased serum phosphorous, decreased serum 1,25-dihydroxycholecalciferol, increased serum alkaline phosphatase, and increased serum intact parathyroid hormone levels.

Answer B is incorrect. A decreased, not increased, serum calcium level (due to decreased gastrointestinal absorption) is characteristic of vitamin D-deficient rickets.

Answer C is incorrect. A decreased, not increased, serum 1,25-dihydroxycholecalciferol (a derivative of vitamin D) level is characteristic of vitamin D-deficient rickets.

Answer D is incorrect. A decreased, not increased, serum 25-hydroxycholecalciferol (the active form of vitamin D) level is characteristic of vitamin D-deficient rickets.

Answer E is incorrect. A decreased, not increased, serum phosphorous level (due to decreased gastrointestinal absorption) is characteristic of vitamin D-deficient rickets.

29. **The correct answer is B.** The patient's inability to abduct his arm and atrophy of the shoulder region suggest that innervation to his deltoid has been compromised. The deltoid is innervated by the axillary nerve, whose fibers originate at levels C5-6. The axillary is a

branch of the posterior cord of the brachial plexus. Because the axillary nerve courses around the surgical neck of the humerus, it is often injured in fractures at this region.

Answer A is incorrect. Nerve root C3 typically does not contribute to the brachial plexus. C4 contributes in about 65% of patients. However, C3-5 roots contribute to the phrenic nerve, which innervates the diaphragm.

Answer C is incorrect. Fibers from C6-7 run together in the lateral cord and are found in the lateral pectoral nerve (innervation to the pectoralis major) and the median nerve (innervation to the forearm, wrist, and hand.)

Answer D is incorrect. Fibers from C7-8 run together in the median nerve, which does not innervate the shoulder region and the thoracodorsal nerve. The thoracodorsal nerve is a branch of the posterior cord, and it innervates the latissimus dorsi. The latissimus dorsi acts through the glenohumeral joint as an adductor of the arm and an extensor of the arm.

Answer E is incorrect. Fibers from C8-T1 are found together in the ulnar nerve, which innervates flexors of the wrist and intrinsic flexors in the hand. These nerve roots also contribute commonly to the radial nerve, which innervates extensors and supinators of the forearm and wrist.

30. **The correct answer is E.** Rheumatoid factor would most likely be positive in this woman, who is suffering from rheumatoid arthritis. Eighty percent of patients with rheumatoid arthritis have positive rheumatoid factor (anti-IgG antibody). This autoimmune condition causes a marked influx of inflammatory cells into the joint synovium, as seen in the image, resulting in destructive change, pannus formation, and eventually joint deformity. The disease is more common in women, and classically symmetrically affects the proximal interphalangeal joints, as described here.

Answer A is incorrect. Anti-centromere antibody is associated with the CREST variant of scleroderma (progressive systemic sclerosis). In this disease patients suffer from Calcinosis,

Raynaud's phenomenon, Esophageal dysmotility, Sclerodactyly, and Telangiectasia. Arthritis is not associated with this syndrome.

Answer B is incorrect. Anti-nuclear antibody is associated with systemic lupus erythematosus, an autoimmune disease with a wide variety of symptoms including fever, rash, joint pain, and photosensitivity. The joint pain in lupus is typically transient, asymmetrical, and non-deforming.

Answer C is incorrect. Borrelia burgdorferi is the cause of Lyme disease. The third stage of Lyme disease can manifest as migratory polyarthritis, but this patient has none of the other signs and symptoms associated with this disease.

Answer D is incorrect. HLA-B27 is strongly associated with arthritides without rheumatoid factor, such as ankylosing spondylitis. This condition most commonly affects men and causes severe stiffening of the spine and sacroiliac joints, as well as uveitis. The hands are not typically involved.

31. **The correct answer is E.** As a child this patient had polio. Patients who develop polio experience injury to the nerve roots that supply the superior gluteal nerve, which innervates the gluteus medius and minimus. These muscles typically abduct and medially rotate the thigh and keep the pelvis level. When these muscles do not function properly, the patient is unable to keep the pelvis level and develops a characteristic limp called the Trendelenburg gait.

Answer A is incorrect. The inferior gluteal nerve innervates the gluteus maximus, which extends and laterally rotates the thigh. It also assists in standing from a sitting position. Individuals with injury to this muscle would have difficulty rising to a standing position.

Answer B is incorrect. Branches of S1 and L5 innervate the quadratus femoris muscle, which laterally rotates the thigh, and the oburator internus, which laterally rotates when the leg is extended and abducts when the thigh is flexed.

Answer C is incorrect. The obturator nerve innervates the obturator externus, which laterally rotates the thigh.

Answer D is incorrect. Branches of S1-S2 innervate the piriformis muscle, which laterally rotates when the leg is extended and abducts when the thigh is flexed.

32. **The correct answer is C.** The syndrome described here is carpal tunnel syndrome, which is compression of the median nerve. This compression is often caused by synovitis, which can manifest in an increased erythrocyte sedimentation rate and WBC count. The median nerve has motor and sensory functions. It supplies the three thenar muscles as well as the following cutaneous regions: the palmar aspect of the lateral hand up to the lateral half of the fourth digit; the areas distal to the (proximal) interphalangeal joints of the first, second, and third digits; and the radial half of the fourth digit. The mnemonic for the three thenar muscles is **Oaf: O**ppose (**O**pponens pollicis), abduct (**Ab**ductor pollicis brevis), and **f**lex (**F**lexor pollicis brevis). The "a" and "f" are lowercase because those muscles are "brevis."

Answer A is incorrect. This area is innervated by the branches of the ulnar nerve, which is unaffected in carpal tunnel syndrome.

Answer B is incorrect. This area is innervated by the branches of the ulnar nerve, which is unaffected in carpal tunnel syndrome.

Answer D is incorrect. This area is innervated by the lateral cutaneous nerve of the forearm, a branch of the musculocutaneous nerve.

Answer E is incorrect. This area is innervated by the medial cutaneous nerve of the forearm.

33. **The correct answer is B.** Paget's disease is abnormal bone remodeling associated with dysfunction of both osteoblasts and osteoclasts. In the early resorptive period of the disease, excessive osteoclast resorption occurs. The cell pictured in the image is an osteoclast, a large multinucleated cell with a ruffled cytoplasmic border frequently found adjacent to bone surfaces undergoing resorption. Osteoclasts are derived from blood or marrow monocytes and are thus of mesodermal origin.

Answer A is incorrect. Endoderm forms gut tube epithelium and derivatives. Osteoclasts are not derived from endoderm.

Answer C is incorrect. Neural crest cells form the autonomic nervous system, melanocytes, dorsal root ganglia, chromaffin cells of the adrenal medulla, enterochromaffin cells, pia, celiac ganglion, Schwann cells, odontoblasts, parafollicular cells of the thyroid, laryngeal cartilage, and aorticopulmonary septum. Osteoclasts are not derived from neural crest cells.

Answer D is incorrect. Neuroectoderm forms the neurohypophysis, central nervous system neurons, oligodendrocytes, astrocytes, and pineal gland. Osteoclasts are not derived from neuroectoderm.

Answer E is incorrect. Surface ectoderm forms the adenohypophysis, the lens of the eye, the epithelial linings, and the epidermis, with the exception of melanocytes. Osteoclasts are not derived from surface ectoderm.

34. **The correct answer is B.** This patient suffers from lateral epicondylitis, better known as tennis elbow. This condition stems from overuse of the superficial extensor muscles of the forearm and wrist, including the extensor carpi radialis muscle. This muscle also inserts at the lateral epicondyle.

Answer A is incorrect. The biceps muscle functions to supinate and flex the forearm.

Answer C is incorrect. The extensor carpi ulnaris muscle functions to extend and adduct the hand at the wrist but does not extend the forearm.

Answer D is incorrect. The flexor carpi ulnaris muscle functions to flex and abduct the hand at the wrist.

Answer E is incorrect. The pronator teres muscle functions to pronate and flex the forearm.

35. **The correct answer is E.** *Yersinia pestis* is the organism responsible for the plague, also known as the Black Death. The bacterium can be spread by fleas. The disease develops after

2–8 days of incubation and is characterized by the presence of exquisitely tender lymph nodes called buboes. Unlike the case in anthrax, the skin ulcers seen in Y. *pestis* infection are painful.

Answer A is incorrect. *Babesia microti* is transmitted to humans through the bite of a tick. It causes a sickness similar to malaria with symptoms of fever and anemia.

Answer B is incorrect. *Bacillus anthracis* can cause cutaneous anthrax, which is characterized by a painless ulcer with a black scab.

Answer C is incorrect. *Leishmania donovani* is transmitted through the bite of a sandfly and causes visceral leishmaniasis. This disease is characterized by abdominal pain and distention, anorexia, weight loss, and fever.

Answer D is incorrect. A person infected with *Trichinella spiralis* presents with fever, periorbital and facial edema, myalgia, and eosinophilia.

36. **The correct answer is B.** The patient's presentation and histology is most consistent with Ewing's sarcoma and is associated with t(11,22) translocations.

Answer A is incorrect. Chronic myelogenous leukemia is associated with t(9,22) translocation (the Philadelphia chromosome) and is not associated with blue cell histology.

Answer C is incorrect. Trisomy 18 is Edwards' syndrome, which is associated with severe mental retardation, rocker bottom feet, micrognathia, and death within the first year of life.

Answer D is incorrect. Trisomy 21 is diagnostic of Down syndrome, a genetic disease associated with mental retardation and characteristic facial features. While individuals with Down syndrome are at a higher risk of acute lymphocytic leukemia, they are not at an increased risk for bone masses or blue cell tumors.

Answer E is incorrect. XXY is Klinefelter's syndrome, a genetic disturbance of the sex chromosomes associated with testicular atrophy, eunuchoid body shape, long extremities, and gynecomastia.

37. **The correct answer is B.** This patient has psoriatic arthritis, which presents with psoriasis (nonpruritic scaly or silvery erythematous plaques with well-defined borders) and joint symptoms that are of acute onset in one-third of patients. Psoriatic arthritis is an inflammatory arthritis and signs of inflammation, such as an elevated erythrocyte sedimentation rate, are commonly seen in patients with this condition. More than 50% of patients have an asymmetric distribution of joint swelling in the distal interphalangeal joints of the hands and feet. Some patients may develop a sausagelike finger from inflammation of the digital tendon sheaths.

Answer A is incorrect. Celiac disease is a malabsorption syndrome in which patients produce autoantibodies to gluten (gliadin). Dermatitis herpetiformis is a skin disorder commonly seen in patients with celiac disease; it causes pruritic papules and vesicles, not scaly plaques. Patients can present with arthralgias; however, the joints do not usually become swollen.

Answer C is incorrect. Gout is characterized by a raised serum uric acid level that leads to uric acid deposition in tissues, particularly the joints. Urate crystal deposition in a joint can cause an inflammatory reaction, leading to joint pain and inflammation. Diagnosis of gout is generally based on clinical symptoms and the presence of urate crystals (which are negatively bifringent and needle-shaped) in the joint fluid. The presence of arthritic symptoms and the absence of elevated uric acid levels make the diagnosis of gouty arthritis unlikely.

Answer D is incorrect. Rheumatoid arthritis is another type of inflammatory arthritis; however, joint involvement is generally bilateral and symmetric. Joint involvement of the hand often leads to ulnar deviation of the wrist, as well as swan-neck and boutonniere deformities of the interphalangeal joints, but generalized swelling and a sausage-like appearance of the digits are not commonly seen. Patients with rheumatoid arthritis can also have cutaneous manifestations, the most characteristic being rheumatoid nodules that are usually located over bony prominences. About 80% of patients with rheumatoid arthritis are positive for rheumatoid factor.

Answer E is incorrect. Pseudogout is a rheumatologic disorder characterized by calcium pyrophosphate dihydrate deposition in connective tissues. The presentation of pseudogout is very similar to that of gout, except the joint fluid contains calcium pyrophosphate dihydrate crystals, which are weakly bifringent and rhomboidal in shape.

38. **The correct answer is A.** The infection caused by *Actinomyces israelii* typically presents as a chronic, slowly progressing mass that eventually evolves into a draining sinus tract. Characteristic sulfur granules are seen in the thick yellow exudate.

Answer B is incorrect. Nocardiosis is caused by *Nocardia asteroides*. This disease begins as a respiratory infection followed by abscess and sinus tract formation. The organism does not produce sulfur granules but is often acid-fast.

Answer C is incorrect. *Prevotella melaninogenica* is part of the normal oral flora and is most commonly responsible for abscess formation in the mouth, pharynx, brain, and lung. It does not produce sulfur granules.

Answer D is incorrect. *Staphylococcus aureus* can also cause abscesses in various body locations but is not associated with the presence of sulfur granules.

Answer E is incorrect. A person infected with *Trichinella spiralis* presents with fever, periorbital and facial edema, myalgia, and eosinophilia.

39. **The correct answer is E.** The white-footed mouse is the main reservoir of *Borrelia burgdorferi*. The bacterium is spread to humans by the *Ixodes* tick. Lyme disease has three characteristic stages. Stage 1 is characterized by erythema chronicum migrans (ECM), arthralgias, and nonspecific flu-like symptoms. Stage 2 is marked by the appearance of multiple small ECM rashes, as well as cardiac and neurologic involvement. Stage 3 involves arthritis, usually of the large joints, and chronic, progressive central nervous system disease.

Answer A is incorrect. Early, localized Lyme is more reliably diagnosed clinically (i.e., on the basis of a tick exposure and rash) due to the delay in the development of antibodies. Serologic tests for Lyme are, however, particularly helpful in evaluating patients for the later stages of Lyme disease.

Answer B is incorrect. Erythema chronicum migrans is the characteristic rash of Lyme disease. It is a circular, macular rash with a clear center that spreads out over time.

Answer C is incorrect. Lyme disease can be treated with doxycycline or any antibiotic from the penicillin family.

Answer D is incorrect. Stage 2, not stage 3, of Lyme disease is characterized by neurologic involvement, including aseptic meningitis and cranial neuropathies, such as Bell's palsy.

40. **The correct answer is C.** C is the epidermis. Pemphigus vulgaris is an autoimmune disorder in which pathogenic antibodies are directed against a cell-cell adhesion protein, desmoglein-3, which is expressed by the keratinocytes of the epidermis. The destruction of desmoglein leads to intraepidermal acantholysis with sparing of the basal layer. Physical exam typically shows flaccid epidermal bullae that easily slough off leaving large denuded areas of skin (Nikolsky's sign), subject to secondary infection. Treatment is usually steroids.

Answer A is incorrect. A is the stratum corneum, which is composed of enucleated, keratinized, flat keratinocytes. The autoantibodies that mediate pemphigus vulgaris are directed against desmoglein-3, a protein involved in cell-cell adhesion within the other layers of the epidermis, not within the stratum corneum.

Answer B is incorrect. B is the dermoepidermal junction. The autoantibodies that mediate this disease are directed against a protein expressed in the epidermis.

Answer D is incorrect. D is the dermis. The autoantibodies that mediate this disease are directed against a protein expressed in the epidermis.

Answer E is incorrect. E is the hypodermis. The autoantibodies that mediate this disease are directed against a protein expressed in the epidermis.

41. **The correct answer is D.** Polyarteritis nodosa is a vasculitis (i.e., inflammation of a blood vessel) characterized by inflammation affecting small to medium-sized arteries, particularly the renal, cardiac, and gastrointestinal tract vessels (usually not the pulmonary vasculature). As many as 30% of patients have been reported to have a history of a prior hepatitis B infection.

Answer A is incorrect. Buerger's disease, also known as thromboangiitis obliterans, is a vasculitis that mostly affects arteries and veins of the extremities. As such, patients often have intermittent claudication and Raynaud's phenomenon. The majority of patients are men who are heavy smokers and show hypersensitivity to tobacco injected into the skin.

Answer B is incorrect. Giant cell (temporal) arteritis is a type of vasculitis that affects the arteries of the head, especially, of course, the temporal arteries. The highlights of this disease can be remembered by the mnemonic **JOE**: patients get **J**aw pain and **O**cular disturbances from ischemia to the arteries supplying them. Patients also often have markedly elevated **E**rythrocyte sedimentation rates. The disease is often associated with the presence of polymyalgia rheumatica.

Answer C is incorrect. Kawasaki's disease is a self-limited vasculitis that normally occurs in infants and children and is characterized by conjunctival and oral erythema, fever, erythema and edema of the palms and soles, generalized rash, and cervical lymph node swelling. About 20% of patients may go on to develop coronary artery inflammation and/or aneurysm.

Answer E is incorrect. Takayasu's arteritis is a vasculitis characterized by fibrotic thickening of the aortic arch (it also affects the pulmonary arteries, the branches of the aortic arch, and the rest of the aorta in up to one-third of patients). Clinically, patients often have lower blood pressure and weaker pulses in the upper extremities than in the lower extremities; some patients have ocular disturbances as well.

42. **The correct answer is C.** This patient has rheumatoid arthritis (RA), which is characterized by systemic symptoms of fever, fatigue, pleuritis, and pericarditis. Women are affected by RA more frequently than men. Patients with RA classically experience symmetric morning stiffness of joints that improves with use. Patients may also have subcutaneous rheumatoid nodules, ulnar deviation of the fingers, and joint subluxation. RA is mediated by a type III hypersensitivity reaction in which antigen-antibody immune complexes form and activate complement. In RA, rheumatoid factor is an IgM autoantibody that is directed against the Fc region of the patient's IgG antibody, leading to immune complex formation and deposition. Rheumatoid factor antibodies are present in a number of asymptomatic patients; more recently, anti-CCP (citrulline-containing protein) antibodies have become more popular as sensitive and specific serological diagnostic indicators of RA.

Answer A is incorrect. The Arthus reaction is a local, subacute, antibody-mediated hypersensitivity reaction. Hypersensitivity pneumonitis from thermophilic actinomycetes, not RA, is explained by the Arthus reaction.

Answer B is incorrect. Delayed, cell-mediated hypersensitivity reactions are also type IV hypersensitivity reactions. In this type of reaction, sensitized T lymphocytes encounter antigen and release lymphokines, leading to macrophage activation. A positive tuberculosis skin test is an example of a type IV hypersensitivity reaction. In rheumatoid arthritis, CD4+ T lymphocytes stimulate the immune cascade, leading to cytokine production such as tumor necrosis factor-α and interleukin-1. However, the main mechanism of injury is believed to be the formation of immune complexes.

Answer D is incorrect. Type I hypersensitivity reactions are characterized by antigens that cross-link IgE antibodies present on presensitized mast cells and basophils. This cross-linking results in the release of vasoactive amines, like histamine.

Answer E is incorrect. Type II hypersensitivity reactions are mediated by antibody binding to a host antigen on a cell, leading to phagocytosis or lysis of the cell by complement. In Graves' disease, an example of a type II hypersensitivity reaction, autoantibodies bind to and activate the thyroid-stimulating hormone receptor on thyroid gland cells, causing increased triiodothyronine and thyroxine production and release.

43. **The correct answer is A.** This patient has ankylosing spondylitis, a chronic inflammatory disease of the spine and sacroiliac joints that often leads to the stiffening or consolidation of the bones that make up the joints. Common findings are low back pain, stiffness for over 3 months, pain and stiffness in the thoracic region, limited movement in the lumbar area, and limited chest expansion. Around 90% of patients are human leukocyte antigen-B27-positive, and common complications include uveitis and aortic regurgitation.

Answer B is incorrect. Osteoarthritis is joint inflammation and destruction secondary to wear and tear. Unlike the symptomatology seen in the above patient, osteoarthritis presents with pain that is worse after use of the joints (i.e., at the end of the day) and tends to present in individuals older than age 50.

Answer C is incorrect. Patients with psoriatic arthritis can have joint pain and be human leukocyte antigen-B27-positive, but the diagnosis requires the presence of psoriasis, which is characterized by nonpruritic scaly or silvery erythematous plaques with well-defined borders.

Answer D is incorrect. While this patient does have sacroiliitis and is human leukocyte antigen-B27-positive, Reiter's syndrome is diagnosed by conjunctivitis in a patient who has had both urethritis (or cervicitis) and arthritis for at least 1 month. It is thought to be caused by an autoimmune reaction within several weeks after a gastrointestinal or genitourinary infection.

Answer E is incorrect. Rheumatoid arthritis is an autoimmune disorder of synovial joints and often presents with morning joint stiffness, subcutaneous joint nodules (particularly in the proximal interphalangeal joints), and symmetric joint involvement. Eighty percent of patients have positive rheumatoid factor in their serum, and the disease may include systemic symptoms (such as fever, pleuritis, and pericarditis).

Answer F is incorrect. Vertebral compression fractures are a complication of osteoporosis and present with acute back pain, loss of height, and kyphosis.

44. **The correct answer is C.** This patient most likely suffers from a "boxer's fracture," which occurs when individuals strike a blow with a closed fist. The most commonly injured sites for experienced boxers are the first and second metacarpals, whereas for inexperienced boxers the fifth metacarpal is the most common site of injury. The metacarpals have a good blood supply and thus heal rapidly.

Answer A is incorrect. A complete transverse fracture of the distal radius is commonly called a Colles' fracture. This occurs most commonly in the elderly following forced dorsiflexion.

Answer B is incorrect. Fracture of the hamate is not common but can be complicated, as the ulnar nerve can often be injured. There are healing difficulties associated with this type of fracture.

Answer D is incorrect. Fracture of the phalanges is a common injury and is often due to crushing or hyperextension injuries.

Answer E is incorrect. Fracture of the scaphoid commonly occurs when individuals fall onto an abducted hand.

45. **The correct answer is A.** Nephritic syndrome is characterized by hematuria, hypertension, oliguria, and azotemia. The patient is exhibiting pathologic findings consistent with poststreptococcal glomerulonephritis. This disease is classically found in children who present 1–2 weeks after recovering from a sore throat

with fever, malaise, oliguria (a pathologically small amount of urine relative to fluid intake), nausea, and hematuria.

Answer B is incorrect. This answer describes the pathologic findings of Goodpasture's syndrome, a type II hypersensitivity against collagen type IV, which is found in the lungs and the kidneys. The disease commonly presents with concurrent hemoptysis and hematuria. Exposure to hydrocarbon solvents such as those found in the dry-cleaning industry as well as cigarette smoking have been associated with an increased risk of developing Goodpasture's syndrome.

Answer C is incorrect. This answer describes the pathologic findings of IgA nephropathy (also known as Berger's nephropathy), one of the most common causes of recurrent gross or microscopic hematuria from glomerulonephritis worldwide.

Answer D is incorrect. This answer describes the pathologic findings of minimal change disease, the most common cause of nephrotic syndrome in children. It tends to respond very well to corticosteroid therapy. Remember, you have to **LEAP** to nephrotic syndrome, as it is characterized by **L**ipiduria/hyper**L**ipidemia, **E**dema (generalized), hypo**A**lbuminemia, and **P**roteinuria.

Answer E is incorrect. This answer describes the pathologic findings of Alport's syndrome, which usually presents between the ages of 5 and 20 years with nerve deafness and ophthalmopathy, accompanied with signs and symptoms of nephritis (such as gross or microscopic hematuria).

CHAPTER 13

Neurology

1. A couple presents to the emergency department with their 5-month-old son. The parents report that their son has never been fussy. However, last night he began to cry incessantly and neither changing his diapers nor feeding was able to calm him. This morning he had become very lethargic and warm, and his temperature reached 39.4° C (103° F). The physician examines the baby and notices some rigidity in his nuchal region. The emergency department physician becomes extremely concerned and orders a lumbar puncture which reveals an elevated opening pressure, elevated protein level, decreased glucose level, and numerous polymorphonuclear cells. What is the most likely cause of this patient's symptoms?

   (A) *Cryptococcus neoformans*
   (B) Cytomegalovirus
   (C) Enterovirus
   (D) *Escherichia coli*
   (E) *Haemophilus influenzae*
   (F) *Neisseria meningitidis*

2. A 27-year-old man presents to his primary care physician for a pre-employment physical examination. The patient states that he has been healthy and has no complaints except that he has been drinking a lot of water for what feels like an unquenchable thirst for the past couple of weeks. He reports that he has also been urinating excessively and is unable to sleep through the night due to his thirst and frequent urination. Urine analysis is significant only for a specific gravity of 1.002. Serum analysis is significant for an osmolality of 320 mOsm/L and a serum glucose level of 120 mg/dL. The patient is admitted to the hospital, where subcutaneous vasopressin is administered. Subsequent urine analysis revealed a specific gravity of 1.009 and serum analysis reveals an osmolality of 300 mOsm/L and a serum glucose level of 124 mg/dL. The patient is most likely to benefit from treatment with which of the following?

   (A) Desmopressin
   (B) Fluid restriction

   (C) Hydrochlorothiazide
   (D) Insulin
   (E) Metformin

3. During the autopsy of a patient who complained of a severe headache shortly before dying, the pathologist removes the calvarium with the dura attached. On the surface of the brain, there is frank blood on visual inspection that she is unable to remove by rubbing or scraping the surface. Which of the following types of hemorrhages most likely caused this finding?

   (A) Epidural hemorrhage
   (B) Intradural hemorrhage
   (C) Parenchymal hemorrhage
   (D) Subarachnoid hemorrhage
   (E) Subdural hemorrhage

4. A 42-year-old woman comes to the physician because of the gradual onset of involuntary limb and facial movements, mood swings, and trouble with her memory. She says that her mother displayed similar symptoms when she was in her 50s. Which of the following changes would most likely be seen in the brain of this patient?

   (A) Accumulation of neuritic plaques
   (B) Copper accumulation in the basal ganglia
   (C) Gliosis of the caudate nucleus
   (D) Loss of pigmentation in substantia nigra
   (E) Scattered plaques of demyelination

5. After a brain tumor resection, a right-handed patient comes to the office with this wife. The wife reports that her husband can no longer balance his checkbook or count his money. Recently he has also had difficulty identifying individual fingers and confuses his left and right sides. Additionally, she reports that although he can read without effort, he has extreme difficulty writing. The damage can be localized to which of the following areas of the brain?

   (A) Left angular gyrus
   (B) Left posterior inferior frontal lobe

(C) Left posterior superior temporal gyrus
(D) Left sylvian region
(E) Left temporoparieto-occipital junction

6. A 40-year-old man was admitted to the neurology service for evaluation of persistent numbness over his left jaw and lower face. MRI reveals a schwannoma, which is compressing a cranial nerve as the nerve exits the skull. The cranial nerve involved in this case exits the skull through which of the following foramina?

(A) Foramen ovale
(B) Foramen rotundum
(C) Foramen spinosum
(D) Jugular foramen
(E) Superior orbital fissure

7. A 47-year-old man presents with dysarthria and progressive muscle weakness of the bilateral upper and lower extremities in the absence of any history of neurologic disease or recent illness, weight loss, or trauma. Physical examination is notable for muscle atrophy and weakness in all extremities. Deep tendon reflexes are absent in the upper extremities but are 3+ in the lower extremities; some fasciculations are present. Babinski's sign is upgoing bilaterally, and cranial nerves are intact. Laboratory and imaging studies are all within normal limits. Which of the following would be expected on microscopic examination of the central nervous system?

(A) Demyelination of axons in the dorsal columns and spinocerebellar tracts in the spinal cord
(B) Demyelination of axons in the posterior limb of the internal capsule in the cerebrum
(C) Neuronal loss in the region of the anterior horn cells and corticospinal tracts in the spinal cord
(D) Neuronal loss in the region of the anterior horn cells and posterior columns in the spinal cord
(E) Neuronal loss only in the region of the anterior horn cells in the spinal cord

8. A 3-week-old infant is noted to have enlargement of the head on a routine physical examination. His birth history is remarkable for an episode of group B streptococcal meningitis that resolved after a course of intravenous antibiotics. Which of the following mechanisms is most likely responsible for this patient's symptoms?

(A) Accumulation of blood in the subarachnoid space
(B) Decreased absorption of cerebrospinal fluid by the arachnoid villi
(C) Increased cerebrospinal fluid reabsorption
(D) Increased production of cerebrospinal fluid
(E) Ventricular obstruction

9. A 19-year-old college student presents to the emergency department with severe vomiting after taking an unknown pill on a night out with her friends. Which of the following labeled areas of the brain is most likely involved in this patient's vomiting?

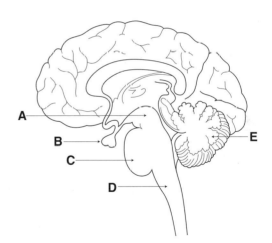

Reproduced, with permission, from USMLERx.com.

(A) A
(B) B
(C) C
(D) D
(E) E

10. A 76-year-old woman dies at home from sudden cardiac arrest after the onset of ventricular fibrillation. The family consents to an autopsy that reveals several small infarcts throughout the basal ganglia. Assuming that the defects arise from a single vessel within the central nervous system, pathology from which artery would be most consistent with this finding?

(A) Anterior cerebral artery
(B) Anterior communicating artery
(C) Lateral striate artery
(D) Posterior cerebral artery
(E) Vertebral cerebral artery

11. A 63-year-old homeless woman is brought to the emergency department by the police, who noted her to be disoriented and confused. On questioning, the patient appears to be having problem with her short-term memory, frequently forgetting what question she had been asked. She provides plausible details of the events prior to her coming to the hospital, but the police report to be untrue. On physical examination she is emaciated and has nystagmus and an unsteady gait. Examination of emergency department records reveals that she has presented multiple times in the past for alcohol withdrawal. The lesion accounting for the patient's symptoms is located in which part of the brain?

(A) Basal ganglia
(B) Broca's area
(C) Cerebellar vermis
(D) Mamillary bodies
(E) Wernicke's area

12. An 82-year-old woman suffers an ischemic stroke with numerous sequelae, including uvular deviation to the right side. Assuming the defect is in the lower motor neuron, damage to which of the following cranial nerves is consistent with this abnormality?

(A) Left IX
(B) Left X
(C) Left XII
(D) Right IX
(E) Right X
(F) Right XII

13. A 26-year-old woman presents to her primary care physician with a 2-month history of difficulty reading, pain in her right eye, and paresthesias in her hands and legs. The patient describes a similar episode that occurred 1 year ago; she assumed that it was a viral illness because it was self-limited. During the physical examination, the patient is noted to have hyperemia and edema of her right optic disc and mild hyperreflexia. The patient undergoes an MRI, which confirms the diagnosis. Histopathology of the lesions would demonstrate which of the following?

(A) Duplication and fragmentation of the internal elastic lamina
(B) Granulomatous inflammatory infiltrate of the adventitial and medial layers with fragmentation of the internal elastic lamina
(C) Inflammation of white matter associated with multinucleate giant cells and aggregates of mononuclear cells
(D) Lymphocyte and macrophage infiltration associated with areas of demyelination
(E) Spongiform degeneration without inflammatory changes

14. A 70-year-old man is referred to a specialist for evaluation because of progressive memory loss and cognitive decline. His wife reports that he gets lost in their neighborhood and that she now pays the bills because he has become unreliable. She also states that the patient's appetite, weight, sleeping pattern, and energy have not changed, but he is less interested in hobbies he used to enjoy. The neurologic examination is normal. He scores 19/30 on the Mini-Mental State Examination, with errors in figure drawing, recall, language, and concentration. Laboratory studies are unremarkable. Which of the following symptoms is most likely to develop in this patient over the next 3 months?

(A) Depression
(B) Gait disturbances
(C) Hyperorality
(D) Stereotyped perseveration
(E) Symmetric muscular weakness

15. A 33-year-old woman presents to the emergency department complaining of right facial weakness and pain behind her right ear since that morning. Neurologic examination confirms complete paralysis of the right side of her face, decreased taste sensation on the right side of her tongue, and increased sensitivity to loud sounds in her right ear. The rest of her neurologic examination is normal. The patient is given a short course of steroids and her facial weakness improved gradually over the next few weeks. In addition to the symptoms described above, which of the following might this patient also develop?

(A) Decreased sensation over her left cheek
(B) Decreased sensation over her right cheek
(C) Deviation of the uvula and soft palate to the left when the patient is asked to say "Ahh"
(D) Deviation of the uvula and soft palate to the right when the patient is asked to say "Ahh"
(E) Dryness in her left eye
(F) Dryness in her right eye

16. During a right temporal craniotomy, the neuronal radiations projecting to the inferior bank of the calcarine sulcus are injured. Which of the following is the most likely visual disturbance to occur in this patient?

(A) Left hemianopia with macular sparing
(B) Left lower quadrantanopia
(C) Left upper quadrantanopia
(D) Right hemianopia with macular sparing
(E) Right lower quadrantanopia
(F) Right upper quadrantanopia

17. The high-power micrograph shown in the image demonstrates a key histologic finding obtained from the brain of a 75-year-old patient at autopsy. The patient had a neurologic illness that was primarily characterized by motor symptoms without evidence of dementia. Which of the following findings might this patient have exhibited?

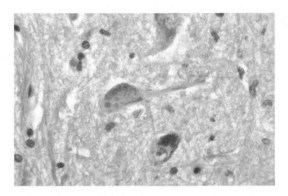

Reproduced, with permission, from PEIR Digital Library (http://peir.net).

(A) Bradykinesia
(B) Grand mal seizures
(C) Myoclonic fasciculations
(D) Symmetric proximal muscle weakness
(E) Tongue fasciculations

18. A 67-year-old woman presents to the physician with right-sided Horner's syndrome and face pain, a hoarse voice, dysarthria, diplopia, numbness, and ataxia with contralateral impairment of pain and temperature sensation in her arm and leg. No other motor or hearing deficits are evident. Which parts of the brain are involved in this patient?

(A) Caudal lateral pontine tegmentum, including cranial nerve VII, the spinal tegmental tract of cranial nerve V, and the inferior surface of the cerebellum
(B) Cochlea and vestibular apparatus
(C) Dorsolateral quadrant of the medulla, including the nucleus ambiguus and the inferior surface of the cerebellum
(D) Internal capsule, caudate nucleus, putamen, and globus pallidus
(E) Lateral geniculate body, globus pallidus, and posterior limb of the internal capsule

19. A 72-year-old woman presents to her physician with worsening low back pain that radiates over her anterior thighs. The pain has affected her for nearly 3 years; it occurs during walking and prolonged standing and is relieved by rest and sitting. The patient also says that she has begun to experience a decreased urinary stream. Physical examination is notable for reduced mobility over the lumbar spine; there is no pain elicited with leg raising in the supine position. Posterior tibial and dorsalis pedis pulses are 2+. Ankle reflexes are 1+ bilaterally. Which of the following represents the most likely process responsible for this patient's back pain?

(A) Conus medullaris syndrome
(B) Lumbar spinal stenosis
(C) Lumbosacral disc herniation
(D) Peripheral vascular disease
(E) Polymyalgia rheumatica

20. A 38-year-old woman comes to the physician with a 4-month history of episodic nausea and a sensation of abnormal motion that lasts for 4–5 minutes. Her symptoms have intensified over the past week, and the episodes now last more than an hour. A particularly severe episode this morning resulted in vomiting and buzzing in her right ear. On physical examination, the patient appears healthy with normal vital signs, mild sensorineural hearing loss in the right ear, and no nystagmus. The patient's laboratory tests are unremarkable. Audiologic testing demonstrates unilateral hearing loss on the right side, most pronounced in the low-frequency range. Which of the following locations is the most likely origin of the abnormality responsible for this patient's symptoms?

(A) Cochlea
(B) Endolymphatic sac
(C) Semicircular canals
(D) Utricle and saccule
(E) Vestibulocochlear nerve

21. The specimen in the image shows the arterial network of the brain. Infarction of the artery designated by the arrow would lead to which of the following deficits?

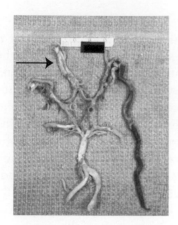

Reproduced, with permission, from PEIR Digital Library (http://peir.net).

(A) Contralateral motor deficits of the arm and hand
(B) Contralateral motor deficits of the face
(C) Contralateral motor deficits of the leg and foot
(D) Ipsilateral motor deficits of the arm and hand
(E) Ipsilateral motor deficits of the face
(F) Ipsilateral motor deficits of the leg and foot

22. A 43-year-old man presents to emergency department complaining of vision problems for the past 2 days. He informs the physicians that he has AIDS and that his last CD4+ cell count 3 months ago was 24/mm^3. He stopped taking antiretroviral therapy 2 years ago. Neurologic examination reveals problems with speech, memory, and coordination. He is admitted to the hospital but his symptoms rapidly worsen, and 3 weeks after admission the patient dies. What is the most likely cause of death in this patient?

(A) *Cryptococcus neoformans*
(B) Herpes simplex virus
(C) JC virus
(D) *Pneumocystis jiroveci*
(E) *Toxoplasma gondii*

23. A 32-year-old woman presents to the physician with worsening anesthesia, weakness of both upper extremities, and headaches. The patient

has no prior significant medical history and cannot recall any recent episodes of trauma. Physical examination is notable for the absence of motor deficits in both upper extremities, but positive for the absence of pain and temperature sensation and reflexes in both upper extremities. Position and vibration sense are intact in the upper extremities and there are no lower extremity abnormalities. An MRI of the spinal column shows dilation within the cervical spinal cord. Which of the following diagnoses is consistent with this patient's findings?

(A) Arnold-Chiari I malformation
(B) Communicating hydrocephalus
(C) Congenital aqueductal stenosis
(D) Dandy-Walker syndrome
(E) Wallenberg's (lateral medullary) syndrome

24. A 7-year-old boy is brought to the emergency department after falling from a tree; an x-ray film shows that he has a midshaft fracture of the humerus. Which of the following structures could be injured with this type of fracture?

(A) Anterior circumflex humeral artery
(B) Axillary nerve
(C) Median nerve
(D) Radial nerve
(E) Ulnar nerve

25. A 42-year-old woman presents to her primary care physician with a chief complaint of paresthesias that started in her fingers and toes about 1 week ago. Since then, her symptoms have progressed to include paresthesias and muscle weakness in her lower legs. A nerve conduction study is performed and shows slowed nerve conduction velocities. As her disease progresses, which of the following acid-base disorders would she be expected to develop?

(A) Metabolic acidosis (anion-gap)
(B) Metabolic acidosis (non-anion-gap)
(C) Metabolic alkalosis
(D) Respiratory acidosis
(E) Respiratory alkalosis

26. A 32-year-old man comes to the physician because of headaches that occur at night and without warning. They begin in his left eye and then generalize to the left side of his face. Alcohol can precipitate the attacks, which last for less than 1 hour. The patient rates the pain as a 10/10, and multiple over-the-counter analgesics have resulted in minimal benefit. He is given a prescription for sumatriptan to treat his symptoms and is prescribed verapamil for prophylaxis. Which of the following is the most likely diagnosis?

(A) Cluster headache
(B) Medication-overuse headache
(C) Migraine headache
(D) Temporomandibular joint dysfunction syndrome
(E) Tension headache

27. A 42-year-old man is brought to the emergency department by police after they found him walking unsteadily in the middle of a busy street harassing other pedestrians. On presentation the patient appears minimally responsive with a respiratory rate of 8/min, heart rate of 54/min, and blood pressure of 101/54 mm Hg. His temperature is normal. The patient is unresponsive to glucose and naloxone administration. An ophthalmology consult is requested after the emergency department physician notes an abnormality on visual examination. Laboratory tests show:

Na^+: 137 mEq/L
Cl^-: 100 mEq/L
Glucose: 69 mg/dL
WBC count: 8000/mm³
Hemoglobin: 14.6 g/dL
Vitamin B_1: 59 pg/dL (normal: 140-820 pg/mL)

Which of the following is the most likely diagnosis?

(A) Diabetic ketoacidosis
(B) Opioid intoxication
(C) Parkinson's disease
(D) Sepsis
(E) Wernicke's encephalopathy

28. A 2-year-old boy is brought to the pediatrician because his mother discovered a large abdominal mass while bathing him. Examination shows that the child has marked hypertension and dark circles around his eyes. Urine catecholamine levels are elevated. A biopsy of the mass reveals small round cells with hyperchromatic nuclei, often forming a pseudorosette pattern around central primitive nerve fibers. Amplification of which of the following oncogenes is associated with this tumor?

    (A) *bcl-2*
    (B) *c-myc*
    (C) *erb*-B2
    (D) n-*myc*
    (E) *ras*

29. A 25-year-old man with a history of intractable seizures has recently been switched to a new antiseizure medication by his neurologist. He subsequently develops a rash on his body, which consists of maculopapular blistering lesions with central erythema surrounded by a halo of erythema. His neurologist also notes that he has developed lesions on his gums and anus. The neurologist discontinues the medication immediately and admits the patient to the hospital. Laboratory test results show:

    Na⁺: 130 mEq/L
    K⁺: 4.2 mEq/L

Cl⁻: 101 mEq/L
Carbon dioxide: 25 mEq/L
Blood urea nitrogen: 10 mg/dL
Careatinine: 0.3 mg/dL
WBC count: 700/mm³
Platelet count: 250,000/mm³
Hematocrit: 39%

Which of the following medication is most likely to have resulted in the patient's symptoms?

(A) Carbamazepine
(B) Gabapentin
(C) Phenytoin
(D) Valproic acid

30. A 2-week-old girl is brought to the pediatrician for her first doctor's appointment. Physical examination reveals a tuft of hair on her lower back; ultrasound shows no herniation of any kind. Which of the following conditions does this baby have?

(A) Anencephaly
(B) Meningocele
(C) Meningomyelocele
(D) Spina bifida cystica
(E) Spina bifida occulta

1. **The correct answer is D.** The concern for this patient is meningitis, which can be caused by bacteria, viruses, or fungi. The classic triad is fever, headache, and nuchal rigidity. Other symptoms such as rash and photophobia are also commonly present. In neonates, though, it may be difficult to identify these symptoms. Inference from the history, such as severe crying in a normally quiet baby, may indicate headache or muscle stiffness. A lumbar puncture and cerebrospinal fluid (CSF) analysis is essential in determining the cause. Classic CSF findings for bacterial meningitis are elevated opening pressure, elevated levels of polymorphonuclear leukocytes, elevated protein levels, and decreased glucose levels, as seen in this patient. In newborns from 0–6 months old, the three most common causes of meningitis are all bacterial and include group B streptococci, *Escherichia coli*, and *Listeria*. Culture and microbiology analysis will be able to differentiate between these species. However, the mortality rate for meningitis is high if untreated, and patients can quickly deteriorate. Therefore, empiric treatment should be initiated prior to obtaining the results of CSF analysis.

Answer A is incorrect. *Cryptococcus* mostly causes meningitis in patients with HIV/AIDS. CSF findings for fungal meningitis are most often an elevated opening pressure, elevated lymphocytes, elevated protein level, and decreased glucose level. The number of polymorphonuclear leukocytes is normal, differentiating it from bacterial etiologies.

Answer B is incorrect. Cytomegalovirus is another pathogen that causes meningitis in patients with HIV/AIDS and immunosuppressed patients. Findings on cerebrospinal fluid analysis are typical for viral meningitis (normal or slightly elevated opening pressure, elevated lymphocytes, normal protein level, and normal glucose level).

Answer C is incorrect. Enterovirus commonly causes viral meningitis in patients 6 months to 60 years old. Clinically, the specific virus causing viral meningitis is not always determined, but the family of enterovirus is most commonly seen. CSF analysis in viral meningitis reveals normal or slightly elevated opening pressure, elevated lymphocytes, normal protein level, and normal glucose level.

Answer E is incorrect. *Haemophilus influenzae* type B used to be a very common cause of bacterial meningitis in children between the ages of 6 months and 6 years. However, the incidence has dramatically decreased in the past 15 years with the introduction of *H. influenzae* type B vaccines.

Answer F is incorrect. *Neisseria meningitidis* is the most common cause of meningitis is patients 6–60 years old. It is also seen less frequently in patients age 6 months to 6 years. It is rarely seen in newborns. Findings of CSF analysis would be consistent with bacterial meningitis.

2. **The correct answer is A.** The patient has central diabetes insipidus, a disorder in which the kidneys fail to concentrate urine due to a lack of ADH (versus nephrogenic diabetes insipidus, in which ADH is present but the kidneys fail detect its presence). This diagnosis is evident from his low urine specific gravity with a high serum osmolality and the increase in urine specific gravity with administration of vasopressin. Desmopressin is an ADH analog that is used intranasally to treat central diabetes insipidus. Patients with nephrogenic diabetes insipidus, however, would not respond to ADH analogs.

Answer B is incorrect. Fluid restriction is not indicated for, and is actually detrimental to, this patient due to the inability of his renal system to reabsorb water.

Answer C is incorrect. Hydrochlorothiazide is a diuretic used to treat nephrogenic diabetes insipidus. Desmopressin is the correct treatment for central diabetes insipidus, such as in this patient.

HIGH-YIELD SYSTEMS

Neurology

Answer D is incorrect. Insulin is used to treat type 1 diabetes mellitus and the later stages of type 2 diabetes mellitus. It has no indication in the treatment of diabetes insipidus.

Answer E is incorrect. Metformin is an oral hypoglycemic agent used to treat type 2 diabetes mellitus by decreasing hepatic gluconeogenesis and increasing peripheral utilization of glucose.

3. **The correct answer is D.** A patient reporting severe headache prior to death along with the finding of blood that cannot be scraped from the surface of the brain is consistent with a subarachnoid hemorrhage, most commonly from a ruptured aneurysm. Blood trapped under the arachnoid mater cannot be scraped off when the dura mater is removed.

Answer A is incorrect. An epidural hemorrhage is generally caused by severe head trauma and damage to the middle meningeal artery. If the bony calvarium with the dura attached is removed, an epidural (above the dura) hemorrhage would be removed, and one would not see blood on the surface of the brain. The blood in an epidural hemorrhage is between the dura and the cranium.

Answer B is incorrect. The dura mater is a thick, fibrous structure of dense connective tissue without space for a significant amount of blood to pool. Blood collects either above or below the dura but not within it.

Answer C is incorrect. An intraparenchymal hemorrhage such as those caused by chronic hypertension would not appear as blood on the surface of the brain. It would likely be deeper in the brain, closer to the cerebral arteries. An intraparenchymal hemorrhage appears more like a bruise of the brain tissue and less like a frank pool of blood, as described in the vignette.

Answer E is incorrect. A subdural hemorrhage is defined as a hemorrhage under the dura mater that is caused by damage to bridging veins. There is a potential space between the dura mater and the arachnoid mater. When the calvarium is removed and the dura is ad-

herent to the bony calvarium, this space is exposed, and any blood there should be readily scraped off. Blood that cannot be scraped off must be under still another layer, and the next layer under the dura is the arachnoid mater.

4. **The correct answer is C.** Huntington's disease is classically characterized by choreiform movements, dystonia, altered behavior, and dementia. It is an autosomal dominant disease involving multiple abnormal CAG triplet repeats on chromosome 4p and demonstrates anticipation (disease severity increases and age of onset becomes earlier with each generation). The caudate and putamen are mainly affected, altering the indirect pathway of the basal ganglia, which results in loss of motor inhibition. Gliosis in these areas results in hyperkinesia. Reserpine has been shown to minimize these unwanted movements.

Answer A is incorrect. Alzheimer's disease is the most common cause of dementia in the elderly. It is marked by progressive memory loss and cognitive impairment. Pathophysiologically, this disease is associated with deposition of neuritic plaques (abnormally cleaved amyloid protein) and neurofibrillary tangles (phosphorylated tau protein) in the cerebral cortex. Donepezil/vitamin E therapy has been shown to slow down but not prevent the progression of the disease.

Answer B is incorrect. Wilson's disease, an autosomal recessive disease, is caused by failure of copper to enter circulation in the form of ceruloplasmin due to a problem with excretion of copper from the liver. This disorder results in copper accumulation in the liver, corneas, and basal ganglia. Symptoms include asterixis, parkinsonian symptoms, cirrhosis, and Kayser-Fleischer rings (deposits of copper in the corneas). Penicillamine, a chelating agent, has been used for treatment with some success. Although Wilson's disease can cause chorea and dementia, it is less likely in this scenario as it is inherited in an autosomal recessive fashion and other expected manifestations are not present.

Answer D is incorrect. Parkinson's disease results from loss of dopaminergic neurons and therefore loss of pigmentation in the substantia nigra. These changes alter the direct pathway of the basal ganglia, resulting in loss of excitation. Parkinson's disease presents with difficulty initiating movement, cogwheel rigidity, shuffling gait, and pill-rolling tremor, not chorea. A levodopa/carbidopa combination is used for treatment.

Answer E is incorrect. Multiple sclerosis is characterized by scattered plaques of demyelination that can occur anywhere in the brain and spinal cord. Patients commonly present with recurring multifocal central nervous system lesions that are separated in time (intervening periods of recovery) and space. Typical symptoms include optic neuritis, internuclear ophthalmoplegia (difficulty with horizontal eye movements), sensory and motor changes, and Lhermitte's sign (an "electric shock" felt down the spine with neck flexion). Treatments are aimed at immunosuppression.

5. **The correct answer is A.** Gerstmann's syndrome is a neurological disorder characterized by four primary symptoms: (1) an inability to distinguish right from left; (2) an inability to identify fingers; (3) a writing disability known as agraphia or dysgraphia; and (4) a lack of understanding the rules for calculation or arithmetic known as acalculia or dyscalculia. Their reading ability remains intact. The syndrome results from damage to the visual association cortex (angular gyrus). Injury to the underlying visual radiations may also result in contralateral homonymous hemianopia or lower quadrantanopia.

Answer B is incorrect. Left posterior inferior frontal lobe injury results in Broca's (expressive) aphasia and possibly brachiofacial weakness.

Answer C is incorrect. Left posterior superior temporal gyrus injury results in Wernicke's (fluent/receptive) aphasia and may involve visual field deficits.

Answer D is incorrect. Injury to the left sylvian region may result in global aphasia as well as hemianopia and hemiplegia. Isolated posterior sylvian region involvement may result in conduction aphasia (poor repetition with good comprehension and fluent speech).

Answer E is incorrect. Injury to the left temporoparieto-occipital junction could result in transcortical sensory aphasia, which involves poor comprehension, good repetition, and nonfluent speech.

6. **The correct answer is A.** The foramina of the trigeminal nerve divisions can be remembered with the mnemonic **S**tanding **R**oom **O**nly (SRO) for the **S**uperior orbital fissure, foramen **R**otundum, and foramen **O**vale, which transmit cranial nerves (CNs) V_1, V_2, and V_3, respectively. This patient has a schwannoma of the mandibular division of the trigeminal nerve (CN V_3) as the nerve exits the skull through the foramen ovale. Compression of V_3 causes numbness over the ipsilateral jaw and lower face.

Answer B is incorrect. The maxillary division of the trigeminal nerve (CN V_2) exits the skull through the foramen rotundum and compression would cause decreased sensation over the cheek and middle face.

Answer C is incorrect. No cranial nerves exit through the foramen spinosum. The middle meningeal artery exits through this opening.

Answer D is incorrect. The jugular foramen transmits the glossopharyngeal (CN IX), vagus (CN X), and the spinal accessory nerve (CN XI).

Answer E is incorrect. CN III, IV, VI, and VI exit the skull through the superior orbital fissure. Lesions of these nerves would lead to ipsilateral extraocular muscle paralysis and numbness of the ipsilateral forehead and upper face.

7. **The correct answer is C.** This patient presents with signs and symptoms consistent with amyotrophic lateral sclerosis (ALS), which affects both anterior horn cells in the spinal cord and upper motor neurons in the spinal cord. ALS results in a combination of upper and lower motor neuron signs, although the deficits may

be asymmetric. More males are affected than females, and the incidence rises after age 40. Riluzole (Rilutek) is the only FDA-approved treatment for the disorder, and it prolongs life by only 3–6 months; it is thought to function by reducing the presynaptic release of glutamate.

Answer A is incorrect. Demyelination of axons in the dorsal columns and spinocerebellar tracts occurs in subacute combined degeneration of the spinal cord, which is also known as vitamin B_{12} neuropathy. It is associated with pernicious anemia and results in loss of vibration and position sense (dorsal columns) and arm/leg ataxia (spinocerebellar tracts).

Answer B is incorrect. Demyelination of axons in the posterior limb of the internal capsule would cause contralateral spastic paralysis secondary to disruption of the descending fibers of the corticospinal tract, resulting in upper motor neuron signs.

Answer D is incorrect. Neuronal loss in the region of the anterior horn cells and posterior columns in the spinal cord occurs in Charcot-Marie-Tooth disease, also known as peroneal muscular atrophy. It results in loss of conscious proprioception (posterior columns) and lower motor neuron signs (anterior horn motor neurons).

Answer E is incorrect. Neuronal loss in the region of the anterior horn cells in the spinal cord occurs in poliomyelitis, an acute inflammatory viral infection that affects the lower motor neurons and results in a flaccid paralysis (pure lower motor neuron disease).

8. **The correct answer is B.** After an episode of meningitis has resolved, meningeal scarring can occur as a complication. Scarring can be severe enough to decrease CSF absorption by arachnoid villi, resulting in hydrocephalus. A CT scan of this patient would show dilatation of the lateral and third ventricles with reduction of the extra-axial spaces. These findings suggest accumulation of CSF in the brain, leading to expansion of the cranial cavity and an increase in intracranial pressure. If left untreated, hydrocephalus can potentially lead to

impairment of mental and muscular functions or even death.

Answer A is incorrect. Accumulation of blood in the subarachnoid space is usually due to trauma or a ruptured berry aneurysm and is not usually a complication of meningitis.

Answer C is incorrect. Increased CSF reabsorption would not cause hydrocephalus, as hydrocephalus is usually a result of increased intracranial pressure in the ventricular system due to mass effect or increased CSF volume.

Answer D is incorrect. Rarely, hydrocephalus can result from increased production of CSF by the choroid plexus. This mechanism is not usually a complication of meningitis.

Answer E is incorrect. Meningeal scarring may lead to narrowing of the passageways between the ventricles, but this would rarely be significant enough to cause hydrocephalus. More commonly, hydrocephalus may be caused by aqueductal stenosis due to subarachnoid hemorrhage or tumors.

9. **The correct answer is D.** The area postrema of the medulla contains a chemoreceptor trigger zone that can initiate vomiting. The medulla also plays a role in cardiovascular and respiratory control and in brain stem reflexes.

Answer A is incorrect. The midbrain helps regulate motor control, control of eye movements, and acoustic relay.

Answer B is incorrect. The hypothalamus plays a role in autonomic and endocrine control.

Answer C is incorrect. The pons plays a role in respiratory and urinary bladder control as well as in vestibular control of eye movements.

Answer E is incorrect. The cerebellum regulates movement and posture and aids in motor learning.

10. **The correct answer is C.** The lateral striate arteries are sometimes referred to as the "arteries of stroke" and are penetrating branches of the middle cerebral artery that supply the internal capsule, caudate, putamen, and globus palli-

dus. Infarcts of this region frequently occur in the setting of long-standing hypertension and are known as lacunar infarcts.

Answer A is incorrect. The anterior cerebral artery supplies the medial surface of the forebrain and supplies the leg-foot area of the motor and sensory homunculus.

Answer B is incorrect. The anterior communicating artery connects the two anterior cerebral arteries and is the most common source of circle of Willis aneurysms, which can lead to bitemporal lower quadrantanopia.

Answer D is incorrect. The posterior cerebral artery supplies the major blood supply to the midbrain and supplies the thalamus, the lateral and medial geniculate bodies, and the occipital lobe. Occlusion of this artery can result in contralateral hemianopia with macular sparing.

Answer E is incorrect. The vertebral cerebral artery gives rise to two other arteries: the anterior spinal artery and the posterior inferior cerebellar artery. The former supplies the anterior two-thirds of the spinal cord and the latter supplies the dorsolateral medulla and inferior cerebellum.

11. **The correct answer is D.** The patient presents with classic signs of Wernicke-Korsakoff encephalopathy, which is associated with thiamine deficiency in chronic alcohol abusers. The classic signs are confusion, disorientation, anterograde amnesia, confabulation, oculomotor dysfunction, and motor ataxia. The lesion is located in the mammillary bodies.

Answer A is incorrect. Lesions in the basal ganglia are associated with movement disorders.

Answer B is incorrect. Lesions in Broca's area are associated with a motor aphasia with good comprehension.

Answer C is incorrect. Lesions in the cerebellar vermis are associated with truncal ataxia and dysarthria.

Answer E is incorrect. Lesions in Wernicke's area are associated with a sensory aphasia with poor comprehension.

12. **The correct answer is B.** Motor innervation of the palatal arches and uvula is mediated by the vagus (X) nerve. Deviation of the uvula to one side implicates a lower motor neuron lesion contralateral to the side to which the uvula is deviating. An upper motor neuron vagus nerve lesion will cause the uvula to deviate toward the side of the lesion.

Answer A is incorrect. The glossopharyngeal nerve mediates taste, salivation, and swallowing, but injury would not cause any uvular, tongue, or palatal deviation.

Answer C is incorrect. The hypoglossal nerve mediates tongue movement. Injury to the left cranial nerve XII would result in deviation to that side because of the unopposed action of the opposite genioglossus muscle.

Answer D is incorrect. The glossopharyngeal nerve mediates taste, salivation, and swallowing, but injury would not cause any uvular, tongue, or palatal deviation.

Answer E is incorrect. A right-sided lower motor neuron injury to the vagus nerve would cause the uvula to deviate towards the intact (left) side.

Answer F is incorrect. The hypoglossal nerve mediates tongue movement. Injury to the right cranial nerve XII would result in deviation to that side because of the unopposed action of the opposite genioglossus muscle.

13. **The correct answer is D.** This patient demonstrates many of the diagnostic features of multiple sclerosis, including optic neuritis and recurrent paresthesias. The pathologic hallmark of this disease consists of small gray plaques of demyelination present in the white matter of the central nervous system; microscopic pathology reveals gliosis and demyelination with associated lipid-laden macrophages.

Answer A is incorrect. Significantly enlarged blood vessels with duplication and fragmentation of the internal elastic lamina are evident in arteriovenous malformations.

Answer B is incorrect. Granulomatous inflammatory infiltrate of the adventitial and medial layers with fragmentation of the internal elastic lamina is consistent with inflammation of blood vessels as seen with arteritis. It does not describe blood vessel changes seen in multiple sclerosis.

Answer C is incorrect. Encephalitis due to infection with HIV is associated with white matter inflammation that includes multinucleate giant cells and mononuclear cells.

Answer E is incorrect. Spongiform degeneration and accumulation of proteinaceous material are associated with prion diseases such as Creutzfeldt-Jacob disease.

14. **The correct answer is A.** Alzheimer's disease is the most likely diagnosis given the patient's age, presentation, and lack of strokelike or parkinsonian symptoms or stepwise progression of illness. Other causes of dementia to consider would include vitamin B_{12} deficiency, thyroid dysfunction, syphilis, and hepatic encephalopathy. It is also unlikely that depression is the primary etiology of the patient's condition. Although this patient does not fulfill the criteria for depression at this point, depression is a significant comorbidity of Alzheimer's disease and should be repeatedly screened for and treated.

Answer B is incorrect. Gait disturbances are uncommon early in the course of Alzheimer's disease and would be much more common in other diagnoses, such as Parkinson's disease.

Answer C is incorrect. Hyperorality and early loss of personal awareness are common signs of frontotemporal dementia as opposed to Alzheimer's disease.

Answer D is incorrect. Stereotyped perseveration is another sign of frontotemporal dementia that is rare in Alzheimer's disease.

Answer E is incorrect. Symmetric muscular weakness can occur in many neurologic diagnoses but is uncommon at this stage of Alzheimer's disease. It is, however, a characteristic sign of amyotrophic lateral sclerosis.

15. **The correct answer is F.** This patient's history and physical exam findings are consistent with Bell's palsy, which is an acute peripheral facial nerve palsy of unknown cause. The symptoms seen in this patient can be easily understood if one remembers the different nerve fibers carried by the facial nerve (cranial nerve VII): afferent taste fibers from the anterior two thirds of the ipsilateral tongue (decreased taste sensation), general touch and pain sensory fibers from a small area around the ipsilateral ear (retroauricular pain), and motor fibers to the muscles of facial expression (ipsilateral facial paralysis) and stapedius muscle (increased sensitivity to noise in the ipsilateral ear due to weakness of the stapedius muscle). This patient may also experience dryness in her ipsilateral (right) eye because the facial nerve carries parasympathetic fibers to the ipsilateral lacrimal gland, which provides lubrication to the eye. In addition, weakness of the facial muscles prevents complete eye closure, exacerbating the eye dryness. Patients with facial nerve paralysis should be given lubricating eye drops and instructed to tape their eye closed at night. While facial nerve paralysis can be caused by head trauma, AIDS, Lyme disease, sarcoidosis, or brain stem lesions, in most cases no cause is discovered and the diagnosis of Bell's palsy is made.

Answer A is incorrect. Decreased sensation of the left cheek could be caused by lesion of the left maxillary division of the trigeminal nerve (cranial nerve V2); however, this patient shows signs of facial nerve palsy and shows no signs of trigeminal nerve involvement.

Answer B is incorrect. Decreased sensation on the right cheek could be caused by lesion of the right maxillary division of the trigeminal nerve (cranial nerve V2); however, this patient shows signs of facial nerve palsy and shows no signs of trigeminal nerve involvement.

Answer C is incorrect. Lesion of the right vagus nerve would lead to deviation of the uvula and soft palate to the left; however, all signs and symptoms in this case suggest damage to the facial nerve (cranial nerve VII) and not the vagus nerve (cranial nerve X).

Answer D is incorrect. Unilateral lesions of the vagus nerve or nucleus ambiguus prevent elevation of the uvula on that side and thus cause the uvula and soft palate to deviate away from the side with the lesion due to unopposed action from the normal side. A lesion of the left vagus nerve would cause the uvula and soft palate to deviate to the right; however, the patient in this case has symptoms indicating palsy of the facial nerve (cranial nerve VII), not the vagus nerve (cranial nerve X).

Answer E is incorrect. The facial nerve carries sensory and motor fibers that innervate the ipsilateral face; thus a lower motor nerve palsy of the facial nerve would cause dryness of the ipsilateral (right), not contralateral (left), eye.

16. **The correct answer is C.** Temporal lobe lesions or injuries can cause damage to the lower division of the geniculocalcarine tract, which is known as Meyer's loop. These radiations contain input from the inferior retinal quadrants and therefore represent the superior visual field quadrants. Since the lesion is behind the optic chiasm, the resulting deficit would be a contralateral upper quadrantanopia.

Answer A is incorrect. Left hemianopia with macular sparing would result from injury to the right visual cortex, which is located on the banks of the calcarine fissure.

Answer B is incorrect. Left lower quadrantanopia would result from injury to the neuronal radiations projecting to the superior bank of the calcarine sulcus.

Answer D is incorrect. Right hemianopia with macular sparing would result from injury to the left visual cortex.

Answer E is incorrect. Right lower quadrantanopia would result from injury of the neuronal projections to the superior bank of the calcarine sulcus on the left side, not the right side, since damage in this region results in contralateral lower quadrantanopia.

Answer F is incorrect. Right upper quadrantanopia would result from injury to Meyer's loop on the left side, not the right side, since damage to the loop results in contralateral upper quadrantanopia.

17. **The correct answer is A.** This specimen is taken from the patient's substantia nigra and demonstrates a typical melanin-containing neuron with pink-staining inclusions known as Lewy bodies. These are aggregations of the protein alpha-synuclein that are primarily seen in two neurologic diseases: Parkinson's disease and Lewy body dementia. Since this patient had no symptoms of dementia, the only remaining option is Parkinson's disease, which is characterized by resting tremor, cogwheel rigidity, bradykinesia, and postural instability.

Answer B is incorrect. Seizures are associated with many neurologic disorders but do not correlate with any particular histopathologic findings, especially Lewy bodies.

Answer C is incorrect. Myoclonic fasciculations are classically seen in Creutzfeldt-Jacob disease.

Answer D is incorrect. Symmetric muscle weakness is seen in Guillain-Barré syndrome and amyotrophic lateral sclerosis; Lewy bodies are not evident in either disease.

Answer E is incorrect. Tongue fasciculations are classically seen in degenerative neurologic diseases such as spinal muscular atrophy and amyotrophic lateral sclerosis.

18. **The correct answer is C.** The stroke syndrome described is the lateral medullary syndrome, also known as the posterior inferior cerebellar artery (PICA) syndrome or Wallenberg's syndrome. This syndrome results in numbness of the ipsilateral face and contralateral limbs, diplopia, dysarthria, and an ipsilateral Horner's syndrome. It classically results from a disruption of the PICA, which provides the blood supply for the dorsolateral quadrant of the medulla, including the nucleus ambiguus and the inferior surface of the cerebellum. The infarcted dorsolateral quadrant of the medulla contains the tract of cranial nerve V (face pain), vestibular nuclei (dysequilibrium), nucleus ambiguus (palate problems and hoarse voice), the spinothalamic tract (contralateral pain and temperature loss), and descending sympathetic fibers (Horner's syndrome). Limb

weakness and reflex changes are not found because corticospinal fibers are in the ventral medulla at this location.

Answer A is incorrect. This vascular territory is supplied by the anterior inferior cerebellar artery. Disruption in blood flow typically causes ipsilateral deafness from involvement of the labyrinthine artery, ipsilateral facial weakness, and ataxia. It is the second most common brainstem stroke syndrome.

Answer B is incorrect. The cochlea and vestibular apparatus are perfused via the labyrinthine artery, and an isolated disruption of this end artery would result in isolated dysfunction of these two structures.

Answer D is incorrect. The internal capsule, caudate nucleus, putamen, and globus pallidus are perfused by the penetrating branches of the middle cerebral artery known as the lateral striate arteries. They are commonly involved with lacunar strokes.

Answer E is incorrect. The lateral geniculate body, globus pallidus, and posterior limb of the internal capsule are supplied by the anterior choroidal artery. Syndromes affecting this artery represent less than 1% of anterior circulation strokes and typically occur in the setting of symptomatic internal carotid artery occlusion.

19. **The correct answer is B.** Lumbar disc degeneration with enlargement of the facet joints can lead to lumbar spinal stenosis in the aging population. Spinal stenosis is characterized by neurogenic claudication: pain in the buttocks or back that is induced by walking or prolonged standing and relieved by rest and forward flexion of the vertebral column. It can mimic vascular claudication symptoms, but the maximal pain is over the anterior thighs as opposed to the legs, as in typical claudication. Patients also have preserved lower extremity pulses without stigmata of peripheral vascular disease. Unlike patients with disc herniation, these patients have pain that is relieved by sitting and have negative leg raises bilaterally. Spinal stenosis can result in focal weakness and potentially alarming signs and should be

aggressively imaged to rule out more ominous causes of back pain.

Answer A is incorrect. Conus medullaris syndrome is a cord compression syndrome that produces perianal numbness and urinary retention with an atonic rectal sphincter, as opposed to the saddle anesthesia more typically found in the cauda equina syndrome, another cord compression syndrome.

Answer C is incorrect. Lumbosacral disc herniation would likely present with positive straight leg raises, and symptoms would not improve upon sitting.

Answer D is incorrect. Peripheral vascular disease (PVD), specifically atherosclerotic narrowing of the iliac and femoral arteries, can mimic symptoms of spinal stenosis. However, if this patient had PVD, her distal pulses would be reduced and her legs would most likely show evidence of stigmata associated with vascular disease.

Answer E is incorrect. Polymyalgia rheumatica (PMR) is a rheumatologic disorder associated with giant cell arteritis. It is characterized by symmetrical, aching proximal muscle pain that is typically most severe in the shoulder girdle, as well as stiffness in the morning and after inactivity. PMR is associated with an elevated erythrocyte sedimentation rate and C-reactive protein.

20. **The correct answer is B.** This patient is suffering from attacks of vertigo that last for more than an hour, which may result from either Meniere's disease or migraine headaches. These can be distinguished based on the presence of auditory dysfunction. Meniere's disease is an idiopathic disorder that typically affects people 30–60 years old and involves episodes of vertigo lasting for a period of hours with associated fluctuation and progressive low-frequency sensorineural hearing loss accompanied by aural fullness or pressure (tinnitus); the disease ultimately affects both ears in nearly half of patients. Meniere's disease is the result of an increase in the volume of the endolymphatic system (hydrops) secondary to mal-

function of the endolymphatic sac, which is responsible for the filtration and excretion of endolymph, the fluid contained in the membranous labyrinth of the inner ear.

Answer A is incorrect. Damage to the cochlea could result in sensorineural hearing loss, as that seen in this patient, but would not result in vertigo.

Answer C is incorrect. Benign paroxysmal positional vertigo (BPPV) is another disease associated with vertiginous symptoms, wherein symptoms are caused by freely moving crystals of calcium carbonate within the semicircular canals. However, the episodes in BPPV last only seconds and are associated with nystagmus.

Answer D is incorrect. The utricle and saccule are responsible for reacting to acceleration and deceleration of the head rather than rotatory movement. Damage to these organs involves the feeling that one is tilted and/or their environment is tilted or even upside down. These patients tend to fall toward the side of the lesion.

Answer E is incorrect. Damage to the vestibulocochlear nerve would also result in sensorineural hearing loss, and potentially equilibrium disturbances, but would not present with the classic triad of Meniere's symptoms (hearing loss, vertigo, and tinnitus, nor would presentation include low-frequency sensorineural hearing loss. Patients with cranial nerve VIII lesions have impairment in the high-frequency range and exhibit problems with speech discrimination.

21. **The correct answer is C.** The specimen in the photo is the circle of Willis. The artery designated by the arrow is the anterior cerebral artery, which supplies the medial surface of the brain, the area responsible for the contralateral leg and foot areas of the motor and sensory cortices. Thus, a lesion in the artery would lead to deficits in contralateral motor function of the leg and foot.

Answer A is incorrect. The artery in question does not supply the arm and hand; the middle cerebral artery does.

Answer B is incorrect. The artery in question does not supply the face; the middle cerebral artery does.

Answer D is incorrect. The artery in question does not supply the arm and hand; the middle cerebral artery does so in a contralateral fashion.

Answer E is incorrect. The artery in question does not supply the face; the middle cerebral artery does so in a contralateral fashion.

Answer F is incorrect. The artery in question supplies the medial side of the brain responsible for contralateral motor function, not ipsilateral leg and foot motor functions.

22. **The correct answer is C.** This patient is presenting with progressive multifocal leukoencephalopathy (PML), which is caused by the JC virus in patients with AIDS. PML is a reactivation of a dormant virus to which the patient has previously been exposed. Initial findings include neurological deficits of speech, memory, and coordination. Vision problems are also common. The disease causes a very rapid decline in neurologic function resulting in coma and death. The 3-week course for this patient is not uncommon. The disease causes multiple areas of demyelination throughout the white matter of the central nervous system. There is no specific treatment for PML, but some patients have shown some clinical improvement with the initiation of highly active antiretroviral therapy.

Answer A is incorrect. *Cryptococcus neoformans* is a common cause of meningitis is patients with HIV/AIDS. The classic meningitis triad of fever, headache, and nuchal rigidity are usually present. Abnormalities on cerebrospinal fluid examination would also be present.

Answer B is incorrect. Herpes simplex virus can cause temporal lobe encephalitis in patients with HIV/AIDS. It is also seen in the general population but at a lower frequency. Rapid onset of fever and focal neurological deficits are the most common presenting features. Deficits often stem from damage to the temporal lobe and can include memory problems, personality changes, and potentially seizures.

Answer D is incorrect. *Pneumocystis jiroveci* is a common cause of pneumonia in patients with HIV whose CD4+ cell counts are <200/mm³. On x-ray of the chest, the classic picture is one of "ground glass," although other radiologic features are also common.

Answer E is incorrect. Toxoplasmosis is the most common cause of encephalitis in patients with HIV/AIDS and is seen mostly in patients with a CD4+ cell count <100/mm³. The most common manifestation of toxoplasmosis is seizures and headache, although other focal neurologic deficits may be seen. The classic radiologic picture is one or more ring-enhancing lesions with surrounding edema.

23. **The correct answer is A.** The history, physical exam, and MRI findings are consistent with the diagnosis of syringomyelia, which may be primary (Arnold-Chiari malformation) or acquired as a result of trauma, tumor, or inflammation. Arnold-Chiari malformations involve downward herniation of the cerebellar tonsils into the foramen magnum and are often associated with syringomyelia. Type II Arnold-Chiari malformations are always associated with spina bifida, whereas type I malformations are not. Syringomyelia consists of an enlargement of the central canal of the spinal cord, most commonly occurring at C8-T1. Crossing fibers of the spinothalamic tract are damaged (loss of pain and temperature sensation) with preserved dorsal column function (intact position and vibration sense).

Answer B is incorrect. Communicating hydrocephalus occurs as a result of a blockage of cerebrospinal fluid outside the brain and is typically associated with malfunctioning arachnoid villi. This diagnosis would show ventricular enlargement on MRI.

Answer C is incorrect. Congenital aqueductal stenosis is a common cause of congenital hydrocephalus and would present very early in life.

Answer D is incorrect. Dandy-Walker syndrome is a congenital noncommunicating hydrocephalus typically associated with a cluster of abnormal findings that include abnormal formation of the cerebellar vermis. This condition leads to obstruction of the outlet foramina of Luschka and Magendie.

Answer E is incorrect. Lateral medullary syndrome, or Wallenberg's syndrome, usually occurs as a result of occlusion of one of the posterior inferior cerebellar arteries. It presents with loss of pain and temperature sensations over the contralateral side of the body and the ipsilateral face. In this case, the patient's symptoms show left-right symmetry.

24. **The correct answer is D.** A midshaft fracture of the humerus could cause injury to the structures found in the radial groove: the radial nerve and the deep brachial artery.

Answer A is incorrect. The anterior and posterior circumflex humeral artery would be damaged by injury to the surgical neck of the humerus.

Answer B is incorrect. The axillary nerve is damaged by injury to the surgical neck of the humerus.

Answer C is incorrect. The median nerve is damaged by injury to the distal end of the humerus.

Answer E is incorrect. The ulnar nerve can be damaged by injury to the medial epicondyle of the humerus.

25. **The correct answer is D.** This patient has Guillain-Barré syndrome. Guillain-Barré syndrome is a demyelinating disease of peripheral nerves causing acute and progressive weakness. A major complication of this syndrome is respiratory paralysis leading to hypoventilation. Hypoventilation leads to an inability of the lungs to excrete the carbon dioxide the body pro-

duces, leading to retention of carbon dioxide. This causes a drop in pH and a compensatory retention of bicarbonate. These acid-base abnormalities are consistent with respiratory acidosis. Hypoventilation (from a variety of etiologies) is a primary cause of respiratory acidosis.

Answer A is incorrect. An increase in anions would be consistent with anion-gap metabolic acidosis. Metabolic acidosis is indicated by the presence of low pH with low plasma bicarbonate and low carbon dioxide and an increased anion gap, measured by ($[Na^+] - [Cl^-] - [HCO_3^-]$), which is normally 10–16 mEq/L. The main causes are lactic acidosis, diabetic ketoacidosis, and renal failure.

Answer B is incorrect. Non-anion-gap metabolic acidosis is the presence of low pH with low plasma bicarbonate without an elevated anion gap. The cause is generally gastrointestinal losses of bicarbonate (i.e., diarrhea, biliary drains, emesis, nasogastric tube losses). Another important and common cause of a metabolic non-anion-gap acidosis is the presence of an ileal conduit or bladder reconstruction from colonic tissue. The gastrointestinal tissue absorbs chloride from the urine in exchange for bicarbonate. Other causes include renal tubular acidosis and hyperchloremia.

Answer C is incorrect. Metabolic alkalosis would present with a high pH, a high bicarbonate, and (with respiratory compensation) a high carbon dioxide. The causes of metabolic alkalosis include vomiting, diuretic therapy, and chloride restriction. The compensation is hypoventilation.

Answer E is incorrect. Respiratory alkalosis can be caused only by an increase in ventilation, leading to excessive loss of carbon dioxide that is balanced by an increased excretion of bicarbonate. Hence, a low carbon dioxide and low bicarbonate indicate respiratory alkalosis. This is caused by hyperventilation.

26. **The correct answer is A.** This patient is suffering from cluster headaches, which are repetitive headaches that occur for weeks to months at a time with intervening periods of remission.

Men are affected more than women, with a peak incidence in persons 25–50 years old. Attacks begin without any prodromal symptoms, typically around the eye or temple, and are excruciating in quality. They are always unilateral and may last for minutes to hours with a mean duration of 45 minutes. In contrast to patients with migraines, who favor remaining in a dark, quiet room, cluster headache patients typically prefer to stay active. Treatment is difficult because of the short duration of symptoms, but effective options include oxygen, intranasal lidocaine, and triptans. Prophylaxis may consist of treatment with prednisone, verapamil, or methysergide for 1–2 months.

Answer B is incorrect. Medication-overuse headaches are secondary to excessive use of analgesia and may occur in patients who have tension, migraine, or cluster headaches. The diagnosis should be considered in patients who have frequent or daily headaches despite the use of medications. Although this patient is taking over-the-counter medications, the periodicity of the headaches precludes the regular administration of analgesia, which would be necessary for the consideration of this diagnosis.

Answer C is incorrect. Migraine headaches can be preceded by prodromal symptoms and can also be bilateral in nature. Typically, the headaches increase in severity and can last from 10–12 hours. They may be associated with nausea and vomiting. Frequently such patients have a family history of migraine. Effective treatment involves use of triptans.

Answer D is incorrect. A headache induced by temporomandibular joint dysfunction syndrome is a result of masticatory system dysfunction and frequently presents with unilateral ear or auricular pain radiating to the jaw. The pain is deep and continuous, is most severe in the morning, and can be associated with jaw dysfunction. Treatment is aimed at the underlying joint malfunction.

Answer E is incorrect. Tension headaches are the most common headache syndrome but typically present with pain that is bifrontal and "squeezing." They may be accompanied by nausea but not by vomiting or photophobia and are not preceded by prodromal symptoms. Acetaminophen and nonsteroidal antiinflammatory drugs are typically effective for relief.

27. **The correct answer is E.** The patient exhibits the classic triad of Wernicke's encephalopathy: encephalopathy, ataxic gait, and some variant of oculomotor dysfunction. However, all three features of the triad are recognized in only about one-third of cases. It is important to consider Wernicke's encephalopathy in the setting of alcohol abuse or malnutrition and acute confusion, decreased level of consciousness, ataxia, ophthalmoplegia, memory disturbance, hypothermia with hypotension, or delirium tremens. Wernicke's encephalopathy is a serious disorder caused by thiamine (vitamin B_1) deficiency.

Answer A is incorrect. Diabetic ketoacidosis (DKA) is a pathophysiologic state of inadequate insulin levels resulting in high blood sugar levels and accumulation of organic acids and ketones in the blood. It is also common in DKA to have severe dehydration and significant laboratory abnormalities, including hyperglycemia, hypernatremia, and anion gap metabolic acidosis. None of these laboratory abnormalities is evident in this patient.

Answer B is incorrect. While the patient demonstrates several signs and symptoms consistent with opioid intoxication (e.g., bradycardia and decreased respiratory rate), the patient was not responsive to naloxone administration. In patients with heroin (or other opioid) intoxication, naloxone (an opioid receptor antagonist) rapidly reverses the effects of opioid intoxication.

Answer C is correct. Parkinson's disease is a disorder of the basal ganglia caused by degeneration of dopaminergic neurons in the substantia nigra. These patients are usually >60 years old and present with a shuffling gait, masked facies, resting pill-rolling tremor, and bradykinesia. This patient is rather young to have Parkinson's disease and does not demonstrate the classic syndrome associated with this disease.

Answer D is incorrect. Sepsis is defined as systemic inflammatory response syndrome (SIRS) in the context of documented infection. The patient does not demonstrate signs consistent with SIRS and there is no evidence of infection (he has a normal temperature and white blood count (WBC).

28. **The correct answer is D.** Neuroblastoma is the most commonly occurring tumor of the adrenal medulla in children, but it can occur anywhere along the sympathetic chain. This rapidly growing tumor is also the most common malignant solid tumor outside of the cranium in children. Wide metastasis and elevated urinary catecholamines are common in these patients. Children diagnosed at <1 year of age have an improved prognosis; in fact, tumors can regress spontaneously in younger patients. The tumors frequently demonstrate areas of necrosis, hemorrhage, and calcification. Microscopic examination reveals malignant small cells in a pseudorosette pattern around nerve fibrils. Amplification of the n-*myc* oncogene can be seen in neuroblastoma. In fact, the greater the gene amplification, the more aggressive the tumor.

Answer A is incorrect. The *bcl-2* oncogene is associated with follicular and undifferentiated lymphomas.

Answer B is incorrect. The c-*myc* oncogene is associated with Burkitt's lymphoma.

Answer C is incorrect. The *erb*-B2 oncogene is associated with breast, ovarian, and gastric carcinomas.

Answer E is incorrect. The *ras* oncogene is associated with a number of cancers, including colon carcinoma.

29. **The correct answer is A.** This patient is experiencing Stevens-Johnson syndrome (SJS), a hypersensitivity reaction with symptoms that include erythema multiforme with mucocutaneous lesions and blisters, systemic symptoms (fever, malaise, headache), and epidermal detachment. The condition is serious and has an associated

mortality rate of approximately 5%. When SJS is related to a pharmacologic etiology, the offending agent must be discontinued immediately. Patients are treated like burn victims and often require aggressive fluid replacement, pain control, and antibiotic therapy. Although many anticonvulsants, particularly phenytoin, are associated with SJS, hyponatremia and agranulocytosis are rare adverse effects characteristically associated with carbamazepine administration.

Answer B is incorrect. Gabapentin is commonly associated with adverse effects including sedation and ataxia.

Answer C is incorrect. Phenytoin is commonly associated with adverse effects including gingival hyperplasia and hirsutism.

Answer D is incorrect. Valproic acid is commonly associated with adverse effects, including tremor, gastrointestinal symptoms (nausea/vomiting), weight loss, hair loss, hepatotoxicity, and, rarely, thrombocytopenia.

30. **The correct answer is E.** Spina bifida occulta is caused by the failure of the posterior vertebral arches to close in utero. Generally there are no associated clinical abnormalities, or a tuft of hair may be present over the site of the defect. Folic acid given before the 28th day of pregnancy can help prevent its occurrence; vitamin A may also have slight protective benefit.

Answer A is incorrect. Anencephaly occurs when the cephalic end of the neural tube fails to close, resulting in the absence of a major portion of the brain, skull, and scalp. Infants with this disorder are born without a forebrain and a cerebrum. The remaining brain tissue is often exposed.

Answer B is incorrect. Meningocele is the herniation of meninges (but no nerve tissue) through a bony defect, often located at the sacrum.

Answer C is incorrect. Meningomyelocele occurs when there is herniation of the meninges and spinal cord through a spinal canal defect.

Answer D is incorrect. Spina bifida cystica is caused by the failure of the posterior vertebral arches to close, along with external protrusion of a saclike structure. This is further classified according to the extent of neural involvement (e.g., meningocele or meningomyelocele).

CHAPTER 14

Psychiatry

1. A psychologist whose first child is now 4 years old is applying the principles of behavioral modification to child-rearing. For instance, if the child throws a temper tantrum in a store because she will not buy him candy, she just picks up the child and leaves the store; however, if the child behaves in the store, she takes him to the zoo. This is an example of which of the following kinds of behavior modification?

(A) Aversive conditioning
(B) Classical conditioning
(C) Learned helplessness
(D) Operant conditioning
(E) Stimulus generalization

2. A 26-year-old African-American woman presents to her primary care physician because of fatigue and insomnia for the past 8 months. She also complains of difficulty concentrating and irritability as well as feeling continually worried. She states that nothing seems to make her feel better or worse; she is still able to perform all of her work duties as a public relations officer and was recently promoted. She denies palpitations and any weight change in this time period and her past medical history is unremarkable. Her vitals signs are within normal range, and physical examination shows no focal findings, but the woman appears markedly agitated. Which of the following is this patient's most likely diagnosis?

(A) Adjustment disorder
(B) Attention deficit/hyperactivity disorder
(C) Generalized anxiety disorder
(D) Hyperthyroidism
(E) Social phobia disorder

3. A 35-year-old woman who was hospitalized for a manic episode 2 weeks ago shows substantial improvement. Her mania has resolved; she is now sleeping through the night. She no longer has delusions of grandeur; her speech is not pressured and does not show flight of ideas. She is ready for discharge. Which of the following drugs could be prescribed as maintenance therapy for this patient?

(A) Bupropion
(B) Carbamazepine
(C) Fluoxetine
(D) Olanzapine
(E) Reserpine

4. A 40-year-old woman presents to a psychiatrist after a referral from her family physician due to the fact that she feels anxious all of the time. Her family physician diagnosed her with generalized anxiety disorder and prescribed buspirone; however, the patient does not report feeling any better. She works as a computer programmer and spends most of her day in a private cubicle. She has no close friends and lives by herself. She says that occasionally people from work invite her out at night, but she never goes (even though she would like to). She is not dating currently and is worried that people won't like her. Which of the following personality disorders best describes this patient?

(A) Avoidant
(B) Dependent
(C) Histrionic
(D) Narcissistic
(E) Schizoid
(F) Schizotypal

5. A 44-year-old schizophrenic patient on a psychiatric ward is interviewed daily as part of her treatment. She has been persistently reporting that she is married to Paul McCartney. This psychotic symptom is a disorder of which of the following?

(A) Affect
(B) Cognition
(C) Perception
(D) Thought content
(E) Thought process

6. A 42-year-old African-American woman is admitted to an in-patient psychiatric unit after police find her exhibiting bizarre and aggressive behavior in a public square. After 10 days on antipsychotic medication, the patient is able to interact more appropriately with other patients on the unit, although she exhibits poor eye contact. Her delusions are incomplete and bizarre. She frequently giggles during her daily interviews and smiles broadly when talking about her delusions. The nurses report that the patient's behavior is childlike, and she has a tendency to expose herself to the other patients. Assuming the patient has schizophrenia, which of the following subtypes would best describe this patient?

(A) Catatonic
(B) Disorganized
(C) Paranoid
(D) Residual
(E) Undifferentiated

7. A 19-year-old inpatient on a psychiatry ward has a contentious relationship with his attending psychiatrist after he was recently diagnosed with major depression and questionable borderline personality disorder. His reactions to the psychiatrist have been aggressive, and most recently the patient spit in the psychiatrist's face. Which of the following is a mature defense mechanism that the psychiatrist might use when talking with other staff members about the patient?

(A) Describing the spitting incident in a matter-of-fact tone without expressing the frustration and disgust he was feeling
(B) Holding in his frustration at the patient and later yelling at his son for being 5 minutes late
(C) Laughing off his unexpected shower
(D) Quitting since all his patients are rude, aggressive, and inappropriate
(E) Telling everyone that he is making progress with the patient

8. A 36-year-old man is brought to the psychiatrist by his wife. She reports that the patient has always been somewhat reclusive and introverted,

but lately he has been refusing to go to friends' houses for dinner. The patient also reports that he has been reluctant to leave the house for any reason for the past few months because he is afraid that he will embarrass himself and others will judge him. The patient is referred for behavioral therapy. What is the best choice of pharmacologic therapy for this patient?

(A) Amitriptyline
(B) Buspirone
(C) Fluoxetine
(D) Propranolol
(E) Valproate

9. A 45-year-old man who has received long-term treatment for schizophrenia has recently been noted to display involuntary movements that include lateral deviations of the jaw and "fly-catching" motions with his tongue. Which of the following agents is the most likely cause of his involuntary movements?

(A) Clozapine
(B) Fluphenazine
(C) Lithium
(D) Risperidone
(E) Selegiline

10. A 35-year-old woman presents to the emergency department with trembling hands and a facial tic. According to her mother, she has been seeing a psychiatrist for the past year. She has no other significant medical history. On examination the patient has repetitive facial grimaces with occasional protrusion of the tongue. She denies that these facial expressions are produced purposefully. Which of the following medications has this patient most likely been taking?

(A) Chlorpromazine
(B) Imipramine
(C) Lithium
(D) Mirtazapine
(E) Sertraline
(F) Trazodone

11. A 35-year-old man with depression presents to the emergency department with flushing, diarrhea, sweating, and muscle rigidity. During the physical examination, he says that he began seeing a new psychiatrist because his sertraline was not working for him. His new doctor gave him a different medication, but he decided to use both medicines to "get rid of the depression." Which of the following medications did the new doctor most likely prescribe for this patient?

(A) Citalopram
(B) Lithium
(C) Nortriptyline
(D) Tranylcypromine
(E) Trazodone

12. A 20-year-old man is seen by a physician for the third time in 3 months. At the first visit he was brought to the emergency department by his mother after swallowing toilet bowel cleaner. He told the doctor that he took the cleaning product to "cleanse his body from the aliens" that had "forced their entry" and "possessed" him. Today the patient appears unclean and disheveled, and his mother reports that he has become progressively withdrawn and expressionless. Four months ago the patient witnessed the gruesome death of his father in a drive-by shooting incident. Prior to this incident, he had a normal and healthy life. Which of the following is the most likely diagnosis?

(A) Factitious disorder
(B) Schizoaffective disorder
(C) Schizophrenia
(D) Schizophreniform disorder
(E) Shared delusional disorder

13. A 60-year-old man comes to the doctor because he has been feeling depressed after the death of his wife 2 months ago. He says he has had a hard time sleeping and even has imagined that she is still in their home with him. He has not been able to return to work yet and has difficulty motivating himself to resume his normal activities. What additional symptom would cause the physician to diagnose the patient with abnormal grieving?

(A) Delusions that his wife is controlling his thoughts
(B) Depressive symptoms
(C) Experiences the "anniversary reaction," in which symptoms of grief reoccur on anniversaries or holidays
(D) Guilt that causes him to blame himself for his wife's death
(E) Initial denial that his wife had died

14. A 28-year-old woman presents to her primary care provider complaining of difficulty sleeping. Although the patient reports trouble falling asleep despite waking up "before the sun" every morning, her major complaint is awakening from sleep multiple times each night. She also complains of decreased energy and motivation to complete tasks at work. Polysomnographic studies reveal >25% of total sleep time is spent in REM sleep and <25% of total sleep time is spent in stages III and IV sleep. Which of the following interventions would be most appropriate in this patient?

(A) Avoidance of caffeine
(B) Continuous positive airway pressure
(C) Fluoxetine
(D) Methylphenidate
(E) No intervention is necessary; these are normal polysomnographic findings in a young adult

15. A 28-year-old woman in the emergency department is receiving an initial evaluation by a third-year medical student because of persistent sore throat and fevers. The student finds the patient's history extremely difficult to follow as she is continuously shifting conversation topics, talking about being from Mars, and claiming she is the president of the United States. The patient's speech is flat and there are few facial expressions. The patient reports her doctor recently prescribed a new medication to "help her mind." Which of the following medications is most likely contributing to the patient's sore throat and fevers?

(A) Clomipramine
(B) Clozapine
(C) Haloperidol

(D) Lithium
(E) Risperidone

16. A 7-year-old boy is brought to his pediatrician by his mother after a troubling parent-teacher conference. The teacher informed the mother that the child is disruptive in class and generally does not finish his homework assignments. The mother reports that the child's room is always messy and that he has difficulty completing chores in a timely fashion. In the office the child is restless and interrupts his mother often. Which of the following is the most likely diagnosis?

(A) Antisocial personality disorder
(B) Attention deficit/hyperactivity disorder
(C) Childhood bipolar disorder
(D) Conduct disorder
(E) Separation anxiety disorder

17. A 15-year-old girl is brought to the emergency department by her mother after experiencing a first-time seizure. The thin-appearing girl has a heart rate of 55/min, signs suggestive of dehydration, and fine, velvety hair covering her arms and legs. The physician calculates her body mass index to be 16.4 kg/m². When the patient's mother leaves the room for a moment, the patient admits to the physician that she has been feeling depressed recently and that for the past week she has been self-medicating with normal daily doses of one of her friend's antidepressant medications. What antidepressant is the patient most likely taking?

(A) Amitriptyline
(B) Bupropion
(C) Fluoxetine
(D) Mirtazapine
(E) Selegiline

18. The image depicts a biochemical pathway occurring in the nervous system. An "X" marks the effect of a certain class of medications on this pathway. For which condition is this class of medications an effective first-line treatment?

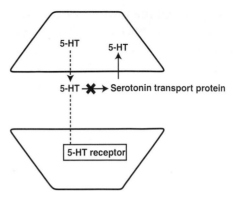

Reproduced, with permission, from USMLERx.com.

(A) Bipolar disorder
(B) Delerium tremens
(C) Dissociative identity disorder
(D) Obsessive-compulsive disorder
(E) Schizophrenia

19. A 42-year-old schizophrenic woman visits her psychiatrist because her caregiver has noticed that she has recently developed involuntary, stereotyped facial grimacing and repetitive thrusting of the tongue. The patient began haloperidol therapy 6 months prior to the visit. Both the patient and her psychiatrist conclude that the patient continues to require treatment for her psychotic symptoms, so the psychiatrist writes a prescription for a different medication. The new medication still has antipsychotic properties, but is less frequently reported to contribute to oromotor symptoms. What is a serious adverse effect of the new medication most likely prescribed by the psychiatrist?

(A) Agranulocytosis
(B) Anorgasmia
(C) Diabetes insipidus
(D) Hypertension
(E) Respiratory depression

20. A 22-year-old man with schizophrenia is being treated as an inpatient with a first-generation antipsychotic medication. Several hours after his initial dose, he develops involuntary muscle spasms, particularly in his facial muscles. To which class of drugs does the indicated treatment for this patient's adverse effects belong?

(A) β-Blockers
(B) Anticholinergic agents
(C) Antiepileptic drugs
(D) Atypical antipsychotic agents
(E) Dopamine agonists
(F) Mood stabilizers

ANSWERS

1. **The correct answer is D.** The basic theory of operant conditioning is that behavior can be modified through reward or punishment. Positive reinforcement is used to increase a desired behavior through a reward system. Negative reinforcement also supports a desired behavior, but instead of a reward, the behavior is encouraged because it allows escape from punishment.

Answer A is incorrect. Aversive conditioning is a part of classical conditioning. Unwanted behaviors are punished by noxious and thus aversive stimuli. A clinical example is the use of the drug disulfiram (which when paired with alcohol results in headache, nausea, and vomiting) to help alcoholics stop drinking.

Answer B is incorrect. Classical conditioning is learning in which a natural response is elicited by a conditioned stimulus that was previously presented in conjunction with an unconditioned stimulus. The classic example is Pavlov's dogs, an experiment in which dogs who salivated (natural response) in response to food (unconditioned stimulus) were taught to salivate (natural response) in response to a bell ringing (conditioned stimulus). This is programming by association, not reward.

Answer C is incorrect. Learned helplessness is created through aversive conditioning, which is an example of classical conditioning.

Answer E is incorrect. Stimulus generalization is part of classical conditioning. This occurs when a new stimulus that is similar to an old stimulus elicits the same response.

2. **The correct answer is C.** Patients with generalized anxiety disorder (GAD) have uncontrollable anxiety unrelated to a specific person, situation, or event. In order for the diagnosis to be made, the patient must have experienced uncontrollable anxiety or worry out of proportion to his or her life events for at least 6 months. They also need three or more of the following symptoms: fatigability, irritability, in-ability to concentrate, insomnia, muscle tension, or restlessness. This patient complains of fatigue, insomnia, difficulty concentrating, and irritability in addition to generalized anxiety. Affected patients respond well to behavioral therapy and treatment with antidepressants and buspirone. Benzodiazepines can be used for short-term management but are not recommended for long-term management because of their addictive potential. GAD is often a chronic disease, but it can be controlled. Comorbid depression is common in GAD.

Answer A is incorrect. Adjustment disorder presents with depression and anxiety in the setting of a psychosocial stressor (e.g., divorce or job loss) in the past 6 months. This patient has been feeling anxiety and worry for 8 months.

Answer B is incorrect. Adult attention deficit/hyperactivity disorder (ADHD) is becoming recognized as an under-diagnosed condition; however, this patient has not developed the degree of impairment that would be expected with ADHD. Symptoms of ADHD include difficulty concentrating and irritability. A hallmark of adult ADHD can be difficulty at work, which this patient is not experiencing.

Answer D is incorrect. Signs and symptoms of hyperthyroidism include tachycardia, palpitations, isolated systolic hypertension (diastolic pressure is normal), anxiety, tremor, atrial fibrillation, diaphoresis, weight loss despite increased appetite, insomnia, fatigue, heat intolerance, exophthalmos, and diarrhea. The fact that this patient denies recent weight change and palpitations, that her vital signs are normal, and her physical exam is normal suggest that she is not suffering from hyperthyroidism.

Answer E is incorrect. Patients with social phobia disorder are anxious and nervous in social situations. This patient has a job with a significant social component in which she has been very successful.

3. **The correct answer is B.** Carbamazepine is an anticonvulsant that is also prescribed for mood stabilization in patients with mania, poor anger management, and lack of impulse control. Valproic acid is another anticonvulsant medication that is used for mood stabilization. Valproic acid and carbamazepine have a wider therapeutic range than lithium, although lithium is typically the first-line maintenance therapy in bipolar disorder.

Answer A is incorrect. Bupropion is an atypical antidepressant. More typical antidepressants, such as selective serotonin reuptake inhibitors (SSRIs), have a place in the treatment of bipolar disorder, but the effect on a patient's mood must be carefully monitored for a cycling into a manic state. Antidepressants are recommended for use in bipolar disorder only in combination with mood stabilizing drugs.

Answer C is incorrect. Fluoxetine is an SSRI that can elevate mood. Antidepressants have a place in the treatment of bipolar disorder, but the effect on a patient's mood must be carefully monitored for a cycling into a manic state. Antidepressants are recommended for use in bipolar disorder only in combination with mood stabilizing drugs.

Answer D is incorrect. Olanzapine is an atypical antipsychotic that can be used in manic patients with severe agitation and psychosis.

Answer E is incorrect. Reserpine depletes central and peripheral catecholamines and depresses sympathetic nerve function, resulting in vasodilation and sedation. This is a drug that can actually cause depression.

4. **The correct answer is A.** Cluster C personality disorders include avoidant, obsessive-compulsive, and dependent; patients with these disorders are characterized as anxious or worried and have abnormal fears about relationships, separation, and control. There is a genetic association with anxiety disorders. Patients with avoidant personality disorder are sensitive to rejection, socially inhibited, and timid, with overwhelming feelings of inadequacy.

Answer B is incorrect. Patients with dependent personality disorder are submissive and clinging; they have low self-esteem and have an excessive need to be taken care of.

Answer C is incorrect. Patients with histrionic personality disorder display excessive emotionality, somatization, and attention-seeking and sexually provocative behavior.

Answer D is incorrect. Patients with narcissistic personality disorder are grandiose and have a sense of entitlement. They frequently demand the best of everything, including physicians and health care.

Answer E is incorrect. Patients with schizoid personality disorder exhibit voluntary social withdrawal and have limited emotional expressions.

Answer F is incorrect. Patients with schizotypal personality disorder demonstrate interpersonal awkwardness, odd thought patterns, and an eccentric appearance.

5. **The correct answer is D.** Disorders of thought content include two types: ideas of reference and delusions. Ideas of reference are false convictions that one is the subject of attention by other people or the media. An example is a patient believing that she is being discussed on a national television program. Delusions are false beliefs not correctable by logic or reason. These beliefs are firmly held by the individual only and not shared by the culture. Delusions of persecution are the most common. Maintaining that one is married to a celebrity is another example of delusional thinking.

Answer A is incorrect. Disorders of affect include flat affect characteristic of schizophrenia and dementia (e.g., the patient is emotionally dull), constricted affect as seen in the narrow range of emotions in obsessive personality disorders (e.g., a patient always talks about his main interest, such as washing hands), and incongruous affect sometimes seen in bipolar disorder (e.g., the patient smiles as she describes a very sad event).

Answer B is incorrect. Disorders of cognition affect a patient's level of alertness and orientation. Cognitive disorders can manifest with problems in memory, calculation, and language.

Answer C is incorrect. Disorders of perception include illusions and hallucinations. Illusions are misperceptions of real external stimuli (e.g., a woman interprets the appearance of a dress in a dark closet as a person). Hallucinations are false sensory perceptions, and are most commonly auditory but can be visual, tactile, gustatory, or olfactory. An example of an auditory hallucination is a patient hearing two voices talking about her when she is alone in the room.

Answer E is incorrect. Disorders of thought process include (1) clang associations, or associating words by their sounds, not because of their logical meaning (e.g., a patient says, "I'm very sure I've got a cure, and I'm not pure."); (2) loose associations, in which ideas shift from one subject to another in an unrelated or only partially related fashion (e.g., a patient begins to answer a question about her parents, then launches into a diatribe about world hunger); (3) neologisms, or inventing new words; (4) perseveration, or repeating the same word or phrase over and over; (5) tangentiality, or beginning a response in a logical fashion but then getting further and further from the point (going off on a tangent); (6) thought blocking, or an abrupt halt in the train of thinking, often because of hallucinations; (7) "word salad," or uttering unrelated combinations of words or phrases (e.g., a patient says, "I'm not so utterly pure that I'm going to anyway to break it.").

6. **The correct answer is B.** Patients with disorganized schizophrenia have disorganized speech and behavior as well as an inappropriate affect. They are frequently childlike and are usually incapable of mustering complete delusions. This subtype is associated with a poor long-term prognosis.

Answer A is incorrect. Patients with catatonic schizophrenia are characterized by extreme stupor (most famously "waxy flexibility"), bi-zarre voluntary movements, and echolalia or echopraxia. This subtype is uncommon.

Answer C is incorrect. Patients with paranoid schizophrenia are characterized primarily by their delusions and hallucinations. In general, they exhibit less thought disorganization and have the best prognosis compared to other subtypes of schizophrenia.

Answer D is incorrect. Patients with residual schizophrenia have met the diagnostic criteria for schizophrenia in the past but are no longer actively psychotic (i.e., not actively delusional). These patients still retain some bizarre behavior patterns, bizarre speech patterns, or negative symptoms such as flat affect, social withdrawal, thought blocking, or lack of motivation.

Answer E is incorrect. Patients with undifferentiated schizophrenia show characteristics that are not exclusive to any one subtype. This is the most common presentation of schizophrenia.

7. **The correct answer is C.** This mature defense mechanism is humor. Humor is appreciating the amusing nature of an anxiety-provoking or adverse situation. The patient attempted to humiliate the doctor, but the situation is relayed to others in an amusing fashion. This is the only **mature** defense mechanism among the answer choices.

Answer A is incorrect. This immature defense mechanism is isolation. Isolation is separation of feelings from ideas and events, such as describing a murder in graphic detail with no emotional response.

Answer B is incorrect. This immature defense mechanism is displacement. He is avoiding his feelings and transferring them to a neutral person, his son.

Answer D is incorrect. This immature defense mechanism is splitting. Splitting is the belief that something is all good or bad. In this case, he is quitting since he believes all his patients are rude.

Answer E is incorrect. This immature defense mechanism is repression. He is withholding his feelings from conscious awareness.

8. **The correct answer is C.** SSRIs such as fluoxetine are the treatment of choice for social phobia disorders. They lack abuse potential and the side effects are generally well tolerated. Social phobia is an irrational fear of social or performance situations that the patient recognizes as irrational. Patients can begin to avoid all social situations in order to avert the unpleasant feelings that are aroused. Social phobia tends to have an insidious onset and remains a chronic problem. Relapse is common after pharmacologic therapy is stopped.

Answer A is incorrect. Tricyclic antidepressants (TCAs) such as amitriptyline are not first-line treatment for social phobia. They are considered to be less effective than the SSRIs.

Answer B is incorrect. Buspirone is not an effective treatment for social phobia. Buspirone is prescribed for patients with generalized anxiety disorder and acts as an anxiolytic.

Answer D is incorrect. Propranolol is a nonspecific β-blocker that is useful in treating patients with performance anxiety but is not as useful in patients with a nonspecific social phobia.

Answer E is incorrect. Valproate is an anticonvulsant that is being investigated for the treatment of social phobia, but no recommendations for its use in social phobia exist.

9. **The correct answer is B.** This patient is displaying signs of tardive dyskinesia, which is a complication of long-term antipsychotic therapy with the older agents. It is thought to result from increased dopamine receptor synthesis in response to long-term receptor blockade, which increases the sensitivity of dopamine at its receptors and causes the dopamine effects to disrupt the balance with cholinergic input. This leads to excessive involuntary movements. Of the drugs listed, fluphenazine, a typical neuroleptic agent, would be the most likely agent to have caused this condition.

Answer A is incorrect. Clozapine, an atypical antipsychotic that modulates both serotoninergic and dopaminergic neurons in the central nervous system, has a much lower risk of tardive dyskinesia than typical antipsychotics such as haloperidol or fluphenazine, which affect dopaminergic 'receptors only'. The most concerning adverse effect of clozapine is agranulocytosis, which can be fatal if untreated.

Answer C is incorrect. Lithium is a mood stabilizer that is primarily used to treat episodes of mania in patients with bipolar disorder. It is not used to treat schizophrenia and does not cause tardive dyskinesia. Adverse effects include nephrogenic diabetes insipidus, nausea, anorexia, and mild diarrhea.

Answer D is incorrect. Risperidone, like clozapine, is an atypical antipsychotic that has a lower incidence of tardive dyskinesia in comparison with typical antipsychotics such as haloperidol, thioridazine, and fluphenazine. More common adverse effects include drowsiness, weight gain, hypotension, elevated prolactin levels, constipation, cough, and diarrhea.

Answer E is incorrect. Selegiline, a monoamine oxidase B inhibitor, is used to treat Parkinson's disease; it has no role in the treatment of schizophrenia. Adverse effects include gastrointestinal upset, nausea, heartburn, and dry mouth.

10. **The correct answer is A.** The patient is exhibiting extrapyramidal adverse effects associated with neuroleptic use. Of the choices listed, only chlorpromazine is a neuroleptic. Typical antipsychotics work by decreasing the amount of dopamine available in the brain; the extrapyramidal adverse effects are the result of blocking the dopamine receptors. Antipsychotics typically associated with extrapyramidal symptoms include, but are not limited to, haloperidol, fluphenazine, perphenazine, and thioridazine.

Answer B is incorrect. Adverse effects include sedation, orthostatic hypotension, weight gain, and sexual disturbances. Severe adverse effects can be remembered by the mnemonic "3 C's": Convulsions, Coma, and Cardiotoxicity (conduction defects and arrhythmias). TCAs primarily have anticholinergic adverse effects as well, including dry mouth, mydriasis, constipation, and urinary retention. These drugs are extremely dangerous in overdose.

Answer C is incorrect. Lithium intake has been associated with tremor, hypothyroidism, and nephrogenic diabetes insipidus. Lithium does not have dopaminergic blockade activity, and thus is not associated with extrapyramidal symptoms.

Answer D is incorrect. Mirtazapine is an antidepressant whose common adverse effects include sedation and weight gain. The hypothesized mechanism of action of mirtazapine combines 5-HT$_2$ receptor and α-adrenoceptor antagonism.

Answer E is incorrect. Sertraline is an SSRI associated with anxiety, insomnia, tremor, and nausea. It may lead to serotonin syndrome that may be characterized by a progression of headaches, dizziness, vomiting, coma, and death if taken with monoamine oxidase inhibitors.

Answer F is incorrect. Trazodone is a heterocyclic associated with sedation, nausea, priapism, and postural hypotension.

11. **The correct answer is D.** Tranylcypromine is a nonselective monoamine oxidase inhibitor and may lead to serotonin syndrome if taken with SSRIs due to an overall increase in serotonin. Serotonin syndrome is characterized by mental status changes, autonomic changes (e.g., fever, diaphoresis, tachycardia), and neuromuscular changes (e.g., tremor or rigidity). The treatment of serotonin syndrome consists of prompt discontinuation of the implicated agent(s) and supportive care including intravenous fluids, benzodiazepines for control of delirium, cooling measure for hyperthermia, and neuromuscular blockers such as dantrolene for hyperthermia, muscle rigidity, and the prevention of rhabdomyolysis.

Answer A is incorrect. Citalopram is an SSRI associated with anxiety, insomnia, tremor, and nausea. While both sertraline and citalopram have serotonergic effects, the combined use of two SSRIs has not been shown to produce serotonin syndrome.

Answer B is incorrect. Lithium intake has been associated with tremor, hypothyroidism, and nephrogenic diabetes insipidus. While lithium is considered as an effective adjunctive therapy for depression in combination with a second antidepressant, lithium prescribed as monotherapy for depression is not recommended.

Answer C is incorrect. Nortriptyline is a TCA associated with the "3 C's": Convulsions, Coma, and Cardiotoxicity (conduction defects and arrhythmias). TCAs primarily have anticholinergic adverse effects as well, including dry mouth, mydriasis, constipation, and urinary retention.

Answer E is incorrect. Trazodone is a heterocyclic associated with sedation, nausea, priapism, and postural hypotension.

12. **The correct answer is D.** Over the course of two visits, the patient has exhibited psychotic and residual symptoms characteristic of schizophrenia and related disorders. A diagnosis of schizophrenia, however, requires active phase ("positive") symptoms, and may include "negative" ones as well, over a period of >6 months. In this case, the patient's symptoms have lasted <4 months, and were potentially incited by a traumatic event and its repercussions. If the symptoms had lasted <1 month, a diagnosis of brief psychotic disorder would be accurate; in such a diagnosis, most patients make a full recovery. In this patient, symptoms with a duration of >1 month but <6 months yield a diagnosis of schizophreniform disorder. Negative symptoms, as seen here, worsen the prognosis of a patient with schizophreniform disorder.

Answer A is incorrect. There is no evidence that either the patient or his mother is actively seeking the attention of medical personnel, or that the symptoms experienced were falsified for secondary gain of tangible items such as food, shelter, or money, as would be the case in malingering.

Answer B is incorrect. The diagnosis of a schizoaffective disorder requires the symptoms of schizophrenia (often both "positive" and "negative" symptoms) as well as those of a mood disorder (i.e., depression, mania). These patients typically have less cognitive impairment than those with strict psychotic disorders.

Answer C is incorrect. Explicit in the diagnosis of schizophrenia is the presence of "positive" and (but not always) "negative" symptoms of >6 months' duration. Many patients with a prior diagnosis of schizophreniform disorder eventually receive a diagnosis of schizophrenia.

Answer E is incorrect. Delusions are fixed, false beliefs or ideas by a patient that are not shared by other individuals. Delusional disorder refers to a pathologic state whereby construct(s) of delusions impair one's social and/or cognitive functioning. Shared delusions are those transmitted from one person to another in a parent-to-child or spouse-to-spouse relationship. There is no evidence presented that the patient's mother shares the false beliefs of her son.

13. **The correct answer is A.** Illusions (misperceptions that the deceased person is still present) can occur during the normal grieving process, but delusions or hallucinations are seen only in abnormal, or pathologic, grieving.

    Answer B is incorrect. The normal grieving process involves signs of depression. However, if these depressive symptoms last >2 years after the death of the loved one, then the survivor is experiencing abnormal (pathologic) grief.

    Answer C is incorrect. Severe symptoms of grief should subside after 2 months, and more moderate symptoms should subside after 1–2 years. Still, it is common for grieving patients to experience feelings of grief on special occasions years after their loved one's death. This "anniversary reaction" is not considered to be pathologic as long as it occurs at these specific times.

    Answer D is incorrect. It is normal for a grieving person to feel some guilt after the death of a loved one. However, extreme guilt or feelings of worthlessness are symptoms of pathologic grief, which needs psychiatric treatment.

Answer E is incorrect. Both normal grief and pathologic grief are characterized by shock, and even denial, after the death has occurred. Although denial typically lasts a few hours in normal grief, it can last for many weeks in pathologic grief.

14. **The correct answer is C.** Depression is often associated with disrupted sleep. Specifically, sleep studies of depressed patients often reveal increased time spent in REM sleep, decreased REM latency, and decreased delta waves, which are characteristic of stages III and IV sleep. Patients with depression often experience decreased daytime energy and motivation to complete tasks; these are commonly misdiagnosed as adverse effects of poor sleep rather than warning signs of depression. Fluoxetine, an SSRI, is an appropriate first-line agent for patients with depression. This provider should also consider referral to a psychiatrist for management of this patient's depression.

    Answer A is incorrect. Avoidance of caffeine is particularly helpful in patients suffering from insomnia, defined as a difficulty falling asleep or staying asleep three times per week for at least 1 month. Although avoidance of caffeine may help this patient with her sleep disturbances, her specific sleep patterns indicate concern for depression, thus further evaluation and treatment with an SSRI should be considered.

    Answer B is incorrect. Continuous positive airway pressure would be helpful in a patient suffering from sleep apnea, which occurs when a person briefly stops breathing during the night and awakens from sleep. Patients with severe sleep apnea might awaken hundreds of times per night. This patient's polysomnographic tracing is not consistent with sleep apnea.

    Answer D is incorrect. Methylphenidate is used to treat narcolepsy, or sudden sleep attacks during the day despite normal nighttime sleep.

    Answer E is incorrect. Normal sleep patterns in young adults include 25% of total sleep time spent in REM sleep and 25% of total sleep time spent in delta wave (stages III and IV) sleep.

15. The correct answer is B. This patient is showing both "positive" and "negative" symptoms of schizophrenia; thus it would have been appropriate for her physician to prescribe a trial dose of an atypical antipsychotic agent. Clozapine, an atypical antipsychotic, may lead to agranulocytosis, most commonly within 6 months of beginning therapy. Agranulocytosis commonly manifests as severe sore throat and fevers, or other risks of infections. If the patients' lab data are consistent with agranulocytosis (severe leukopenia), clozapine should be replaced by an alternative antipsychotic agent such as risperidone.

Answer A is incorrect. Clomipramine, a tricyclic antidepressant, is commonly prescribed to treat obsessive compulsive disorder. Its adverse effects includes sedation and dry mouth (anticholinergic effects), potential for increased cardiac conduction intervals and arrhythmias with risk of ventricular tachycardia/ventricular fibrillation in extreme dosing, and risk of seizure in overdose.

Answer C is incorrect. Haloperidol, a dopamine receptor antagonist, was previously commonly prescribed to treat schizophrenia. Haloperidol's first-line use has largely been replaced by atypical antipsychotics because of its adverse effects, including acute dystonia, akinesia, akathisia, tardive dyskinesia, gynecomastia, dry mouth, and sedation.

Answer D is incorrect. Lithium is a mood stabilizer commonly prescribed for patients with bipolar affective disorder. This patient's symptoms are not consistent with bipolar disorder, which requires both mania and depression or both hypomania and depression for diagnosis. Adverse effects of lithium include nephrogenic diabetes insipidus, tremor, and hypothyroidism.

Answer E is incorrect. Risperidone, an atypical antipsychotic agent, would be appropriate for the treatment of schizophrenia. It is not associated with agranulocytosis.

16. The correct answer is B. Children with ADHD demonstrate persistent symptoms of inattention, hyperactivity, and impulsivity that have persisted for at least 6 months and are maladaptive and disruptive to the child's life. These children are often difficult to control in the classroom.

Answer A is incorrect. Patients with antisocial personality disorder show a disregard for and violation of the rights of others, including a proclivity for criminal behavior. To receive this diagnosis, patients must be >18 years old; minors with similar behavior are considered to have conduct disorder. This is the only personality disorder in which males outnumber females.

Answer C is incorrect. Bipolar disorder can be diagnosed in children; however, this patient is not exhibiting characteristics of bipolar disorder. These characteristics include periods of mania followed by depression. Mania commonly manifests as irritability and belligerence in children, which differs from the euphoria often seen in manic adults. This child is not experiencing cyclical changes in mood.

Answer D is incorrect. Conduct disorder can exist in children with attention deficit/hyperactivity disorder, but at this point the patient is not exhibiting diagnostic characteristics such as aggression, inflicting harm on animals, destruction of property, deceitfulness, or serious violations of rules.

Answer E is incorrect. Children with separation anxiety disorder display signs of distress such as acting out or crying when they are forced to leave people they are attached to (usually parents). The mean age of onset is around 6–7 years, which is consistent with this patient's age. However, problems with following through on tasks are not characteristic of separation anxiety disorder.

17. The correct answer is B. This patient has physical signs consistent with anorexia nervosa, most notably a low body mass index, bradycardia, evidence of hypotension, lanugo, and concomitant depression. Anorexia nervosa is a serious condition that requires intensive mental health care, as well as close medical monitoring of weight, electrolyte levels, and hydration status. The mainstay of therapy is a combination of cognitive behavioral therapy and SSRIs. Use of the antidepressant bupropion is contraindicated in patients with anorexia nervosa because it increases the risk of seizure in this population.

Answer A is incorrect. Amitriptyline is a TCA. TCAs, although effective, are not first-line therapy in the management of anorexia nervosa, given the potential for cardiac adverse effects in anorexic patients already suffering from bradycardia and electrolyte abnormalities. TCAs are not known to increase the risk of seizure in anorexic patients.

Answer C is incorrect. Fluoxetine is an SSRI most commonly used as an antidepressant. It has also been used to treat anorexia nervosa, although with questionable efficacy. SSRIs are not known to increase the risk of seizure in anorexic patients.

Answer D is incorrect. Mirtazapine in an atypical antidepressant that induces weight gain, which may be beneficial in patients with weight control issues, although this has not yet been studied rigorously. Mirtazapine is not known to increase the risk of seizure in anorexic patients.

Answer E is incorrect. Selegiline is a monoamine oxidase inhibitor most commonly used as an antidepressant; it is not typically used to manage anorexia nervosa. Monoamine oxidase inhibitors are not known to increase the risk of seizure in anorexic patients.

18. **The correct answer is D.** SSRIs block the reuptake of serotonin (5-hydroxytryptamine [5-HT]) by the serotonin transport protein (STP) in presynaptic neurons; the result is an effective increase in serotonin within the synaptic space. SSRIs act at the "X" in the image by inhibiting the binding of 5-HT to STP. SSRIs have demonstrated efficacy for numerous medical and psychiatric conditions, most notably depression, anxiety, obsessive-compulsive disorder, and eating disorders.

Answer A is incorrect. SSRIs are not first-line treatment for bipolar disorder; a mood stabilizing agent (e.g., lithium or valproic acid) would be the treatment of choice.

Answer B is incorrect. SSRIs are not first-line treatment for delirium tremens; a long-acting benzodiazepine (e.g., chlordiazepoxide) would be the treatment of choice.

Answer C is incorrect. SSRIs are not first-line treatment for multiple personality disorder; an antipsychotic (e.g., haloperidol or risperidone) would be the treatment of choice.

Answer E is incorrect. SSRIs are not first-line treatment for schizophrenia; an antipsychotic (e.g., haloperidol or risperidone) would be the treatment of choice.

19. **The correct answer is A.** This patient is suffering from tardive dyskinesia, which is a known extrapyramidal adverse effect of antipsychotics, usually occurring after **4 months** of therapy; it is usually irreversible. Other extrapyramidal adverse effects of antipsychotic agents include acute dystonia (after **4 hours**), akinesia (after **4 days**), and akathisia (after **4 weeks**). Tardive dyskinesia commonly manifests as involuntary, stereotyped movements of the trunk, extremities, face, or lips, along with repetitive thrusting or protrusion of the tongue. It is believed to be due to sensitization and/or upregulation of dopamine receptors. Discontinuing the responsible antipsychotic is the preferred treatment. However, if therapy must continue, an atypical antipsychotic may cause fewer extrapyramidal adverse effects. Clozapine has been demonstrated to be particularly effective, although it has the serious adverse effect of causing agranulocytosis.

Answer B is incorrect. Anorgasmia is an adverse effect of SSRI therapy. SSRIs are commonly used to treat depression and anxiety disorders; they are not indicated for the treatment of psychotic symptoms.

Answer C is incorrect. Diabetes insipidus is an adverse effect of lithium therapy. Lithium is a mood stabilizer commonly used to treat bipolar disorder; it is not indicated for the treatment of psychotic symptoms.

Answer D is incorrect. Hypertension is an adverse effect of venlafaxine, which inhibits the reuptake of serotonin, as well as norepinephrine and dopamine. It is commonly used to treat depression and anxiety disorders; it is not indicated for the treatment of psychotic symptoms.

Answer E is incorrect. Respiratory depression is an adverse effect of benzodiazepines and barbiturates, which are used to treat anxiety disorder; they are not indicated for the treatment of psychotic symptoms.

20. **The correct answer is B.** This patient has acute dystonia, which is an extrapyramidal adverse effect of antipsychotics, usually occurring after **4 hours** of therapy; it is easily treatable. Other extrapyramidal adverse effects of antipsychotic agents include akinesia (after **4 days**), akathisia (after **4 weeks**), and tardive dyskinesia (after **4 months**). Acute dystonia is usually most pronounced in the facial muscles and involves involuntary, sustained, and repetitive muscle spasms, which may manifest as torticollis or oculogyric crisis. Anticholinergic medications (e.g., benztropine) rapidly relieve the symptoms; anticholinergics may be given prophylactically with the initial administration of antipsychotics to prevent the onset of acute dystonia.

Answer A is incorrect. β-Blockers are used to treat extrapyramidal symptoms, particularly in patients with akathisia. They will not remedy the patient's acute dystonic symptoms.

Answer C is incorrect. Antiepileptics are used to treat seizure disorders. Acute dystonia is not related to seizure activity; therefore, antiepileptic therapy will not remedy the patient's acute dystonic symptoms.

Answer D is incorrect. Atypical antipsychotics have a lower associated incidence of extrapyramidal adverse effects. However, switching antipsychotics will not remedy the patient's acute dystonic symptoms.

Answer E is incorrect. Dopamine agonists are used to treat extrapyramidal symptoms, particularly in patients with dyskinesia. They will not relieve the patient's acute dystonic symptoms.

Answer F is incorrect. Mood stabilizers are often concurrently administered in psychiatric patients with schizoaffective disorders. However, they will not remedy the patient's acute dystonic symptoms.

CHAPTER 15

Renal

QUESTIONS

1. Patients with renal artery stenosis may present with very high blood pressures due to increased renin secretion. Which of the following structures in the kidney is responsible for sensing inadequate perfusion and secreting renin?

   (A) Afferent arteriole
   (B) Collecting duct
   (C) Distal convoluted tubule
   (D) Efferent arteriole
   (E) Loop of Henle

2. A 48-year-old man is hospitalized for shock after massive blood loss in a motor vehicle accident. On the patient's second day in the hospital, his blood urea nitrogen (BUN) and creatinine levels begin to rise and he develops pitting edema to his knees. A subsequent urinalysis shows numerous granular casts. Which of the following is the most appropriate treatment?

   (A) Angioplasty
   (B) Broad-spectrum antibiotics
   (C) Corticosteroids
   (D) Fluids and dialysis
   (E) Use of ultrasound to remove blockage

3. A 64-year-old man with a medical history significant for hypertension, hypercholesterolemia, and coronary artery disease comes to the emergency department because of blood in his urine, nausea, and vomiting. Urinalysis reveals reddish-colored urine with no RBCs, but is positive for granular casts and protein. A basic metabolic panel shows highly elevated BUN and creatinine levels with a BUN:creatinine ratio of 10:1, as well as severe uremia. He is declared to be in acute renal failure and placed on dialysis. This patient has recently started a new drug prescribed by his family physician. Which of the following is the most likely cause of this patient's renal failure?

   (A) A β-blocker
   (B) An autoimmune reaction
   (C) A statin drug
   (D) Trauma

4. Respiratory acidosis is a major complication in morphine overdoses. Which of the following laboratory data correspond to a pure respiratory acidosis?

Choice	pH	P_{CO_2} (mm Hg)	HCO_3^- (mEq/L)	Na^+ (mEq/L)	Cl^- (mEq/L)
A	7.2	42	15	140	89
B	7.2	42	15	140	114
C	7.2	68	15	140	104
D	7.2	68	25	140	104
E	7.4	68	12	140	89
F	7.6	42	20	140	104
G	7.6	68	18	140	104

   (A) A
   (B) B
   (C) C
   (D) D
   (E) E
   (F) F
   (G) G

5. Monitoring acid-base status is very important in individuals with kidney pathology. Which of the following diuretics causes metabolic alkalosis?

   (A) Acetazolamide and potassium-sparing diuretics
   (B) Loop diuretics and acetazolamide
   (C) Loop diuretics and potassium-sparing diuretics
   (D) Loop diuretics and thiazides
   (E) Thiazides and acetazolamide
   (F) Thiazides and potassium-sparing diuretics

6. A 25-year-old man comes to the emergency department with bloody sputum. A few weeks later he progresses to renal failure with significant hematuria and hypertension. A renal biopsy shows linear immunofluorescence. Which of the following types of hypersensitivity reaction is this patient experiencing?

(A) Type I hypersensitivity
(B) Type II hypersensitivity
(C) Type III hypersensitivity
(D) Type IV hypersensitivity

7. A 7-year-old boy with nephrotic syndrome is brought by ambulance to the emergency department with altered mental status. His mother reports that this morning he had difficulty moving the right side of his body, and that she couldn't arouse him from an afternoon nap. On physical examination the patient is obtunded and has absent right-sided movement. His prothrombin time is 12 seconds. CT of the brain is shown in the image. What is the most likely etiology of this patient's symptoms?

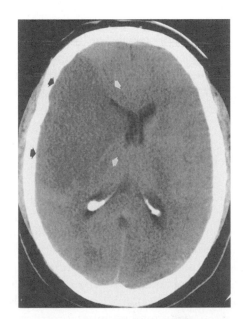

Reproduced, with permission, from Chen MYM, Pope TL, Ott DJ. *Basic Radiology.* New York: McGraw-Hill, 2004: Figure 12-17, A.

(A) Decreased antithrombin III levels
(B) Decreased factor II levels
(C) Decreased fibrinogen levels
(D) Increased protein S levels
(E) Increased protein C levels

8. A 28-year-old woman who is 6 months pregnant presents to the emergency department with a temperature of 38.2° C (100.8° F) and complains of shaking chills and pain on her right side, which she locates by pointing to the area above her right iliac crest. During the examination she is tender to percussion at the junction of the lower ribs and the thoracic vertebrae. Urinalysis reveals WBC casts. Which of the following is the most likely diagnosis?

(A) Abdominal aortic aneurysm
(B) Appendicitis
(C) Ectopic pregnancy
(D) Localized cystitis
(E) Premature labor
(F) Pyelonephritis

9. A 64-year-old man presents to his primary care physician for a routine physical. He is in good health, smokes half a pack of cigarettes a day, and has no concomitant medical problems. However, he tells the physician that he has been diagnosed with hypertension in the past. In the course of the physical examination, the physician notes a blood pressure of 160/100 mm Hg and 1+ pitting edema to his knees. The physician also notes bilateral bruits when auscultating the abdomen. Which of the following is contraindicated in this patient's care?

(A) Angioplasty
(B) Angiotensin-converting enzyme inhibitor
(C) Diuretics
(D) Smoking cessation
(E) Surgical management

10. A 2-month-old infant is found to have a horse-shoe kidney. Which structure prevents this abnormal kidney from occupying its appropriate position?

(A) Aorta
(B) Celiac trunk
(C) Inferior mesenteric artery
(D) Inferior vena cava
(E) Superior mesenteric artery

11. A 23-year-old man is beginning chemotherapy for leukemia when he develops severe intermittent left flank pain that soon migrates to the pelvis. Three days later, the patient's creatinine level rises and he is diagnosed with acute renal failure. His fractional excretion of sodium is >4% with a urine osmolality of <350 mOsm/kg. Blood and urine cultures are negative for bacteria and eosinophilia. An abdominal radiograph fails to locate any pathology. Which of the following is the most likely location of the lesion causing this patient's renal failure?

(A) Glomeruli
(B) Interstitium of the kidney
(C) Kidney tubules
(D) Spleen
(E) Urethra

12. A 68-year-old white woman recovering from a total hip replacement following a fall at home is administered ketorolac for the management of pain. Twenty-four hours later, her urine production decreases, and her serum BUN and creatinine levels rise to 44 mg/dL and 3.1 mg/dL, respectively. Which of the following describes the mechanism through which nonsteroidal anti-inflammatory drugs, such as ketorolac, cause acute renal failure?

(A) Inhibition of renal prostaglandin production and constriction of the afferent arteriole
(B) Inhibition of renal prostaglandin production and constriction of the efferent arteriole
(C) Inhibition of renal prostaglandin production and significant dilation of glomerular efferent arterioles
(D) Stimulation of renal prostaglandin produc-

tion and reflex arteriolar vasoconstriction
(E) Stimulation of renal prostaglandin production and reflex arteriolar vasodilation

13. A 56-year-old man with a 60 pack-year smoking history and normal fluid intake presents to his physician with 2 months of fatigue and weakness accompanied by cough and mild dyspnea. The patient's vital signs are normal, but a lower left lobe mass is noted on x-ray of the chest. Biopsy leads to the diagnosis of small cell carcinoma. Laboratory tests show:

Plasma Na$^+$: 125 mEq/L
Plasma K$^+$: 3.9 mEq/L
Plasma CO$_2$: 24 mEq/L
Plasma osmolality: 253 mOsm/L
Urine Na$^+$: 48 mEq/L
Urine osmolality: 280 mOsm/L

The hormone most likely responsible for this patient's abnormal laboratory values has which of the following direct effects?

(A) Activation of G-protein coupled receptors in the adrenal cortex elevates cAMP levels and leads to increased production and secretion of corticosteroids
(B) Activation of G-protein coupled receptors in the hypothalamus results in elevated cAMP levels and inhibition of hypothalamic-induced thirst mechanism
(C) Cleavage of angiotensinogen to angiotensin I leads to an increase in both aldosterone levels and total peripheral resistance
(D) Activation of V2 receptors leads to an increase in total peripheral resistance; activation of V1 receptors results in the concentration of urine
(E) Activation of V2 receptors results in the insertion of aquaporins into the collecting duct; activation of V1 receptors leads to a decrease in total peripheral resistance
(F) Activation of V2 receptors results in the insertion of aquaporins into the renal collecting duct; activation of V1 receptors leads to an increase in total peripheral resistance

14. A 24-year-old man who is in the hospital for treatment of a severe gram-negative infection subsequently becomes oliguric. He is also having difficulty hearing the hospital staff. Laboratory studies show elevated BUN and creatinine levels. Which of the following is the most likely cause of this patient's symptoms?

Alports

(A) Chloramphenicol
(B) Doxycycline
(C) Erythromycin
(D) Gentamicin
(E) Imipenem

15. A 50-year-old man with a history of large bowel obstruction is diagnosed with colon cancer and undergoes resection of his colon. He returns to his physician for his regular checkup and complains that in the past 3 weeks he has not been feeling well and has noticed significant swelling of his legs. On physical examination, the physician notes 2+ pitting edema and a blood pressure of 155/94 mm Hg. Urinalysis shows 4+ protein with no RBCs or casts. The patient has otherwise been healthy. Which of the following would most likely be present on a kidney biopsy from this patient?

(A) A spike-and-dome pattern of deposition on electron microscopy
(B) A tram-track pattern on light microscopy
(C) Lumpy subepithelial deposits on light microscopy
(D) Nonlinear mesangial staining with IgA immunofluorescence
(E) "Splintering" of the lamina densa

16. A 35-year-old woman presents to the emergency department after experiencing the acute onset of right flank pain and fever. Laboratory results show white cell casts in the urine. Which of the following is the most prominent cell type found in the infiltrate of the involved organ?

(A) Macrophage
(B) Monocyte
(C) Plasma cell
(D) Polymorphonuclear leukocytes
(E) T lymphocyte

17. A 67-year-old woman with osteoporosis is given a diuretic to treat her hypertension. This particular diuretic has the adverse effect of limiting calcium excretion by the kidney. Referring to the image, where along the nephron does this drug act?

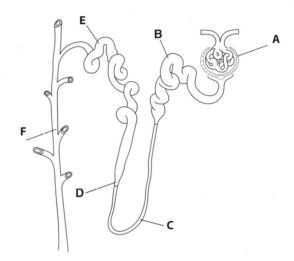

Reproduced, with permission, from USMLERx.com.

(A) A
(B) B
(C) C
(D) D
(E) E
(F) F

18. A 22-year-old college student is brought to the emergency department after he began complaining of ants crawling over his body and his friends noted increasing agitation and threatening gestures. On physical examination he is febrile, restless, and tachycardic, and his pupils are markedly dilated. Appropriate treatment would most likely include which of the following?

(A) Acidifying urine to increase renal clearance

(B) Alkalinizing urine to increase renal clearance

(C) Treating with flumazenil

(D) Treating with naloxone

(E) Treating with water to dilute drug effects

19. A 19-year-old woman with a severe gastrointestinal infection presents to the emergency department with a 5-day history of vomiting and diarrhea. Serum chemistry tests show:

Na⁺: 138 mEq/L
K⁺: 3.0 mEq/L
Cl⁻: 88 mEq/L
HCO₃⁻: 21 mEq/L;
BUN: 10 mg/dL
Creatinine: 0.8 mg/dL
Glucose: 101 mg/dL

Arterial blood gas analyses shows a pH of 7.38, partial arterial carbon dioxide pressure of 37 mm Hg, partial arterial oxygen pressure of 82 mm Hg, and an oxygen saturation of 96% on room air. Which of the following statements is most accurate regarding this patient's acid-base status?

(A) She has a metabolic acidosis

(B) She has a mixed metabolic alkalosis and metabolic acidosis

(C) She has a mixed respiratory alkalosis and respiratory acidosis

(D) She has no acid-base disturbances

(E) She has a respiratory alkalosis

20. A 59-year-old woman with type 2 diabetes mellitus comes to her primary care physician for a routine visit. Her creatinine level has been slowly increasing over the last decade due to poor compliance with her medical regimen. If her renal disease were to progress, she would be at risk for developing which of the following conditions?

(A) Bacteriuria

(B) Hypokalemia

(C) Hypotension

(D) Metabolic alkalosis

(E) Osteomalacia

(F) Polycythemia

21. A 16-year-old boy comes to the physician with a 1-year history of intermittent, painless hematuria without dysuria or increased frequency of micturition. He says he has also had several respiratory infections and adds that the hematuria increased within several days of the infections. Which of the following is most likely to be found if the boy is diagnosed with IgA nephropathy (Berger's disease)?

(A) Increased antistreptolysin O titer

(B) Lumpy-bumpy electron-dense deposits

(C) Mesangial deposits

(D) Proteinuria exceeding 3.5 gm/24 h

(E) Subepithelial deposits

22. A 34-year-old woman comes to the hospital to deliver a full-term infant. The labor is complicated by an amniotic fluid embolism, and subsequent blood tests show the presence of fibrin split products. The next day the patient abruptly develops anuria, gross hematuria, and flank pain accompanied by rapidly increasing BUN and creatinine levels and a new cardiac friction rub. The patient's CT scan demonstrates hypodensities within the renal cortex. Which of the following is the correct treatment?

(A) Aggressive fluid support

(B) Biopsy to evaluate for malignancy

(C) Broad-spectrum antibiotics

(D) Dialysis

(E) No treatment is necessary at this time

23. A 40-year-old man presents to his physician with sharp, sudden, sporadic pain in his lower back and hematuria. His blood pressure is normal and his physical examination is significant for flank pain. A plain film of the pelvis does

not show any renal calculi. Which of the following is the most likely cause of this man's symptoms?

(A) Hyperparathyroidism
(B) Hyperuricemia
(C) Infection with *Proteus vulgaris*
(D) Prostate cancer
(E) Staphylococcal infection

24. Angiotensin II (AT II) stimulates the Na⁺-H⁺ exchanger in the proximal tubule. How does this affect the handling of HCO_3^- and H^+ in the proximal tubule?

CHOICE	NET HCO_3^- RESORPTION	NET H^+ RESORPTION
A	↓	↓
B	no effect	no effect
C	no effect	↑
D	↑	no effect
E	↑	↑

(A) A
(B) B
(C) C
(D) D
(E) E

25. A patient is recovering at the hospital from a suspected bacterial pneumonia. Over the course of a few days he develops fever, rash, dysuria, and urinary urgency. Urinalysis shows a specific gravity of 1.001 with hematuria and mild proteinuria. Renal biopsy shows partial effacement of the tubulointerstitial structures with pronounced edema and infiltration of the interstitium with polymorphonuclear leukocytes, eosinophils, and lymphocytes with papil-

lary necrosis. What is most likely to have caused this condition?

(A) Antibiotics
(B) Chronic hypertension
(C) Lead ingestion
(D) Multiple myeloma
(E) Wegener's granulomatosis

26. A 56-year-old woman who has been taking cefoxitin for treatment of *Klebsiella* pneumonia is found to still have *Klebsiella* organisms in her blood 1 week after beginning treatment. Another drug is added to the patient's regimen. Two days later, laboratory tests show:

Na⁺: 141 mEq/L
K⁺: 4.3 mEq/L
Cl⁻: 102 mEq/L
HCO_3^-: 24 mEq/L
BUN: 65 mg/dL
Creatinine: 4.4 mEq/L

Which of the following medications was most likely added to this patient's regimen?

(A) Azithromycin
(B) Aztreonam
(C) Clindamycin
(D) Piperacillin
(E) Tobramycin

27. A 2-year-old boy is brought to the emergency department with complaints of fever, chills, and flank pain. His immunizations are up to date and his mother states that this is the second time he has been seen because of these symptoms. His temperature is 39.1° C (102.2° F) and physical examination is unremarkable except for costovertebral angle tenderness on the right. A complete blood cell count shows leukocytosis, and urinalysis demonstrates the presence of WBCs and RBCs in the urine. What is the most likely mechanism of this patient's recurrent complaints?

(A) Immunoglobulin deficiency
(B) Nephroblastoma
(C) Poststreptococcal glomerulonephritis
(D) Vesicoureteral reflux

28. ADH exerts its effects on the collecting ducts of the kidney. Which of the following best characterizes ADH activity, as depicted in the image?

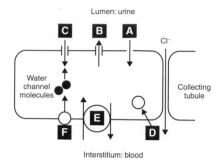

Reproduced, with permission, from USMLERx.com.

(A) Binds and blocks A
(B) Binds and blocks C
(C) Binds at F and activates G_i-mediated cyclic adenosine monophosphate cascade
(D) Binds at F and activates G_s-mediated cyclic adenosine monophosphate cascade
(E) Stimulates D

29. A 40-year-old woman presents to the emergency department after a 5-day course of profuse vomiting. She has a history of rheumatoid arthritis, which is treated with celecoxib. She complains of joint pain at present. Which of the reasons below describes why celecoxib would be contraindicated in this patient at presentation?

(A) Because of its effects on platelet function
(B) Because of its effects on the arterioles of the kidney
(C) Because of its effects on the gastrointestinal mucosa
(D) Because of its effects on the macula densa
(E) Because of its effects on the production of inflammatory cytokines

30. A medical student is doing research to measure the effects of newly bioengineered molecules on the function of the glomerulus. Which of the following mechanisms is likely to result in an overall increase in renal blood flow?

(A) Stimulation of afferent α-adrenergic receptors alone
(B) Stimulation of afferent AT II receptors alone
(C) Stimulation of AT II receptors and opening of vascular smooth muscle stretch-activated calcium channels
(D) Stimulation of renal dopamine and bradykinin receptors
(E) Stimulation of renal α-adrenergic and AT II receptors

31. An 18-year-old woman presents to the emergency department with a 3-day history of worsening fever and redness in her right foot. On examination, the patient is found to have erythema around a puncture wound in her foot. The patient is admitted to the hospital and given intravenous penicillin and nonsteroidal anti-inflammatory drugs, which decrease the erythema, pain, and swelling. Three days later the patient develops new onset of weakness, fatigue, rash, and fever. Significant laboratory findings include a BUN level of 45 mg/dL and a creatinine level of 2.8 mg/dL. Urinalysis shows WBC casts, eosinophils, and a fractional excretion of sodium of 2.5%. Which of the following is the most likely cause of her new onset of illness?

(A) Intravenous antibiotics
(B) Poststreptococcal glomerulonephritis
(C) Septic shock
(D) Systemic lupus erythematosus
(E) Urolithiasis

32. A diet high in sodium can contribute to hypertension. Which of the following is a mechanism of how the kidney responds to high sodium intake?

(A) Decrease in atrial natriuretic peptide and constriction of glomerular afferent arterioles
(B) Decrease in sympathetic activity in stretch baroreceptors and dilation of glomerular afferent arterioles
(C) Increase in atrial natriuretic peptide and dilation of glomerular afferent arterioles

(D) Increase in sympathetic activity in stretch baroreceptors and constriction of glomerular afferent arterioles

(E) Increase in the renin-angiotensin-aldosterone axis

33. During gynecologic surgery, it is always necessary to identify and isolate the ureters to prevent damage to these important structures during a procedure. Which of the following best describes the course of the ureters in the female pelvis?

(A) Anterior to both the external iliac and uterine arteries

(B) Anterior to the external iliac artery and posterior to the uterine artery

(C) Posterior to both the external iliac and uterine arteries

(D) Posterior to the external iliac artery and anterior to the uterine artery

(E) Running along with the ovarian artery

34. The nephrotic syndrome is characterized by severe proteinuria, decreased serum albumin level, and edema. This results from damage to one or more components of the glomerular capillary wall. In particular, the glomerular basement membrane is essential for maintaining serum oncotic pressure. In nonpathologic states, which of the following properties of the glomerular basement membrane prevent albumin from being freely filtered into the urine?

(A) A combination of small pore size and negatively charged pore-forming molecules prevents albumin filtration

(B) A combination of small pore size and positively charged pore-forming molecules prevents albumin filtration

(C) Albumin is freely filtered across the basement membrane but is readily reabsorbed along the nephron

(D) The positive charge of proteoglycans in the basement membrane repels albumin

(E) The small size of the glomerular basement membrane pores excludes albumin molecules

35. A 54-year-old homeless woman is found unconscious on the street. Upon admission to the emergency department, her laboratory tests show:

Na^+: 137 mEq/L
K^+: 3.3 mEq/L
Cl^-: 112 mEq/L
HCO_3^-: 15 mEq/L
Arterial blood gas on room air: pH 7.28
Partial carbon dioxide pressure: 28 mm Hg
Partial oxygen pressure: 90 mm Hg

Which of the following most likely caused her acidosis?

(A) An aspirin overdose

(B) Diabetic ketoacidosis

(C) Severe diarrhea

(D) Severe underperfusion of her peripheral muscles

(E) Uremia

36. A patient with hepatocellular carcinoma develops severe ascites such that 3–5 L of fluid must be drained from her peritoneal cavity every 3 days. This procedure may have detrimental effects on kidney function that necessitates monitoring of the glomerular filtration rate (GFR). Laboratory tests show:

Creatinine clearance: 120 mL/min
Glomerular capillary hydrostatic pressure: 40 mm Hg
Plasma inulin: 1.5 mg/mL
Urinary inulin: 50 mg/mL

Which of the following is her urine flow rate?

(A) 1.6 mL/min

(B) 3.6 mL/min

(C) 4.5 mL/min

(D) 36 mL/h

(E) 450 mL/d

37. Diuretics are medications that increase the amount of urine flow by inhibiting transport proteins or enzymes in the nephron. Different classes of diuretics affect different parts of the nephron. Which of the following diuretics will also decrease the amount of calcium excreted from the kidney?

    (A) Acetazolamide
    (B) Amiloride
    (C) Furosemide
    (D) Hydrochlorothiazide
    (E) Spironolactone

38. Mannitol, an osmotic diuretic, is sometimes used to lower intracranial pressure. Where along the nephron is the primary site of action of mannitol?

    (A) Collecting tubule
    (B) Distal tubule
    (C) Loop of Henle
    (D) Thick ascending limb of loop of Henle

39. An 18-year-old African-American man has had increasing lethargy, proteinuria, and edema following a bout of the flu 3 weeks ago. At that time, the patient visited his primary care physician, who prescribed corticosteroids for 3 weeks without improvement of his condition. His physician then referred him to a nephrologist, who performed a renal biopsy and diagnosed him with focal segmental glomerulosclerosis. Which of the following was the most likely histologic description in this patient's biopsy report?

    (A) Entire glomerular tufts show obliterated capillaries; >50% of glomeruli affected
    (B) Entire glomerular tufts show obliterated capillaries with cellular proliferation
    (C) Parts of the glomerular tufts show obliterated capillaries; <50% of glomeruli affected
    (D) Parts of the glomerular tufts show obliterated capillaries; >50% of glomeruli affected
    (E) Parts of the glomerular tufts show obliterated capillaries with cellular proliferation

40. Mr. Jones has type 1 diabetes mellitus and forgot to take his insulin. Although his serum glucose level begins to rise rapidly, sugars are not detectable in his urine for hours. Which molecules are responsible for this phenomenon?

    (A) Glucose-chloride cotransporters in the thick ascending limb
    (B) Negatively charged proteins in the glomerular wall
    (C) Occludin proteins in the tight junctions of glomerular capillary endothelial cells
    (D) Sodium-glucose cotransporters in the proximal tubule
    (E) Sodium-potassium exchange pump in the distal convoluted tubule

41. A 72-year-old man presents to his physician complaining of pain in his lower abdomen, increased difficulty urinating, and decreased urine output for the past couple days. The physician notes an enlarged prostate on digital rectal examination. Serum creatinine level is 2.5 mg/dL. Results of cystography are shown in the image. Which of the following would most likely be seen on urinalysis?

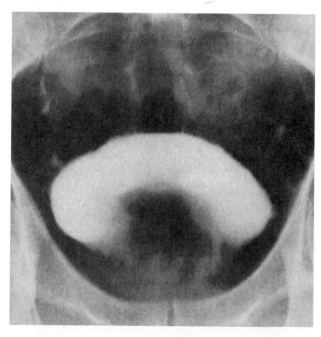

Reproduced, with permission, from Tanagho EA, McAninch JW. *Smith's General Urology*, 17th ed. New York: McGraw-Hill, 2008: Figure 6-12, A.

(A) Epithelial casts
(B) BUN:creatinine ratio <15
(C) Fractional excretion of sodium <1%
(D) Urine Na+ <10 mmol/L
(E) Urine osmolality <350 mmol/kg

42. A 53-year-old woman is undergoing renal function testing to evaluate proteinuria detected by her primary care physician at a routine visit. The patient's GFR is initially estimated at 100 mL/min by inulin clearance. Subsequently, as part of a research study, the patient's GFR is determined using a novel marker (compound X) and is found to be 125 mL/min. Which mechanism most likely explains the difference noted between these two GFR estimates?

(A) Compound X is not freely filtered at the glomerulus
(B) Compound X is reabsorbed in the descending limb of the loop of Henle
(C) Compound X is reabsorbed in the proximal convoluted tubule
(D) Compound X is secreted in the proximal convoluted tubule
(E) Inulin is reabsorbed in the proximal convoluted tubule

43. A 43-year-old man has had type 1 diabetes mellitus for 30 years. He uses insulin to treat his diabetes, but his blood glucose levels are poorly controlled. Over the years, he has developed painful peripheral neuropathy and a nonhealing diabetic foot ulcer. Recently he has experienced increased urinary frequency, which prompted his visit to the physician. His temperature is 37.6° C (99.7° F), blood pressure is 155/95 mm Hg, heart rate is 72/min, and respiratory rate is 16/min. Which of the following would most likely be found on a biopsy of this man's kidney?

(A) Crescent-shaped lesions in the glomeruli
(B) Nodular glomerular changes
(C) Proliferation of the mesangial membranes
(D) Segmental sclerosis and hyaline casts
(E) Tram-track appearance on light microscopy

44. What is the primary driving force for calcium reabsorption in the thick ascending limb of the loop of Henle?

(A) Action of parathyroid hormone
(B) A functioning sodium-potassium-chloride cotransporter
(C) Calcium delivery to the loop of Henle
(D) Maintenance of negative charge in the lumen
(E) Sodium-calcium cotransport

45. A 67-year-old man with a history of hypertension has a severe heart attack while walking to his car after a night drinking with his friends. When he arrives at the emergency department, he is pale and cold and his friends notice that "he seems to be sweating a lot." He is tachycardic and hypotensive, and is admitted to the cardiac intensive care unit. The next day, he has low urine output, his BUN level is 35 mg/dL, his creatinine level is 1.3 mg/dL, and his blood pressure is 85/55 mm Hg. His baseline blood pressure due to his hypertension was around 145/90 mm Hg. Which of the following is the most likely cause of his low urine input?

(A) A blockage of the ureters or urethra
(B) Acute tubular necrosis
(C) Decrease in perfusion of the kidney
(D) Ethanol-induced reduction in urine output
(E) Low urine output is normal in times of stress

46. A 13-year-old boy is brought to the emergency department with periorbital edema, hypertension, and tea-colored urine. His parents say that he had a sore throat about 3 weeks ago. Urinalysis shows RBCs with casts. A positive antistreptolysin O titer and decreased levels of complement are also noted. What findings would be expected in this patient's glomeruli?

(A) Granular subendothelial deposits
(B) Linear subendothelial pattern
(C) Mesangial deposits
(D) Subendothelial deposits
(E) Subepithelial humps

47. Two weeks after initiation of diuretic therapy to control essential hypertension, a 51-year-old man presents to his physician for a check-up. Physical examination reveals a blood pressure of 130/85 mm Hg. Laboratory tests show a pH of 7.48, partial arterial carbon dioxide pressure of 50 mm Hg, and a bicarbonate of 41 mEq/L. Which of the following etiologies is most consistent with this clinical situation?

(A) Acetazolamide-induced metabolic alkalosis
(B) Acetazolamide-induced respiratory alkalosis
(C) Hydrochlorothiazide-induced metabolic alkalosis
(D) Hydrochlorothiazide-induced respiratory alkalosis
(E) Spironolactone-induced metabolic alkalosis
(F) Spironolactone-induced respiratory alkalosis

48. A 17-year-old girl develops severe diarrhea after eating an undercooked hamburger at a family picnic. After 3 days of experiencing diarrhea, she presents to the emergency department with moderate dehydration and orthostatic hypotension. Which of the following acid-base states is most probable in this patient?

Choice	Na$^+$ (mEq/L)	Cl$^-$ (mEq/L)	K$^+$ (mEq/L)	HCO$_3^-$ (mEq/L)	Pco$_2$ (mm Hg)	pH
A	135	90	3.0	15	38	7.31
B	138	110	3.5	22	60	7.32
C	140	105	3.7	35	40	7.49
D	140	110	3.5	18	39	7.30
E	140	110	3.5	24	40	7.42
F	141	100	3.8	24	25	7.48

(A) A
(B) B
(C) C
(D) D
(E) E
(F) F

49. An 8-year-old girl presents to the emergency department complaining of frequent urination, constant thirst, and new, strange "staining" of her teeth. She recently had a cold, and her pediatrician prescribed an antibiotic that she said may hurt her kidneys. She did not bring the bottle with her. Which of the following medications was this patient most likely prescribed?

(A) Demeclocycline
(B) Neomycin
(C) Norfloxacin
(D) Penicillin G
(E) Vancomycin

50. A newborn with hypercalciuria and hypokalemic alkalosis is diagnosed with neonatal Bartter's syndrome, a rare inherited dysfunction of the thick ascending limb of the nephron. Which diuretic may mimic these symptoms by blocking a cotransporter found in this part of the nephron?

(A) Acetazolamide
(B) Ethacrynic acid
(C) Hydrochlorothiazide
(D) Mannitol
(E) Triamterene

1. **The correct answer is A.** The juxtaglomerular (JG) cells in the afferent arteriole and the macula densa in the distal convoluted tubule together make up the JG apparatus, which is responsible for controlling renal blood flow via renin release. In renal artery stenosis, the blood flow to the kidney is low. This low pressure is detected by JG cells in the afferent arteriole that secrete renin to raise blood pressure and renal perfusion through the renin-angiotensin system.

Answer B is incorrect. The collecting duct is strongly influenced by hormones such as ADH and aldosterone and aids in concentrating or diluting urine. It does not have a role in sensing perfusion pressure or secreting renin.

Answer C is incorrect. The distal convoluted tubule contains the macula densa cells that sense low Na$^+$ flow inside the nephron, another sign that the kidney is not well perfused. The macula densa cells are in intimate contact with the JG cells, and although the macula densa cells help in sensing low perfusion, it is the JG cells that actually secrete renin.

Answer D is incorrect. The efferent arteriole carries blood flow away from the glomerulus. The JG cells that sense blood pressure are in the afferent arteriole. The words "afferent" and "efferent" are also used in nerves, and it may help to remember the mnemonic "SAME" (**S**ensory **A**fferent, **M**otor **E**fferent) to remember the direction of flow in the afferent (toward the kidney) and efferent (away from the kidney) systems.

Answer E is incorrect. The loop of Henle is primarily responsible for concentrating urine, not for sensing perfusion or secreting renin.

2. **The correct answer is D.** This man's history indicates that he is suffering from acute tubular necrosis secondary to ischemia of the epithelial cells of the proximal convoluted tubule. Granular casts on urinalysis is also a significant sign that this is acute tubular necrosis. These cells, given their high metabolic rate, are par-

ticularly sensitive to a drop in blood pressure such as that experienced in hemorrhagic shock. In this patient, the immediate therapeutic plan is to correct the fluid and electrolyte imbalance. The fluid replacement should include both crystalloid (eg, normal saline, lactated Ringer's) and blood products due to the severity of blood loss. If recovery of renal function is delayed or if the kidneys never fully recover, dialysis is indicated. The epithelium will usually regenerate in a few weeks.

Answer A is incorrect. Angioplasty is a minimally invasive procedure that involves eliminating the renal artery occlusion by placing intravascular stents in the renal artery and thereby restoring proper blood flow to the kidney. This patient is not suffering from acute renal failure due to stenosis/occlusion of the renal artery, so angioplasty is not indicated as an appropriate treatment.

Answer B is incorrect. Broad-spectrum antibiotics are indicated in cases of shock due to sepsis or in pyelonephritis. This patient is in hemodynamic shock caused by massive blood loss. Since there is no infection, antibiotics will not be beneficial. Additionally, because the patient is experiencing renal failure, any drug that is metabolized by the kidney should be used with caution.

Answer C is incorrect. Immune-mediated disease can also cause acute renal failure. Corticosteroids are indicated in immune-mediated disease. Since that is not the mechanism of this patient's renal failure, it is not indicated.

Answer E is incorrect. This treatment is reserved primarily for renal stones obstructing the outflow of urine and causing postrenal acute renal failure.

3. **The correct answer is C.** This man is suffering from acute tubular necrosis (ATN), which is shown by the granular casts in his urine. A documented adverse effect of statin drugs is that they can cause rhabdomyolysis, or the destruction of skeletal muscle with subsequent

excretion of myoglobin by the kidneys. Myoglobin is nephrotoxic and, in significant amounts, may lead to ATN (also a common complication of crush injuries). There is no hemoglobin in the urine; myoglobin is causing the urine to turn red.

Answer A is incorrect. β-Blockers do not cause ATN. The adverse effects commonly seen with β-blockers include impotence, exacerbation of asthma, bradycardia, atrioventricular block, and sedation. In patients with diabetes, there is an increased risk of hypoglycemia both because the drugs inhibit glucose formation and because they mask the signs of symptoms of the hypoglycemic event so that the patient may not realize that his/her sugar is low. Metoprolol can cause a dyslipidemia.

Answer B is incorrect. Hemolytic-uremic syndrome or thrombotic thrombocytopenic purpura could cause acute renal failure, but there is no other evidence of this type of process.

Answer D is incorrect. A crush injury could cause this scenario, but any injury large enough to cause kidney failure would certainly be noticeable to the patient and/or doctors.

4. **The correct answer is D.** Hypoventilation causes an inability on the part of the lungs to excrete the CO_2 the body produces, leading to retention of CO_2. This causes a drop in pH and a compensatory retention of bicarbonate. These acid-base abnormalities are consistent with respiratory acidosis. Hypoventilation (from a variety of etiologies) is a primary cause of respiratory acidosis.

Answer A is incorrect. An increase in anions would be consistent with anion-gap metabolic acidosis. Metabolic acidosis is indicated by the presence of low pH with low plasma bicarbonate and low carbon dioxide and an increased anion gap, measured by $([Na^+] - [Cl^-] - [HCO_3^-])$, which is normally 10–16 mEq/L. The main causes are lactic acidosis, diabetic ketoacidosis, and renal failure.

Answer B is incorrect. Non-anion-gap metabolic acidosis is the presence of low pH with low plasma bicarbonate without an elevated

anion gap. The cause is generally gastrointestinal losses of bicarbonate (i.e., diarrhea, biliary drains, emesis, nasogastric tube losses). Another important and common cause of a metabolic non-anion-gap acidosis is the presence of an ileal conduit or bladder reconstruction from colonic tissue. The gastrointestinal tissue absorbs Cl^- from the urine in exchange for bicarbonate. Other causes include renal tubular acidosis, or hypochloremia.

Answer C is incorrect. The pH in this answer is low, which corresponds to an acidosis. The PcO_2 is high, which is consistent with a respiratory acidosis, however the HCO_3^- is low, which is consistent with a metabolic acidosis. Thus this patient has a mixed respiratory and metabolic acidosis.

Answer E is incorrect. The pH in this instance is normal, while there is an increased anion gap. An anion gap usually indicates that the patient has an acidosis. Since the pH of the blood is normal and not lowered, it indicates that this is a mixed acid-base disorder, in which a metabolic or respiratory alkalosis is counteracting a metabolic anion-gap acidosis.

Answer F is incorrect. Respiratory alkalosis can be caused only by an increase in ventilation leading to excessive loss of carbon dioxide, which is balanced by an increased excretion of bicarbonate. Hence, a high pH, a low CO_2, and a low bicarbonate indicate respiratory alkalosis. This is caused by hyperventilation.

Answer G is incorrect. Metabolic alkalosis would present with a high pH, a high bicarbonate, and (with respiratory compensation) a high CO_2. The causes of metabolic alkalosis include vomiting, diuretic therapy, and chloride restriction. The compensation is hypoventilation.

5. **The correct answer is D.** Thiazides and furosemide lead to metabolic alkalosis. There are two components to the development of metabolic alkalosis: volume depletion and electrolyte imbalance; specifically hypochloremia and hypokalemia. Volume contraction leads to increased sodium reabsorption and bicarbonate

retention. The diuretic-induced hypochloremia and hypokalemia lead to persistence of the alkalosis because the hypokalemia causes hydrogen to be exchanged for sodium rather than potassium at the distal convoluted tubule.

Answer A is incorrect. Neither potassium-sparing diuretics nor acetazolamide cause metabolic alkalosis. Potassium-sparing diuretics cause metabolic acidosis by inhibiting sodium-hydrogen exchange channels, and acetazolamide promotes the loss of bicarbonate in the urine, causing metabolic acidosis.

Answer B is incorrect. Acetazolamide inhibits the enzyme carbonic anhydrase, which is important in the reabsorption of sodium, bicarbonate, and chloride at the proximal tubule. Since it promotes the loss of bicarbonate in the urine, it tends to cause metabolic acidosis.

Answer C is incorrect. The potassium-sparing diuretics, such as spironolactone, inhibit aldosterone-sensitive sodium channels that excrete hydrogen or potassium in exchange for sodium. Inhibition of these channels may lead to hyperkalemia and metabolic acidosis.

Answer E is incorrect. Thiazides do cause metabolic alkalosis by causing volume depletion, hypochloremia, and hypokalemia. However, acetazolamide promotes the loss of bicarbonate in the urine, causing metabolic acidosis.

Answer F is incorrect. Thiazides do cause metabolic alkalosis by causing volume depletion, hypochloremia, and hypokalemia. However, potassium-sparing diuretics cause metabolic acidosis by inhibiting sodium-hydrogen exchange channels.

6. **The correct answer is B.** This patient has Goodpasture's syndrome, which is an autoimmune disease involving the formation of antibodies to the alveolar and glomerular basement membranes. This is an example of a type II hypersensitivity reaction in which antibody binds to antigen on a cell, leading to lysis by complement or phagocytosis. It is one of the several forms of rapidly progressive (or crescentic) glomerulonephritis. Patients are usually men

in their 20s presenting with a history of hemoptysis and nephritic renal failure that is associated with crescent formation. Since the damage in this disease is caused by the actions of antibodies to the basement membrane, diagnosis is made by immunofluorescence, which shows a smooth linear staining along the basement membrane.

Answer A is incorrect. Type I hypersensitivity reactions are those in which antigen cross-links pre-formed IgE on presensitized mast cells and basophils, triggering the release of vasoactive amines. Examples of this type of reaction are asthma and anaphylaxis.

Answer C is incorrect. Type III hypersensitivity reactions are those involving immune complex deposition. Antigen-antibody complexes are deposited and activate complement, which attracts neutrophils, which then release lysosomal enzymes. Serum sickness and Arthus reaction are variants of the type III hypersensitivity reaction. Examples include rheumatoid arthritis and polyarteritis nodosa.

Answer D is incorrect. Type IV hypersensitivity reactions are delayed cell-mediated reactions. Sensitized T-lymphocytes encounter antigen and then release lymphokines, which leads to macrophage activation. Examples include skin tests for tuberculosis and transplant rejection.

7. **The correct answer is A.** This patient is suffering from a massive left-sided stroke that occurred secondary to a hypercoagulable state. Patients with nephrotic syndrome are at increased risk for thromboembolic events due to renal losses of antithrombin III, protein C, and protein S, all of which normally function as anticoagulants. Patients with nephrotic syndrome also commonly have other factors contributing to a hypercoagulable state, including hemoconcentration, increased fibrinogen, and thrombocytosis. Mental status or neurologic changes in patients with nephritic syndrome should be taken very seriously.

Answer B is incorrect. Patients with decreased factor II levels have an increased risk of hemorrhagic events; nephrotic syndrome is not associated with decreased factor II levels.

Answer C is incorrect. Patients with nephrotic syndrome have increased fibrinogen levels, which predispose them to thromboembolic events.

Answer D is incorrect. Patients with nephrotic syndrome have decreased protein S levels, which predispose them to thromboembolic events.

Answer E is incorrect. Patients with nephrotic syndrome have decreased protein C levels, which predispose them to thromboembolic events.

8. **The correct answer is F.** Pyelonephritis is infection of the kidneys by an ascending infection from the lower urinary tract, most often caused by *Escherichia coli* from the periurethral/perianal area. The classic symptoms are fever, chills, flank pain, and costovertebral angle tenderness, all of which are demonstrated by this patient. Casts indicate that the origin of the WBCs is the kidney, which confirms the clinical suspicion of pyelonephritis.

Answer A is incorrect. An abdominal aortic aneurysm may present with back and abdominal pain and/or pulsations of the abdomen. This condition may often be asymptomatic for years as the dilation of the aorta worsens. Fever and urinary casts would not be a part of the clinical picture.

Answer B is incorrect. Appendicitis is an acute inflammation of the appendix and a surgical emergency. Depending on the location of the appendix, appendicitis can present with back pain. The more classical presentation is abdominal pain that is at first generalized, but then localizes to the right lower quadrant as the peritoneum becomes irritated. Peritoneal irritation is indicated by the localization of the pain, as well as by rebound tenderness and guarding.

Answer C is incorrect. An ectopic pregnancy may present with back, abdominal, and/or pelvic pain. Classically, the patients presents with abdominal pain and irregular vaginal bleeding.

Diagnosis of ectopic pregnancy is extremely important as the pregnancy can rupture, leading to internal hemorrhage and shock.

Answer D is incorrect. Localized cystitis is not usually accompanied by systemic symptoms, such as fever. However, cystitis may be present in conjunction with the pyelonephritis, as it is an ascending infection. Symptoms of cystitis include urinary frequency and dysuria. Casts would not be seen if the infection were localized to the urinary bladder.

Answer E is incorrect. Premature labor involves regular uterine contractions that dilate the cervix. The labor does not cause fever, but back pain may be present.

9. **The correct answer is B.** This patient is most likely suffering from bilateral renal artery stenosis, which is indicated on physical exam by renal bruits. Stenosis of the renal arteries leads to a decrease in perfusion of the kidney and therefore a drop in intraglomerular pressure and glomerular filtration rate (GFR). The underperfused kidneys respond by the activation of the renin-angiotensin-aldosterone system. With angiotensin-converting enzyme (ACE) inhibitors, the vasoconstrictive effect of angiotensin II on the ability of the efferent arterioles to increase effective GFR will be abolished. ACE inhibitors should be avoided in patients with renal stenosis due to deterioration of renal function.

Answer A is incorrect. Angioplasty is a minimally invasive procedure that involves eliminating the occlusion by placing intravascular stents in the renal artery, thereby restoring blood flow to the kidney. This form of therapy is the primary indication for renal stenosis in symptomatic patients. Patency rates after angioplasty are strongly dependent on the size of the vessel treated and the quality of inflow and outflow through the vessel.

Answer C is incorrect. In patients with bilateral renal artery stenosis leading to hypertension, both kidneys will be underperfused, so both kidneys will retain sodium and water by activation of the renin-angiotensin-aldosterone system. Diuretics can counteract this effect and control blood pressure; therefore, this treatment is appropriate in this clinical scenario.

Answer D is incorrect. Smoking is a risk factor for developing atherosclerotic plaques that may occlude vessels such as the renal arteries. Quitting may lower the rate of atherosclerotic buildup. This recommendation is appropriate for this patient.

Answer E is incorrect. Surgery is another therapeutic option for renal stenosis. It is particularly indicated if angioplasty cannot be performed, as in completely occluded renal vessels.

10. **The correct answer is C.** A horseshoe kidney forms when the inferior poles of two kidneys fuse during development. As the kidneys rise from the pelvis, they encounter the inferior mesenteric artery and cannot rise to the normal level in the abdomen. These patients are typically asymptomatic if they have no other abnormalities.

Answer A is incorrect. The aorta would not obstruct the path of a rising horseshoe kidney during development.

Answer B is incorrect. The celiac trunk leaves the aorta at a level above the location of normally developed kidneys, and thus cannot be responsible for the low location of a horseshoe kidney.

Answer D is incorrect. The inferior vena cava would not obstruct the path of a rising horseshoe kidney during development.

Answer E is incorrect. The superior mesenteric artery leaves the aorta at the level where normally developing kidneys are located, and thus it cannot be responsible for the low level of a horseshoe kidney.

11. **The correct answer is E.** The history of being started on chemotherapy for leukemia is strongly suggestive of tumor lysis syndrome, which occurs when leukemic cells are lysed, releasing potentially toxic contents including potassium, phosphate, and uric acid. Uric acid stones are radiolucent, so they may not appear on x-ray films. It is likely that this patient's presentation has been caused by a kidney stone

that has passed into the left ureter and now into the urethra, causing postrenal failure. The FENa >4% is consistent with postrenal failure.

Answer A is incorrect. Kidney failure as a result of glomerular dysfunction presents with a prerenal azotemia. There is an effective decrease in GFR, and Na^+/H_2O are retained by the kidney. The fractional excretion of sodium in prerenal failure is normally less than 1% with an osmolality that is >350 mOsm/kg.

Answer B is incorrect. Acute interstitial disease of the kidney is commonly caused by an allergic reaction to medicine (e.g., penicillin, nonsteroidal anti-inflammatory drugs) or infection. In an acute setting, it presents with an intrinsic renal picture as is seen in this patient. In the setting of an infection, urine cultures are usually positive; in the setting of an allergic reaction, eosinophilia is common.

Answer C is incorrect. Kidney failure as a result of tubular dysfunction presents with an intrinsic renal picture. This is most commonly due to acute tubular necrosis or ischemia/toxins. Patchy necrosis leads to debris obstructing the tubules and fluid backflow, leading to a drop in GFR. The fractional excretion of sodium in intrinsic renal failure is normally >2% with an osmolality that is >350 mOsm/kg (similar to postrenal). However, the presentation of severe intermittent pelvic pain in the context of leukemia therapy is more likely to be caused by a kidney stone.

Answer D is incorrect. The spleen can be involved in leukemia, but the presence of acute renal failure in this case makes a urethral obstruction more likely.

12. **The correct answer is A.** Renal prostaglandin synthesis produces a vasodilatory effect on the afferent arterioles, while angiotensin II vasoconstricts primarily efferent arterioles. Nonsteroidal anti-inflammatory drugs (NSAIDs) inhibit renal prostaglandin synthesis, resulting in an inability of afferent arterioles to dilate. Without adequate afferent arteriolar vasodilation, the GFR is reduced and acute renal failure ensues. The BUN:creatinine (BUN:Cr) ra-

tio in the question stem is consistent with an intrinsic cause of renal failure, which would also be consistent with renal failure secondary to NSAIDs.

Answer B is incorrect. Inhibition of prostaglandin synthesis causes excessive vasoconstriction of the afferent arterioles, leading to decreased GFR. Constriction of the efferent arteriole would serve to increase GFR.

Answer C is incorrect. Prostaglandins act to dilate the afferent arterioles, with less significant effect on the efferent arterioles.

Answer D is incorrect. NSAIDs act to inhibit, not stimulate, renal prostaglandin synthesis, leading to excessive constriction of the afferent arteriole and a decrease in the GFR.

Answer E is incorrect. NSAIDs act to inhibit, not stimulate, renal prostaglandin synthesis, leading to excessive constriction of the afferent arteriole and a decrease in the GFR.

13. **The correct answer is F.** In healthy people, osmoreceptors in the wall of the third ventricle sense increased body fluid osmolarity and trigger the release of ADH from the posterior pituitary. ADH exerts its main effects on the V2 receptors located in the principal cells of the late distal tubule and collecting duct, where a G_s protein-coupled mechanism directs the insertion of aquaporin water channels into the luminal wall. These channels are permeable only to water and result in a reabsorption of water, concentration of urine, and dilution of body fluids. Activation of the V1 receptor found in the vascular smooth muscles results in activation of G_q protein second-messenger cascade and contraction of vascular smooth muscle, leading to an increase in total peripheral resistance. In patients with the syndrome of inappropriate ADH secretion (SIADH), which can be caused by central nervous system disturbances (e.g., stroke, hemorrhage, infection), small cell lung carcinoma, intracranial neoplasms, and occasionally by pancreatic tumors, the unregulated release of ADH leads to the persistent excretion of concentrated urine high in sodium. This causes hyponatremia and decreased serum osmolality without potassium or acid-base disturbances.

Answer A is incorrect. ACTH is secreted by the anterior pituitary in response to the presence of corticotropin releasing hormone produced in the hypothalamus. It can also be secreted by pituitary tumors or small cell lung carcinomas, but would present with Cushing's syndrome (hypertension, weight gain, buffalo hump, truncal obesity, striae, hyperglycemia, and osteoporosis) rather than hyponatremia.

Answer B is incorrect. Neuronal signals from the osmoreceptors of the third ventricle stimulate the production of ADH as well as stimulate the sensation of thirst.

Answer C is incorrect. Renin is secreted by smooth muscle cells in the afferent arteriole and acts to cleave angiotensinogen to angiotensin I. This activates the renin-angiotensin-aldosterone axis, leading to increased salt and water retention. A patient with persistent activation of this axis would present primarily with hypertension and edema with relatively low urine sodium levels.

Answer D is incorrect. V2 receptors are coupled to the insertion of aquaporins; V1 receptors are coupled to the contraction of vascular smooth muscle.

Answer E is incorrect. Activation of V1 receptors leads to an increase in total peripheral resistance.

14. **The correct answer is D.** This patient is in the early stages of renal failure with symptoms of oliguria and elevated BUN and creatinine levels. Combined with the patient's reduced hearing, these symptoms represent the ototoxicity and nephrotoxicity seen with aminoglycoside administration. Gentamicin is a type of aminoglycoside.

Answer A is incorrect. Chloramphenicol toxicity is associated with anemia, aplastic anemia, and gray baby syndrome.

Answer B is incorrect. Doxycycline toxicity includes gastrointestinal distress, tooth discoloration and inhibition of bone growth in children, and photosensitivity reactions.

Answer C is incorrect. Erythromycin toxicity includes gastrointestinal discomfort, acute cholestatic hepatitis, eosinophilia, and skin rashes. It is not generally associated with nephrotoxicity.

Answer E is incorrect. Imipenem is a broad-spectrum antibiotic that can cause gastrointestinal distress, skin rash, and seizures at higher doses.

15. **The correct answer is A.** This vignette describes a nephrotic syndrome. Spike-and-dome deposits are only found in membranous glomerulonephritis. Membranous glomerulonephritis is an immune complex-mediated disease. Immunofluorescence shows a granular pattern of IgG and complement along the basement membrane. Membranous glomerulonephritis is the most common cause of adult-onset nephrotic syndrome. Patients with this disease normally present with a nephrotic picture of generalized edema due to massive loss of albumin and proteins.

Answer B is incorrect. This is a finding of membranoproliferative glomerulonephritis, an uncommon autoimmune renal disorder that normally affects young individuals (8–30 years of age). The diagnosis is based on a histologic presentation that includes mesangial proliferation and a tram-track appearance on light microscopy. As this patient is 50 years old, this diagnosis is less likely.

Answer C is incorrect. This is a description of the findings in acute poststreptococcal glomerulonephritis, an autoimmune disease most frequently seen in children. It normally presents a few weeks after a streptococcal infection (throat or skin) with peripheral and periorbital edema, dark, "smoky" urine, and proteinuria. These symptoms are caused by circulating antistreptococcal antibody-antigen complexes that deposit in the glomerular basement membrane, leading to complement activation and glomerular damage. As this patient has otherwise been healthy and is 50 years old, this diagnosis is unlikely.

Answer D is incorrect. This is the main finding in IgA nephropathy (Berger's disease). This disease presents within several days of an infection (as opposed to poststreptococcal glomerulonephritis, which presents weeks after) with a nephritic picture due to IgA deposition in the mesangium. It is the most common global nephropathy, but it is a mild disease with minimal clinical significance. As this patient has not had a recent infection, this diagnosis is unlikely.

Answer E is incorrect. This is a finding of Alport's syndrome, a heterogeneous (although most commonly X-linked) genetic disorder with either absent or mutated collagen IV, which leads to a nephritic renal disease, as well as nervous system and ocular disorders. This patient has no other complaints and the edema is a fairly recent finding, making this diagnosis less likely.

16. **The correct answer is D.** The presence of white cell casts in the urine indicates that this is acute pyelonephritis and not just a lower urinary tract infection (UTI). Pyelonephritis is an acute infection of the renal parenchyma that most often results from an ascending progression of a UTI from the bladder. This most frequently involves *Escherichia coli*. Other clinical manifestations of a UTI include dysuria, urinary frequency, hematuria, bacteriuria, and pyuria. If white blood cell casts are seen, implying involvement of the kidney, the clinician can be sure that the UTI has ascended, making it a case of pyelonephritis. Acute pyelonephritis, like most acute phases of inflammation, is characterized by a predominance of polymorphonuclear leukocytes.

Answer A is incorrect. After 2–3 days, neutrophils are replaced by monocytes, macrophages, plasma cells, and lymphocytes as part of chronic inflammation. Macrophages are longer-lived than neutrophils and are capable of proliferating and phagocytosing larger particles.

Answer B is incorrect. A monocyte has a kidney-shaped nucleus and differentiates into a macrophage in tissue; it is seen in chronic inflammation.

Answer C is incorrect. A plasma cell has a clock-faced chromatin distribution. B lymphocytes differentiate into plasma cells, which then produce large amounts of antibody. They are a component of humoral immunity.

Answer E is incorrect. T lymphocytes are the key component of cell-mediated immunity and are not the primary cell in acute inflammation.

17. **The correct answer is E.** The only diuretics that specifically limit calcium loss are the thiazides. They act in the early distal tubule, which is marked as region E in the image.

Answer A is incorrect. There are no diuretics that act at the glomerulus.

Answer B is incorrect. Carbonic anhydrase inhibitors, which act in the proximal convoluted tubule, do not affect calcium excretion.

Answer C is incorrect. Osmotic diuretics act in the loop of Henle (as well as the proximal convoluted tubule and collecting duct), but they do not affect ion channels.

Answer D is incorrect. Loop diuretics, which encourage calcium excretion, act in the thick ascending limb.

Answer F is incorrect. Potassium-sparing diuretics and ADH antagonists such as lithium and demeclocycline act along the collecting tubule, although neither class affects calcium excretion.

18. **The correct answer is A.** This patient is suffering an acute overdose of amphetamine. He should be treated with ammonium chloride to acidify his urine and increase renal clearance of the weak base. This phenomenon, called ion trapping, occurs because increasing the ratio of ionized to nonionized drug species in the renal tubule allows more of the drug to be retained in the urine and excreted. Weak bases in acidic environments have high ratios of ionized species, which are water soluble and do not cross membranes. When urine is acidified, the levels of ionized amphetamine are high, and therefore more drug is trapped in the renal tubule.

Answer B is incorrect. Alkalinization with bicarbonate is used to increase renal clearance of weak acids such as phenobarbital, methotrexate, tricyclic antidepressants, and aspirin.

Answer C is incorrect. Flumazenil is a treatment for acute benzodiazepine overdose.

Answer D is incorrect. Naloxone is a treatment for opioid overdose.

Answer E is incorrect. Treatment with water would have no effect on this patient's acute intoxication.

19. **The correct answer is B.** While this patient's pH, bicarbonate, and carbon dioxide levels are all very close to normal, it is always important to look more closely before concluding that there is no disorder. Vomiting is a common cause of a metabolic alkalosis, while diarrhea is a common cause of non-anion-gap metabolic acidosis. The patient has had gastrointestinal symptoms that have led to acute dehydration, which indicates that these symptoms are probably quite severe. It is also important to look at the serum chemistry. One would expect a hypokalemic hypochloremic metabolic alkalosis from vomiting, but only the electrolyte deficiencies are present. The equalized pH suggests that the patient is losing an equal amount of acid through vomiting as she is base through diarrhea. Therefore, it is more likely that she has a mixed acid-base disorder than no electrolyte imbalances at all.

Answer A is incorrect. Non-anion-gap metabolic acidosis is the presence of a low pH with a low plasma bicarbonate level and without an elevated anion gap. It is characterized by a compensatory retention of the other main body anions, which results in hyperchloremia. The cause is generally diarrhea and renal tubular acidosis.

Answer C is incorrect. While a mixed respiratory disorder could lead to this electrolyte profile, the patient has no respiratory pathology. Therefore, it is more likely that her acid-base status is being determined by a metabolic process.

Answer D is incorrect. Although this patient's pH, bicarbonate, and carbon dioxide levels are close to normal, the gastrointestinal symptoms (vomiting, diarrhea) suggest that she has a mixed acid-base disorder than no electrolyte imbalances at all.

Answer E is incorrect. Respiratory alkalosis can be caused only by an increase in ventilation leading to excessive loss of carbon dioxide, which is balanced by an increased excretion of bicarbonate. Hence, a high pH and low carbon dioxide and bicarbonate levels indicate respiratory alkalosis.

20. **The correct answer is E.** Osteomalacia occurs in renal failure due to the kidney's inability to maintain its normal vitamin D production. Chronic renal failure is a common complication in noncompliant diabetic patients. Chronic renal failure results in the progressive loss of renal function, eventually leading to end-stage renal disease. In chronic renal failure, the kidneys are unable to keep up their normal excretory, metabolic, and endocrine functions. The abnormalities include accumulation of toxins, underproduction of hormones (vitamin D and erythropoietin), and increased release of renin. Symptoms and clinical abnormalities associated with chronic renal failure include edema, hyperkalemia, metabolic acidosis, hyperphosphatemia, hypocalcemia, renal osteodystrophy, hypertension, pulmonary edema, congestive heart failure, uremia, anemia, nausea, vomiting, peripheral neuropathy, and pruritus. The pathogenesis of osteomalacia in patients with chronic renal disease is caused by failure of the kidney to turn $25(OH)D$ into the active form $1,25(OH)_2D$. Without active vitamin D, there is impaired mineralization of bone, leading to renal osteodystrophy.

Answer A is incorrect. Bacteriuria is the presence of bacteria in the urine. This is associated with urinary tract infections, not renal failure.

Answer B is incorrect. In end-stage renal disease, the kidneys are unable to regulate and excrete potassium, leading to hyperkalemia, not hypokalemia. Cardiac arrhythmias are a common complication of hyperkalemia.

Answer C is incorrect. Hypotension is not caused by renal failure. Excess retention of sodium and water leads to fluid overload and results in hypertension, congestive heart failure, and pulmonary edema.

Answer D is incorrect. Metabolic acidosis, not alkalosis, occurs due to a decrease in acid secretion and a decrease in bicarbonate production.

Answer F is incorrect. Anemia, not polycythemia, will result in renal failure as the kidneys become unable to produce erythropoietin. Some renal cancers can lead to overexpression of erythropoietin and lead to polycythemia, but renal failure leads to anemia.

21. **The correct answer is C.** IgA nephropathy (Berger's disease) presents within several days of an infection (as opposed to poststreptococcal glomerulonephritis, which presents weeks after) with a nephritic picture due to IgA deposition in the mesangium. It is the most common global nephropathy, but it is a mild disease. It is common in children and presents as a recurrent hematuria with minimal clinical significance. On immunofluorescence, it presents with nonlinear mesangial deposits of IgA. Treatment is with angiotensin-converting enzyme inhibitors and corticosteroids. Patients with IgA nephropathy have a risk of recurrence of the disease.

Answer A is incorrect. Increased antistreptolysin O titers are associated with acute poststreptococcal glomerulonephritis rather than IgA nephropathy. The classic findings include RBCs and casts in the urine (causing the tea-colored appearance), elevated antistreptolysin O titers, decreased complement levels, and "lumpy-bumpy" electron-dense deposits in the glomerulus.

Answer B is incorrect. Acute poststreptococcal glomerulonephritis is an autoimmune disease most frequently seen in children. It normally presents a few weeks after a streptococcal with a nephritic picture of peripheral and periorbital edema, dark urine, and proteinuria. These symptoms are caused by circulating antistreptococcal antibody-antigen complexes that deposit in the glomerular basement membrane, leading to complement activation and glomerular damage. The classic findings are RBCs and casts in the urine (which cause the characteristic tea-colored urine), a positive antistreptolysin O titer, decreased levels of complement, and "lumpy-bumpy" electron-dense deposits in the subepithelium of the glomerulus. Recovery is spontaneous and treatment is supportive.

Answer D is incorrect. IgA nephropathy usually presents with a nephritic picture, which does not involve the massive proteinuria that is seen in nephrotic syndromes.

Answer E is incorrect. IgA deposition in Berger's disease is primarily in the mesangium and not the subepithelium.

22. **The correct answer is D.** This patient has diffuse cortical necrosis: generalized infarctions of the cortices of both kidneys, which is a common complication of disseminated intravascular coagulation (DIC). DIC commonly occurs after a complication of pregnancy such as amniotic fluid embolus and placental abruption, and affected patients develop the abrupt onset of the triad of anuria, gross hematuria, and flank pain. The diagnosis can usually be established by ultrasonography, which will demonstrate hypodense areas in the renal cortex. Although many patients can be sustained on dialysis, only 20%–40% have partial recovery of kidney function. Indications for acute dialysis in DIC include (1) acidosis refractory to bicarbonate, (2) severe electrolyte abnormalities refractory to medical intervention (especially high potassium levels), (3) intoxication with some drugs, (4) volume overload refractory to diuretics, and (5) uremic symptoms (e.g., cardiac friction run, altered mental status). The fact that this patient has a new-onset pericardial friction rub indicates uremia and makes dialysis imperative.

Answer A is incorrect. Aggressive fluid support is not beneficial for kidney recovery after the development of diffuse cortical necrosis. The kidney has been severely damaged by the microthrombi of disseminated intravascular coag-

ulation. Aggressive fluid resuscitation is contraindicated due to (1) the lack of hypotension, and (2) the renal failure. Fluids will only cause volume overload if they cannot be excreted.

Answer B is incorrect. While renal malignancy can cause hematuria, it is less likely to cause renal failure. In this case a biopsy to look for renal malignancy is not necessary because the cause of the patient's symptoms is already known. The first treatment should be dialysis to counteract renal failure and allow any remaining renal tissue to recover.

Answer C is incorrect. Broad-spectrum antibiotics are indicated in cases of shock due to sepsis. This patient has disseminated intravascular coagulation caused by an amniotic embolus, and since there is no infection, antibiotics will not be beneficial. Additionally, as the patient is experiencing renal failure, any antibiotic that is renally metabolized should be renally dosed to account for the patient's creatinine clearance rate.

Answer E is incorrect. This patient is in severe acute renal failure. Failure to treat will result in death.

23. **The correct answer is B.** Normally hyperuricemia leads to kidney stones that are radiolucent and therefore not seen on x-ray. These stones are often seen in the setting of diseases with increased cell proliferation and turnover, such as leukemia and myeloproliferative disorders. Remember that uric acid is a metabolite of nucleic acid turnover, which is heightened in the setting of cell destruction.

Answer A is incorrect. Calcium stones are the most common cause of kidney stones (80%–85%). Therefore, states that lead to increased calcium (e.g., hyperparathyroidism, destructive bone diseases) can lead to their formation. The stones are made of calcium oxalate or calcium phosphate and are radiopaque. Other risk factors are increased vitamin D and milk-alkali syndrome.

Answer C is incorrect. Urinary tract infection with urease-positive microorganisms such as *Proteus vulgaris* and *Staphylococcus saprophyti-*

cus can form large struvite calculi (ammonium, magnesium, and phosphate) that are usually (80%) radiopaque. This is the second most common cause of kidney stones.

Answer D is incorrect. Prostate cancer commonly sends metastases to the bone, the destruction of which leads to a hypercalcemic state and the production of radiopaque calcium-based stones.

Answer E is incorrect. Urinary tract infection with urease-positive microorganisms such as *Staphylococcus saprophyticus* can form large struvite calculi that are radiopaque.

24. **The correct answer is D.** Angiotensin II (AT II) increases the activity of the Na^+-H^+ exchanger in the proximal tubule to facilitate salt and water resorption. As a result, increased H^+ is pumped into the tubular lumen. Luminal H^+ is then returned to the tubular cell in the process of HCO_3^- resorption as H^+ and HCO_3^- join and form water and carbon dioxide after catalysis by brush border carbonic anhydrase. Water and carbon dioxide diffuse back into the tubular cell and again liberate H^+ and HCO_3^- after carbonic anhydrase catalysis. Here, the HCO_3^- is transported into the bloodstream while the H^+ is free to participate in another round of HCO_3^- resorption via the Na^+-H^+ exchanger. Thus, the net result of increased Na^+-H^+ exchange is an increase in HCO_3^- resorption and no net change in H^+ secretion. Increased HCO_3^- reabsorption after AT II stimulation accounts for the contraction alkalosis that occurs as a result of volume depletion.

Answer A is incorrect. Increased Na^+-H^+ exchange in the proximal tubule leads to increased delivery of H^+ to the tubular lumen, which is then used to shuttle HCO_3^- back into the tubular cell. Hence, HCO_3^- resorption is increased while net H^+ secretion remains unchanged.

Answer B is incorrect. Increased Na^+-H^+ exchange in the proximal tubule leads to increased delivery of H^+ to the tubular lumen, which is then used to shuttle HCO_3^- back into the tubular cells. Hence, HCO_3^- resorption is

increased while net H^+ secretion remains unchanged.

Answer C is incorrect. Increased Na^+-H^+ exchange in the proximal tubule leads to increased delivery of H^+ to the tubular lumen, which is then used to shuttle HCO_3^- back into the tubular cells. Hence, HCO_3^- resorption is increased while net H^+ secretion remains unchanged. There is no net increase in H^+ secretion, as the H^+ in the lumen is returned to the cell in the process of HCO_3^- resorption.

Answer E is incorrect. Increased Na^+-H^+ exchange in the proximal tubule leads to increased delivery of H^+ to the tubular lumen. However, there is no net increase in H^+ secretion, as the H^+ in the lumen is returned to the tubular cell in the process of HCO_3^- resorption.

25. **The correct answer is A.** Given the patient's fever, rash, loss of urine concentrating ability (low specific gravity of urine), and biopsy findings, this patient most likely has acute interstitial nephritis. Acute interstitial nephritis has a variety of causes, but by far the most common is drugs, which include antibiotics such as β-lactams, sulfonamides, quinolones, and rifampin; anticonvulsant drugs; infection with certain strains of bacteria (*Streptococcus, Staphylococcus, Legionella*); and viruses (Epstein-Barr virus, cytomegalovirus, HIV).

Answer B is incorrect. Chronic hypertension can cause hypertensive glomerulosclerosis, but not interstitial inflammation and papillary necrosis. Also, renal damage due to hypertension does not present with fever and rash.

Answer C is incorrect. Lead ingestion can produce tubulointerstitial damage, but the progression of renal disease due to lead toxicity takes a prolonged, chronic course and is not consistent with the acute clinical picture seen in this patient.

Answer D is incorrect. Multiple myeloma and other plasma cell dyscrasias can cause renal lesions known as myeloma kidney, characterized by atrophic tubules, eosinophilic casts, and multinucleated giant cells, which are not seen in this patient. Furthermore, the cause of renal damage due to multiple myeloma is the accumulation of Bence-Jones protein, which causes the formation of proteinaceous casts and Bence-Jones proteinuria.

Answer E is incorrect. Wegener's granulomatosis causes renal damage, but this disease presents with focal, segmental glomerulonephritis with crescent formation and concomitant pulmonary disease. These symptoms and this pathologic picture are not seen in this patient.

26. **The correct answer is E.** On its own, tobramycin, an aminoglycoside, can cause nephrotoxicity. However, when combined with a cephalosporin (such as cefoxitin), the nephrotoxic effects are greatly increased. Renal failure is reflected by the elevated creatinine level.

    Answer A is incorrect. Azithromycin is not an appropriate treatment for *Klebsiella pneumoniae* infection and is not associated with nephrotoxicity.

    Answer B is incorrect. Aztreonam is not associated with nephrotoxicity.

    Answer C is incorrect. Clindamycin can cause pseudomembranous colitis but does not cause nephrotoxicity.

    Answer D is incorrect. Piperacillin is associated with hypersensitivity reactions and not nephrotoxicity.

27. **The correct answer is D.** This patient presents with pyelonephritis, which is characterized by costovertebral angle tenderness, fever, and chills. Symptoms of lower UTI may also be present, such as dysuria, increased frequency of urination, and urgency. The onset of symptoms of pyelonephritis often occurs approximately 1 week after the onset of a lower UTI. In children, recurrent UTIs suggest an anatomic abnormality and warrant further investigation. Lower UTIs may ascend to the kidneys through incompetent ureterovesical sphincters, leading to pyelonephritis, dilatation of the ureters, and renal pelves, potentially causing renal scarring. Thus urologic repair is often recom-

mended to prevent renal damage in children with vesicoureteral reflux.

Answer A is incorrect. Immunoglobulin deficiency, such as Bruton's X-linked agammaglobulinemia, is associated with recurrent bacterial infections that in this age group typically affect the lungs, ears, skin, and sinuses.

Answer B is incorrect. Nephroblastoma, or Wilms' tumor, is the most common solid renal tumor in children and usually presents with a palpable abdominal mass. Vesicoureteral reflux is more prevalent than nephroblastoma.

Answer C is incorrect. Poststreptococcal glomerulonephritis typically presents 1–2 weeks after an infection with Group A β-hemolytic streptococci. The vignette does not provide any evidence of a recent streptococcal infection.

28. **The correct answer is D.** ADH binds V_2 receptors on the basolateral side of the principal cell and activates a G_s-mediated cyclic adenosine monophosphate cascade. The final result is that aquaporin transmembrane channels, previously sequestered within intracellular vesicles, are mobilized to the luminal surface of the cells. Net water movement may now occur from the collecting duct lumen to the hyperosmolar interstitium, decreasing urine output and conserving volume.

    Answer A is incorrect. A represents the apical sodium channel, which reabsorbs sodium from the collecting duct lumen. The potassium sparing diuretics amiloride and triamterene bind and block this channel.

    Answer B is incorrect. C represents luminal aquaporins. While ADH indirectly mobilizes these proteins, it does not bind them directly.

    Answer C is incorrect. ADH is coupled to G_s, not G_i.

    Answer E is incorrect. D represents intracellular mineralocorticoid receptors, which are stimulated by aldosterone.

29. **The correct answer is B.** When the amount of fluids in the body contracts, the body attempts to compensate by releasing angio-

tensin II, a potent vasoconstrictor. In order to protect the kidney from losing its perfusion due to this vasoconstriction, the kidney simultaneously releases prostaglandins at both the afferent and efferent arterioles, where they act as vasodilators. By inhibiting cyclooxygenase (COX)-1 and/or (COX)-2 enzymes, the pathway that produces the prostaglandins that keep the kidneys perfused becomes blocked, leading to decreased blood flow to the kidneys and resulting in a prerenal cause of renal failure. Celecoxib is a selective COX-2 inhibitor that affects the arterioles of the kidney and can cause renal failure in dehydrated patients.

Answer A is incorrect. Inhibition of the COX-2 enzyme will lead to a decrease in the production of thromboxane, causing a decrease in platelet aggregation. Thus, COX-2 inhibitors are used to prevent thrombosis in patients with a history of myocardial infarction or in patients with an increased likelihood of clotting. This effect is not contraindicated in the context of volume contraction.

Answer C is incorrect. Celecoxib is a selective COX-2 inhibitor that is effective because it spares the gastric mucosa the damaging effects of COX-1 inhibition.

Answer D is incorrect. The macula densa is a specialized portion of the thick ascending limb adjacent to the hilus of the glomerulus. The cells of the macula densa sense changes in sodium and chloride concentrations. Inhibition of COX-2 enzymes prevents macula densa stimulation of renin secretion. However, in times of dehydration, the body upregulates secretion of renin.

Answer E is incorrect. Inhibition of the COX-2 enzyme will lead to a decrease in the production of prostaglandins, thromboxane, and prostacyclins, which affect platelet function and small vessel diameter. This effect is not contraindicated in the context of volume contraction.

30. **The correct answer is D.** Renal blood flow is determined by the equation: flow = change in pressure/resistance. In the kidney, resistance is provided by the glomerular afferent and efferent arterioles. These arterioles can be modified by a number of endogenous substances and physiologic actions. Dopamine has a selective action such that low levels dilate cerebral, cardiac, splanchnic, and renal arterioles. Similarly, bradykinin induces the vasodilation of arterioles. The combined actions of these substances act to reduce resistance and thus increase renal blood flow.

Answer A is incorrect. Stimulation of afferent α_1-adrenergic receptors acts to vasoconstrict the arteriole.

Answer B is incorrect. Stimulation of afferent angiotensin II receptors acts to vasoconstrict the arteriole.

Answer C is incorrect. In autoregulation of renal blood flow, the myogenic hypothesis suggests that increased stimulation of stretch-activated calcium channels in the vascular smooth muscle causes an increase in intracellular calcium and a contraction of the muscle. This increase in resistance produces a reduction in flow.

Answer E is incorrect. α_1-Adrenergic receptors are found on both the afferent and efferent arterioles, but there are far more receptors on the afferent vessels. AT II is a potent constrictor of both afferent and efferent arterioles, but the efferent arterioles are more sensitive to low levels of AT II. Activating both receptors causes vasoconstriction, thereby increasing vascular resistance and decreasing flow.

31. **The correct answer is A.** The patient's urinalysis indicates that her renal failure is intrarenal in origin (shown by her fractional excretion of sodium of between 2% and 4%) and that interstitial nephritis is occurring (as seen by the WBC casts). Allergic interstitial nephritis is an inflammatory process that results in infiltration of the interstitium of the kidney with polymorphonuclear leukocytes and lymphocytes. The cause of interstitial nephritis is usually an allergic reaction to medications, but infections and immunologic disorders occasionally precipitate the disorder. Medications commonly associated with allergic reaction include penicillins

(particularly methicillin and nafcillin), cephalosporins, and sulfonamides. Clinical findings include fever, rash, and eosinophilia. The most likely culprit in this case is the penicillin she was given for the foot infection.

Answer B is incorrect. Poststreptococcal glomerulonephritis is a type of immune-complex glomerulonephritis. This condition usually presents about 10 days after pharyngitis or 2 weeks after skin infection and is usually seen in children. Most patients test positive for antistreptolysin O, which can be helpful in making the diagnosis. While this is possible given her skin infection, it classically presents with a nephritic picture. Eosinophils and rash would not be seen.

Answer C is incorrect. While it is theoretically possible that the infection in this patient's puncture wound entered the bloodstream and led to septic shock, causing hypoperfusion of the kidney and prerenal acute renal failure, it is unlikely. First, the patient's infection responded well to antibiotics. Second, the pattern of acute renal failure suggests a parenchymal rather than prerenal etiology. In prerenal failure, typically the ratio of BUN to creatinine is >20 and the fractional excretion of sodium is <1%, indicating volume depletion with normally functioning glomeruli and tubules. In addition, prerenal failure is not associated with eosinophilia.

Answer D is incorrect. Systemic lupus erythematosus (SLE) is a chronic autoimmune disease that affects multiple organ systems, including the kidney. SLE affects young adults (women almost three times more than men) and usually presents with a glomerular nephritis rather than with interstitial nephritis. Eosinophilia is not typically found in lupus nephropathy.

Answer E is incorrect. Urolithiasis (kidney stones) will present with postrenal failure and a fractional excretion of sodium of >4%. The complications of urolithiasis are hydronephrosis due to obstruction and interstitial nephritis if the stone is secondary to a bacterial infec-

tion. On clinical presentation, some patients present with excruciating flank pain.

32. **The correct answer is B.** Increased sodium intake leads to volume expansion and increased stretch in baroreceptors located in the afferent arteriole. The baroreceptor response to increased plasma volume is decreased sympathetic activity producing vasodilation of glomerular afferent arterioles. This increases the GFR while also decreasing sodium reabsorption in the proximal tubule.

Answer A is incorrect. Atrial natriuretic peptide is secreted by the atria in response to increased extracellular fluid volume and causes dilation, not constriction, of the glomerular afferent arterioles.

Answer C is incorrect. Atrial natriuretic peptide is secreted by the atria in response to increased extracellular fluid volume and causes dilation of the glomerular afferent arterioles. However, this is a physiologic response by cells in the atria of the heart to high sodium intake and volume expansion, not a response intrinsic to the kidney.

Answer D is incorrect. This is the opposite response to the correct answer. High sodium intake leads to volume expansion and increased stretch in baroreceptors, which leads to decreased sympathetic activity, not increased activity. Additionally, constriction of the afferent arteriole would cause a decrease in GFR.

Answer E is incorrect. Increased plasma sodium and water leads to increased sodium chloride delivery to the macula densa, leading to the suppression (not the increase) of renin release by the JG apparatus.

33. **The correct answer is B.** The ureter crosses the iliac artery anteriorly at its bifurcation. It then continues into the pelvis, where is passes posteriorly to the uterine artery. One way to remember the location of the ureter with relation to the uterine artery is "water under the bridge."

Answer A is incorrect. The ureter does cross over (anterior to) the iliac artery but crosses the uterine artery posteriorly.

Answer C is incorrect. The ureter does cross the uterine artery on the posterior aspect, but it passes over (anterior to) the iliac artery.

Answer D is incorrect. The ureter crosses over (anterior to) the iliac artery and under (posterior to) the uterine artery.

Answer E is incorrect. The ovarian artery is found posterior to the psoas muscle, while the ureter runs along the anterior surface of the psoas muscle.

34. **The correct answer is A.** The glomerular basement membrane is composed of endothelial fenestrae with filtration slits lined with anionic glycoproteins on the lamina rara interna and externa. The small diameter of the filtration slits partially blocks albumin filtration, but the charge selectivity of the barrier provides the largest obstacle to filtration by electrostatically repelling the negatively charged albumin molecules.

Answer B is incorrect. This choice is incorrect, as the filtration slits are lined with negatively charged anionic glycoproteins and are not positively charged.

Answer C is incorrect. Albumin is neither freely filtered by the glomerulus nor reabsorbed along the nephron.

Answer D is incorrect. Basement membrane proteoglycans are negatively charged, as is albumin.

Answer E is incorrect. The size selectivity of the endothelial filtration slits provides an obstacle to albumin filtration, but size selectivity alone does not account for the complete absence of albumin filtration in nonpathologic states.

35. **The correct answer is C.** To understand the metabolic abnormality of this woman, one must first look at the pH and then the HCO_3^- and partial carbon dioxide pressure. Her pH is 7.28, so she is suffering from a form of acidosis.

Metabolic acidosis is the presence of low pH with low plasma HCO_3^- level; her level is 15 mEq/L (normal = 23 mEq/L), thus she is suffering from metabolic acidosis. Her lungs are blowing off more CO_2 in order to raise the pH. The causes of metabolic acidosis are events that either increase acid levels (e.g., diabetic ketoacidosis, uremia, hypovolemic shock) or decrease the amount of base present (e.g., diarrhea, kidney failure). Metabolic acidosis can be further subdivided into non-anion-gap and anion-gap metabolic acidosis. The serum anion gap ($[Na^+]$ – $[Cl^-]$ – $[HCO_3^-]$) is usually within 10–16 mEq/L. If the primary cause of acidosis is a loss of HCO_3^-, there will be an increase in Cl^- and the anion gap will be normal, as seen in the case of severe diarrhea. However, in the case of high serum anion gap, the metabolic acidosis is caused by an increase of an "unmeasured" anion (e.g., lactate in the case of lactic acidosis): (Na^+) – (Cl^-) – (HCO_3^-) = unmeasured anions – unmeasured cations. In this case the patient's anion gap is 137 – 112 – 15 = 10, thus she has a non-anion gap acidosis. Of the answers listed, only diarrhea can cause a non-anion gap acidosis.

Answer A is incorrect. Salicylate overdose is one of the causes of anion-gap acidosis (ingested salicylic acid is the unmeasured anion). Note that severe salicylate toxicity can cause respiratory depression, which would cause a high partial arterial carbon dioxide pressure.

Answer B is incorrect. Diabetic ketoacidosis causes a severe anion-gap acidosis (the unmeasured anions in this case are ketoacids). One way to remember all of the causes of anion gap acidosis is the mnemonic **MUDPILES**: Methanol, Uremia, Diabetic ketoacidosis, Paraldehyde or Phenformin, Iron tablets or Isoniazid, Lactic acidosis, Ethylene glycol, Salicylates.

Answer D is incorrect. Underperfusion causes anion-gap acidosis (the anion in this case is lactic acid). The patient has a non-anion gap acidosis, so this answer is incorrect.

Answer E is incorrect. Uremia indicates renal failure. The inability of the kidney to excrete organic acids leads to an anion-gap acidosis. Renal failure also causes hyperkalemia because the kidney is unable to excrete potassium.

36. **The correct answer is B.** Inulin is freely filtered across the glomerular capillary wall and is neither reabsorbed nor secreted. It is therefore used to calculate the GFR, otherwise known as clearance of inulin. Creatinine clearance can also be used as a physiologic approximation of GFR. GFR is calculated as: urinary concentration of inulin × urinary flow rate/plasma concentration of inulin. Using this equation, urine flow rate = GFR × plasma concentration of inulin/urinary inulin concentration = 120 mL/min × 1.5 mg/mL ÷ 50 mg/mL = 3.6 mL/min. Note that glomerular capillary hydrostatic pressure listed in the table of laboratory values is a distracter that is not used in the equation.

    Answer A is incorrect. This answer underestimates the patient's urine flow rate, which is 3.6 mL/min.

    Answer C is incorrect. This answer overestimates the patient's urine flow rate, which is 3.6 mL/min.

    Answer D is incorrect. This answer translates into a value of 0.6 mL/min, which underestimates the patient's urine flow rate, which is 3.6 mL/min.

    Answer E is incorrect. This answer translates into a value of 0.3 mL/min, which underestimates the patient's urine flow rate, which is 3.6 mL/min.

37. **The correct answer is D.** Hydrochlorothiazide is a diuretic that inhibits NaCl reabsorption at the distal tubule and also reduces the excretion of calcium. The inhibition of the NaCl symporter on the luminal side of the cell results in decreased Na^+ transport into the cells of the distal convoluted tubule. This results in an increased Na^+ electrochemical gradient. On the interstitial side of the distal convoluted tubule cells, there is a Na^+/Ca^{2+} antiporter, which responds to this change in the Na^+ gradient by transporting more Na^+ into the cell, while transporting more Ca^{2+} into the interstitium. Ca^{2+} is transported on the luminal side of the cell by a parathyroid hormone-controlled chan-

nel, which is not inhibited by the thiazide diuretics. Thus thiazide diuretics are often used to treat chronic renal stone formation (due to hypercalciuria).

Answer A is incorrect. Acetazolamide inhibits carbonic anhydrase at the proximal convoluted tubule to cause increased excretion of HCO_3^-. It has no effect on calcium excretion.

Answer B is incorrect. Amiloride is also a potassium-sparing diuretic that directly inhibits the Na^+ reabsorption transport ion at the cortical collecting duct and thus reduces the K^+ secretion at the same site. Amiloride has no effect on calcium excretion.

Answer C is incorrect. Furosemide is a loop diuretic that reduces the medullary concentration gradient by inhibiting the co-transport of ions (Na^+, K^+, and $2Cl^-$) in the thick ascending loop of Henle. Because of the blockade of this cotransporter and its creation of the lumen-positive potential, there is decreased reabsorption of divalent cations, including calcium. Therefore, furosemide actually increases calcium excretion from the kidney.

Answer E is incorrect. Spironolactone is a potassium-sparing diuretic that functions as an aldosterone antagonist so that Na^+ reabsorption and K^+ secretion are inhibited at the cortical collecting duct. It does not affect calcium excretion.

38. **The correct answer is C.** Osmotic diuretics are filtered but not reabsorbed and thus serve to increase the osmolarity of tubular fluid, drawing water into the lumen and increasing urine production. Although osmotic diuretics are functional at many locations along the nephron, their primary site of action is in the descending loop of Henle, where the tubule is permeable to water but impermeable to solutes.

Answer A is incorrect. The collecting tubule is the site of action for potassium-sparing diuretics.

Answer B is incorrect. The distal tubule is the site of action for thiazide diuretics.

Answer D is incorrect. The thick ascending limb of the loop of Henle is the site of action for furosemide and other loop diuretics.

39. **The correct answer is C.** Focal segmental glomerulosclerosis is a nephrotic disease and generally presents in African-Americans between 18–30 years of age; it is three to four times more common in men than in women. Other risk factors include obesity and HIV-positive status. Nephrotic syndrome is a renal disorder that is characterized by massive proteinuria (>3.5 g/24 h protein in urine). This is due to, hypoalbuminemia, generalized edema, and hyperlipidemia (thought to be secondary to elevated hepatic activity, which is meant to replace the lost albumin and clotting factors). Simply put, this is considered a "leaky" kidney without active inflammation. The name of the disease describes the pattern of glomerular damage, which is glomerular sclerosis (obliteration of capillary lumen) with focal (<50% of glomeruli affected) and segmental (only parts of glomerulus effected) patterns. The cause of focal segmental glomerulosclerosis is unknown. Typically it is resistant to steroid treatment.

Answer A is incorrect. Focal segmental glomerulosclerosis means that <50% of the glomeruli are affected (focal) and that only parts of the glomerular tuft are affected (segmental). This answer is not consistent with this definition.

Answer B is incorrect. Focal segmental glomerulosclerosis means that <50% of the glomeruli are affected (focal) and that only parts of the glomerular tuft are affected (segmental). This answer is not consistent with this definition.

Answer D is incorrect. Focal segmental glomerulosclerosis means that <50% of the glomeruli are affected (focal) and that only parts of the glomerular tuft are affected (segmental). This answer is not consistent with this definition.

Answer E is incorrect. There is no cellular proliferation seen in focal segmental glomerulosclerosis.

40. **The correct answer is D.** Glucose is reabsorbed from the proximal tubule by a sodium-glucose cotransport system. These transporters are able to handle filtered glucose concentrations in the healthy physiologic range. Glucose transporters are able to reabsorb all glucose up to 200 mg/dL. At 200 mg/dL, however, the transporters begin to become saturated and glucose starts to spill into the urine. At 350 mg/dL, all transporters are occupied and all filtered glucose above that concentration is excreted. Glucose will therefore not begin to spill into Mr. Jones' urine until his glucose level is elevated to at least 200 mg/dL.

Answer A is incorrect. Glucose is normally resorbed completely by the proximal tubule. There are no glucose transporters elsewhere in the renal tubules.

Answer B is incorrect. Negatively charged proteins in the glomerular wall help form the glomerular filtration barrier. In particular, they impede the filtration of large negatively charged molecules such as albumin and other plasma proteins. Glucose, a small neutral molecule, is not affected by this barrier.

Answer C is incorrect. Glomerular capillaries are made up of fenestrated epithelial cells that do not contain tight junctions. Tight junctions are normally found in the blood-brain barrier of the brain and retina.

Answer E is incorrect. The sodium-potassium exchange pump indirectly provides the energy for glucose resorption in the proximal convoluted tubule; the sodium gradient is necessary for the sodium-glucose cotransporters to function. Glucose is only resorbed in the proximal tubule, not in the distal tubule.

41. **The correct answer is E.** This clinical presentation is classic for benign prostatic hyperplasia obstructing the urethra and causing bilateral hydronephrosis. The cystogram shows gross enlargement of the prostate gland that is elevating the bladder base. This obstruction can lead to renal failure. Renal failure can be divided into prerenal (due to lack of perfusion of the kidney), intrinsic renal (due to acute tubular necrosis from ischemia or toxins), and postre-

nal (due to obstruction of outflow). Each type of renal failure has distinct characteristics, allowing differentiation by urinalysis. In postrenal failure, the kidneys are unable to effectively concentrate the urine, so the urine osmolality would be <350 mmol/kg.

Answer A is incorrect. Epithelial casts are seen in acute tubular necrosis, a cause of intrinsic renal failure.

Answer B is incorrect. A BUN:Cr ratio <15 is seen with intrinsic renal failure because renal damage causes decreased BUN reabsorption. In postrenal failure, reduced flow causes increased BUN reabsorption without increased Cr reabsorption, therefore the BUN:Cr ratio is >15.

Answer C is incorrect. The fractional excretion of sodium is a measure of the amount of sodium in the urine compared to the amount of sodium in the plasma, and can be calculated by $[(U_{Na} \times P_{Cr}) / (P_{Na} \times U_{Cr})] \times 100$. A value <1% would be expected in prerenal failure, where the kidney is working to reabsorb as much sodium as possible to increase plasma volume and thereby improve perfusion. In postrenal failure, the kidney is unable to effectively reabsorb sodium, and therefore the fractional excretion of sodium would commonly be >4%.

Answer D is incorrect. A urine sodium level of <10 mmol/L would be expected in prerenal failure, where the kidney is working to reabsorb as much sodium as possible to increase plasma volume and thereby improve perfusion. In postrenal failure, the kidney is unable to effectively reabsorb sodium, and therefore the urine sodium level would commonly be >40 mmol/L.

42. **The correct answer is D.** Inulin clearance is an accurate estimate of GFR because it is freely filtered and neither reabsorbed nor secreted in the nephron. Because it overestimates true GFR, compound X must therefore undergo net secretion in the nephron. That is, more compound X is excreted in the urine

than is filtered at the glomerulus. Indeed, it is precisely this mechanism that is responsible for the characteristic overestimation of GFR by measuring creatinine clearance.

Answer A is incorrect. If compound X were not freely filtered at the glomerulus, its clearance would underestimate GFR.

Answer B is incorrect. The descending limb of the loop of Henle is poorly permeable to solute and instead allows passive efflux of water from the filtrate. Furthermore, compound X cannot undergo net reabsorption in the nephron.

Answer C is incorrect. The proximal convoluted tubule is responsible for most ultrafiltrate reabsorption. However, if compound X underwent net reabsorption, its clearance would underestimate, not overestimate, the inulin-calculated GFR.

Answer E is incorrect. Inulin is freely filtered and neither reabsorbed nor secreted in the nephron. It is these characteristics that allow its use as an accurate measure of GFR.

43. **The correct answer is B.** In diabetic nephropathy, diagnostic tests are important in the treatment and control of the progression of the disease. The histologic morphology is characterized by an increase in mesangial matrix by marked nodular accumulations known as Kimmelstiel-Wilson nodules and diffuse glomerulosclerosis.

Answer A is incorrect. Rapidly progressive (crescentic) glomerulonephritis is a renal disease that has a rapid course (weeks to months) to renal failure. It is characterized by extensive capillary damage that leads to accumulation of cells and fibrinous changes in Bowman's space, leading to the characteristic "crescent" seen on biopsy.

Answer C is incorrect. Membranoproliferative glomerulonephritis is an uncommon autoimmune renal disorder that normally affects young individuals (8–30 years of age). The diagnosis is based on a histologic presentation that includes mesangial proliferation, thickening of the peripheral capillary walls by subendothelial immune deposits, and mesangial interposition into the capillary wall, giving rise to a tram-track appearance on light microscopy.

Answer D is incorrect. Focal segmental glomerulosclerosis is a nephrotic disease and generally presents in young, hypertensive African-American males (obesity and HIV-positive status are also risk factors). The name of the disease describes the pattern of glomerular damage, which is glomerular sclerosis (obliteration of capillary lumen) with focal patterns (some glomeruli affected) and segmental patterns (only parts of glomerulus).

Answer E is incorrect. Membranoproliferative glomerulonephritis is characterized by a tram-track appearance on light microscopy due to mesangial interposition into the capillary wall.

44. **The correct answer is B.** Calcium is reabsorbed in three areas along the nephron: the proximal tubule, the thick ascending limb of the loop of Henle, and the distal tubule. In the proximal tubule, calcium reabsorption is coupled to sodium reabsorption. In the distal tubule, calcium reabsorption is controlled by parathyroid hormone. In the thick ascending limb, however, calcium reabsorption is dependent on the function of the sodium-potassium-chloride cotransporter (NKCC). Calcium reabsorption occurs paracellularly, driven by the electrochemical gradient created by NKCC. Because the sodium potassium pump (ATPase) causes sodium to exit the cell and potassium to enter, it creates the sodium-generated driving force for the NKCC. The potassium that enters from the basolateral (through the ATPase) and luminal (through NKCC) cell surfaces is passed passively through both the basolateral and luminal membranes by specific channels. Because the cotransporter brings in two cations and two anions and the ATPase exchanges three cations for two cations, the potassium exiting the luminal membrane creates an electronegative environment inside the cell. This +7-mV positive luminal charge difference drives the reabsorption of calcium (and magnesium) by a paracellular route.

Answer A is incorrect. Parathyroid hormone controls calcium reabsorption in the distal tubule.

Answer C is incorrect. Calcium delivery plays a role in driving calcium reabsorption, but the transluminal gradient established by the NKCC is more important.

Answer D is incorrect. The triple transporter maintains a lumen positive charge; positive ions are reabsorbed to maintain electroneutrality.

Answer E is incorrect. Sodium and calcium are not cotransported in the thick ascending loop of Henle.

45. **The correct answer is C.** This patient is in cardiogenic shock, which is shown by his hypotension with a systolic blood pressure of <90 mm Hg. This has led to a loss of perfusion in his kidneys, which has, in turn, led to prerenal failure. Prerenal failure is defined by a BUN:Cr ratio of >20:1. When the GFR drops, there is an increase in sodium and water reabsorption in the proximal tubule. This leads to an increase in tubular urea concentration, which favors increased reabsorption of urea. This will raise the BUN (remember, this is urea in the blood) and therefore, the BUN:Cr ratio will rise.

Answer A is incorrect. Blockage of the ureters is a postrenal cause of renal failure. It would present with pain on urination and is unlikely in the setting of cardiogenic shock.

Answer B is incorrect. This patient's BUN:Cr ratio of >20:1 indicates that this is a prerenal process, not an intrarenal one. An acute tubular necrosis would present with renal failure in the setting of a BUN:Cr ratio of 10–15:1 with many hyaline casts and cellular debris in the urine.

Answer D is incorrect. Ethanol actually causes diuresis. By inhibiting the release of anti-diuretic hormone from the posterior pituitary, alcohol consumption leads to increased urine output. The volume load that accompanies alcohol ingestion also contributes to increased urine output.

Answer E is incorrect. Urine output is controlled mainly by two factors: the hydration state of the body and the level of kidney function. Therefore, low urine output is seen only in the setting of dehydration or kidney dysfunction. Stress by itself will not cause low urine output unless it is coupled with dehydration or an acute renal disease process.

46. **The correct answer is E.** Acute poststreptococcal glomerulonephritis is an autoimmune disease most frequently seen in children. Under light microscopy, the glomeruli appear enlarged and hypercellular, with neutrophils and subepithelial immune complex depositions described as "lumpy-bumpy." Under electron microscopy, the large irregular deposits are observed in the subepithelium of the glomerulus. This condition normally presents a few weeks after a streptococcal infection with peripheral and periorbital edema, dark urine, and proteinuria. These symptoms are caused by circulating antistreptococcal antibody-antigen complexes that deposit in the glomerular basement membrane, leading to complement activation and glomerular damage. The classic findings are RBCs and casts in the urine (which cause the characteristic tea-colored urine), a positive antistreptolysin O titer, and decreased levels of complement.

Answer A is incorrect. Granular subendothelial deposits are usually seen in systemic lupus erythematosus.

Answer B is incorrect. Linear subendothelial patterns are seen in vasculitides such as Goodpasture's syndrome.

Answer C is incorrect. Mesangial deposits are usually seen in IgA nephropathy.

Answer D is incorrect. A "spike-and-dome" pattern of deposition is a pattern seen in membranous glomerulonephritis.

47. **The correct answer is C.** Hydrochlorothiazide and furosemide cause metabolic alkalosis. Note that the laboratory values have elevated pH, partial arterial carbon dioxide pressure, and bicarbonate, indicating a metabolic alkalosis with partial respiratory compensation. Both thiazides and loop diuretics inhibit sodium uptake and thus increase distal delivery of sodium to the late distal tubule and collecting duct. An increased amount of sodium is taken into these distal cells from the luminal surface and exchanged for potassium and protons to maintain electroneutrality. This creates a condition of hypokalemia (too little potassium in the blood), kaluresis (urination of excess potassium), and excess urinary acid secretion. This loss of acid promotes metabolic alkalosis. In addition, hypokalemia induces the movement of potassium from its vast storehouse within tissues to the extracellular compartment in exchange for protons. This movement of potassium from tissues into blood and protons from the blood into tissues further promotes metabolic alkalosis.

Answer A is incorrect. Acetazolamide impairs reuptake of bicarbonate and secretion of acid in the proximal tubule. The loss of bicarbonate in the urine leads to metabolic acidosis.

Answer B is incorrect. Diuretics do not cause respiratory alkalosis.

Answer D is incorrect. Diuretics do not cause respiratory alkalosis.

Answer E is incorrect. Spironolactone inhibits the absorption of sodium in the distal convoluted tubule and proximal collecting duct, resulting in a decrease in secretion of other cations (potassium and protons) into the lumen. Decreased acid secretion can result in metabolic acidosis.

Answer F is incorrect. Diuretics do not cause respiratory alkalosis.

48. **The correct answer is D.** The lab values given show low pH with low plasma bicarbonate and lack of an anion gap. Anion gap can be calculated by: $Na^+ - (Cl^- + HCO_3^-)$, where normal is within 10–16 mEq/L. This patient has a nonanion gap metabolic acidosis. The cause of metabolic acidosis is generally either an increase in acid (e.g., diabetic ketoacidosis, hypovolemic shock via generation of lactic acid) or a decrease in base (e.g., diarrhea, kidney failure). Metabolic acidosis can be further subdivided into nonanion-gap and anion-gap metabolic ac-

idosis. If the primary cause of acidosis is a loss of HCO_3^-, there will be an increase in Cl^- and the anion gap will be normal, as seen in the case of severe diarrhea. However, in the case of high serum anion gap, the metabolic acidosis is caused by an increase of an "unmeasured" anion such as lactate (e.g., lactic acidosis).

Answer A is incorrect. The lab values in this choice are consistent with an anion gap metabolic acidosis. However, the patient's anion gap will be normal. The primary cause of her metabolic acidosis is loss in HCO_3^- due to her diarrhea. Increased anion-gap metabolic acidosis is caused by an increase in "unmeasured" anion. A useful mnemonic is **MUDPILES**: **M**ethanol, **U**remia, **D**iabetic ketoacidosis/ EtOH ketoacidosis, **P**araldehyde, **I**soniazid/ Iron toxicity, **L**actic acidosis, **E**thylene glycol, and **S**alicylates. Rhabdomyolysis is also a cause of metabolic acidosis but traditionally is not included in this mnemonic.

Answer B is incorrect. Respiratory acidosis is the presence of low pH due to a decrease in ventilation and an increase in serum carbon dioxide. This occurs in cases of inadequate ventilation (e.g., depressed respiration by drugs or neurologic injury) or impaired gas exchange (e.g., pulmonary edema). This would not be caused by diarrhea.

Answer C is incorrect. Metabolic alkalosis is the presence of high pH with increased plasma bicarbonate. This occurs with addition of alkaline compounds (antacid ingestion) or loss of acid (vomiting). This would not be caused by diarrhea.

Answer E is incorrect. In severe diarrhea with significant loss of fluids and electrolytes, especially bicarbonate, it is unlikely that the patient will have a normal acid-base state.

Answer F is incorrect. Respiratory alkalosis is the presence of high pH due to an increase in ventilation leading to a decrease in serum carbon dioxide. This occurs in cases of increased respiratory drive (e.g., by drugs or central nervous system disorders, anxiety, and fear). This would not be caused by diarrhea.

49. **The correct answer is A.** Demeclocycline is a tetracycline that is associated with nephrotoxicity, hepatotoxicity, and tooth discoloration.

Answer B is incorrect. Neomycin is an aminoglycoside that is associated with nephrotoxicity, ototoxicity, and a myasthenialike syndrome.

Answer C is incorrect. Norfloxacin is a fluoroquinolone and is associated with tendinitis and tendon rupture.

Answer D is incorrect. Penicillin is associated with hypersensitivity reactions and hemolytic anemia in sensitive individuals.

Answer E is incorrect. Vancomycin is associated with nephrotoxicity, ototoxicity, and thrombophlebitis. It is also known to cause a diffuse flushing known as "red man" syndrome.

50. **The correct answer is B.** The only diuretics acting along the thick ascending limb of the nephron are loop agents (e.g., furosemide, torsemide, ethacrynic acid). These drugs work by inhibiting the NKCC. It is worth noting that ethacrynic acid is unique because it is not a sulfonamide and therefore can be used in individuals with an allergy to sulfa drugs.

Answer A is incorrect. Acetazolamide, which acts in the proximal convoluted tubule, blocks resorption of sodium bicarbonate.

Answer C is incorrect. Hydrochlorothiazide inhibits sodium chloride resorption in the early distal tubule.

Answer D is incorrect. Osmotic agents act in three places along the nephron: the proximal convoluted tubule, the thin descending limb, and the collecting tubule. They do not, however, act on any of the ion pumps.

Answer E is incorrect. Triamterene, a potassium-sparing diuretic, blocks sodium channels in the cortical collecting tubule.

CHAPTER 16

Reproductive

QUESTIONS

1. A 53-year-old woman experiences hot flashes associated with menopause. She calls her primary care physician to ask for advice about the risks and benefits of hormone replacement therapy (HRT). Which of the following is a potential benefit of HRT?

   (A) Decreased risk of breast cancer
   (B) Decreased risk of deep venous thrombosis
   (C) Decreased risk of hip fracture
   (D) Decreased risk of myocardial infarction
   (E) Decreased risk of stroke

2. A 38-year-old nulliparous woman comes to the physician for an annual check-up. She reports a 10-pack-year smoking history and a family history of early mastectomy. Physical examination is notable for a scaly patch on her right nipple. On palpation, there is a firm mass and a clear discharge from the nipple. Which of the following would most likely be seen on a histological examination of this mass?

   (A) Intralobular clusters of tumor cells
   (B) Large cells with clear halos
   (C) Lymphocytic infiltration
   (D) Necrosis
   (E) Pools of mucus
   (F) Proliferation of normal epithelial cells
   (G) Proliferation of normal glands and ducts

3. During hernia surgeries, it is important to isolate important structures in the inguinal canal so that they do not become damaged and cause a functional deficit. Which of the following structures lies inside the inguinal canal but outside of the spermatic cord?

   (A) Ductus deferens
   (B) Ilioinguinal nerve
   (C) Pampiniform plexus
   (D) Testicular artery
   (E) Testicular lymphatic vessels

4. A 23-year-old sexually active woman presents to her physician with a high temperature, pelvic pain, purulent cervical discharge, and cervical motion tenderness. A Gram's stain prepared from a swab of the discharge is shown in the image. Which of the following is the most likely infectious organism?

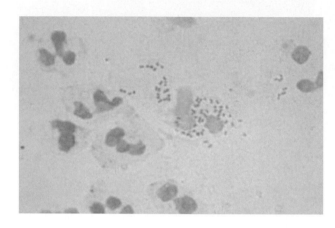

Reproduced, with permission, from Wolff K, Johnson RA, Suurmond D. *Fitzpatrick's Color Atlas & Synopsis of Clinical Dermatology*, 5th ed. New York: McGraw-Hill, 2005: Figure 27.15.

   (A) *Candida albicans*
   (B) *Chlamydia trachomatis*
   (C) *Gardnerella vaginalis*
   (D) *Neisseria gonorrhoeae*
   (E) *Trichomonas vaginalis*

5. A woman who is 31 weeks' pregnant comes to the emergency department with symptoms of preeclampsia. The presence of which of the following signs would change this initial diagnosis?

   (A) Edema
   (B) Hyperreflexia
   (C) Hypertension
   (D) Proteinuria
   (E) Seizure

6. CT imaging of the pelvis performed on a 29-year-old African-American woman with dysmenorrhea reveals uterine masses similar to those seen in the image. Biopsy shows a whorled pattern of smooth muscle. These masses are most commonly associated with which of the following conditions?

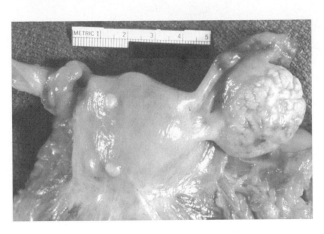

Reproduced, with permission, from PEIR Digital Library (http://peir.net).

(A) Enlargement with menopause
(B) Enlargement with pregnancy
(C) Formation of chocolate cysts
(D) Malignant transformation
(E) Necrosis and hemorrhage

7. An endocrine research laboratory is investigating the regulation of the hypothalamic-pituitary axis both through pharmacologic means and by direct ablation of different regions of the brains of chimpanzees. They find that extremely high doses of chlorpromazine as well as destruction of the hypothalamus causes the levels of a certain hormone to rise. Levels of what hormone were found to be elevated?

(A) ADH
(B) Growth hormone
(C) Luteinizing hormone
(D) Oxytocin
(E) Prolactin
(F) Testosterone
(G) Thyroid-releasing hormone

8. A patient with a testicular tumor has blood work done that shows a serum α-fetoprotein level of 30 μg/mL (normal: <10 μg/mL). Which of the following is the most likely age range of this patient?

(A) 0–3 years
(B) 10–20 years
(C) 20–30 years
(D) 30–40 years
(E) 40–50 years

9. A 25-year-old woman with a history of recurrent upper respiratory infections presents to her physician with her fifth such infection in the past year. She mentions that she may be getting sick due to increased stress at home; she and her husband have been trying to conceive unsuccessfully for several years. The patient's WBC count, immunoglobulin, and platelet levels are within normal limits. Which organizational unit represents the structure most likely to be defective in this patient?

(A) Central pair with nine peripheral pairs of microtubules
(B) Collagen α chains in triplets
(C) Multilobular nucleus with enzyme-filled granules
(D) Numerous adjoining e-cadherin molecules with actin filaments
(E) Two longer heavy chains and two shorter light chains linked by disulfide bonds

10. A young couple is having trouble conceiving and decides to undergo in vitro fertilization. The woman begins treatment to stimulate ovulation prior to ova collection and fertilization. Which of the following hormones is most directly responsible for ovulation?

(A) Estrogen
(B) Follicle-stimulating hormone
(C) Gonadotropin-releasing hormone
(D) Human chorionic gonadotropin
(E) Luteinizing hormone
(F) Progesterone

11. A 57-year-old woman is scheduled for elective hysterectomy. Severing which of the following structures during surgery would disrupt the most blood flow to the ipsilateral ovary?

(A) Cardinal ligament
(B) Fallopian tube
(C) Round ligament
(D) Suspensory ligament
(E) Ureter

12. Which of the following is the function of the androgen-binding globulin?

(A) Binding of inhibin
(B) Binding of testosterone
(C) Conversion of testosterone into estrogen
(D) Inhibition of androgen secretion
(E) Testosterone transport

13. A 23-year-old woman who works as a prostitute comes to the clinic for a follow-up appointment because the results of her Pap smear showed a high-grade squamous intraepithelial lesion. Which of the following strains of the human papillomavirus (HPV) is this condition most often associated with?

(A) Strain L1-3
(B) Strains 1 and 2
(C) Strains 6 and 11
(D) Strain 8
(E) Strains 16 and 18

14. Following a normal pregnancy and labor, a baby is born to a young couple. The baby cries immediately and has Apgar scores of 9 at both 1 and 5 minutes. While examining the baby, the pediatrician at delivery notes that the baby has some labial scrotal fusion and a phallus-like organ. The baby is also hypotensive and hypovolemic. Genotyping reveals a karyotype of 46,XX. Which of the following is the most likely cause of the patient's physical findings and symptoms?

(A) 11α-Hydroxylase deficiency
(B) 17β-Hydroxylase deficiency
(C) 21α-Hydroxylase deficiency
(D) Mutation in the androgen receptor gene
(E) 5α-Reductase deficiency

15. A 50-year-old woman tells her physician that she is concerned about her risk for developing endometrial cancer. Which of the following factors poses the largest risk for developing endometrial cancer?

(A) Alcoholism
(B) Early sexual activity
(C) Low-fiber diet
(D) Multiparity
(E) Prolonged unopposed estrogen use

16. A 64-year-old man visits his physician for an annual examination. He complains of a recent 9.1-kg (20-lb) unintentional weight loss and pain in his back and pelvis. Otherwise, he has no complaints. His examination is notable for point tenderness along his spine and pelvis. He also had firm prostate nodules palpated on digital rectal examination. Which of the following laboratory values would be expected in this patient?

Choice	Prostate Specific Antigen	Calcium	Alkaline Phosphatase
A	↓	↓	↓
B	↓	↓	↑
C	↑	↓	↓
D	↑	↓	↑
E	↑	↑	↓

(A) A
(B) B
(C) C
(D) D
(E) E

17. A 57-year-old man with erectile dysfunction has cavernosography prior to surgery. Cavernosography demonstrates a leak from the dorsal vein to the saphenous vein. Which of the following is the most likely cause of this patient's impotence?

(A) Arterial insufficiency
(B) Hormonal impotence
(C) Psychogenic impotence
(D) Somatosensory defect
(E) Venous outflow

18. A 26-year-old primigravida presents to her obstetrician for a check-up. One week earlier she underwent a cesarean section because of failure to progress. She says that she has been crying a lot over the past week and is worried that

it is not normal to feel like this. Which of the following symptoms would make one more suspicious about postpartum depression instead of postpartum blues?

(A) Anxiety about the infant
(B) Easily fatigued
(C) Easily irritated
(D) Emotional lability
(E) Feeling hopeless

19. A 28-year-old woman presents to her physician with concerns that she is unable to produce breast milk, despite having given birth approximately 1 month ago. On further questioning she indicates she has been exceptionally thirsty lately, and describes feelings of fatigue and cold intolerance. Physical examination reveals no abnormalities except a scarcity of axillary hair. Laboratory tests reveal a serum sodium level of 150 mEq/L and urinalysis reveals a urine osmolality of 220 mOsm/kg. Which of the following most likely increased the patient's risk of developing this condition?

(A) Abnormalities of the placenta
(B) Alcohol intake during pregnancy
(C) Endometriosis
(D) Gestational diabetes
(E) Incorrect use of tampons
(F) Multiple sexual partners
(G) Pelvic inflammatory disease

20. A 46,XY infant is born with a nonsense mutation in the SRY gene. Which of the following will be the symptomatic manifestation of this mutation?

(A) Female phenotype
(B) Female pseudohermaphrodite
(C) Male phenotype
(D) Male pseudohermaphrodite
(E) True hermaphrodite

21. Biopsy of a bilateral ovarian mass reveals round, mucin-secreting cells, as seen in the image. Which of the following other physical findings might be found in a patient with this condition?

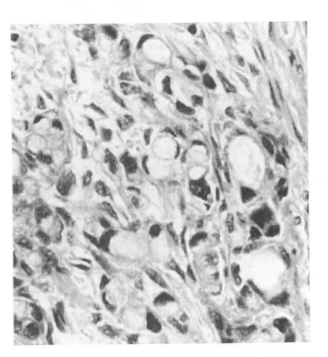

Reproduced, with permission, from Chandrasoma P, Taylor CR. *Concise Pathology*, 3rd ed. New York: McGraw-Hill, 1998: Figure 52-16.

(A) Galactorrhea
(B) Melena
(C) Palpable gallbladder
(D) Pearly papules on face
(E) Supraclavicular lymphadenopathy

22. A 25-year-old married woman who has been trying to become pregnant for the past 5 months presents to the emergency department with sudden and severe abdominal pain. Ultrasonography shows a mass in her left fallopian tube with free fluid in the cul-de-sac. Previous infection by which of the following agents most likely put this patient at a higher risk for developing this complication?

(A) *Chlamydia trachomatis*
(B) *Escherichia coli*
(C) Herpes simplex virus
(D) Human papilloma virus
(E) *Streptococcus agalactiae*

23. A woman in her seventh month of pregnancy asks her obstetrician why her breasts are enlarging. In which of the following locations is the hormone responsible for breast milk production synthesized?

(A) Adenohypophysis
(B) Corpus luteum
(C) Hypothalamus
(D) Placenta
(E) Syncytiotrophoblast

24. A 29-year-old sexually active woman presents to the clinic complaining of a malodorous, fishy vaginal discharge for the past 2 weeks. She notices the smell most after sexual activity and does not complain of any pelvic pain. On examination there is a thin, homogeneous, grayish discharge coating her vaginal wall. Vaginal pH is 6.0, and urinalysis for β-human chorionic gonadotropin (β-hCG) is negative. A saline wet mount of the vaginal fluid is shown in the image. What is the mechanism of action of the antibiotic indicated for this condition?

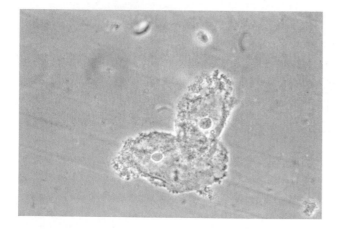

Image courtesy of the Centers for Disease Control and Prevention's Public Heath Image Library; content provider M. Rein.

(A) Binds to the 30S subunit of the ribosome and prevents attachment of aminoacyl-tRNA
(B) Inhibits DNA-dependent RNA polymerase
(C) Inhibits ergosterol synthesis
(D) Inhibits topoisomerase II
(E) Interacts with DNA to form toxic metabolites in the bacterial cell

25. A 14-year-old boy is brought to the clinic by his parents who are concerned because he has not yet begun puberty. Laboratory results indicate hypogonadism secondary to failure of the hypothalamic-pituitary-gonadal axis. Which of the following are possible adverse effects of the treatment for this patient's condition?

(A) Decreased serum LDL cholesterol levels
(B) Growth of scalp hair
(C) Increased spermatogenesis
(D) Nausea and vomiting
(E) Premature closing of the epiphyseal plates

26. A 26-year-old woman presents to her gynecologist with a purulent vaginal discharge, lower abdominal pain, and fever. She reports having unprotected sexual intercourse about 1 month ago. On physical examination, she demonstrates cervical motion tenderness. What type of organism is the most likely cause of this patient's infection?

(A) Budding yeast with pseudohyphae
(B) Coccobacillus often seen with clue cells
(C) Gram-positive, catalase-negative, bacitracin-resistant cocci
(D) Obligate intracellular parasite
(E) Trophozoites seen on wet mount

27. A 34-year-old woman is 35 weeks pregnant and comes to the emergency department because she is unable to walk secondary to swelling in her legs. Physical examination shows a temperature of 36.5° C (97.7° F), a pulse of 95/min, and a blood pressure of 150/90 mm Hg. The patient complains of a severe headache but has no other symptoms. Which of the following tests would help most in the initial diagnosis of this patient?

(A) Electroencephalogram
(B) 24-hour urine collection
(C) Liver panel
(D) Papanicolaou smear
(E) Peripheral blood smear

28. An 80-year-old woman sustains a broken hip after a minor fall from a chair. The only medications she takes are multivitamins. Which of the following is the most likely hormonal profile of this woman?

CHOICE	ESTROGEN	LUTEINIZING HORMONE	FOLLICLE-STIMULATING HORMONE	GONADOTROPIN-RELEASING HORMONE
A	↓	↓	↓	↑
B	↓	↓	↓	↓
C	↓	↑	↑	↑
D	↑	↑	↑	↑
E	↑	↑	↑	↓

(A) A
(B) B
(C) C
(D) D
(E) E

29. A 23-year-old woman comes to the physician with vaginal candidiasis and is placed on an antifungal medication. Shortly thereafter, she experiences amenorrhea. Which of the following antifungal drugs did this patient most likely use?

(A) Amphotericin B
(B) Fluconazole
(C) Flucytosine
(D) Itraconazole
(E) Ketoconazole

30. A 26-year-old man presents to a urologist after he and his wife failed to conceive for 14 months. His testosterone levels are normal, and initial semen analysis shows significantly decreased volume and no detectable sperm. Testicular fine-needle biopsy demonstrates normal sperm motility and normal sperm morphology. His past surgical history includes an inguinal repair. Which of the following is the most likely cause of the patient's infertility?

(A) Disordered sperm transport
(B) Primary gonadal deficiency
(C) Secondary hypogonadism
(D) Sperm dysfunction
(E) Y-chromosome abnormality

31. A 73-year-old patient has been hospitalized for 6 days due to complications from surgery. The patient had a urinary catheter in place, which was removed on the fourth hospital day. Now she is complaining of painful and frequent urination and has a fever of 38.9° C (102° F). Urinalysis results are positive for nitrites and leukocyte esterase. A urine culture grows a gram-negative rod that produces a red pigment. Which of the following organisms is the most likely cause of this patient's symptoms?

(A) *Candida albicans*
(B) *Escherichia coli*
(C) *Klebsiella pneumoniae*
(D) *Proteus mirabilis*
(E) *Pseudomonas aeruginosa*
(F) *Serratia marcescens*
(G) *Staphylococcus saprophyticus*

32. A 25-year-old woman comes to her physician complaining of cyclic dysmenorrhea and pain with intercourse. A sonogram reveals bilateral adnexal masses, and a laparoscopy shows chocolate cysts. This patient at risk for developing which of the following conditions?

(A) Carcinoma
(B) Infertility
(C) Masculinization
(D) Obesity

33. A new mother calls her obstetrician to say that she is having trouble breast-feeding. She is unable to produce enough milk to sate her baby even though her breasts are aching with stored milk. What is the name of the specialized intracellular organelle where the hormone this patient is lacking is stored?

    (A) Birbeck granules
    (B) Ferruginous bodies
    (C) Herring bodies
    (D) Lewy bodies
    (E) Negri bodies

34. A previously healthy 25-year-old sexually active man comes to the physician because of a painful genital rash for the past 5 days. Physical examination reveals grouped vesicles on an erythematous base. Tzanck smear shows multinucleated giant cells. Which of the following mechanisms is involved in the pathogenesis of this patient's infective agent?

    (A) Direct invasion into the bloodstream
    (B) Invasion of CD4+ cells
    (C) Migration to the central nervous system by retrograde axonal transport
    (D) Migration to the peripheral nervous system by anterograde axonal transport
    (E) Migration to the peripheral nervous system by retrograde axonal transport

35. A 2-month-old boy is brought to the pediatrician by his mother for a well-baby visit for the first time since his birth. On examination, the doctor notes that the patient has cryptorchidism, with both testicles remaining undescended. This patient is at increased risk for developing which of the following conditions?

    (A) Hypogonadotropic hypogonadism
    (B) Indirect inguinal hernia
    (C) Retractile testis
    (D) Testicular cancer
    (E) Torsion of the spermatic cord

36. A 45-year-old man presents to his physician complaining of erectile dysfunction. Which of the following is the mechanism of action of the oral agents approved for the treatment of erectile dysfunction?

    (A) Androgen supplementation
    (B) Antiandrogen action via receptor site interference
    (C) Binding to G proteins to stimulate adenylyl cyclase
    (D) Inhibition of cAMP phosphodiesterase
    (E) Inhibition of cGMP phosphodiesterase

37. A 35-year-old man comes to the physician complaining of painful genital vesicles. On further questioning, he admits to unprotected sex with multiple partners. To confirm the diagnosis, the physician performs a Tzanck test; results are shown in the image. Which of the following is the pathognomonic finding on this patient's Tzanck smear?

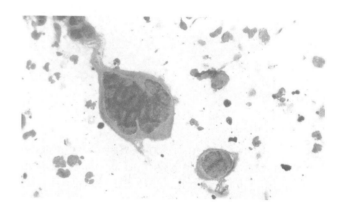

Reproduced, with permission, from Wolff K, Johnson RA, Suurmond D. *Fitzpatrick's Color Atlas & Synopsis of Clinical Dermatolgy*, 5th ed. New York: McGraw-Hill, 2005: Figure 25-23.

    (A) Auer rods
    (B) Call-Exner bodies
    (C) Lewy bodies
    (D) Mallory bodies
    (E) Multinucleated giant cell

38. A woman at 32 weeks' gestation comes to the emergency department with painless vaginal bleeding. Her temperature is 37.1° C (98.8° F), pulse is 76/min, and blood pressure is 126/90 mm Hg. The fetal heart rate is 155/min. She has no other symptoms. Urinalysis

shows no blood cells or bacteria and a normally elevated β-hCG level. Which of the following diagnoses should the emergency department physician consider before performing a gynecologic examination?

(A) Abruptio placentae
(B) Eclampsia
(C) Hydatidiform mole
(D) Placenta previa
(E) Preeclampsia

39. Abnormal opening of the urethra on the ventral penis is caused by the failure of a certain urogenital structure to complete normal development in the fetus. This structure is present in both male and female infants, but has a different fate in each. What structure in the female infant is derived from the fetal structure described here?

(A) Glans clitoris
(B) Greater vestibular glands (of Bartholin)
(C) Labia majora
(D) Labia minora
(E) Urethral and paraurethral glands (of Skene)
(F) Vestibular bulbs

40. A 66-year-old woman visits her primary care physician because she has been having vaginal bleeding for several days. Her last menstrual period was 10 years ago. Her physical examination and review of systems are otherwise normal, with the exception of blood seen within the cervical os. Which of the following is a risk factor for this condition?

(A) Alcohol consumption
(B) Late onset of menarche
(C) Multiparity
(D) Oral contraceptive pills
(E) Polycystic ovarian syndrome
(F) Smoking

41. A 24-year-old bartender returning from Panama presents to the clinic because of a painful penile lesion that appeared about 1 week after having unprotected sex with a new female partner. On examination the ulcer is 1.5 cm in diameter with an erythematous base and clearly demarcated borders. The base of the ulcer is covered with a yellow purulent exudate and bleeds when scraped. Gram stain of the exudates shows gram-negative rods in chains in a school-of-fish appearance. Otherwise, examination is notable only for tender inguinal lymphadenopathy. Which of the following is the most appropriate treatment at this time?

(A) A 10-day course of oral acyclovir
(B) Highly active retroviral therapy until the lesion resolves
(C) Nystatin powder to the lesion daily for at least 1 week
(D) One high dose of intramuscular penicillin G
(E) One high dose of oral azithromycin

42. A 32-year-old woman who is at 30 weeks of gestation presents to the emergency department with vaginal bleeding and painful abdominal cramps. Her blood pressure is 125/80 mm Hg. A urinalysis shows no protein, leukocytes, or bacteria with few RBCs. A peripheral blood smear shows a decreased number of normocytic, normochromatic RBCs with many schistocytes. Which of the following is the most likely diagnosis?

(A) Abruptio placentae
(B) Amniotic fluid embolism
(C) Hydrops fetalis
(D) Placenta previa
(E) Preeclampsia

43. A 30-year-old woman finds a lump in her breast during a self-examination. A biopsy indicates malignancy, and a lumpectomy is performed. The pathology report states that the malignant tissue is a primary breast cancer that is Her-2/neu-positive, but estrogen and progesterone receptor-negative. Which of the following therapies would fail in treating this patient's breast cancer?

(A) Cyclophosphamide
(B) Doxorubicin
(C) Paclitaxel
(D) Tamoxifen
(E) Trastuzumab

44. A 65-year-old man visits his physician because of increasingly difficult urination. He has trouble initiating a stream and experiences postvoid dribbling. He wakes from sleep three times per night to urinate. His baseline creatinine level was 1.0 mg/dL, and it is now 1.5 mg/dL. Which treatment is most feasible to immediately improve this patient's creatinine level?

(A) Administration of fluid boluses
(B) Dialysis
(C) Placement of a Foley catheter
(D) Treatment with terazosin

45. An infant is born with ambiguous genitalia. On initial laboratory testing, the infant has a testosterone level of 482 ng/dL (normal 437–707 ng/dL), an estrogen level of 12 pg/mL (normal 10–60 pg/mL) and a LH level of 8 U/L (normal 7–24 U/L). Testes are present. Supposing this child's genitalia masculinize at puberty, which of the following disorders does this infant most likely have?

(A) Complete androgen insensitivity
(B) Double Y syndrome
(C) Female pseudohermaphroditism
(D) 5α-Reductase deficiency
(E) True hermaphroditism

46. A 27-year-old woman presents to her primary care physician with breast pain, nonbloody nipple discharge, and multiple bilateral breast masses. She denies any history of breast cancer in her family. Which of the following would most likely confirm that a breast mass is benign?

(A) Central necrosis
(B) Lymphocytic infiltration
(C) Lymphatic involvement
(D) Overlying eczema
(E) Sclerosis

47. A 22-year-old obese woman presents to her gynecologist with amenorrhea and hirsutism. Ultrasonography reveals polycystic ovaries. Which of the following is a likely pathophysiologic mechanism of this disorder?

(A) Decreased estrogen
(B) Decreased testosterone
(C) Excess follicle-stimulating hormone
(D) Excess luteinizing hormone
(E) Excess progesterone

48. A 23-year-old woman is brought to the emergency department with vaginal bleeding. The patient says that she is in her ninth week of pregnancy. Laboratory studies show a β-hCG level of 153 IU/L. The sample shown in the image is retrieved from the patient's uterus. There are no recognizable fetal parts. Which of the following describes the most likely genotype and parental source of DNA in this mass?

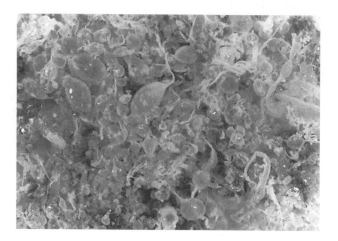

Image courtesy of Armed Forces Institute of Pathology.

(A) 46,XX; maternal
(B) 46,XX; maternal and paternal
(C) 46,XX; paternal
(D) 69,XXX; maternal and paternal
(E) 69,XXY; maternal and paternal

49. After fertilization of the ovum, implantation occurs in the endometrium and the developing placenta begins to produce a hormone necessary for embryonic viability. Which of the following is the action of this hormone?

(A) To initiate parturition
(B) To increase the threshold for uterine contraction

(C) To stimulate the corpus luteum to produce estriol and progesterone

(D) To stimulate the uterus to produce estriol and progesterone

50. A 38-year-old woman comes to the physician complaining of vaginal burning and itching. On physical examination a whitish, curd-like vaginal discharge and inflammation of the walls of the vagina and vulva are observed. Laboratory results indicate the infection is not bacterial. Which of the following clinically significant symptoms could also result from infection with this organism?

(A) Blood-tinged sputum, loss of appetite, weight loss, painful red rash on the legs, and change in mental status

(B) Chronic lung disease resembling tuberculosis

(C) Lung cavity lesions

(D) Meningoencephalitis

(E) Thrush, "diaper rash," disseminated infection, chronic mucocutaneous disease

HIGH-YIELD SYSTEMS

Reproductive

1. **The correct answer is C.** Menopause occurs when a woman has no menstrual cycles for 1 year. The 2–8 years leading up to this time are called perimenopause. During this time, hormones fluctuate tremendously, eventually leading to a decrease in estrogen, an increase in follicle-stimulating hormone (FSH), an increase in luteinizing hormone (LH), and an increase in gonadotropin-releasing hormone (GnRH). Associated symptoms include hot flashes, vaginal atrophy, osteoporosis, and coronary artery disease. (Remember, menopause causes **HAVOC: H**ot flashes, **A**trophy of the **V**agina, **O**steoporosis, and **C**oronary artery disease.) Combinations of estrogen and progestin are used as HRT to decrease hot flashes, vaginal dryness, mood swings, and postmenopausal osteoporosis. Unfortunately, HRT has recently been associated with an increased risk of breast cancer, stroke, myocardial infarction in the first year after starting therapy, and deep venous thrombosis leading to pulmonary embolism. However, HRT has also been associated with potential benefits including decreased risks of hip fracture and colorectal cancer.

Answer A is incorrect. The risk of breast cancer is increased by 26% in women receiving HRT. Breast cancer has been shown to be an estrogen-dependent disease. Women who have never been exposed to estrogen, through a lack of ovarian function and absence of hormone treatment, do not develop breast cancer.

Answer B is incorrect. The risk of deep venous thrombosis and pulmonary embolism is doubled in women receiving HRT. While no conclusive evidence has been found to date, it is surmised that the progestin component of HRT may counteract the beneficial effects of estrogen on the cardiovascular system.

Answer D is incorrect. The risk of myocardial infarction is increased by 29% in women receiving HRT. While no conclusive evidence has been found to date, it is surmised that the progestin component of HRT may counteract

the beneficial effects of estrogen on the cardiovascular system.

Answer E is incorrect. The risk of stroke is increased by 41% in women receiving hormone replacement therapy. While no conclusive evidence has been found to date, it is surmised that the progestin component of HRT may counteract the beneficial effects of estrogen on the cardiovascular system.

2. **The correct answer is B.** Paget's disease is an eczematous patch on the nipple or areola, often with underlying ductal carcinomas that are firm and fibrous on breast examination. On histologic examination, there are large cells with surrounding halos in the epidermis, with underlying islands of tumor cells embedded in fibrosis. Risk factors for breast cancer include nulliparity, early menarche, late menopause, obesity, high-fat diet, and a positive family history.

Answer A is incorrect. Paget's disease is almost always associated with intraductal carcinoma, not intralobular. Infiltrating lobular carcinomas are often bilateral, made up of cells in clusters or in "Indian file" within ductules.

Answer C is incorrect. Medullary carcinoma involves lymphocytic infiltration and scant stroma. The tumors are often soft and fleshy, not firm. Medullary carcinomas are not associated with Paget's disease.

Answer D is incorrect. Comedocarcinoma is a tumor with a "cheesy" consistency and central necrosis. While this is also an intraductal carcinoma in situ, it is not associated with Paget's disease.

Answer E is incorrect. Mucinous (colloid) carcinomas have a gelatinous consistency and show pools of extracellular mucus surrounding clusters of tumor cells. These are not associated with Paget's disease.

Answer F is incorrect. Proliferation of normal-looking epithelial cells describes epithelial hyperplasia; it poses no increased risk of carcinoma. This is an example of a fibrocystic change that often occurs in women older than 30 years. These tumors are benign and are not associated with Paget's disease or malignancy.

Answer G is incorrect. Proliferation of normal-looking glands and ducts suggests intraductal papilloma, which can often present with nipple discharge. These tumors are benign and are not associated with Paget's disease or malignancy.

3. **The correct answer is B.** The spermatic cord is a thick cord containing the structures that run to and from the testes. It is covered by three layers: external spermatic fascia derived from the external oblique muscle, cremasteric muscle and fascia derived from the internal oblique muscle, and internal spermatic fascia derived from the transversalis fascia. The ilioinguinal nerve arises from L1, passes through the inguinal ligament on top of the spermatic cord, and supplies cutaneous sensation to the scrotum/labia and medial aspect of the thigh. It is not a part of the spermatic cord and must be isolated separately from the cord during hernia surgeries to ensure that there is no loss of sensation to these areas.

Answer A is incorrect. The ductus deferens is the tube that carries sperm from the testes to the ejaculatory duct. It is at the center of the spermatic cord.

Answer C is incorrect. The pampiniform plexus, or testicular venous plexus, drains blood from the testes and is a part of the spermatic cord.

Answer D is incorrect. The testicular artery supplies blood to the testes and epididymis and runs in the spermatic cord. Remember that anything running to or from the testes will be a part of the spermatic cord. Even if you don't know the layers of the cord, you can eliminate structures that you know have something to do with testicular function.

Answer E is incorrect. The testes, as vascular organs, do produce lymph that needs to be drained by lymphatic vessels. Since the spermatic cord contains structures that run away from the testes, the testicular lymph vessels are a part of the spermatic cord.

4. **The correct answer is D.** This clinical picture of acute reproductive tract pain and tenderness is consistent with pelvic inflammatory disease (PID). Of the bacteria that cause PID, *Neisseria gonorrhoeae* is most likely to cause acute high fever and purulent discharge. The Gram's stain of the gram-negative diplococci in the vaginal discharge is diagnostic of gonococcal PID. Complications of PID include tubo-ovarian abscesses, infertility, ectopic pregnancy, and the development of scar tissue leading to chronic pain.

Answer A is incorrect. *Candida albicans* is another cause of vulvovaginitis, diagnosed by visualization of pseudohyphae on potassium hydroxide preparation.

Answer B is incorrect. Chlamydial PID is more subacute, and these intracellular organisms are not accessible to gram staining nor easily appreciated through light microscopy. Polymerase chain reaction- or immunology-based tests are more likely to accurately diagnose *Chlamydia trachomatis*.

Answer C is incorrect. *Gardnerella vaginalis* is a cause of bacterial vaginosis, resulting in vaginal discharge with a fishy odor. *Gardnerella* species are pleomorphic bacilli with variable gram staining. The classic histological picture for vulvovaginitis is clue cells (vaginal epithelial cells covered with adherent offending bacteria).

Answer E is incorrect. *Trichomonas vaginalis* is a motile protozoan (seen on a wet mount) that causes yellow-green vaginal discharge upon vulvovaginal infection.

5. **The correct answer is E.** Preeclampsia usually presents with the triad of hypertension, proteinuria, and edema. Preeclampsia affects 7% of pregnant women in their third trimester. Other symptoms include headache, blurry vision, abdominal pain, edema, and hyperreflexia. Definitive treatment is delivery of the fetus. If a

patient has a seizure in the setting of preeclampsia, her diagnosis changes to eclampsia, a potentially life-threatening emergency.

Answer A is incorrect. Edema of the face and extremities is one of the triad of symptoms that classify preeclampsia and would not change the initial diagnosis.

Answer B is incorrect. Hyperreflexia is a common symptom of preeclampsia and would not change the initial diagnosis.

Answer C is incorrect. Hypertension is one of the triad of symptoms that classify preeclampsia and would not change the initial diagnosis.

Answer D is incorrect. Proteinuria is one of the triad of symptoms that classify preeclampsia and would not change the initial diagnosis.

6. **The correct answer is B.** Leiomyomas, or fibroids, are common smooth muscle tumors that are most often seen in African-American women and present with multiple masses. These tumors are benign and can be associated with menstrual pain and menorrhagia (increased bleeding). Since they are estrogen-sensitive, they tend to increase in size during pregnancy and decrease in size after menopause.

Answer A is incorrect. Leiomyomas, or fibroids, are common smooth muscle tumors that are most often seen in African-American women and present with multiple masses. These tumors are benign and are usually associated with menstrual pain and menorrhagia (increased bleeding). Since they are estrogen-sensitive, they tend to increase in size during pregnancy and decrease (not increase) in size after menopause.

Answer C is incorrect. Chocolate cysts and "powder burns" are most often associated with endometriosis (non-neoplastic endometrial tissue outside the uterus). Endometriosis is often associated with severe menstrual-related pain and infertility.

Answer D is incorrect. Leiomyomas are benign tumors that are very rarely associated with malignant transformation. Malignant leiomyo-

sarcomas most typically arise de novo with areas of necrosis and hemorrhage, not from leiomyomas.

Answer E is incorrect. Leiomyomas are benign tumors that are very rarely associated with malignant transformation, necrosis, or hemorrhage. Malignant leiomyosarcomas most typically arise de novo, not from leiomyomas.

7. **The correct answer is E.** The hypothalamus regulates prolactin release by the anterior pituitary. Thyroid-releasing hormone stimulates prolactin release, while dopamine inhibits it. Prolactin stimulates milk production and breast development while inhibiting ovulation and spermatogenesis. Destruction of the hypothalamus would cause a reduction in dopamine secretion, increasing prolactin release. The antipsychotic chlorpromazine is a dopamine receptor antagonist, and would therefore also cause an increase in prolactin release.

Answer A is incorrect. ADH is released by the posterior pituitary by neurons arising from the hypothalamus. ADH increases water permeability in the late distal tubules and collecting ducts and constricts vascular smooth muscle. Destruction of the neuron bodies in the hypothalamus would reduce ADH secretion.

Answer B is incorrect. Growth hormone (GH) is released by the anterior pituitary in response to hypothalamus growth hormone releasing hormone (GHRH). GH decreases glucose uptake into cells, increases lipolysis, increases protein synthesis, and stimulates insulin-like growth factor. Destruction of the hypothalamus would reduce GHRH, thereby reducing GH.

Answer C is incorrect. LH is released by the anterior pituitary in response to hypothalamic GnRH. LH increases testosterone synthesis by stimulating cholesterol desmolase. Destruction of the hypothalamus would reduce GnRH, thereby reducing LH.

Answer D is incorrect. Oxytocin is also released by the posterior pituitary by neurons arising from the hypothalamus. Oxytocin causes ejection of milk from the breast in response to suckling by contracting myoepithelial cells; oxytocin also contracts the uterus during labor. Destruction of the neuron bodies in the hypothalamus would reduce oxytocin secretion.

Answer F is incorrect. Testosterone is released by the testes and adrenal glands in response to LH from the anterior pituitary. Testosterone has many functions, including prenatal differentiation of wolffian ducts, development of male secondary sex characteristics, stimulating the pubertal growth spurt, spermatogenesis, and increasing libido. Destruction of the hypothalamus would reduce GnRH secretion, thereby reducing LH and testosterone levels.

Answer G is incorrect. Thyroid-releasing hormone is released by the hypothalamus and stimulates the anterior pituitary to release thyroid-stimulating hormone (TSH); thus, prolactin levels would decrease with its destruction.

8. **The correct answer is A.** The only testicular tumor that has an elevated serum α-fetoprotein level is a yolk sac tumor, which has a peak incidence in infancy and early childhood. The yolk sac tumor is thought to be derived from endodermal cells. Symptoms include a lump or swelling in the testicle accompanied by pain.

Answer B is incorrect. This patient has a yolk sac tumor, which most often develops during infancy and early childhood rather than adolescence.

Answer C is incorrect. Embryonal carcinoma accounts for up to one third of all germ cell tumors. It tends to form glands or spaces. Typically, embryonal carcinoma presents with pain in the third decade of life.

Answer D is incorrect. Choriocarcinoma is a rare germ cell tumor that can cause an increase in serum β-hCG but not α-fetoprotein. It requires intensive chemotherapy and can metastasize via the bloodstream to the lungs and central nervous system. Testicular choriocarcinoma is extremely rare, or even nonexistent in prepubescent males.

Answer E is incorrect. Seminomas, which present as a painless enlargement of the testes, have a peak incidence in the fourth decade of life. Seminomas are tumors of the germ cells in the testes and are highly sensitive to radiation therapy.

9. **The correct answer is A.** This woman has Kartagener's syndrome, which is a caused by a defect in microtubule dynein, resulting in immotile cilia. Loss of ciliary "sweeping" renders women infertile because eggs are not advanced through the fallopian tubes; it also results in an increased incidence of upper respiratory infections as the loss of mucociliary clearance allows debris to accumulate in the airway. Cilia have a distinct organization, with a central pair of microtubules and nine surrounding pairs, allowing them to bend and sway by differential sliding of the pairs.

Answer B is incorrect. Collagen fibrils are made up of many staggered collagen molecules, each composed of triplets of collagen α chains. A defect in collagen structure results in connective tissue diseases such as scurvy, which is characterized by easy bruising and bleeding gums and is associated with vitamin C deficiency. A defect in collagen would not cause infertility or urinary tract infections (UTIs).

Answer C is incorrect. Neutrophils usually have a multilobular nucleus with granules filled with hydrolytic enzymes, lysozymes, myeloperoxidase, and lactoferrin. Neutrophils are part of the acute inflammatory response with phagocytic capabilities. A defect in neutrophils can result in conditions such as chronic granulomatous disease and Chédiak-Higashi syndrome, both of which affect immunity. However, this patient's normal WBC suggests that this is not the case. Moreover, a defect in neutrophils would not cause infertility.

Answer D is incorrect. Zona adherens is an example of an epithelial cell junction; it consists of adjoining e-cadherin between cells and far-reaching actin filaments around the perimeter of the cells. A defect in cell junctions would not cause infertility or UTIs.

Answer E is incorrect. Antibodies have two heavy chains and two light chains connected by disulfide bonds. The variable parts of the chains recognize antigens, while the constant part of the heavy chain can fix complement (e.g., IgM and IgG). A defect in antibody structure may affect immunity, but the patient's normal immunoglobulin levels suggest that this is not the case. Moreover, a defect in antibodies would not cause infertility.

10. **The correct answer is E.** During the follicular phase leading up to ovulation, estradiol levels are increasing, causing proliferation of the uterus. The estradiol levels suppress FSH and LH levels by negative feedback inhibition. At the end of the follicular phase, there is a burst of estradiol, resulting in positive feedback on the pituitary and a burst of LH production. This LH surge causes ovulation.

Answer A is incorrect. Estrogen is not directly responsible for ovulation. It induces a surge in LH that causes ovulation.

Answer B is incorrect. FSH is suppressed by estradiol levels during the follicular phase. Along with the LH surge, there is an increase in FSH production that stimulates steroid hormone synthesis by the corpus luteum. It does not affect ovulation.

Answer C is incorrect. GnRH is suppressed by the negative feedback of estradiol levels during the follicular phase. With the burst of estradiol synthesis at the end, GnRH is positively reinforced, producing a LH surge. It does not directly cause ovulation, however.

Answer D is incorrect. Human chorionic gonadotropin is produced by the syncytiotrophoblast after conception. It is not part of the normal menstrual cycle and has no effect on ovulation.

Answer F is incorrect. After ovulation, the corpus luteum begins to grow, secreting progesterone. Progesterone is not secreted until after ovulation and is therefore not responsible for ovulation.

11. **The correct answer is D.** The suspensory ligaments (also known as the infundibulopelvic ligaments) contain the ovarian arteries that give direct blood supply to the ovaries. The ovaries also receive collateral flow from the uterine arteries that travel in the transverse ligament within the broad ligament.

Answer A is incorrect. The cardinal ligament carries descending branches of the uterine artery. Severing the cardinal ligament should not significantly decrease blood flow to the ovary.

Answer B is incorrect. The fallopian tubes carry the ova from the ovary to the uterus during ovulation. Severing this structure would disrupt normal fertilization but would not significantly affect blood flow to the ovary.

Answer C is incorrect. The round ligament runs inferior to the ovary before attaching to the uterus. It is not a direct source of blood supply for the ovary.

Answer E is incorrect. The ureters run directly inferior to the uterine arteries before feeding into the bladder. Remember: "Water under the bridge." Severing this structure would not affect ovarian blood flow.

12. **The correct answer is B.** Androgen-binding proteins are produced in the Sertoli cells in response to FSH. These proteins play a role in sequestering testosterone near the spermatocytes, whose maturation is androgen-dependent.

Answer A is incorrect. Inhibin is a hormone produced by the Sertoli cells in response to FSH that functions as a negative feedback inhibitor of FSH secretion by the anterior pituitary gland. It is not bound by androgen-binding globulin.

Answer C is incorrect. Testosterone is converted into estrogen by the enzyme aromatase, not by androgen-binding globulin.

Answer D is incorrect. Androgen-binding globulin does not feed back on the Sertoli cell or the Leydig cell and does not affect androgen production.

Answer E is incorrect. Testosterone is transported in the blood bound to sex hormone-binding globulin or albumin, not androgen-binding globulin.

13. **The correct answer is E.** Cervical cancer is associated with HPV strains 16 and 18. Cervical cancers arise from disordered epithelial growth, classified as cervical intraepithelial neoplasia (CIN) 1, 2, or 3, depending on the extent of epithelial involvement from the basal layer. An important risk factor for cervical cancer includes early sexual activity and multiple sex partners, making the incidence especially high in prostitutes. Pap smears have reduced the mortality of these cancers. HPV strains 31 and 33 are also associated with malignancy.

Answer A is incorrect. There are no HPV strains L1-3. However, *Chlamydia trachomatis* types L1-3 are associated with lymphogranuloma venereum, an acute lymphadenitis most often occurring in the inguinal area.

Answer B is incorrect. HPV strains 1 and 2 are not associated with cervical cancer. However, herpes simplex virus (HSV) can cause oral (HSV-1) and genital (HSV-2) vesicular lesions.

Answer C is incorrect. HPV strains 6 and 11 are associated with benign warts.

Answer D is incorrect. HPV strain 8 is not associated with cervical cancer. Human herpesvirus 8 is associated with malignant Kaposi's sarcoma, often found in HIV and immunosuppressed patients.

14. **The correct answer is C.** This female baby has masculinization of her external genitalia due to congenital adrenal hyperplasia (CAH). CAH is caused by deficiencies in enzymes required for adrenocortical steroid synthesis, such as 21α-hydroxylase and 11β-hydroxylase. 21α-Hydroxylase deficiency results in a total lack of synthesis of aldosterone or cortisol, so that all intermediates generate androgen synthesis, leading to elevation of androgen levels and masculinization of tissue. The lack of aldosterone leads to salt wasting, and the infant can present with hypovolemia and hypotension. Treatment includes intravenous saline and steroid hormone replacement.

Answer A is incorrect. 11β-Hydroxylase deficiency can cause CAH but does not result in hypotension or hypovolemia. Instead, it can re-

sult in hypertension because one of the intermediates that is not blocked by this deficiency but is blocked by 21α-hydroxylase deficiency acts as a mineralocorticoid to cause salt retention and hypervolemia.

Answer B is incorrect. 17α-Hydroxylase deficiency is a cause of male pseudointersexuality, not female intersexuality. This enzyme usually converts androstenedione to testosterone. This deficiency, and the resulting lack of testosterone, causes underdevelopment of the penis and scrotum with normal male reproductive internal organs. Clinically it appears very similar to 5α-reductase deficiency until puberty.

Answer D is incorrect. Complete androgen insensitivity is a result of a mutation in the androgen receptor gene. These 46,XY patients develop testes and female external genitalia and vagina with no internal reproductive organs. They typically present as normal-appearing girls who consult their physician when they do not begin menstruation.

Answer E is incorrect. 5α-Reductase deficiency is a cause of male pseudointersexuality, not female intersexuality, so that patients have an XY genotype. Normally, 5α-reductase converts testosterone to dihydrotestosterone (DHT). DHT is essential in the development of the external genitalia, and a lack of DHT results in feminization of the penis and scrotum with normal internal male reproductive organs. At puberty, these patients may suddenly experience virilization of the external organs due to the increase in testosterone.

15. **The correct answer is E.** Prolonged unopposed estrogen use is a risk factor for developing endometrial carcinoma; it stimulates endometrial gland proliferation and manifests as vaginal bleeding. Other risk factors for endometrial cancer include obesity, diabetes, and hypertension. Curiously, tobacco use is actually protective against endometrial cancer.

Answer A is incorrect. Alcoholism has little relation to endometrial cancer but is strongly associated with chronic pancreatitis and pancreatic adenocarcinoma. Smoking is also a risk factor for these conditions.

Answer B is incorrect. Early sexual activity has little relation to endometrial cancer but is a major risk factor for cervical cancer. Other risk factors for cervical cancer include early sexual activity, multiple sex partners, HPV infection, smoking, and low socioeconomic status.

Answer C is incorrect. A low-fiber diet has little relation to endometrial cancer, but it is a risk factor for colorectal cancer. Other risk factors include villous adenomas, familial adenomatous polyposis, hereditary nonpolyposis colorectal cancer, inflammatory bowel disease, and a positive personal or family history.

Answer D is incorrect. Although nulliparity is a risk factor of endometrial cancer, multiparity is protective.

16. **The correct answer is D.** The firm prostate nodules and weight loss suggest prostate cancer. The prostate-specific antigen level is typically elevated in prostate cancer. Calcium levels should be low because calcium is being used to build new bone in the areas of metastases. The alkaline phosphatase level should be increased because this is a marker of bone formation.

    Answer A is incorrect. Prostate-specific antigen should be elevated in prostate cancer, and the alkaline phosphatase level should be high.

    Answer B is incorrect. Prostate-specific antigen should be elevated in prostate cancer.

    Answer C is incorrect. In prostate cancer, because bone is being made, the alkaline phosphatase level should increase.

    Answer E is incorrect. The calcium level should be low in prostate cancer because it is being used to make new bone. The alkaline phosphatase level should be elevated as a marker of bone formation.

17. **The correct answer is E.** A leak into the dorsal and saphenous vein, demonstrating venous outflow, is typically due to insufficient relaxation of the smooth muscle resulting from excessive adrenergic tone or damaged parasympathetic innervation.

Answer A is incorrect. Arterial insufficiency due to atherosclerotic change or trauma can decrease blood flow to the lacunar spaces, resulting in decreased rigidity. This patient, however, has leakage into veins, not arteries.

Answer B is incorrect. Normal levels of testosterone are important for erectile function, as is demonstrated in studies showing that testosterone therapy for erectile dysfunction increases libido weeks before it has an effect on erection, but the exact role of androgens in libido is unclear.

Answer C is incorrect. Cavernosography demonstrates an organic etiology. Some common causes of psychogenic impotence are anxiety, depression, and relationship conflict.

Answer D is incorrect. Cavernosography does not test somatosensory deficits. Intact sensory nerves are required for erection because sensory nerves that originate from receptors in the penile skin travel to the S2–S4 dorsal root ganglia in order to elicit the proper parasympathetic response.

18. **The correct answer is E.** A feeling of hopelessness would make one more suspicious of postpartum depression, which is a more serious disorder than postpartum blues. Women with postpartum depression present with symptoms more suggestive of a major depression, such as feelings of hopelessness and helplessness, anhedonia, and poor grooming. Without treatment, postpartum depression can last up to 1 year.

    Answer A is incorrect. Women with postpartum blues may be very anxious about their infant and can worry excessively about the infant's care and health. Similarly, depression may present with anxiety symptoms, but hopelessness is a more prominent feature.

    Answer B is incorrect. Fatigue is a common complaint of women with postpartum blues. Although it may be a part of postpartum depression, hopelessness is more consistent with depression.

    Answer C is incorrect. Irritability is a common complaint of women with postpartum blues.

Although it may be a part of postpartum depression, hopelessness is more consistent with depression.

Answer D is incorrect. Weeping is a common complaint of women with postpartum blues. A striking characteristic of postpartum blues is emotional lability. Crying and laughing can occur at the same time.

19. **The correct answer is A.** This patient is presenting with Sheehan's syndrome or postpartum pituitary necrosis, caused by hemorrhage during delivery. Risk factors include pregnancy with multiples (twins or triplets) and abnormalities of the placenta. Peripartum hemorrhage predisposes the already enlarged pituitary to ischemia, leading to necrosis of parts of the anterior and/or posterior pituitary. The most common clinical feature of Sheehan's syndrome is an inability to lactate, caused by damage to the anterior pituitary and decreased prolactin production. Other symptoms include those associated with hypothyroidism (as seen by the patient's cold intolerance), along with central diabetes insipidus caused by decreased production of ADH. Diabetes insipidus presents with polyuria and dilute urine in the presence of elevated serum sodium levels. Decreased FSH and LH levels often lead to amenorrhea and scant pubic and axillary hair growth. Treatment involves lifelong hormone replacement therapy of all deficient hormones, along with estrogen and progesterone supplementation.

Answer B is incorrect. Alcohol intake during pregnancy is not associated with any of the symptoms seen in this patient. Instead, it is associated with growth and developmental defects in the offspring, such as microcephaly, facial dysmorphism, and malformations of the brain, cardiovascular system, and genitourinary system. Fetal alcohol syndrome is the leading cause of mental retardation and is easily preventable by maternal abstinence from alcohol during pregnancy.

Answer C is incorrect. Endometriosis is a common condition characterized by growth of ectopic endometrial tissue outside the uterus. It generally presents in women 20–40 years old, but its pathogenesis is poorly understood. Although its clinical presentation varies, endometriosis can present with pelvic pain associated with the menstrual cycle, dysmenorrhea, and dyspareunia, or it can be asymptomatic. Endometriosis is a risk factor for ectopic pregnancy and infertility, and many women who have endometriosis first present with problems getting pregnant. It is not associated with Sheehan's syndrome.

Answer D is incorrect. Gestational diabetes is a form of diabetes that is present during pregnancy and is often transient, although overt nongestational diabetes may later develop. Gestational diabetes is associated with increased fetal birth weight, increased fetal mortality, and increased incidence of neonatal respiratory distress syndrome. In addition, increased fetal insulin levels created in response to maternal glucose levels can cause a hypoglycemic crisis after birth, when the maternal supply of glucose is no longer present. Gestational diabetes is not a known risk factor for Sheehan's syndrome and would not cause this patient to present with the symptoms seen.

Answer E is incorrect. Incorrect use of tampons is associated with toxic shock syndrome (TSS), originally associated with the use of highly absorbent tampons left in the vagina for long periods of time. TSS is caused by an exotoxin produced by *Staphylococcus aureus*, which grows on the tampon. This toxin is a superantigen that allows nonspecific binding of major histocompatibility complex class II with T-lymphocyte receptors, resulting in polyclonal T-lymphocyte activation and systemic symptoms. TSS generally presents acutely with fever, hypotension, and desquamation of the palms and soles, nausea, vomiting, and diarrhea.

Answer F is incorrect. Having multiple sexual partners is associated with an increased risk of various sexually transmitted diseases (STDs), including HIV and HPV, the virus associated with cervical cancer. STDs present with various symptoms depending on the underlying infectious agent, but none would cause the symptoms seen in this patient.

Answer G is incorrect. PID is most commonly caused by infection with *Chlamydia trachomatis* or *Neisseria gonorrhea*, the latter presenting more acutely. Symptoms include fever, cervical motion tenderness, lower abdominal pain, and painful intercourse, although PID is often asymptomatic. Treatment of the underlying cause is important because PID is a risk factor for ectopic pregnancy and infertility. It is not associated with Sheehan's syndrome.

20. **The correct answer is A.** Without a functional sex-determining region of the Y chromosome (*SRY*) gene, no symptoms will be noticed, and the embryo will develop as a phenotypical female. Normally, the *SRY* gene encodes the testis-determining factor (TDF), which is responsible for the differentiation of the indifferent gonads into testes. In the testes, Leydig cells produce testosterone and Sertoli cells produce müllerian-inhibiting substance (MIS). Testosterone causes the development of the mesonephric (wolffian) duct into male internal sex organs (remember the mnemonic **SEED:** **S**eminal vesicles, **E**pididymis, **E**jaculatory duct, and **D**uctus deferens), and the development of male external organs after conversion to 5-hydroxytestosterone. MIS causes regression of the paramesonephric (müllerian) duct, preventing development of female organs. In the absence of TDF, whether due to a destructive mutation of *SRY* or to a normal 46,XX karyotype, the wolffian duct regresses spontaneously; the müllerian duct develops into the fallopian tubes, uterus, and upper vagina; and the external genitalia feminize. This condition will likely be discovered incidentally if a karyotype is performed for an unrelated reason.

Answer B is incorrect. By definition, a female pseudohermaphrodite has ovaries but ambiguous genitalia. A common cause of this condition is CAH, often due to 21-α-hydroxylase deficiency.

Answer C is incorrect. A functional *SRY* gene is critical for the development of the male phenotype.

Answer D is incorrect. A male pseudohermaphrodite has testes but ambiguous genitalia.

Common causes of this condition include partial androgen insensitivity, 5-α-reductase deficiency, and defects in testosterone production.

Answer E is incorrect. A true hermaphrodite has both testes and ovaries with ambiguous external genitalia. This condition is quite rare but may be the product of the fertilization of a binucleated ovum by two sperm (one X and one Y).

21. **The correct answer is E.** Krukenberg's tumors are stomach cancer metastases to both ovaries that are described as mucin-secreting "signet-ring" cells. Stomach cancer is often adenocarcinoma that can spread aggressively to lymph nodes and the liver. A classic sign of metastatic stomach cancer is involvement of the supraclavicular lymph nodes, called Virchow's nodes.

Answer A is incorrect. Galactorrhea is leakage from the breasts that is not associated with normal lactation but is associated with elevated prolactin levels secondary to prolactinomas in the anterior pituitary. Prolactin stimulates breast development and milk production while also inhibiting ovulation and spermatogenesis by inhibiting the release of GnRH and subsequently suppressing LH and FSHs. Galactorrhea is not associated with stomach or ovarian cancers. Prolactinomas rarely metastasize.

Answer B is incorrect. Melena is bloody stool and is often an early sign of colorectal carcinoma. Risk factors for colorectal carcinoma include villous adenomas, inflammatory bowel disease, low-fiber diet, familial adenomatous polyposis, hereditary nonpolyposis colorectal cancer, and a positive history. Melena is not associated with stomach or ovarian cancers. Colorectal carcinomas usually metastasize to the liver.

Answer C is incorrect. A palpable gallbladder (Courvoisier's sign) is associated with pancreatic duct obstruction secondary to pancreatic adenocarcinoma. Other signs and symptoms of pancreatic cancer include abdominal pain radiating to the back, weight loss, anorexia, and migratory thrombophlebitis (Trousseau's syndrome). A palpable gallbladder is not associated with stomach or ovarian cancers.

Answer D is incorrect. Basal cell carcinoma often presents as "pearly papules" on sun-exposed areas, such as the face and arms. Papules are not associated with stomach or ovarian cancers. This type of cancer is locally invasive but almost never metastasizes.

22. **The correct answer is A.** Ectopic pregnancies often occur in one of the fallopian tubes or occasionally in the ovary, abdominal cavity, or cervix. Ectopic pregnancies can be complicated by rupture and can develop into a life-threatening condition. Risk factors include a history of PID, endometriosis, postoperative adhesions, and chronic salpingitis.

Answer B is incorrect. *Escherichia coli* is part of the normal flora of the vagina, along with group B streptococcus. It is also one of the most common causes of UTI (UTI) in ambulatory young women, along with *Staphylococcus saprophyticus*. UTIs are not associated with PID or ectopic pregnancies.

Answer C is incorrect. HSV type 2 is a sexually transmitted, enveloped DNA herpes virus. Genital herpes presents with painful penile, vulvar, or cervical ulcers. HSV is also one of the ToRCHeS organisms that can cross the placenta and negatively affect the fetus. However, HSV is not associated with PID or ectopic pregnancies.

Answer D is incorrect. HPV is associated with cervical and anal carcinomas. It is not associated with PID or ectopic pregnancies.

Answer E is incorrect. *Streptococcus agalactiae* is a group B streptococcus that is part of the normal flora in the vagina and would not increase the risk of developing PID or an ectopic pregnancy.

23. **The correct answer is A.** Prolactin is a protein hormone produced by the adenohypophysis, or anterior pituitary, to prepare mammary glands for lactation. Prolactin also increases dopamine synthesis and secretion from the hypothalamus and inhibits the secretion of GnRH, preventing ovulation. Other hormones released from the anterior pituitary include LH, FSH, TSH, GH, and ACTH.

Answer B is incorrect. Progesterone is secreted by the corpus luteum for the first 8 weeks of pregnancy. It acts on the endometrium to maintain the pregnancy and decrease uterine contractions. It is also used by the fetus as a precursor for steroid hormone synthesis.

Answer C is incorrect. Oxytocin is produced by the hypothalamus and stored in the posterior pituitary. It acts on the mammary glands to stimulate milk letdown, not milk production, as prolactin does. The other hormone secreted by the posterior pituitary is ADH.

Answer D is incorrect. Human placental lactogen and progesterone are secreted by the placenta. Human placental lactogen induces lipolysis, raising the level of free fatty acids and acting as a growth hormone for the fetus. Progesterone is secreted by the placenta to maintain the endometrium after week 8 of pregnancy.

Answer E is incorrect. Human chorionic gonadotropin is produced by the syncytiotrophoblast during the first trimester of pregnancy. Its action is to stimulate the production of progesterone by the corpus luteum until the 8th week of pregnancy, at which point the placenta begins secreting progesterone on its own.

24. **The correct answer is E.** This patient has bacterial vaginosis, a condition characterized by malodorous discharge after sexual activity. Bacterial vaginosis is a noninflammatory condition caused by a number of organisms, most notably *Gardnerella vaginalis*. Diagnosis is supported by a positive whiff or amine test (reproduction of the fishy odor by the application of 10% potassium hydroxide to a sample of the vaginal discharge) or by the visualization of clue cells on saline wet mount, as shown here. Clue cells are vaginal epithelial cells studded by adherent bacteria. Metronidazole is standard first-line therapy for this condition, although some physicians avoid this drug in pregnancy because it crosses the placenta. The

mechanism of action of metronidazole is still incompletely understood but involves direct DNA damage by the antibiotic, causing the accumulation of toxic metabolites within bacterial species.

Answer A is incorrect. Tetracycline antibiotics work by binding to the 30S subunit of the ribosome and preventing attachment of aminoacyl-tRNA. Tetracyclines are also contraindicated in pregnancy. Common toxicities include gastrointestinal distress, discoloration of teeth, inhibition of bone growth in children, and photosensitivity.

Answer B is incorrect. The antimycobacterial drug rifampin works by inhibiting DNA-dependent RNA polymerase. Rifampin toxicities include hepatotoxicity, increasing expression of cytochrome P-450 enzymes and causing bodily fluids to turn red/orange.

Answer C is incorrect. The azole class of antifungal drugs works by inhibiting ergosterol synthesis. Although vaginal candidiasis is associated with reduced vaginal acidity and malodorous discharge, clue cells are not seen in this condition. Toxicities of azole antifungals include hormone synthesis inhibition, liver dysfunction, fever, and chills.

Answer D is incorrect. Fluoroquinolone antibiotics work by inhibiting topoisomerase II, also known as DNA gyrase. These drugs are also contraindicated in pregnancy. Common toxicities include gastrointestinal upset, super-infections, rash, headache, and dizziness.

25. **The correct answer is E.** Androgenic steroids are used to treat hypogonadism due to failure of the hypothalamic-pituitary-gonadal axis or due to Leydig cell dysfunction. Androgens cause premature closing of the epiphyseal plates by promoting calcium deposition in the bones.

Answer A is incorrect. Some androgenic steroids increase, rather than decrease, LDL cholesterol levels. The lipid profile disturbance increases the possibility of atherosclerotic change and raises the risk of coronary artery disease.

Answer B is incorrect. Androgenic steroids cause male-pattern baldness in both men and women because of increased production of DHT from the excess testosterone. Androgens cause growth of facial hair in women but not growth of hair on the scalp.

Answer C is incorrect. Excess androgens can cause decreased spermatogenesis by down-regulating GnRH. Decreased GnRH causes decreased release of luteinizing and FSHs, which are necessary for spermatogenesis.

Answer D is incorrect. Nausea and vomiting are common adverse effects of estrogen therapy, not androgenic steroids.

26. **The correct answer is D.** This patient presents with PID. The vast majority of cases of PID are caused by *Chlamydia trachomatis* and/or *Neisseria gonorrhoeae*. *C. trachomatis*, an obligate intracellular parasite, is the most common sexually transmitted disease in the United States and the world. It is usually treated with doxycycline. Morphologic features of *C. trachomatis* urethritis are nearly identical to those of gonorrhea. Primary infection manifests as a mucopurulent discharge with many neutrophils. Organisms are not visible by Gram stain.

Answer A is incorrect. A budding yeast with pseudohyphae, *Candida albicans* is the causative agent in the common yeast infection, which is a fairly common cause of vulvovaginitis. Symptoms include vaginal itching and a thick, copious, cottage cheese-like vaginal discharge. *C. albicans* is not a known cause of PID and is treated with fluconazole.

Answer B is incorrect. *Gardnerella vaginalis*, a coccobacillus often seen with clue cells under the microscope, is the most common cause of vulvovaginitis. It is a potential etiologic agent in PID but is not the most common cause.

Answer C is incorrect. A gram-positive, catalase-negative, bacitracin-resistant cocci, *Streptococcus agalactiae* (group B streptococcus) has been implicated as a causative agent in PID, but it is not a very common cause. It is, however, the most common cause of neonatal meningitis. Women who are pregnant and positive for group B streptococcus must be treated with antibiotics before giving birth.

Answer E is incorrect. *Trichomonas vaginalis* can cause vaginal itching, burning, or pain (vulvovaginitis) with a foul-smelling, frothy green vaginal discharge. *T. vaginalis* infection is not a known cause of PID, but it is somewhat common as a cause of nongonococcal urethritis. On wet mount, trophozoites without cysts can be seen. Many women who carry this organism are asymptomatic.

27. **The correct answer is B.** Preeclampsia usually presents with the triad of hypertension, proteinuria, and edema. Preeclampsia affects 7% of pregnant women in their third trimester, with increased incidence in patients with preexisting hypertension, diabetes, chronic renal disease, and autoimmune disorders such as lupus. Other symptoms include headache, blurry vision, abdominal pain, and hyperreflexia. Definitive treatment is delivery of the baby. The patient in this vignette presents with edema and hypertension. A 24-hour urine collection would test for proteinuria, completing the triad for the diagnosis of preeclampsia.

Answer A is incorrect. An electroencephalogram looks at electrical brain activity and is especially useful for looking at waveforms during a seizure. Eclampsia is essentially the symptoms and signs of preeclampsia with seizures. Preeclampsia by definition does not involve seizures, and thus an electroencephalogram would not help in a definitive initial diagnosis.

Answer C is incorrect. Elevated liver enzymes are associated with the **HELLP** syndrome (Hemolysis, Elevated Liver function tests, and Low Platelets). A liver panel would reveal any elevated liver enzymes. Preeclampsia may or may not involve elevated liver enzymes, and thus a panel would not help in a definitive initial diagnosis.

Answer D is incorrect. A Pap smear allows a physician to identify dysplastic cervical koilocytes by scraping off cells from the cervix and mounting them onto a slide to be viewed under a microscope. This is useful in diagnosing disordered epithelial growth that is possibly associated with cervical carcinoma. Preeclampsia does not involve dysplastic cervical cells, and thus a Pap smear would not help in a definitive initial diagnosis.

Answer E is incorrect. Hemolysis is associated with the **HELLP** syndrome (Hemolysis, Elevated Liver function tests, and Low Platelets). A blood smear would help identify RBC fragments, indicative of hemolysis. Preeclampsia may or may not involve hemolysis, and thus a smear would not help in a definitive initial diagnosis.

28. **The correct answer is C.** This patient most likely suffers from osteoporosis, or weakened bones, as a complication of menopause. Estrogen regulates bone resorption, maintaining proper bone mass in women. Menopause, whose average age of onset is 50 years, is a cessation of estrogen production due to a decreased number of ovarian follicles, resulting in increased bone resorption. Postmenopausal women would have low estrogen levels but high levels of LH, FSH, and GnRH due to the lack of negative feedback on the anterior pituitary and hypothalamus.

Answer A is incorrect. While estrogen is indeed low in postmenopausal women, levels of LH and FSH would be high due to the lack of negative feedback on the anterior pituitary. This profile suggests that the problem is in the anterior pituitary, which is receiving high GnRH but is unable to produce enough LH and FSH to stimulate the ovaries. Menopause is a primary dysfunction of estrogen production in the ovaries.

Answer B is incorrect. While estrogen is indeed low in postmenopausal women, LH, FSH, and GnRH levels would be high due to the lack of negative feedback on the anterior pituitary and hypothalamus. This profile suggests that the problem is in the hypothalamus, releasing low GnRH and suboptimally stimulating the anterior pituitary and ovaries. Menopause is a primary dysfunction of estrogen production in the ovaries.

Answer D is incorrect. Menopause is a primary dysfunction of estrogen production in the ovaries. Thus, estrogen levels would be low.

Answer E is incorrect. Menopause is a primary dysfunction of estrogen production in the ovaries. Thus, estrogen levels would be low.

29. **The correct answer is E.** Ketoconazole is an antifungal drug used to treat mucocutaneous candidiasis that acts by blocking formation of fungal membrane sterols. It also has an endocrine effect because it blocks enzymes necessary for testosterone and cortisol synthesis. Other endocrine effects include decreased libido, impotence, and gynecomastia in men. Remember that testosterone is converted into estrogen.

   Answer A is incorrect. Amphotericin B is an antifungal drug used to treat systemic mycoses. It acts by disrupting fungal wall synthesis by binding to ergosterol (a component of the cell wall). Adverse effects include fever and chills, decreased creatinine clearance, hypotension, and anemia.

   Answer B is incorrect. Fluconazole is an antifungal drug with the same mechanism of action as ketoconazole, but without the endocrine side effects. It has good penetration into the cerebrospinal fluid and is used to treat *Cryptococcus neoformans*. Adverse effects include nausea and vomiting.

   Answer C is incorrect. Flucytosine is an antifungal drug used solely in combination with amphotericin B to treat systemic *Cryptococcus neoformans* and systemic *Candida*. Adverse effects include pancytopenia, elevated liver function tests, and nausea and vomiting.

   Answer D is incorrect. Itraconazole is an antifungal that lacks the endocrine effects of ketoconazole. It is used to treat blastomycosis and AIDS-associated histoplasmosis. Adverse effects include nausea and vomiting, as well as rash in immunocompromised patients.

30. **The correct answer is A.** The history of a past inguinal repair strongly suggests an obstructive abnormality of the vas deferens, leading to disordered sperm transport. The vas deferens can be accidentally ligated, or scar tissue can make passage through the vas deferens impossible. In the case of vas deferens obstruction, the semen volume will be low with decreased or absent sperm. In these cases, testicular biopsy can confirm normal sperm production, and sperm can be collected for intracytoplasmic sperm injection in vitro fertilization.

   Answer B is incorrect. Primary gonadal deficiency is unlikely given the husband's normal testosterone level. Typically, gonadal deficiency results in low testosterone with high LH and FSH levels.

   Answer C is incorrect. Secondary hypogonadism is unlikely given the husband's normal testosterone level. A low testosterone level in association with low LH and low FSH levels would suggest pituitary or hypothalamic dysfunction.

   Answer D is incorrect. The results from the testicular biopsy demonstrate sperm within normal parameters. Normal fertility is associated with sperm motility exceeding 63% and more than 12% of sperm exhibiting normal morphology.

   Answer E is incorrect. A Y-chromosome deletion has been associated with azoospermia (no sperm) or oligospermia (low sperm count). In this case, the husband has normal sperm on testicular biopsy, making it unlikely that he has a Y-chromosome abnormality.

31. **The correct answer is F.** This patient presents with symptoms of a UTI, most likely caused by prolonged urethral catheterization. Nosocomial UTI is most often associated with *Escherichia coli, Proteus mirabilis, Pseudomonas aeruginosa, Klebsiella pneumoniae, Serratia marcescens*, staphylococci, enterococci, and *Candida albicans*. Although the patient's symptoms are not specific for any of these organisms, the urine culture tells us that (1) the organism is a gram-negative rod, and (2) the organism produces a red pigment. *S. marcescens* is a gram-negative rod that produces a red pigment called prodigiosin.

Answer A is incorrect. The presence of *Candida albicans* in an otherwise normal female usually represents colonization rather than infection. UTI with *Candida* usually can be attributed to structural abnormalities, metabolic or hormonal abnormalities, or impaired host defenses. *C. albicans* is a yeast.

Answer B is incorrect. *Escherichia coli* is the most common cause of UTI. Although it is a gram-negative rod, it does not produce any pigments.

Answer C is incorrect. *Klebsiella pneumoniae* is a gram-negative rod and is responsible for approximately 8% of nosocomial infections. It is a significant cause of UTI and pneumonia in hospitalized and ambulatory patients. *K. pneumoniae* does not produce any pigments.

Answer D is incorrect. *Proteus mirabilis* is a gram-negative bacillus and is a frequent cause of nosocomial UTI. It produces the enzyme urease, which serves to create a more alkaline environment for itself (urea → ammonia + carbon dioxide) but does not produce any pigments.

Answer E is incorrect. *Pseudomonas aeruginosa* has been known to cause catheter associated UTI. Although it is a gram-negative rod, it produces a blue-green pigment called pyocyanin.

Answer G is incorrect. *Staphylococcus saprophyticus* is the second most common cause of UTI in young women. It is a gram-positive coccus and does not produce any pigments.

32. **The correct answer is B.** A blood-filled chocolate cyst is characteristic of endometriosis, a condition that results in non-neoplastic endometrial glands/stroma abnormally located outside the uterus. The ovary is one of the most common sites, and the cysts are formed from cyclic bleeding from the tissue, mimicking menstruation. Severe menstrual-related pain and infertility are possible complications of endometriosis.

Answer A is incorrect. Common cancers in the reproductive tract include endometrial carcinoma, which can arise from endometrial hyperplasia caused by excess estrogen stimulation, and cervical carcinoma, associated with HPV infection. Endometriosis does not progress to cancer.

Answer C is incorrect. Polycystic ovarian syndrome (PCOS) (Stein-Leventhal syndrome) manifests with amenorrhea, infertility, obesity, and hirsutism due to increased androgen production from theca cells secondary to increased LH levels. Endometriosis is not associated with masculinization.

Answer D is incorrect. PCOS manifests with amenorrhea, infertility, obesity, and hirsutism due to increased androgen production from theca cells secondary to increased LH levels. Endometriosis is not associated with obesity.

33. **The correct answer is C.** Milk letdown is a reflex that causes milk ejection from the breast. Typically, milk letdown is induced by infant suckling. Oxytocin is produced by the posterior pituitary in response to suckling and, when produced synthetically, is used to induce labor or promote milk letdown in nursing mothers. It causes milk letdown by stimulating contraction of the myoepithelial cells around the mammary alveoli, causing ejection of the milk. Oxytocin is produced in the cell bodies of hypothalamic neurons in the paraventricular nucleus. After synthesis, it is stored in terminal swellings of these neurons in the posterior pituitary known as Herring bodies.

Answer A is incorrect. Birbeck granules are tennis racket-like structures visualized by electron microscopy in Langerhans cells in the skin. These are also seen in malignant histiocytosis, a tumor originating from Langerhans cells.

Answer B is incorrect. Ferruginous bodies are found in the lungs of patients with asbestosis. They represent inhaled asbestos fibers ingested by macrophages and stained by Prussian blue iron stain.

Answer D is incorrect. Lewy bodies are neural inclusions seen in the substantia nigra in Parkinson's disease.

Answer E is incorrect. Negri bodies are neuronal inclusion bodies diagnostic of rabies virus infection.

34. **The correct answer is E.** The grouped vesicles along with a Tzanck smear positive for multinucleated giant cells indicate that this young man has an active herpes infection. HSV is an enveloped virus with a double-stranded linear DNA genome. After the primary outbreak, the virus travels in a retrograde fashion along the axon via microtubular-dependent transport and remains latent in dorsal root ganglia such as the trigeminal ganglia of cranial nerve V. Over time, the virus can be reactivated, causing recurrent outbreaks that are usually less severe in symptoms, duration, and viral shedding than the primary infection.

Answer A is incorrect. HSV could disseminate and cause systemic illness; however, it is very unlikely in immunocompetent individuals.

Answer B is incorrect. HSV does not infect CD4 cells. This is characteristic of HIV, which can initially present with an acute illness somewhat resembling infectious mononucleosis. This might be followed by complete resolution followed by an asymptomatic carrier state for many years before development of full-blown AIDS.

Answer C is incorrect. HSV does not transport itself to the central nervous system (CNS). An example of a virus that can enter the CNS from the periphery is rabies. However, this would be a very uncommon clinical presentation for rabies. Rabies is usually acquired from animal bites (skunks, raccoons) and has a long incubation period (weeks to 3 months) followed by fatal encephalitis with seizures and hydrophobia.

Answer D is incorrect. After the primary outbreak of genital herpes, HSV travels via retrograde, not anterograde, transport to the cell body of the peripheral nervous system. The microtubules of the cytoskeleton serve as tracks for the movement of synaptic vesicles, organelles, and other material from the neuronal cell body to the axon terminal in an anterograde direction.

35. **The correct answer is D.** Cryptorchid testicles are undescended or completely absent. An absent testicle may be due to agenesis or to intrauterine vascular compromise (e.g., torsion). Most cryptorchid testicles are undescended. True undescended testicles have stopped short along their normal path of descent into the scrotum and may remain in the abdominal cavity or be palpable in the inguinal canal or just outside the external ring. Cancer is 35–48 times more likely in cryptorchidism than in the normally descended testis. About 5% of full-term babies and one-third of premature babies have one undescended testis at birth, but descent is typically complete by the end of the first few weeks of life. Treatment for cryptorchidism can be hormonal, surgical, or a combination of the two.

Answer A is incorrect. Hypogonadotropic hypogonadism is due to congenital or acquired causes, not cryptorchidism. Impaired secretion of LH and FSH due to congenital GnRH deficiency results in secondary hypogonadism, characterized by low testosterone in the setting of low LH and FSH.

Answer B is incorrect. An indirect inguinal hernia is a protrusion of bowel through the deep inguinal ring that is unrelated to cryptorchidism. The bowel may descend all the way into the scrotum. Clinical signs include a tender mass in the inguinal region that cannot be reduced with pressure.

Answer C is incorrect. Retractile testes are a physiologic retraction of the testes into the abdominal cavity in response to cold, a benign condition requiring no treatment.

Answer E is incorrect. Torsion of the spermatic cord is rarely seen in cryptorchidism. The incidence of testicular torsion is increased, however, in males in whom the tunica vaginalis is attached high on the spermatic cord.

36. **The correct answer is E.** Sildenafil acts by inhibiting cGMP phosphodiesterase, which increases cGMP levels and thereby leads to smooth muscle relaxation in the corpus cavernosum. The muscle relaxation allows increased

blood flow. Some of the adverse effects include headache, flushing, and disturbances in color vision.

Answer A is incorrect. Testosterone cannot be given orally due to issues of hepatotoxicity. It can be administered intramuscularly, topically, or buccally but is rarely effective in the setting of normal testosterone levels and is discouraged because of the adverse effects of decreased spermatogenesis, gynecomastia, and possible impotence.

Answer B is incorrect. Clomiphene is an example of a selective estrogen receptor modulator. A partial agonist, it interferes with estrogen's binding site on the hypothalamus and the pituitary, thus increasing the secretion of GnRH. It is used to treat women with infertility associated with anovulatory cycles.

Answer C is incorrect. Alprostadil is an intraurethral prostaglandin pellet that increases arterial inflow and decreases venous outflow, thereby increasing erection by binding G proteins and stimulating adenylyl cyclase. It is also available as an intracavernosal injection, but this form is associated with a higher risk of priapism.

Answer D is incorrect. Sildenafil works via inhibition of cGMP phosphodiesterase, not cAMP phosphodiesterase.

37. **The correct answer is E.** A Tzanck test is a smear of an opened skin lesion to detect multinucleated giant cells and assay for the HSV. The Tzanck test can detect HSV-1 and -2 and the varicella-zoster virus. Epidermal cells in the vesicles sometimes develop eosinophilic intranuclear viral inclusions, or several cells may fuse to produce giant cells (multinucleate polykaryons), changes that are demonstrated by the diagnostic Tzanck test based on microscopic evaluation of the vesicle fluid. The vesicles usually clear within 3–4 weeks, but the virus travels along the regional nerves and become dormant in the local ganglia.

Answer A is incorrect. Auer rods are rod-shaped bodies in myeloid cells. They are found in acute myelogenous leukemia. They represent abnormal azurophilic granules and are particularly numerous in acute myelogenous leukemia associated with the t(15;17) translocation.

Answer B is incorrect. Call-Exner bodies are spaces between granulosa cells in ovarian follicles and in granulosa cell tumors.

Answer C is incorrect. Lewy bodies are abnormal aggregates of protein that develop inside nerve cells. On microscopy of affected brain tissue, these spherical masses displace other cell components. The main disease associated with the presence of Lewy bodies is Parkinson's disease. Lewy bodies are also present in patients with dementia with Lewy bodies.

Answer D is incorrect. Mallory bodies are eosinophilic intracytoplasmic inclusions found in hepatic cells and seen in a variety of diseases, including alcoholic liver disease.

38. **The correct answer is D.** Placenta previa occurs when the placenta overlies the cervical os. This can be asymptomatic, or it may present with vaginal bleeding. Classically, the bleeding is painless; however, it may be associated with contractions. If a digital vaginal examination is performed and the placenta is disrupted, it can result in massive vaginal bleeding. Prior to pelvic examination, a sonogram should be performed to verify placental location in all pregnant patients with vaginal bleeding in the second or third trimesters.

Answer A is incorrect. Abruptio placentae is the premature separation of the placenta from the uterine wall, usually during the third trimester of pregnancy. It is usually associated with **painful** vaginal bleeding. Severe abruption may result in fetal death and disseminated intravascular coagulation.

Answer B is incorrect. Eclampsia is characterized by a seizure in the second or third trimester in a patient who has not been previously diagnosed with a seizure disorder. Eclampsia is not usually associated with independent painless vaginal bleeding.

Answer C is incorrect. A hydatidiform mole is a pathologic ovum that causes swelling of chorionic villi and proliferation of chorionic epithelium, resulting in a "honeycombed uterus" or "cluster of grapes." This is associated with extremely elevated β-hCG. Complete moles would present earlier in pregnancy and would not have fetal heart tones.

Answer E is incorrect. Preeclampsia is characterized by hypertension, edema, and proteinuria, which this patient does not display. There is an increased incidence in patients with pre-existing hypertension, diabetes, chronic renal disease, and autoimmune diseases. Preeclampsia is not usually associated with independent painless vaginal bleeding.

39. **The correct answer is D.** This infant has a hypospadias, in which the penile urethra opens on the ventral surface of the penis rather than the tip. Hypospadias are caused by incomplete closure of the urethral folds. In the male, the urethral folds give rise to the ventral shaft of the penis; in the female, they give rise to the labia minora.

Answer A is incorrect. The glans clitoris arises from the genital tubercle, which produces the glans penis in the male.

Answer B is incorrect. The glands of Bartholin are derived from the urogenital sinus. The urogenital sinus produces the corpus spongiosum, the bulbourethral glands, and the prostate gland in the male.

Answer C is incorrect. The labia majora are derived from the labioscrotal swelling, which gives rise to the scrotum in the male.

Answer E is incorrect. The urethral and paraurethral glands of Skene are derived from the urogenital sinus. The urogenital sinus produces the corpus spongiosum, the bulbourethral glands, and the prostate gland in the male.

Answer F is incorrect. The urogenital sinus produces the vestibular bulbs, the glands of Bartholin, and the glands of Skene in the female. It produces the corpus spongiosum, the bulbourethral glands, and the prostate gland in the male.

40. **The correct answer is E.** Postmenopausal bleeding is a sign of endometrial cancer until proven otherwise by biopsy. PCOS is a risk factor for endometrial. Women with PCOS have adequate amounts of circulating estrogen, but lack progesterone secretion seen in the luteal phase of the menstrual cycle. Unopposed estrogen leads to stimulation of the endometrium and can be a risk factor for endometrial cancer.

Answer A is incorrect. Alcohol consumption has not been linked to endometrial cancer.

Answer B is incorrect. Late onset of menarche is believed to be a protective factor because there is less estrogen stimulation of the endometrium.

Answer C is incorrect. Multiparity is not a risk factor, but epidemiologic studies have shown that nulliparity is a risk factor for endometrial cancer.

Answer D is incorrect. Oral contraceptive pills are a protective factor for endometrial cancer, likely because the progestin component prevents endometrial stimulation.

Answer F is incorrect. Smoking has been shown to be protective against endometrial cancer, although its other adverse effects far outweigh this benefit.

41. **The correct answer is E.** This patient has chancroid, a painful genital ulcer caused by *Haemophilus ducreyi*. Chancroid is relatively uncommon in the United States, but is more common in sub-Saharan Africa and Latin America. Chancroid presents with a painful exudative ulcer with lymphadenitis. The most appropriate treatment is single-dose azithromycin.

Answer A is incorrect. A 10-day course of oral acyclovir would be appropriate treatment for genital herpes viral infection. Herpes lesions are also painful, but are commonly multiple, and microscopic examination (Tzanck test) shows multinucleated giant cells with viral inclusion bodies.

Answer B is incorrect. Highly active antiretroviral therapy is appropriate treatment for HIV infection in the absence of fulminant concomitant opportunistic infections. Although chancroid and HIV are often found in the same patients, chancroid also frequently occurs in immunocompetent hosts. This particular patient shows no evidence of immunodeficiency, and highly active antiretroviral therapy will not be effective for his penile lesion. However, he is clearly at high risk for HIV infection, and his HIV status should be further discussed.

Answer C is incorrect. Nystatin powder is effective treatment for candidal intertrigo in moist areas such as inguinal folds. Although this patient has inguinal lymphadenopathy, he has no reported skin changes in this area consistent with candidal intertrigo.

Answer D is incorrect. Intramuscular penicillin G is appropriate treatment for syphilis. However, genital ulcers in syphilis are typically painless, and Gram stain is unrevealing.

42. **The correct answer is A.** Abruptio placentae is premature separation of the placenta during the third trimester, resulting in painful vaginal bleeding, uterine contractions, and possible fetal death secondary to decreased blood flow. This complication of pregnancy may be associated with disseminated intravascular coagulation secondary to hemorrhage, illustrated in this patient by the partially hemolyzed schistocytes.

Answer B is incorrect. Amniotic fluid embolism is also referred to as anaphylactoid syndrome of pregnancy and is characterized by hypoxia, respiratory distress, cardiogenic shock, and disseminated intravascular coagulation. It occurs with tearing of maternal vessels and can result in maternal respiratory distress.

Answer C is incorrect. Hydrops fetalis is diagnosed with two or more of the following findings: fetal skin edema, pleural effusion, pericardial effusion, or ascites. It can be a complication of parvovirus B19 infection but is not associated with hemolysis or vaginal bleeding.

Answer D is incorrect. Placenta previa is atypical implantation of the placenta inferiorly, partially or completely covering the cervical os. This can present with painless bleeding, especially near the time of delivery, and cervical dilatation. This condition is not associated with infection or hemolysis.

Answer E is incorrect. Preeclampsia usually presents during the third trimester of pregnancy with hypertension, proteinuria, and edema. It can also be associated with **HELLP** syndrome (**H**emolysis, **E**levated **L**iver function tests, and **L**ow **P**latelets). This patient does not have hypertension or proteinuria. Few RBCs in the urine are normal, considering vaginal bleeding.

43. **The correct answer is D.** Tamoxifen as a chemotherapeutic agent is useful only in estrogen receptor-positive breast cancer. It is an estrogen antagonist whose mechanism of action relies on binding estrogen receptors to impede the production of estrogen-responsive genes. Tamoxifen is not useful in a breast cancer that is estrogen receptor-negative.

Answer A is incorrect. Cyclophosphamide is an alkylating agent that cross-links DNA leading to apoptosis. Cyclophosphamide is commonly used to treat non-Hodgkin's lymphoma and breast/ovarian cancer.

Answer B is incorrect. Doxorubicin is an anti-tumor antibiotic commonly used to treat breast cancer. It acts by intercalation into DNA, inhibiting topoisomerase II and resulting in DNA damage and cell death. Doxorubicin is associated with congestive heart failure.

Answer C is incorrect. Paclitaxel and other taxanes act by inhibiting depolymerization of microtubules leading to cell cycle arrest in mitosis. Paclitaxel is commonly used in breast cancer chemotherapy.

Answer E is incorrect. Trastuzumab is a monoclonal antibody against HER-2 that can kill breast cancer cells overexpressing HER-2. This patient's breast cancer is HER-2/neu-positive, thus she is likely to have a positive response to the chemotherapeutic agent trastuzumab (Herceptin).

44. **The correct answer is C.** This patient has symptoms consistent with benign prostatic hypertrophy, including difficulty initiating a stream, postvoid dribbling, and frequent nighttime urination. In this case, the large prostate encasing the prostatic urethra caused urinary obstruction, leading to a decline in renal function reflected by an increase in creatinine level. On ultrasound one may be able to see dilation of the urinary collection system. A well-placed Foley catheter definitively relieves the obstruction.

Answer A is incorrect. Giving fluids would improve renal function if the patient were hypovolemic. The patient's symptoms point to an obstructive reason for his rise in creatinine level rather than to a prerenal cause.

Answer B is incorrect. Dialysis would be appropriate if the patient were in renal failure. However, his creatinine level is not severely elevated, and he is still making urine. Placing a Foley catheter directly addresses the cause of the patient's declining renal function.

Answer D is incorrect. Terazosin is an α_1-blocker that relaxes prostatic smooth muscle surrounding the prostatic urethra. This does improve the obstruction, but does not have the immediate effect of relieving it.

45. **The correct answer is D.** 5α-Reductase converts testosterone to DHT. DHT is required for the development of the penis and scrotum before birth. The infant has testes and normal levels of testosterone, estrogen, and LH. The dramatic increase in testosterone levels during puberty causes the genitalia to be masculinized.

Answer A is incorrect. Complete androgen insensitivity, or testicular feminization syndrome, is usually caused by defect in the androgen receptor. These XY individuals have female phenotype, except that testes are present. Levels of testosterone, estrogen, and LH are all high.

Answer B is incorrect. Males with the genotype XYY are phenotypically normal, so their genitalia are unambiguous.

Answer C is incorrect. Female pseudohermaphroditism occurs when ovaries are present and the external genitalia are ambiguous. This condition is usually due to exposure to androgens early in gestation.

Answer E is incorrect. True hermaphroditism occurs only when both ovary and testicular tissue is present; this is rare in humans.

46. **The correct answer is E.** Fibrocystic disease is benign and presents with diffuse breast pain and multiple bilateral masses. Fibrocystic changes can be characterized histologically and include fibrosis, cysts, sclerosis, and epithelial hyperplasia. Without the presence of atypia, these lesions are not usually associated with an increased risk of carcinoma.

Answer A is incorrect. Central necrosis is characteristic of comedocarcinoma, often resulting in a cheesy consistency. Comedocarcinomas are malignant.

Answer B is incorrect. Lymphocytic infiltration of mammary ducts and/or glands indicates medullary carcinoma. These lesions are well circumscribed, soft, and histologically cellular with scant stroma. Medullary carcinomas are malignant.

Answer C is incorrect. Lymphatic involvement of breast tissue is indicative of inflammatory carcinoma, which is malignant with a poor prognosis.

Answer D is incorrect. Paget's disease is an eczematous patch on the nipple or areola, often with underlying ductal carcinomas that are firm and fibrous on breast examination. On histology, there are large cells with surrounding halos in the epidermis, with underlying islands of tumor cells embedded in fibrosis. Paget's disease is a type of malignant breast carcinoma.

47. **The correct answer is D.** The disorder described is Stein-Leventhal syndrome, or PCOS. Although there is a great deal of variation in clinical presentation in this syndrome, a subset of patients have elevated serum LH levels and elevated LH:FSH ratios. Consistently high levels of LH can lead to anovulation due to down-

regulation of the LH receptors at the ovaries. Elevated LH also stimulates the thecal cells of the ovaries to secrete excess androstenedione, which can be converted into testosterone by most peripheral tissues, leading to hirsutism, acne, or male-patterned alopecia.

Answer A is incorrect. The majority of patients with PCOS have elevated or normal estrone and estradiol levels.

Answer B is incorrect. Serum androgen levels, including testosterone, androstenedione, and dehydroepiandrosterone sulfate, are increased in the majority of patients with PCOS.

Answer C is incorrect. FSH levels may be normal or low in PCOS, contributing to the elevated LH/FSH ratio seen in many patients.

Answer E is incorrect. Elevated LH levels and reduced ovulation leads to deficient ovarian progesterone secretion. Patients with PCOS are at an increased risk for endometrial hyperplasia and carcinoma due to the unopposed estrogen stimulation of the endometrium.

48. **The correct answer is C.** A hydatidiform mole is a pathologic ovum with no DNA that causes cystic swelling of chorionic villi and proliferation of the trophoblast, resulting in a mass that can look like a "cluster of grapes," as seen in the image. The genotype of a complete mole is 46,XX, completely consisting of paternal DNA. There is no associated fetus with this entity despite the elevated β-hCG.

Answer A is incorrect. Maternally derived 46,XX would not cause a hydatidiform mole. Moles are derived from "empty" ova that are then fertilized by sperm.

Answer B is incorrect. 46,XX describes the genotype of a normal fetus, receiving one set of chromosomes from each parent.

Answer D is incorrect. Paternally derived 69,XXX describes another possible DNA make-up of a partial mole. A partial mole contains more than two sets of chromosomes that usually consist of two paternal and one maternal set of chromosomes, resulting in triploidy or tetraploidy. Partial moles may present with a

similar grapelike mass but are also associated with fetal parts.

Answer E is incorrect. Maternally and paternally derived 69,XXY describes one possible DNA make-up of a partial mole. A partial mole contains more than two sets of chromosomes that usually consist of both paternal and maternal sets, resulting in triploidy or tetraploidy. Partial moles may present with a similar grapelike mass but are associated with fetal parts

49. **The correct answer is C.** β-hCG is produced by the placenta immediately after implantation in the endometrium of the uterus. β-hCG acts on the corpus luteum to rescue it from regression. The corpus luteum then goes on to produce estriol and progesterone to maintain the pregnancy until the placenta takes over this role in the second and third trimesters. β-hCG levels peak at week 9 of gestation and then start to decline until reaching a steady state around week 25.

Answer A is incorrect. β-hCG does not initiate parturition at the end of pregnancy. The actual initiating event is unknown.

Answer B is incorrect. Progesterone, not β-hCG, raises the threshold for uterine contraction. This helps prevent spontaneous abortion of the fetus.

Answer D is incorrect. Estrogen and progesterone, produced by the corpus luteum in the first trimester and by the placenta in the second and third trimesters, stimulate the growth of breasts during pregnancy.

50. **The correct answer is E.** *Candida albicans* infection can cause thrush in immunocompromised patients. It can also cause vulvovaginitis, disseminated candidiasis (to any organ), and chronic mucocutaneous candidiasis. Diagnosis is made through cultures and tissue biopsy for invasive systemic disease.

Answer A is incorrect. Coccidioidomycosis is the second most common fungal infection encountered in the United States. About 60% of these infections cause no symptoms, and in the remaining 40% of cases the symptoms range from mild to severe. Severe forms of the infection can present with blood-tinged sputum, loss of appetite, weight loss, a painful red rash on the legs, and change in mental status.

Answer B is incorrect. Histoplasmosis does not typically lead to any symptomatic presentation. When symptoms are present, they usually present as a flu-like illness with fever, cough, headaches, and myalgias. Histoplasmosis can result in lung disease resembling tuberculosis and widespread disseminated infection affecting the liver, spleen, adrenal glands, mucosal surfaces, and meninges. Histoplasmosis occurs most commonly in the Mississippi and Ohio river valleys.

Answer C is incorrect. *Aspergillus fumigatus* infection can present with bronchopulmonary

aspergillosis, lung cavity aspergillomas ("fungus balls"), and invasive aspergillosis. A. *fumigatus* is a mold with septate hyphae that branch at a V-shaped 45-degree angle. A. *fumigatus* is not dimorphic.

Answer D is incorrect. *Cryptococcus neoformans* infection does not often present with any symptoms in an immunocompetent host. However, in an immunocompromised individual, it can present with meningoencephalitis. *Cryptococcus* is a heavily encapsulated yeast that is not dimorphic. The fungus is found in soil and pigeon droppings.

CHAPTER 17

Respiratory

1. A 25-year-old woman with asthma presents to the emergency department in severe cardiovascular distress after taking a theophylline overdose in an attempt to commit suicide. At presentation, she is convulsing, her blood pressure is 80/40 mm Hg, and she has developed a cardiac arrhythmia. Considering the mechanism of action of theophylline, which of the following drugs may be used to counteract its effects?

(A) Albuterol
(B) β-Blockers
(C) Digoxin
(D) Epinephrine
(E) Furosemide

·2. On a routine check-up, a 65-year-old woman with recently diagnosed adenocarcinoma of the lung is found to have drooping of the right eyelid. Pupillary examination reveals anisocoria with the right pupil smaller than the left. Upon further questioning she reveals that after exerting herself she has to mop the sweat off of her left brow, but does not notice any sweat on her right side. Which of the following is the most likely etiology of the patient's symptoms?

(A) Apical lung tumor
(B) Graves' disease
(C) Myasthenia gravis
(D) Paraneoplastic endocrine hormone production
(E) Superior vena cava obstruction

3. A 50-year-old man is treated for septic shock with multiple antibiotics. Seven days later, the patient is alert and oriented, and his tissue perfusion has returned to normal. However, he describes a terrible feeling that "the world is spinning." Which of the following therapeutic agents is most likely responsible for this patient's symptom?

(A) Erythromycin
(B) Gentamicin
(C) Imipenem
(D) Metronidazole
(E) Piperacillin-tazobactam

4. A homeless man who is an alcoholic is brought to the emergency department after being found unconscious by the side of the road. Films taken on arrival show some old trauma to the jaw. X-ray of the chest and CT of the chest reveal a mass lesion in the right lower lobe with spiculation, which appears to extend into the pleural space and involve an adjacent rib. A biopsy specimen of the mass-like lesion is shown in the image. Histologic specimens of bronchial lavage fluid after biopsy contain numerous hyphae but no malignant cells. What should be included in the treatment regimen for this man's condition?

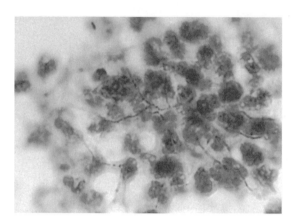

Reproduced, with permission, from Brooks GF, Carroll KC, Butel JS, Morse SA. *Jawetz, Melnick, & Adelberg's Medical Microbiology*, 24th ed. New York: McGraw-Hill, 2007: Figure 13-2.

(A) Amphotericin B
(B) Ciprofloxacin
(C) Fluconazole
(D) Isoniazid
(E) Penicillin G

5. A 55-year-old woman with a history of schizophrenia presents to the emergency department with paranoia and active hallucinations. Her agitation is so severe that she has to be restrained for several days. She is started on haloperidol. A few days later she becomes tachy-

cardic and complains of sharp right-sided chest pain. What step should be taken next in the care of this patient?

(A) Discontinue the haloperidol
(B) Start a β-blocker
(C) Start broad-spectrum antibiotics
(D) Start intravenous heparin
(E) Watchful waiting

6. A 25-year-old medical student presents with a nonproductive cough, low-grade fever, and malaise of 3 weeks' duration. He says that a few of the people he studies with have been feeling the same way. Sputum cultures come back negative. The patient denies exposure to farm animals, travel, or HIV. The physician decides to treat for an atypical pneumonia. Which of the following methods could identify the organism responsible for such a pneumonia?

(A) Acid-fast stain
(B) Cold agglutinin testing
(C) Gram stain
(D) India ink stain
(E) Polymerase chain reaction

7. A 50-year-old man complains of shortness of breath on exertion of a few months' duration. On inspection there is an increased anteroposterior diameter of the chest, pursed lips, and dyspnea with no scleral icterus or jaundice. The patient has a 75-pack-year history of smoking. On physical examination, the patient is tachycardic and has hyperresonant lungs with decreased breath sounds. There is no evidence of hepatomegaly or liver nodules on palpation. Which of the following is the most likely diagnosis?

(A) α₁-Antitrypsin deficiency
(B) Asthma
(C) Bronchiectasis
(D) Centriacinar emphysema
(E) Chronic bronchitis
(F) Panacinar emphysema

8. A 13-year-old white girl with a past medical history of nasal polyps develops severe bronchoconstriction and wheezing after taking a large dose of aspirin, having mistaken it for a cold medication. After presenting to the emergency department, she is found to have a past history of aspirin allergy. Which of the following medications can be used effectively to stop the bronchoconstriction resulting from her aspirin allergy?

(A) Cromolyn
(B) Dopamine
(C) Methylxanthines
(D) Prednisone
(E) Zileuton

9. A 60-year-old white man presents to his physician with a productive cough of a few months' duration. The patient reports having three of these episodes over the past 2 years, with each episode lasting 4 months. On physical examination the patient is cyanotic, wheezing, and has crackles in the lungs upon auscultation. Lung biopsy reveals hypertrophy of mucus-secreting glands in the bronchioles, with a Reid index >50%. Which of the following is associated with the most likely diagnosis?

(A) Air pollution
(B) Alcohol intake
(C) Cold climate
(D) Hypertension
(E) Intravenous drug abuse
(F) Seasonal allergies

10. During dental procedures, it is possible that small fragments may be aspirated into the trachea and cause aspiration pneumonia. If the patient is sitting upright during the procedure, which of the following is the most common site of aspiration pneumonia?

(A) Left lower lobe
(B) Left upper lobe
(C) Lingula
(D) Right lower lobe
(E) Right upper lobe

11. A 57-year-old man with a 40-year history of smoking has chronic obstructive lung disease. He presents to the physician with a blood pressure of 150/95 mm Hg. Which of the following antihypertensive agents is contraindicated in this patient?

(A) Acebutolol
(B) Atenolol
(C) Esmolol
(D) Metoprolol
(E) Nadolol

12. Gas exchange in the lungs occurs in the alveoli. There are two components to this exchange, diffusion and perfusion. Either of these components can limit the exchange of oxygen from the air into the bloodstream. Which of the following describes perfusion-limited exchange?

(A) CO and O_2 exchange in the lungs during strenuous exercise
(B) Disease states such as fibrosis and emphysema
(C) Exchanges that are not affected by changes in blood flow
(D) Gas equilibrating early along the length of the pulmonary capillary
(E) Gas exchange in the lungs other than N_2O and CO_2 under healthy, resting conditions
(F) Maintenance of the oxygen partial pressure difference between alveolar air and pulmonary capillary blood

13. While examining a patient, the physician notices decreased breath sounds at the right lower lobe, dullness on percussion, and decreased tactile fremitus without tracheal deviation. These findings most likely represent which of the following?

(A) Bronchial obstruction
(B) Intestinal infiltration
(C) Lobar pneumonia
(D) Pleural effusion
(E) Pneumothorax

14. A 65-year-old man with an 80-pack-year history of smoking presents with a cough and increasing dyspnea over the past 6 weeks. A 2-cm diameter mass is seen in the left lower lobe on x-ray of the chest. A sample of nonneoplastic tissue from the lung biopsy is shown in the image. Which of the following types of epithelium not normally present in the lung lines the bronchus shown in this image?

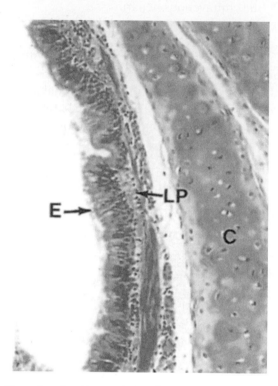

Reproduced, with permission, from Berman I. *Color Atlas of Basic Histology*, 3rd ed. New York: McGraw-Hill, 2003: 220, Figure 14-11 .

(A) Pseudostratified columnar
(B) Simple squamous
(C) Stratified columnar
(D) Stratified squamous
(E) Transitional

15. The oxygen-hemoglobin dissociation curve represents the percent saturation of hemoglobin with oxygen as a function of the partial pressure of oxygen in the blood. This curve is sigmoidal in shape due to the change in affinity of heme groups for oxygen as each successive oxygen molecule binds. Which of the following in an adult would cause a shift in the curve so that it resembles that of a neonate?

(A) High altitude
(B) Increased 2,3-diphosphoglycerate
(C) Increased partial pressure of carbon dioxide in the blood
(D) Increased pH
(E) Increased temperature

16. A 45-year-old African-American woman presents to her physician because of dyspnea and fatigue that has worsened over the past 6 weeks. Over the past week she has noticed the appearance of subcutaneous nodules on her lower extremities. Physical examination reveals dry rales and flat, elevated lesions on the lower extremities bilaterally. X-ray of the chest shows bilateral hilar lymphadenopathy. Laboratory tests are performed. Which result, although not diagnostic, is most commonly associated with this patient's condition?

(A) Elevated angiotensin-converting enzyme level
(B) Elevated cardiac enzyme levels
(C) Elevated serum amylase levels
(D) Hypocalcemia
(E) Hypouricemia

17. A 7-year-old boy is brought to the pediatrician because of a chronic cough, fatty diarrhea, and failure to thrive. *Pseudomonas aeruginosa* is cultured from his respiratory tract. The physician informs the patient's parents that their son has a disease that is caused by a mutation in a specific ion transporter. This patient has a mutation in the ion transporter of which of the following electrolytes?

(A) Bicarbonate
(B) Calcium
(C) Chloride
(D) Potassium
(E) Sodium

18. An 18-year-old man comes to the physician complaining of a runny nose, sneezing, and

difficulty breathing for the past 2 days. On questioning, the patient says that his younger sister received a baby kitten as a birthday present 2 days ago. The response seen in this patient is mediated by which of the following?

(A) Antigen-antibody complexes activating complement
(B) Antigen cross-linking IgE on presensitized mast cells and basophils
(C) IgM and IgG binding to antigens on enemy cells
(D) Sensitized T lymphocytes releasing lymphokines
(E) Serum sickness

19. Inspiration during vigorous exercise involves rapid and deep breathing, which may damage the lungs without mechanisms to prevent overinflation of lung tissue. Which of the following is critical to prevent lung damage due to overinflation?

(A) Decreased discharge frequency of slowly adapting pulmonary stretch receptors in the lungs during maximal blood flow to the lungs
(B) Decreased discharge frequency of slowly adapting pulmonary stretch receptors in the lungs during maximal expansion of the parenchyma
(C) Increased discharge frequency of slowly adapting pulmonary stretch receptors in the lungs during maximal blood flow to the lungs
(D) Increased discharge frequency of slowly adapting pulmonary stretch receptors in the lungs during maximal expansion of the parenchyma
(E) Maintenance of discharge frequency of slowly adapting pulmonary stretch receptors in the lungs during both inspiration and expiration

20. A 5-year-old girl is brought to the emergency department by her aunt because of a sore throat. The patient is visiting from Nicaragua and has had very few immunizations. Physical examination reveals a grayish-white membrane on the pharynx with marked cervical lymphadenopathy and edema of the throat and neck area. The girl is, however, afebrile. Definitive diagnosis is made by gram-positive rods growing on which of the following media?

(A) Bordet-Gengou agar
(B) Chocolate agar with factors V and X
(C) Sabouraud's agar
(D) Tellurite agar
(E) Thayer-Martin agar

21. A 57-year-old man from Colombia presents to the emergency department with fever, night sweats, and a productive cough. A sputum smear shows acid-fast bacilli, and the patient is started on several medications. Three months later, the patient returns to the emergency department with reduced visual acuity and an inability to see the color green. Which of the following is the most likely cause of this patient's change in visual acuity?

(A) Ethambutol toxicity
(B) Isoniazid toxicity
(C) Pyrazinamide toxicity
(D) Rifampin toxicity
(E) Tuberculous eye infection

22. A 12-year-old boy is found unconscious in his bedroom by his parents and is taken to the emergency department. On arrival the patient's skin is pale and lacks turgor, and there is a sweet scent on his breath. His parents report constant urination and weight loss in the 2 weeks prior to presentation. Laboratory tests show a glucose level of 610 mg/dL, sodium of 130 mEq/L, bicarbonate of 9 mEq/L, and chloride of 95 mEq/L. Which of the following would most likely be associated with this patient's condition at presentation?

(A) Calcium oxalate crystals in the urine
(B) Decreased anion gap
(C) Decreased blood partial pressure of carbon dioxide
(D) Elevated blood partial pressure of carbon dioxide
(E) Hypokalemia

23. Atelectasis (the collapse of alveoli) is a common complication of surgical procedures, especially those requiring general anesthesia, due to impaired surfactant activity and its corresponding effects on alveolar compliance. Which of the following is a characteristic of alveolar compliance?

(A) Decreased surfactant production results in increased airway compliance
(B) Increasing the radius of alveoli increases the pressure required to collapse the alveoli
(C) Increasing the surface tension of alveoli increases the pressure required to collapse the alveoli
(D) Large, surfactant-lined alveoli have the highest probability of collapse
(E) Small alveoli have increased compliance relative to large alveoli

24. A 7-year-old girl is brought to the pediatrician because of a fever of 39.7° C (103.5° F), trouble swallowing, and drooling. Within a few minutes of arriving at the office, she develops inspiratory stridor and respiratory distress. An x-ray film of her neck is shown in the image. Which of the following is most likely responsible for this patient's condition?

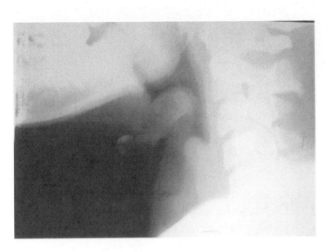

Reproduced, with permission, from Stone CK, Humphries RL. *Current Diagnosis & Treatment: Emergency Medicine*, 6th ed. New York: McGraw-Hill, 2008: Figure 48-4.

(A) *Haemophilus influenzae*
(B) *Mycoplasma pneumoniae*
(C) Parainfluenza virus
(D) Respiratory syncytial virus
(E) *Streptococcus pyogenes*

25. An 8-year-old boy comes to the physician with his mother, who wants to discuss respiratory problems that have arisen since an upper respiratory infection 4 months ago. The mother says that the patient has attacks characterized by wheezing and shortness of breath that usually resolve after an hour. On one occasion, an attack required a visit to the emergency department, and the mother remembers the treating physician saying something about an abnormally high level of eosinophils in the patient's blood. Which cytokine is involved in the pathogenesis of this disease?

(A) Interferon-γ
(B) Interleukin-2
(C) Interleukin-4
(D) Tumor necrosis factor–α
(E) Tumor growth factor–β

26. A 46-year-old woman presents to the emergency department with a 4-week history of worsening nausea and lethargy. While she is waiting to see the doctor, the patient experiences a seizure. Her past medical history is significant for hypertension and tuberculosis. Laboratory tests show:

Serum Na$^+$: 125 mEq/L
Serum osmolality: 255 mOsm/kg
Urine osmolality: 1550 mOsm/kg
Hematocrit: 27%

Which of the following is the most likely diagnosis?

(A) Central diabetes insipidus
(B) Epilepsy
(C) Nephrogenic diabetes insipidus
(D) Psychogenic polydipsia
(E) Syndrome of inappropriate ADH secretion

27. A 17-year-old girl involved in a car accident presents to the emergency department with penetrating chest trauma to her left side. She is having difficulty breathing and has an oxygen saturation of 86%. After x-ray of the chest is performed, a chest tube is placed, and her oxygen saturation improves. Which of the following is responsible for her difficulty breathing upon presentation?

(A) Her intrapleural pressure is greater than atmospheric pressure during inspiration
(B) Her intrapleural pressure is less than atmospheric pressure during inspiration
(C) Her intrapleural space is open to the atmosphere
(D) Pain from the trauma has made it difficult to breathe
(E) The elastic force of the chest wall is pulling it inward

28. An HIV-positive 24-year-old man from Southern California comes in to his physician's office with a dry cough, headache, mild wheezing, and slight fever. A complete blood cell count shows elevated eosinophils, and a potassium hydroxide sputum smear is positive for microorganisms. The infectious form of the organism causing the patient's symptoms possesses which of the following key components?

(A) Dipicolinic acid
(B) Hemagglutinin
(C) Lipopolysaccharide
(D) Polysaccharide
(E) Teichoic acid

29. A 74-year-old patient presents with increased shortness of breath. A sputum sample reveals golden-brown beaded fibers, which result from iron- and protein-coated fibers. On CT scan, dense fibrocalcific plaques of the parietal pleura are seen. A particular pneumoconiosis is suspected. Which of the following is the likely etiology of the patient's condition?

(A) Autoimmune attack of lung parenchyma
(B) Idiopathic (unknown) etiology
(C) Living in a polluted city for years
(D) Long-term complication of steroid abuse
(E) Reactivation of a contained primary disease
(F) Working in a coal mine for 40 years
(G) Working in a shipyard for 40 years

30. A 158.8-kg (350-lb) man with a body mass index of 40 kg/m^2 comes to the physician complaining of frequent fatigue, shortness of breath, general sleepiness, and an inability to concentrate. Physical examination shows an extremely obese, tired-looking man with hypertension and an elongated uvula. Which of the following metabolic findings is most likely?

(A) Decreased serum glucose
(B) Increased HDL cholesterol
(C) Increased renal HCO$_3^-$ reabsorption
(D) Increased renal HCO$_3^-$ secretion
(E) Increased renal H$^+$ reabsorption

31. A 55-year-old woman presents with a painless mass at the angle of the mandible 1 week after undergoing a dental procedure. On physical examination, her physician notes that the mass is draining pus and yellowish granules. A stained sample from the abscess shows branching gram-positive rods. She is treated with penicillin. What is the most likely causative organism?

(A) *Actinomyces israelii*
(B) *Candida albicans*
(C) *Clostridium perfringens*
(D) *Nocardia asteroides*
(E) *Staphylococcus epidermidis*

32. Respiratory rate changes dynamically according to input from many different sources. There are central control mechanisms, chemoreceptors, and other receptors responsible for respiration. What is one mechanism by which the body exerts control over respiration?

(A) Central chemoreceptors affect breathing by directly detecting blood levels of H$^+$ ions
(B) Breathing is centrally regulated via the hypothalamus and amygdala
(C) Peripheral chemoreceptors stimulate breathing when the partial pressure of oxygen dips below 60 mm Hg
(D) Stretch, irritant, and J receptors all function outside the lung to regulate breathing
(E) The aortic and carotid bodies are considered central chemoreceptors

33. A 21-year-old college student presents to his student health center with complaints of malaise, headaches, fever up to 38.3° C (101° F), chills, and a nonproductive cough for the past week. His temperature is 38.1° C (100.6° F), heart rate is 90/min, respiratory rate is 20/min, and blood pressure is 118/75 mm Hg. On physical examination the patient appears fatigued. Auscultation of the lungs reveals bilateral diffuse wheezes and rales. X-ray of the chest reveals bilateral infiltrates. The doctor prescribed ceftriaxone, but the patient failed to show any improvement over the subsequent week. Which antibiotic should the physicians prescribe instead?

(A) Ampicillin
(B) Azithromycin
(C) Clindamycin
(D) Fourth-generation cephalosporin
(E) Penicillin

34. A previously healthy, tall, thin 23-year-old man comes to the emergency department complaining of sudden pleuritic chest pain and shortness of breath. X-ray of the chest is shown in the image. Which of the following is the most likely diagnosis?

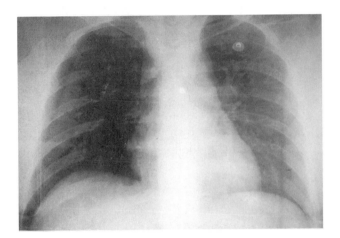

Reproduced, with permission, from Stone CK, Humphries RL. *Current Diagnosis & Treatment: Emergency Medicine*, 6th ed. New York: McGraw-Hill, 2008: Figure 11-3.

(A) Asbestosis
(B) Asthma
(C) Bronchiectasis
(D) Bronchitis
(E) Emphysema
(F) Oat cell carcinoma
(G) Pneumothorax

35. A 40-year-old patient with AIDS presents to the clinic with fatigue and weakness. X-ray of the chest is shown in the image. A methenamine silver stain of a bronchoalveolar lavage specimen reveals multiple organisms. Treatment with trimethoprim-sulfamethoxazole is contraindicated because the patient has a sulfa allergy. Which of the following agents should be used to treat this patient's infection?

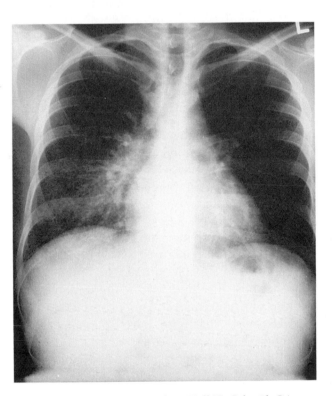

Reproduced, with permission, from Hall JB, Schmidt GA, Wood LDH. *Principles of Critical Care*, 3rd ed. New York: McGraw-Hill, 2005: Figure 48-1.

(A) Ivermectin
(B) Metronidazole
(C) Penicillin
(D) Pentamidine
(E) Protamine

36. A 71-year-old man is brought to the emergency department by ambulance after he was found by his neighbor walking around his garden confused and unable to answer questions. He is confused and oriented only to person. His temperature is 37.6° C (99.7° F), heart rate is 110/min, respiratory rate is 20/min, and blood pressure is 130/92 mm Hg. While in the emergency department the patient has a seizure. Laboratory tests show a serum sodium level of 115 mEq/L, potassium of 3.8 mEq/L, glucose of 100 mg/dL, and osmolality of 250 mOsm/kg. Urine electrolyte testing show a urine osmolality of 500 mOsm/kg. X-ray of the chest shows a mass in the lung. Which of the following is the most likely etiology of the mass?

(A) Foreign body aspiration
(B) Metastatic brain cancer
(C) Prostate cancer
(D) Small cell carcinoma
(E) Tuberculosis

37. Public health investigators looking into several cases of pneumonia that have occurred in a community are able to trace the outbreak to a water-mist machine used in the produce section of a supermarket. Patients exposed to the water-mist machine have presented with cough, high fever, headache, and abdominal pain. Elderly patients present with more severe disease. Which of the following is most likely to have caused this outbreak?

(A) *Bordetella pertussis*
(B) *Haemophilus influenzae* type B
(C) *Legionella pneumophila*
(D) *Mycobacterium tuberculosis*
(E) *Streptococcus pneumoniae*

38. Medium-sized bronchi are the major site of airway resistance in the lungs. Bronchial smooth muscle can change bronchial diameter by contracting or relaxing. Which of the following conditions is associated with dilation of airways?

(A) Asthma
(B) Atelectasis
(C) Bronchiectasis
(D) Idiopathic pulmonary fibrosis
(E) Neonatal respiratory distress syndrome

39. A mother brings her 10-year-old son with fever, cough, and difficulty breathing to the emergency department. Approximately 2 days ago she noted the development of a rash on his face that spread downward over his body. Physical examination reveals a toxic-appearing child with a temperature of 40° C (104° F), rapid pulse, and rapid respiratory rate. The physician notes the appearance of a reddish-brown blotchy rash throughout the child's body. In his mouth he has small red spots with blue-white centers. Chest examination reveals clear breath sounds with poor inspiratory effort. CT of the chest shows diffuse interstitial involvement. Which of the following would the physician most likely see in this child's sputum?

(A) Acid-fast bacilli
(B) Cells with nuclei surrounded by halo and clear cytoplasm
(C) Cowdry-type inclusions in cells
(D) Gram-negative coccobacilli and polymorphonuclear leukocytes
(E) Gram-positive diplococci and polymorphonuclear leukocytes
(F) Multinucleated giant cells

40. At a check-up during her 22nd week of pregnancy, a woman tells her doctor that she feels like she is "abnormally large" considering how long she has been pregnant. Her doctor agrees, and performs an ultrasound, which reveals an excess of fluid in the uterus. In addition, the stomach, spleen, and a portion of the small intestine are visible in the fetus' thorax. What structure(s) most likely failed to form completely in the fetal thorax?

(A) Dorsal mesentery of the esophagus
(B) Foregut
(C) Lateral body wall
(D) Pleuroperitoneal folds
(E) Septum transversum

41. Which of the following letter choices represents the residual volume?

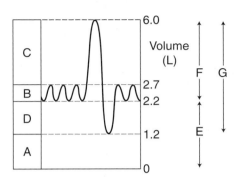

Reproduced, with permission, from USMLERx.com.

(A) A
(B) B
(C) C
(D) D
(E) E
(F) F
(G) G

42. A woman presents to the emergency department in labor. She is only at 29 weeks' gestation. The fetus is large for gestational age. The mother was diagnosed with gestational diabetes by her gynecologist earlier in the pregnancy. The infant is at increased risk for which of the following?

(A) Diffuse alveolar damage
(B) Hyaline membrane disease
(C) Hypersensitivity pneumonitis
(D) Neonatal pneumonia
(E) Noncaseating granulomatous disease
(F) Panacinar emphysema
(G) Patent foramen ovale

43. A 37-year-old man is brought to the emergency department after he is stabbed immediately superior the right nipple with an unknown object. His blood pressure is 100/60 mm Hg, heart rate is 126/min, respiratory rate is 26/min, and oxygen saturation is 94% on 100% oxygen face mask. The wound is small but is bubbling, and the skin immediately around the wound is moving in and out with respirations. Which of the following will most likely be found on x-ray of this patient's chest?

(A) Right hemothorax
(B) Right ninth and tenth rib fractures
(C) Right pleural effusion
(D) Right pneumothorax
(E) Right upper lobe consolidation

44. A 67-year-old homeless man reports to the physician with a 1-week history of a productive cough, shortness of breath and high fever. He denies alcohol, drug, or tobacco use. The patient says that the onset of symptoms was sudden. X-ray of the chest shows a large left lower lobe opacity. Which of the following antibiotics would best initially treat this patient's infection?

(A) Ceftriaxone
(B) Clindamycin
(C) Doxycycline
(D) Erythromycin
(E) Trimethoprim-sulfamethoxazole

45. A 26-year-old recent immigrant from China presents to the emergency department with a 3-week history of fevers accompanied by night sweats and chills, weight loss of 2.3 kg (5 lb), and cough that is often productive of blood-tinged sputum. Bronchoalveolar lavage is performed and an acid-fast stain of the sample reveals the organism shown in the image. Which of the following should be included in this patient's therapy to prevent a common toxicity of treatment?

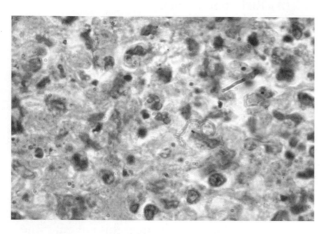

Reproduced, with permission, from PEIR Digital Library (http://peir.net).

(A) Vitamin B_1
(B) Vitamin B_6
(C) Vitamin B_{12}
(D) Vitamin C
(E) Vitamin E

46. A 15-year-old boy with a history of severe asthma presents to the emergency department in obvious respiratory distress. After admission and multiple nebulizer treatments, he develops nausea, vomiting, and weakness. Studies reveal a potassium level of 2.6 mEq/L and U waves on ECG. Which of the following medications most likely would have elicited these symptoms?

(A) Albuterol
(B) Ipratropium
(C) Theophylline
(D) Zileuton

47. A 32-year-old woman presents to her physician complaining of "swollen lymph nodes" under her chin. Further questioning reveals that she has had a cough for the past 2 months and some increased shortness of breath. After completing a full physical examination, her physician orders an x-ray of the chest, which shows an abnormality. A lung biopsy is ordered, and a micrograph of the biopsy is shown in the image. What is her most likely diagnosis?

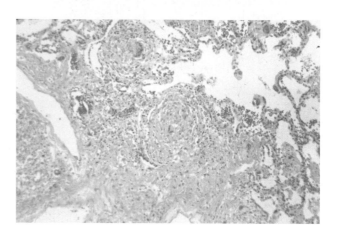

Reproduced, with permission, from PEIR Digital Library (http://peir.net).

(A) Goodpasture's syndrome
(B) Sarcoidosis
(C) Small cell lung cancer
(D) Systemic lupus erythematosus
(E) Tuberculosis

48. A tourist visits a cattle ranch and 5 days later develops fever, malaise, a dry cough, and pressure in his chest. These symptoms resolve after a few days. He then develops high fever, severe shortness of breath, chest pain, cyanosis, and diaphoresis, and is rushed to the emergency department, where work-up reveals hemorrhagic mediastinitis and bloody pleural effusions. Within a few hours, the patient develops septic shock and dies. Which of the following organisms is most likely responsible for this patient's symptoms?

(A) *Bacillus anthracis*
(B) *Brucella abortus*

(C) *Francisella tularensis*

(D) *Legionella pneumophila*

(E) *Nocardia asteroides*

49. A 44-year-old man with a recent history of community-acquired pneumonia treated with doxycycline and clarithromycin arrives at the clinic for follow-up. The patient is hypoxic with an oxygen saturation of 92%. Arterial blood gas analyses reveal hypercapnia. With regard to CO_2 trafficking, which of the following physiologic processes is taking place?

(A) All of the dissolved CO_2 becomes converted to bicarbonate, which binds to hemoglobin

(B) Bicarbonate travels in the RBCs until it reaches the lung, where it gets exhaled as CO_2

(C) Carbaminohemoglobin (CO_2 bound to hemoglobin) becomes the primary CO_2 transport carrier

(D) More chloride is entering the RBCs peripherally to compensate for increased carbonic anhydrase activity

(E) The acidic environment of the lungs shifts the hemoglobin-oxygen curve to the right and causes the release of CO_2 from hemoglobin

50. A 65-year-old patient comes in for an insurance physical that requires pulmonary function tests to ensure he does not have underlying restrictive or obstructive lung disease before the insurance company will cover him. The patient has a 55-pack-year history of smoking. Laboratory testing reveals an arterial carbon dioxide pressure of 40 mm Hg and his expired carbon dioxide pressure is 30 mm Hg. His physiologic dead space is determined to be 0.125 L. What is the patient's tidal volume?

(A) 0.01 L

(B) 0.05 L

(C) 0.1 L

(D) 0.5 L

(E) 1 L

(F) 5 L

HIGH-YIELD SYSTEMS

Respiratory

1. **The correct answer is B.** An overdose of theophylline will cause a decrease in the hydrolysis of cAMP to adenosine monophosphate, resulting in an increasing and potentially toxic level of cAMP. β-Agonists activate adenylate cyclase, which converts ATP to cAMP, so β-blockers may be given to stop this process and reduce cAMP levels.

Answer A is incorrect. Albuterol would potentiate the effects of theophylline by increasing cAMP.

Answer C is incorrect. Digoxin inhibits the Na^+-K^+-ATPase pump. It is used to increase myocardial contractility in patients with congestive heart failure. It is unrelated to theophylline overdose.

Answer D is incorrect. Epinephrine would potentiate the effects of theophylline by increasing cAMP.

Answer E is incorrect. Furosemide, a diuretic, is unrelated to theophylline overdose. It works by inhibiting the Na^+-K^+-$2Cl^-$ cotransport system of the thick ascending loop of Henle.

2. **The correct answer is A.** A tumor at the apex of the lung, or superior sulcus, is known as a Pancoast's tumor. Due to its location, it can sometimes compress the cervical sympathetic plexus, resulting in Horner's syndrome (ptosis, miosis, enophthalmos, and anhidrosis), as seen in this patient.

Answer B is incorrect. Graves' disease, an autoimmune reaction involving antibodies that stimulate the thyroid-stimulating hormone receptor, often presents with unilateral exophthalmos, which may appear similar to ptosis. However, miosis and anhidrosis are not associated with Graves' disease.

Answer C is incorrect. Myasthenia gravis, an autoimmune process involving the production of antibodies to the acetylcholine receptor, is associated with lung cancer and often presents with ptosis, but not with miosis or anhidrosis.

Answer D is incorrect. A paraneoplastic endocrine syndrome would be a lung carcinoma that secretes products similar to ACTH, ADH, or parathyroid hormone (PTH). These would cause Cushing's syndrome, the syndrome of inappropriate ADH secretion, or hypercalcemia, respectively, but not the symptoms this patient is experiencing.

Answer E is incorrect. Superior vena cava syndrome results when a tumor compresses the superior vena cava. Clinically one would see facial swelling, cyanosis, and dilation of the veins of the head, neck, and upper extremities, not eyelid droop and hemianhidrosis.

3. **The correct answer is B.** Gentamicin is an aminoglycoside antibiotic used in the treatment of gram-negative rod infections. It is often combined with β-lactam antibiotics because it acts synergistically. Aminoglycosides can cause nephrotoxicity and nonoliguric acute tubular necrosis, or ototoxicity, which can present as either vestibular or cochlear damage. Vestibular toxicity may result in vertigo, nausea, vomiting, or ataxia, whereas cochlear damage causes tinnitus or hearing loss. The patient in this question is experiencing vertigo.

Answer A is incorrect. Erythromycin is a macrolide antibiotic used to treat atypical pneumonias and upper respiratory infections caused by *Legionella*, *Chlamydia*, *Mycoplasma*, and *Neisseria* species. Erythromycin toxicity causes gastrointestinal discomfort, acute cholestatic hepatitis, eosinophilia, and skin rash.

Answer C is incorrect. Imipenem is a β-lactamase-resistant agent that has a wide spectrum of activity. It is not effective for treating methicillin-resistant *Staphylococcus aureus*, vancomycin-resistant enterococcus, or some strains of *Pseudomonas* species infections. Adverse effects of imipenem include gastrointestinal distress and seizures.

Answer D is incorrect. Metronidazole is a nitroimidazole antibiotic that has antibacterial activity against anaerobes and antiprotozoal activity. Toxicity can cause nausea, diarrhea, stomatitis, peripheral neuropathy, and disulfiram-like effects.

Answer E is incorrect. Piperacillin-tazobactam is used to treat *Pseudomonas* species infections, resistant *Staphylococcus aureus* infections, and many gram-negative infections. Adverse reactions include hypersensitivity reactions and diarrhea.

4. **The correct answer is E.** This man likely has actinomycosis from infection with *Actinomyces israelii*, a gram-positive anaerobic bacterium with a branching filamentous appearance. The image shows what is known as a "sulfur granule" formed by a colony of *Actinomyces* filaments solidified with tissue exudates. The bacteria are generally normal inhabitants of the oral cavity and are found in dental caries. Poor oral hygiene coupled with trauma increases the risk of aspiration of the organism leading to infection. Infections with *Actinomyces* tend to be chronic and extend through multiple tissue planes. *Actinomyces* species appear to be susceptible to a wide range of β-lactam agents, which are regarded as agents of first choice in treatment.

Answer A is incorrect. Amphotericin B is an antifungal agent believed to interact with membrane sterols to produce an aggregate that forms a transmembrane channel. It would not be appropriate treatment of actinomycosis.

Answer B is incorrect. Ciprofloxacin is a fluoroquinolone drug and generally has little effect on *Actinomyces*. β-Lactam agents are first-line treatment.

Answer C is incorrect. Although *Actinomyces* exhibit some features typical of fungus, such as branching mycelia formation, they are gram-positive bacteria. They lack nuclear membranes and mitochondria, and have cell walls characteristic of bacteria. In addition, they reproduce by bacterial fission rather than sporogenic or filamentous budding. Fluconazole is an antifungal agent that inhibits the enzyme 14 α-demethylase, preventing the conversion of lanosterol to ergosterol. It would not be appropriate treatment for a bacterial infection.

Answer D is incorrect. Isoniazid is a first-line medication used in the prevention and treatment of tuberculosis, along with rifampicin, pyrazinamide, and ethambutol. The image shows a sulfur granule, not a caseating granuloma, bordered by giant multinucleated cells.

5. **The correct answer is D.** Her symptoms of tachycardia and sharp chest pain make it most likely that the patient has developed a pulmonary embolism secondary to being restrained for several days. The best treatment for this would be an anticoagulant.

Answer A is incorrect. Extrapyramidal adverse effects are usually the complications seen with typical antipsychotic agents. These include acute dystonia (in the first several hours after starting dosing), akinesia (in the first several days), akathisia (in the first several weeks), and tardive dyskinesia (after several months). Neuroleptic malignant syndrome is an emergency that can result with this class of medications. However, this condition presents with elevated blood pressure and temperature and not with chest pain.

Answer B is incorrect. A β-blocker would be a good choice if she were having a myocardial infarction (MI). However, her main risk factor is that she was restrained for several days, which makes it more likely that she has suffered a pulmonary embolism (PE). Also, right-sided chest pain is less common (although not unheard of) with a MI.

Answer C is incorrect. Pneumonia can present with pleuritic chest pain and shortness of breath. However, the onset is usually more gradual and is accompanied by constitutional symptoms (i.e., fever and chills). Furthermore, this patient does not have any specific risk factors to develop pneumonia, whereas the restraints put her at risk for developing a PE.

Answer E is incorrect. A PE can be life-threatening, and treatment should be started as soon as possible.

6. **The correct answer is B.** *Mycoplasma pneumoniae* is the most common cause of interstitial (atypical) pneumonia, along with viruses. It cannot be cultured and is diagnosed by the cold agglutinin test, which measures the agglutination of immunoglobulins when they are cooled.

Answer A is incorrect. The acid-fast stain is used to diagnose mycobacterial illness, specifically *Mycobacterium tuberculosis*.

Answer C is incorrect. Gram stains are used to visualize gram-positive or gram-negative bacteria. *Mycoplasma* will not be visualized on a Gram stain.

Answer D is incorrect. The India ink stain can be used to visualize mucoid encapsulated yeasts such as *Cryptococcus*.

Answer E is incorrect. Polymerase chain reaction can be used to diagnose viral illnesses, such as HIV.

7. **The correct answer is D.** The patient presents as a classic "pink puffer," making emphysema the most likely diagnosis. Because smoking is closely linked to centriacinar emphysema, this is the best answer choice. The stem mentions an absence of jaundice and liver problems, making α_1-antitrypsin deficiency, and the associated panacinar emphysema, unlikely.

Answer A is incorrect. α_1-Antitrypsin deficiency usually presents with emphysema and liver cirrhosis (jaundice).

Answer B is incorrect. Asthma would present with wheezing after exposure to a trigger. However, asthma is reversible most of the time, and would not produce a barrel chest or pursed lips.

Answer C is incorrect. Bronchiectasis is permanent abnormal bronchial dilation caused by chronic infection. This is characterized by copious purulent sputum.

Answer E is incorrect. Patients with chronic bronchitis are often called "blue bloaters." To be diagnosed with chronic bronchitis, a patient must have a productive cough for at least 3 consecutive months for at least 2 years.

Answer F is incorrect. Panacinar emphysema is a result of α_1-antitrypsin deficiency.

8. **The correct answer is E.** Aspirin serves to inhibit the cyclooxygenase enzymes. An allergy to aspirin is thought to result from the diversion of arachidonic acid to the leukotriene pathway when the cyclooxygenase-catalyzed prostaglandin pathway is blocked. The resulting increase in leukotriene synthesis leads to the bronchoconstriction that is typical of an aspirin allergy. Zileuton is an effective inhibitor of the 5-lipoxygenase pathway and thus blocks the conversion of arachidonic acid to leukotrienes. Because of this, zileuton can be used in the treatment of aspirin allergy.

Answer A is incorrect. Cromolyn may be used as prophylactic treatment for aspirin allergy because it inhibits the release of inflammatory mediators from mast cells. However, it cannot be used to treat active aspirin allergy because the mast cell mediators have already been released.

Answer B is incorrect. Dopamine, which is used in shock and heart failure, is not used for aspirin allergy.

Answer C is incorrect. Methylxanthines such as theophylline are not effective in treating aspirin allergy because they affect the phosphodiesterase pathway rather than the leukotriene pathway.

Answer D is incorrect. Prednisone is not effective in treating aspirin allergy.

9. **The correct answer is A.** Although cigarette smoking is the most common cause of chronic bronchitis, air pollution is also associated with this diagnosis.

Answer B is incorrect. Alcohol intake is not directly associated with chronic bronchitis.

Answer C is incorrect. A cold climate is not associated with chronic bronchitis.

Answer D is incorrect. Hypertension is not associated with chronic bronchitis.

Answer E is incorrect. Intravenous drug abuse is not associated with chronic bronchitis.

Answer F is incorrect. Seasonal allergies are not associated with chronic bronchitis.

10. **The correct answer is D.** The right main bronchus is more vertical and wider than the left, and aspirated particles are more likely to lodge at the junction of the right inferior and right middle bronchi. Because of this, aspiration pneumonia contracted when an individual is in an upright position is most common in the right lower and middle lobes.

Answer A is incorrect. The left main bronchus is narrower and less vertical than the right main bronchus. The right main bronchus is more vertical and wider than the left, and aspirated particles are more likely to lodge at the junction of the right inferior and right middle bronchi.

Answer B is incorrect. The left main bronchus is narrower and less vertical than the right main bronchus. The right main bronchus is more vertical and wider than the left, and aspirated particles are more likely to lodge at the junction of the right inferior and right middle bronchi.

Answer C is incorrect. The lingula is in the left lung, and the left main bronchus is narrower and less vertical than the right main bronchus. The right main bronchus is more vertical and wider than the left, and aspirated particles are more likely to lodge at the junction of the right inferior and right middle bronchi.

Answer E is incorrect. When a person is supine, aspiration pneumonia may affect the upper lobes and posterior segments of the lungs, since they become the gravity-dependent regions when a person lies flat.

11. **The correct answer is E.** Nonselective β-blockers are contraindicated in patients with lung disease because they can cause bronchoconstriction by blocking the β_2 receptors responsible for relaxation of bronchial smooth muscle. β_2 Agonists are a mainstay of asthma therapy. Acebutolol, atenolol, esmolol, metoprolol, and betaxolol are all cardioselective β_1-blockers that could be used in a patient with lung/ airway disease. Nadolol is a nonselective β-blocker and should **not** be used in a patient with lung disease. Other nonselective β-blockers include timolol and pindolol.

Answer A is incorrect. Acebutolol is cardioselective and can be used in patients with asthma or other obstructive lung diseases.

Answer B is incorrect. Atenolol is cardioselective and can be used in patients with asthma or other obstructive lung diseases.

Answer C is incorrect. Esmolol is cardioselective and can be used in patients with asthma or other obstructive lung diseases.

Answer D is incorrect. Metoprolol is cardioselective and can be used in patients with asthma or other obstructive lung diseases

12. **The correct answer is D.** In perfusion-limited exchange, gas equilibrates early along the length of the pulmonary capillary, so gas exchange can only increase or decrease with increased or decreased blood flow, respectively.

Answer A is incorrect. Diffusion-limited exchange is illustrated by CO and O_2 during strenuous exercise.

Answer B is incorrect. Diffusion-limited exchange is illustrated in disease states such as fibrosis and emphysema, because the diseased lung interstitium causes difficulty in gas diffusion even if blood is flowing to the region at a maximal rate.

Answer C is incorrect. Perfusion-limited exchange is increased only if blood flow increases, and it decreases when blood flow decreases.

Answer E is incorrect. Perfusion-limited exchange is illustrated by N_2O and CO_2 under normal conditions, along with O_2 under normal conditions.

Answer F is incorrect. The partial pressure of the gas in the pulmonary capillary blood becomes equal to the partial pressure in the alveolar air. It is maintained in diffusion-limited exchange.

13. **The correct answer is D.** Small to moderate pleural effusions can present without tracheal deviation, decreased breath sounds over the effusion, dullness to percussion, and decreased tactile fremitus.

Answer A is incorrect. Bronchial obstruction would present with absent breath sounds over the area, decreased resonance, decreased tactile fremitus, and tracheal deviation toward the side of the lesion.

Answer B is incorrect. Intestines can appear in the thoracic cavity if there is a diaphragmatic hernia. There would be no breath sounds at all, and the patient could have tracheal deviation.

Answer C is incorrect. Lobar pneumonia may have bronchial breath sounds over the lesion, dullness to percussion, increased tactile fremitus, and no tracheal deviation.

Answer E is incorrect. Pneumothorax presents with decreased breath sounds, hyperresonant lungs to percussion, absent tactile fremitus, and tracheal deviation away from the side of the lesion.

14. **The correct answer is D.** The letter *E* in the image points to pseudostratified ciliated columnar epithelium, *LP* refers to the lamina propria, and *C* refers to hyaline cartilage. In smokers, pseudostratified ciliated columnar epithelium lining the bronchi can undergo metaplasia and transform into stratified squamous epithelium. Stratified squamous epithelium is classified by the flattened shape of the cells in the surface layer. Examples of tissues with stratified squamous epithelium include the skin, mouth, anus, vagina, and esophagus.

Answer A is incorrect. Pseudostratified columnar epithelium is the normal respiratory epithelium on the right that is undergoing metaplasia. This type of epithelium only appears stratified; however, all cells are in contact with basal lamina and only some cells reach the surface of epithelium.

Answer B is incorrect. Simple squamous epithelium lines alveoli, loops of Henle, and en-

dothelial linings of blood vessels. Simple epithelium indicates that the epithelial membrane is composed of a single layer of cells. Under the microscope, simple squamous epithelium is characterized by a single sheet of flattened cells lying on a basal lamina. It does not play a role in this case.

Answer C is incorrect. Stratified columnar epithelium is found in only a few places in the body, namely, the conjunctivae of the eye and regions of the male urethra. It is composed of a low polyhedral to cuboidal deeper layer in contact with the basal lamina along with a superficial layer of columnar cells.

Answer E is incorrect. The bladder is lined by transitional epithelium, not the lung. Transitional epithelium is characterized by several layers of cuboidal cells, with the surface layer being large and dome-shaped.

15. **The correct answer is D.** Neonates have high concentrations of fetal hemoglobin in their blood. Fetal hemoglobin has a higher affinity for oxygen than adult hemoglobin (to allow fetuses to extract oxygen from mother's blood), therefore fetal oxygen-hemoglobin dissociation curves are left-shifted. Other physiologic conditions that cause left shifts in the curve include increased pH (or reduced H^+ concentration), decreased temperature, 2,3-diphosphoglycerate levels, and arterial carbon dioxide pressure.

Answer A is incorrect. High altitude causes a shift in the curve to the right, reducing the affinity of RBCs for oxygen, thereby allowing them to deliver more oxygen to tissues.

Answer B is incorrect. An increase in 2,3-diphosphoglycerate binds to deoxygenated hemoglobin in RBCs, allosterically upregulating the ability of RBCs to release oxygen. Because it reduces RBC affinity for oxygen, it right-shifts the oxygen-hemoglobin dissociation curve.

Answer C is incorrect. An increase in the partial pressure of carbon dioxide in the blood right-shift the curve, allowing increased delivery of oxygen to tissues because of decreased affinity for oxygen by RBCs.

Answer E is incorrect. Increased temperature is an indicator of metabolic activity (and therefore increased oxygen demand). At high temperatures, the curve shifts to the right, indicating a decreased affinity for oxygen by RBCs.

16. **The correct answer is A.** This patient has sarcoidosis involving the lungs and skin. Sarcoidosis is characterized by noncaseating granulomas, and hilar lymphadenopathy is one of the most common findings in this condition. Skin involvement occurs in approximately 25% of patients. Angiotensin-converting enzyme levels are elevated in sarcoidosis due to its overproduction by immune cells comprising the granulomas.

Answer B is incorrect. Elevated cardiac enzyme levels may be detected in rare cases of heart involvement in sarcoidosis, but this is not the best answer.

Answer C is incorrect. Serum amylase levels are elevated in conditions such as pancreatitis and are not associated with sarcoidosis.

Answer D is incorrect. Hypercalcemia often occurs in sarcoidosis, but not hypocalcemia. Infiltrating macrophages produce excess $1,25(OH)_2$ vitamin D, which is normally produced primarily in the kidney. $1,25(OH)_2$ vitamin D is the most biologically active metabolite of vitamin D, leading to elevated blood levels of calcium.

Answer E is incorrect. Hypouricemia is not associated with sarcoidosis. Hyperuricemia is often associated with gout, which can cause subcutaneous nodules, but does not cause dyspnea.

17. **The correct answer is C.** Cystic fibrosis (CF) is an autosomal recessive disease that most commonly occurs in the white population. It is usually caused by a mutation in the CF transmembrane conductance regulator (CFTR) protein, a protein that functions as a Cl^- channel and is regulated by cAMP. The delta F508 mutation is the most common gene abnormality associated with the disease; it involves the deletion of three base pairs from the gene and the consequent loss of a phenylalanine from the protein. Because three base pairs are deleted, there is no frameshift. Dysfunction of this channel causes abnormal chloride conductance with associated water transport abnormalities, leading to viscous secretions in exocrine glands. Failure to clear secretions in the respiratory tract, pancreas, sweat glands, and other exocrine tissues results in recurrent pneumonias, exocrine pancreatic insufficiency, abnormal sweat gland function, urogenital dysfunction, and, ultimately, failure to thrive.

Answer A is incorrect. Bicarbonate transporters are not affected in CF.

Answer B is incorrect. Calcium transporters are not affected in CF.

Answer D is incorrect. Potassium transporters are not affected in CF.

Answer E is incorrect. Sodium transporters are not affected in CF.

18. **The correct answer is B.** This response is an example of a type I hypersensitivity reaction. In these reactions, an allergen cross-links antigen-specific IgE on the surface of mast cells and basophils. Subsequently, the mast cells and basophils release vasoactive amines. Since antibodies are preformed in this type of hypersensitivity, the reaction develops quite rapidly.

Answer A is incorrect. Antigen-antibody complexes activate complement in a type III hypersensitivity reaction. This reaction would not present with sneezing and a runny nose but rather with local inflammation.

Answer C is incorrect. IgM and IgG binding occurs in a type II hypersensitivity reaction, which leads to a cytotoxic response to the allergen in the serum. This reaction would not present with sneezing and a runny nose, but rather with local inflammation.

Answer D is incorrect. In type IV hypersensitivity, or delayed-type hypersensitivity, one sees sensitized T lymphocytes releasing cytokines. This reaction would not present with sneezing and a runny nose but rather with local inflammation such as that associated with contact dermatitis from poison ivy. In addition, the clinical response occurs several days after antigen exposure.

Answer E is incorrect. Serum sickness is a type III hypersensitivity reaction in which antibodies to foreign proteins are formed. It presents a few days after an immunologic insult with urticaria, fever, arthralgia, and proteinuria.

19. **The correct answer is B.** The Hering-Breuer reflex prevents lung tissue damage during active, rapid breathing. The smooth muscle of the tracheobronchial tree contains slowly adapting pulmonary stretch receptors that become active during heavy breathing, but have no effect during rest. The discharge frequency decreases when the lungs have maximally expanded and increases when the lungs are deflated (when the reflex is activated).

Answer A is incorrect. Blood flow does not affect stretch receptor activation.

Answer C is incorrect. Blood flow does not affect stretch receptor activation.

Answer D is incorrect. Stretch receptor activation would decrease, not increase, during maximal lung expansion.

Answer E is incorrect. If the discharge frequency of the stretch receptors remained constant during heavy breathing, the lack of negative feedback would lead to lung damage.

20. **The correct answer is D.** The disease described in this vignette is diphtheria, which is caused by the gram-positive rod *Corynebacterium diphtheriae*. Diphtheria classically presents with a grayish-white pseudomembrane on the pharynx or tonsils. Underlying tissue of the throat and neck becomes edematous, and lymphadenopathy develops. Fever is usually mild or absent. It is seen very rarely in vaccinated populations but is endemic to certain parts of the world. Culture of *C. diphtheriae* requires tellurite to prevent growth of normal upper respiratory tract flora.

Answer A is incorrect. Bordet-Gengou agar is used to culture *Bordetella pertussis*. Pertussis presents with paroxysmal coughing spells and whooping sounds on inspiration.

Answer B is incorrect. Chocolate agar is used to grow *Haemophilus influenzae*. Encapsulated strains of *H. influenzae* cause invasive diseases such as septicemia, meningitis, cellulitis, septic arthritis, epiglottitis, and pneumonia. Nonencapsulated strains are likely to cause otitis media, conjunctivitis, bronchitis, and sinusitis.

Answer C is incorrect. Sabouraud's agar is used to grow fungi.

Answer E is incorrect. Thayer-Martin agar is a chocolate agar plate which has VCN antibiotics (vancomycin, colistin, and nystatin) that suppress the growth of endogenous flora while supporting *Neisseria gonorrhoeae* growth. This patient does not have symptoms of gonorrhea.

21. **The correct answer is A.** Ethambutol is active only against *Mycobacterium tuberculosis*, and it is among the first-line agents used to treat tuberculosis (TB) infection (others are isoniazid, rifampin, and pyrazinamide). Ethambutol's mechanism of action appears to be the inhibition of polymerization of cell wall precursors. Although the drug is generally well tolerated, its most common adverse effects involve ocular toxicity such as the kind described in this question, which usually appears several months after the initiation of treatment. Ethambutol is usually used in an anti-TB regimen with rifampin for patients who either cannot tolerate isoniazid or are infected with isoniazid-resistant *M. tuberculosis*.

Answer B is incorrect. Although rifampin is considered the best antituberculous agent, isoniazid is used for prophylaxis in asymptomatic patients with a positive purified protein derivative (PPD) test. A 6-month course of isoniazid prevents active TB in 90% of patients for at least 20 years. Isoniazid blocks mycolic acid cell wall synthesis and is bactericidal for rapidly multiplying organisms. Major adverse effects include hepatotoxicity and peripheral neuropathy, but many other adverse effects occur, such as lupus-like syndrome and optic atrophy.

Answer C is incorrect. Like isoniazid, the spectrum of action of pyrazinamide is limited to *Mycobacterium tuberculosis*. The site of activity for pyrazinamide is thought to be a fatty acid synthase gene. The major adverse effect of pyrazinamide therapy is hepatotoxicity, but it is rare at recommended dosages. Another major adverse effect is hyperuricemia and subsequent gout.

Answer D is incorrect. Rifampin is the most potent antituberculous agent available. Rifampin blocks DNA-dependent RNA polymerase, preventing RNA synthesis. Although it is a better agent than isoniazid for preventing active tuberculosis infection, it has a significant risk of liver toxicity that outweighs its benefits as a preventive medicine.

Answer E is incorrect. *Mycobacterium tuberculosis* can have extrapulmonary manifestations, but the eye is not commonly involved. Miliary TB infection can affect the eye and cause chorioretinitis, uveitis, and conjunctivitis, but these manifestations are rare. Color blindness would not be associated with such an infection.

22. **The correct answer is C.** This patient most likely has type 1 diabetes mellitus and a resulting ketoacidosis. He has a metabolic acidosis with a large anion gap (>10 mEq) as calculated by the following formula: Anion gap = Na^+ − [HCO_3^- + Cl^-]. This leads to respiratory compensation by deep respiration (Kussmaul's respiration), resulting in a decrease in blood partial pressure of carbon dioxide. The large anion gap is due to the overproduction of ketones in the absence of insulin production.

Answer A is incorrect. Calcium oxalate crystals may be seen in ethylene glycol poisoning, which can be another cause of metabolic acidosis with an increased anion gap.

Answer B is incorrect. This case of metabolic acidosis involves an increased anion gap. Normal-gap acidosis is caused by renal loss of bicarbonate due to tubular dysfunction (caused by drug toxicity, systemic lupus erythematous) or gastrointestinal loss of bicarbonate through vomiting or diarrhea.

Answer D is incorrect. In metabolic acidosis, respiratory compensation occurs and reduces blood partial pressure of carbon dioxide through deep respiration. Elevated blood partial pressure of carbon dioxide is seen in patients with metabolic alkalosis with respiratory compensation or respiratory acidosis.

Answer E is incorrect. Hyperkalemia, not hypokalemia, is associated with diabetic ketoacidosis.

23. **The correct answer is B.** To answer this question, one must remember that the collapsing pressure (the pressure required to keep an alveolus open) is directly related to surface tension and inversely related to the radius of alveoli. This is described by LaPlace's law, where pressure equals 2 times the surface tension divided by the radius (P = 2T / r). Thus, a larger alveolus will require more pressure to collapse. Surfactant, a substance produced by type II alveolar cells that contains mainly phospholipids and apoproteins, coats alveoli and small airways and serves to reduce surface tension over the air-water interface.

Answer A is incorrect. Surfactant decreases surface tension, which increases compliance.

Answer C is incorrect. From LaPlace's law, increasing the surface tension increases the pressure required to keep alveoli open. This results in decreased pressure required to collapse the alveoli.

Answer D is incorrect. Small alveoli without surfactant have the greatest chance of collapsing.

Answer E is incorrect. From LaPlace's law, small alveoli are more likely to collapse, so they have decreased compliance compared to larger alveoli.

24. **The correct answer is A.** High fever, dysphagia, drooling, inspiratory stridor, and respiratory distress are all consistent with the diagnosis of epiglottitis. The x-ray film shows thickening of the epiglottic (thumbprint sign) and aryepiglottic folds. The most common etiologic agent associated with epiglottitis is *Haemophilus influenzae*.

Answer B is incorrect. *Mycoplasma pneumoniae* causes atypical pneumonia that presents with cough and shortness of breath, and bilateral diffuse infiltrates are visible on an x-ray film. This patient's symptoms and x-ray findings are not consistent with this disease.

Answer C is incorrect. Parainfluenza virus is associated with croup. This disease can present with inspiratory stridor, seal-like barking cough, retractions, and coryza. The x-ray film in this case would show a characteristic steeple sign.

Answer D is incorrect. Respiratory syncytial virus is an etiologic agent of bronchiolitis that is characterized by gradually developing respiratory distress and paroxysmal wheezing.

Answer E is incorrect. *Streptococcus pyogenes* (group A) can cause pharyngitis. Patients with this illness present with headache, abdominal pain, and vomiting. The patient's symptoms are not consistent with this diagnosis.

25. **The correct answer is C.** This boy suffers from asthma, which is characterized by airway hyperresponsiveness and airflow obstruction. This condition can be precipitated by several factors, including allergens, upper respiratory infections, drugs, and stress. Clinically, asthmatics experience episodes of wheezing, coughing, and dyspnea. Sputum samples may demonstrate Curschmann's spirals and Charcot-Leyden crystals. Blood tests will typically reveal eosinophilia. Other causes of eosinophilia include neoplasms, parasites, collagen vascular diseases, and allergic processes. Asthma is thought to be driven by hyperresponsive T lymphocytes in the lung, producing Th_2-type cytokines IL-4, IL-5, and IL-13.

Answer A is incorrect. Interferon-γ is the signature Th_1 cytokine. It is involved in tuberculous granuloma formation and priming macrophages to eliminate intracellular pathogens.

Answer B is incorrect. IL-2 is a T lymphocyte-derived autocrine T cell growth factor. Recombinant IL-2 is used to promote antitumor immunity in end-stage melanoma.

Answer D is incorrect. Tumor necrosis factor-α (TNF-α) is a central cytokine involved in inflammation. Biological therapy targeted at TNF-α is used to treat autoimmune diseases such as rheumatoid arthritis, ankylosing spondylitis, psoriasis and psoriatic arthritis, Crohn's disease, and ulcerative colitis.

Answer E is incorrect. Tumor growth factor-β is a pleiotropic cytokine involved in, among other things, promoting tissue fibrosis. It is thought that excessive levels in the skin are involved in the pathogenesis of systemic sclerosis.

26. **The correct answer is E.** The patient is suffering from the syndrome of inappropriate ADH secretion (SIADH), a condition in which excessive ADH is secreted independent of serum osmolality; this can be seen in pulmonary diseases such as TB. SIADH is caused by central nervous system disturbances, such as strokes; certain drugs, such as cyclophosphamide; and ectopic secretion by certain carcinomas, such as small cell lung carcinoma, as a part of a paraneoplastic syndrome. Excessive ADH secretion can lead to nausea, lethargy, seizures, and even coma. The patient's laboratory values are typical of someone with SIADH, showing hyponatremia, serum hypo-osmolality, urine hyperosmolarity, and decreased hematocrit secondary to dilution.

Answer A is incorrect. In central diabetes insipidus (DI), there is deficient secretion of ADH by the posterior pituitary, resulting in a clinical picture opposite from SIADH. Patients with central DI present with large quantities of dilute urine, serum hyperosmolality, and hypernatremia, and will report polydipsia and polyuria. Central DI can be caused by posterior pituitary tumors, meningitis, sarcoid and skull-based trauma or surgery, and can be corrected with administration of exogenous ADH.

Answer B is incorrect. Hyponatremia and glucose abnormalities can be found following epileptic seizures; however, the presence of serum hypoosmolality, urine hyperosmolality, and decreased hematocrit secondary to dilution would be unlikely if epilepsy were the diagnosis.

Answer C is incorrect. The signs and symptoms of nephrogenic DI are similar to those of central DI; however, unlike central DI, nephrogenic DI cannot be corrected with exogenous ADH because it results from ADH receptor dysfunction at the kidneys. Nephrogenic DI is a potential adverse effect of demeclocycline and lithium.

Answer D is incorrect. Although patients with psychogenic polydipsia drink excessive amounts of fluid and may present with decreased serum osmolality, they will have appropriate ADH suppression and will thus have a large volume of hypotonic, not hypertonic urine, as seen in this patient.

27. **The correct answer is C.** The patient's penetrating chest wound opened her intrapleural space to the atmosphere. Therefore, as she attempts to inhale, her thoracic cavity expands but air enters through the wound, equalizing the pressure; this prevents the normal expansion of the lungs.

Answer A is incorrect. Intrapleural pressure greater than atmospheric pressure could occur with a pleural effusion, but with a penetrating injury allowing communication between the intrapleural space and the atmosphere it is unlikely in this case.

Answer B is incorrect. Intrapleural pressure should be less than atmospheric pressure during inspiration, allowing air entry.

Answer D is incorrect. Pain with inspiration is a frequent complication of traumatic injury. While it may decrease the tidal volume, it would also increase breathing frequency, resulting in an oxygen saturation closer to normal.

Answer E is incorrect. The elastic properties of the chest wall would tend to spring out, but the negative intrapleural pressure normally created during inspiration opposes this tendency. After the penetrating injury equalized the pressure of the intrapleural space and the atmosphere, the chest wall will spring out, not pull inward.

28. **The correct answer is A.** The description is a typical presentation of coccidioidomycosis, which is endemic to the southwestern United States. This infection causes disseminated disease in immunocompromised patients and forms spherules in tissue. Infection is caused by inhalation of spores of the fungus, Coccidioides immitis. Dipicolinic acid is a key component of fungal spores, which provide the fungus with resistance to dehydration, heat, and chemicals.

Answer B is incorrect. Hemagglutinin is an influenza virus antigen.

Answer C is incorrect. Lipopolysaccharide is an antigen located in the cell wall of most gram-negative bacteria.

Answer D is incorrect. Encapsulated bacteria and yeast have capsules made of polysaccharide; one exception is *Bacillus anthracis*, whose capsule contains D-glutamate.

Answer E is incorrect. Teichoic acid is a bacterial surface antigen that induces tumor necrosis factor-α and interleukin-1.

29. **The correct answer is G.** Working in a shipyard is associated with asbestos exposure. Chronic inhalation of asbestos fibers can result in asbestosis, which is marked histologically by ferruginous bodies that stain positively with Prussian blue. Asbestosis, unlike most other pneumoconioses, results in marked predisposition to bronchogenic carcinoma and to malignant mesothelioma. Smoking and asbestos exposure together greatly increase one's risk of developing bronchogenic carcinoma.

Answer A is incorrect. Asbestosis is not related to an autoimmune phenomenon.

Answer B is incorrect. The cause of asbestosis is the inhalation of asbestos fibers into the lungs. Idiopathic restrictive lung diseases include sarcoidosis and idiopathic pulmonary fibrosis.

Answer C is incorrect. Living in an urban area for years can cause anthracosis, which is a result of inhalation of carbon dust. It is characterized histologically by carbon-carrying macrophages and results in irregular black patches visible on gross inspection. Anthracosis is harmless.

Answer D is incorrect. Ferruginous bodies and ivory-white pleural plaques are not long-term sequelae of steroid abuse.

Answer E is incorrect. Tuberculosis has Ghon's complexes in primary infection. Cavitary lesions are present in secondary reactivation.

Answer F is incorrect. Working in a coal mine can cause "coal workers' pneumoconiosis" or silicosis. It involves inhalation of coal dust, which contains both carbon and silica. It is marked histologically by macrophages containing coal dust particles located around the bronchioles.

30. **The correct answer is C.** This man is likely suffering from obstructive sleep apnea (OSA) secondary to extreme obesity (pickwickian syndrome). During the night he has intermittent cessation of airflow at the nose and mouth. During this progressive asphyxia, he has a brief arousal, restores airway patency, and returns to sleep. This patient's obesity and elongated uvula are very good indicators of OSA, as are his daytime sleepiness, inability to concentrate, and hypertension. Periodic, recurrent asphyxia has the effect of causing a respiratory acidosis that, when present chronically, is compensated for by renal retention of HCO_3^-.

Answer A is incorrect. If anything, this patient's glucose is likely elevated.

Answer B is incorrect. This patient likely has a decreased HDL level.

Answer D is incorrect. Renal secretion of HCO_3^- would worsen acidosis.

Answer E is incorrect. Increased reabsorption of H^+ would worsen acidosis.

31. **The correct answer is A.** *Actinomyces israelii* is a microaerophilic organism that causes oral and facial abscesses, with characteristic "sulfur granules" that may drain through sinus tracts in skin.

Answer B is incorrect. *Actinomyces'* long branched filaments can resemble fungi, such as *Candida albicans*. The oral lesions caused by *Candida*, known as thrush, usually occur on the mucous membranes such as the throat and tongue in immunocompromised patients and appear white. It would be an unlikely cause of an oral abscess in a patient with a healthy immune system.

Answer C is incorrect. *Clostridium perfringens* is also a gram-positive anaerobic rod; however, it typically causes food poisoning from meat dishes or myonecrosis (gas gangrene), not dental abscesses.

Answer D is incorrect. Like *Actinomyces*, *Nocardia* is a filamentous, beaded, gram-positive bacterium. Unlike *Actinomyces*, *Nocardia* is not considered normal flora. It causes pulmonary infections in immunocompromised patients.

Answer E is incorrect. *Staphylococcus epidermidis* is a gram-positive clustering coccus, not a rod. It is part of the normal skin flora and usually pathologic only in immunocompromised patients.

32. **The correct answer is C.** Peripheral, not central, chemoreceptors stimulate breathing in response to oxygen levels <60 mm Hg.

Answer A is incorrect. Central chemoreceptors do affect breathing with varying levels of H^+ in the blood, but they do not directly detect levels of H^+ in the blood. The H^+ in blood cannot cross the blood-brain barrier. Thus, CO_2 in the blood crosses the cerebrospinal fluid and combines with H_2O to form H^+ and HCO_3^-. The resulting H^+ acts directly on the receptors.

Answer B is incorrect. Central control is located in the brainstem and cerebral cortex. The most important structures include the medullary respiratory center located in the reticular formation, the apneustic center in the lower pons, the pneumotaxic center in the upper pons, and the cerebral cortex.

Answer D is incorrect. Stretch, irritant, and J (juxtacapillary) receptors all function within the lung to regulate breathing. Stretch receptors are located in the smooth muscle, irritant receptors are located in the airway epithelial cells, and the J receptors are located in the alveolar walls close to the capillaries.

Answer E is incorrect. The aortic and carotid bodies are not central chemoreceptors. They are the peripheral chemoreceptors that are able to respond to decreased partial pressure of oxygen in arterial blood.

33. **The correct answer is B.** The patient's presentation is most consistent with an atypical pneumonia likely caused by *Mycoplasma pneumoniae*. Macrolide antibiotics such as azithromycin are effective in treating this disease. *Mycoplasma* has no cell wall, so it is not sensitive to the penicillins or cephalosporins, which act by inhibiting cell wall synthesis.

Answer A is incorrect. *Mycoplasma* is not sensitive to ampicillin. Some cases of pneumococcal pneumonia are sensitive to and can be treated effectively with ampicillin.

Answer C is incorrect. Clindamycin is used in the treatment of anaerobic bacterial infections, not *Mycoplasma* infections.

Answer D is incorrect. All cephalosporins are ineffective against *Mycoplasma*.

Answer E is incorrect. *Mycoplasma* is not sensitive to penicillins. Some cases of pneumococcal pneumonia are sensitive to penicillin and can be treated effectively with this drug.

34. **The correct answer is G.** Pneumothorax typically presents as acute-onset pleuritic chest pain, often in otherwise young, healthy men. On physical exam, pneumothorax would present with an increasingly resonant chest cavity after collapse of the lung, decreased breath sounds secondary to decreased ventilation, and decreased fremitus secondary to less solid tissue transmitting vibration. On x-ray of the chest, the trachea would deviate away from the affected side. The other pathology that commonly presents with sudden pleuritic chest pain and shortness of breath is a PE, though this usually also presents with tachycardia.

Pneumonia can also present this way, but it is usually accompanied by constitutional symptoms (i.e., fever, chills).

Answer A is incorrect. Asbestosis presents with dyspnea and is associated with a history of exposure to asbestos, persistent bibasilar crackles, reduced lung volumes, and fibrosis on the radiograph.

Answer B is incorrect. Asthma is characterized by hyperreactivity of the airways and obstruction. It is a chronic illness, so one would not expect it to suddenly present in a previously healthy man. It also usually does not present with pleuritic chest pain.

Answer C is incorrect. Bronchiectasis is dilation of the bronchial tree secondary to mucus plugging. It does not present with pleuritic chest pain and it commonly seen in patients with a history of repeated lung infections (as in patients with cystic fibrosis).

Answer D is incorrect. Bronchitis presents with productive cough and an increased Reid index, not with pleuritic chest pain.

Answer E is incorrect. Emphysema typically is found in an older smoker who is barrel-chested. Also, there is no tracheal deviation.

Answer F is incorrect. Oat cell carcinoma would present in an older person with cough, hemoptysis, and possibly with a paraneoplastic endocrine syndrome.

35. **The correct answer is D.** Diffuse, patchy infiltrate is consistent with *Pneumocystis jiroveci* pneumonia, which is confirmed by methenamine silver stain of lavage or biopsy sample. The first-line treatment of this condition is trimethoprim-sulfamethoxazole for patients with no contraindications to sulfa drugs. In the case of a patient with a sulfa allergy, the first-line treatment is pentamidine.

Answer A is incorrect. Ivermectin is used to treat onchocerciasis (river blindness). It is thought to block the release of microfilariae from gravid female worms. One dose reduces microfilarial counts by up to 95%.

Answer B is incorrect. Metronidazole is used to treat a wide variety of anaerobic bacterial infections. It is also effective against parasitic infections such as *Giardia lamblia, Entamoeba histolytica, Gardnerella vaginalis,* and *Trichomonas vaginalis.*

Answer C is incorrect. Penicillin is used to treat a variety of bacterial infections but is not effective in the treatment of *Pneumocystis jiroveci* pneumonia.

Answer E is incorrect. Protamine is used to treat heparin overdose. It binds to heparin to form a stable complex that has no anticoagulant activity. Used alone, protamine has anticoagulant properties.

36. **The correct answer is D.** The patient's presentation is consistent with syndrome of inappropriate ADH secretion (low serum osmolality and sodium, with high urine osmolarity), which can be caused by the secretion of ADH from small cell carcinomas of the lung. This type of carcinoma is clearly associated with cigarette smoking.

    Answer A is incorrect. An aspirated foreign body can be associated with confusion if it is associated with a decreased gag reflex. However, it is unlikely to cause the electrolyte abnormalities seen in this patient.

    Answer B is incorrect. Brain cancer could cause the altered mental status, but would not be associated with the observed electrolyte abnormalities.

    Answer C is incorrect. Prostate cancer is most likely to metastasize to the bone, and is unlikely to cause the electrolyte abnormalities seen in this patient.

    Answer E is incorrect. TB would not cause the electrolyte abnormality seen in this patient.

37. **The correct answer is C.** *Legionella pneumophila* is a gram-negative rod that causes Legionnaires' disease, a condition in which patients develop pneumonia and a high fever. Other signs and symptoms include hyponatremia and central nervous system changes. The organism is present only in water sources (e.g., air-conditioning systems, whirlpools, mist sprayers) and can cause infection when aerosolized water droplets are inhaled. The organism is not transmitted by person-to-person contact.

    Answer A is incorrect. *Bordetella pertussis* is a gram-negative rod, but it causes an upper respiratory infection or whooping cough. It is transmitted by person-to-person contact, not through infected water sources.

    Answer B is incorrect. *Haemophilus influenzae* type B is a gram-negative rod, but it is more likely to be associated with acute epiglottitis or meningitis. It is an exclusively human pathogen that is transmitted by aerosolized droplets or direct contact with secretions. The Hib vaccine has rendered these infections far less common.

    Answer D is incorrect. *Mycobacterium tuberculosis* is an acid-fast mycobacterium that causes TB. It would not present this acutely, and the organism is not transmitted via water sources.

    Answer E is incorrect. *Streptococcus pneumoniae* is a significant cause of bacterial pneumonia, but it is a gram-positive cocci. It is transmitted by person-to-person contact.

38. **The correct answer is C.** Bronchiectasis can be caused by a chronic necrotizing infection of the bronchi leading to dilated airways. In addition to bronchopulmonary infections, bronchiectasis can be caused by bronchial obstructions or congenital abnormalities (bronchial cysts, tracheobroncial fistulas).

    Answer A is incorrect. Asthma is a condition associated with airway constriction, marked by wheezing.

    Answer B is incorrect. Atelectasis is alveolar collapse, not associated with airway dilation.

    Answer D is incorrect. Idiopathic pulmonary fibrosis causes restrictive lung disease and does not involve the major airways.

Answer E is incorrect. Neonatal respiratory distress syndrome is related to surfactant deficiency, causing alveolar collapse. Dilated airways are not a feature of the syndrome.

39. **The correct answer is F.** This child has measles complicated by pneumonia. Pneumonia complicates approximately 4% of measles cases in the United States and as many as 50% of cases abroad. Clinically, this child has a high fever, Koplik's spots, maculopapular rash, and CT of the chest showing diffuse interstitial involvement. Measles-infected respiratory cells will fuse and form multinucleated giant cells, which can be detected in sputum samples. Measles is a member of the Paramyxoviridae family, a group of negative-sense, single-stranded RNA viruses. In immunocompromised hosts, measles pneumonia may evolve to giant cell pneumonia, which is often fatal.

Answer A is incorrect. Acid-fast bacilli would be expected in the sputum of a child infected with mycobacteria such as *Mycobacterium tuberculosis*.

Answer B is incorrect. Cells with nuclei surrounded by a halo and clear cytoplasm are koilocytes and would be found in cells infected with human papillomavirus. This child has measles, which will form multinucleated giant cells.

Answer C is incorrect. Cowdry-type inclusions in cells is suggestive of infection with cytomegalovirus (CMV). Although CMV can cause pneumonia, it does so more commonly in immunocompromised hosts.

Answer D is incorrect. Gram-negative coccobacilli and polymorphonuclear leukocytes are commonly associated with *Haemophilus influenzae*, which is a common cause of pneumonia in children. However, this child is likely infected with measles.

Answer E is incorrect. Gram-positive diplococci and polymorphonuclear leukocytes are often seen in pneumococcal pneumonia, which would more likely present with a dense lobar pneumonia. This child has other signs and symptoms characteristic of measles.

40. **The correct answer is D.** The ultrasound reveals a congenital diaphragmatic hernia (CDH) in the fetus. The diaphragm is derived from four embryological structures: the septum transversum, the pleuroperitoneal folds, the dorsal mesentery of the esophagus, and a muscular outgrowth of the lateral body wall. The pleuroperitoneal folds form a large portion of the fetal diaphragm; if they fail to form completely, the thorax and the abdomen are incompletely separated posterolaterally and the abdominal contents often herniate into the thorax (known as a Bochdalek hernia). Pressure from abdominal organs results in lung hypoplasia. The polyhydramnios could result either from mechanical compression of the esophagus by the herniated viscera (most likely), and/or from the lung hypoplasia, as the lungs may offer a resorbtive surface for the recycling of amniotic fluid. Newborns with CDH typically have a flat stomach and a heart displaced to the right.

Answer A is incorrect. The dorsal mesentery of the esophagus forms the central part of the fetal diaphragm. Post-embryonically, this structure becomes the crura of the diaphragm. It is not normally defective in CDH.

Answer B is incorrect. Although the foregut is displaced from the abdomen into the thorax in the presence of a CDH, its formation is normal.

Answer C is incorrect. Muscular outgrowths of the lateral body wall form the lateral edge of the diaphragm, bordering the left and right costodiaphragmatic recesses. These structures are not commonly defective in CDH.

Answer E is incorrect. The septum transversum grows out from the ventrolateral body wall and separates the heart from the liver in the embryo. Ultimately, it gives rise to the central tendon of the diaphragm. However, defects in the septum transversum are rarely the cause of CDH.

HIGH-YIELD SYSTEMS

Respiratory

41. The correct answer is D. Choice D represents the residual volume, which is the volume that remains in the lungs after a maximal expiration.

Answer A is incorrect. Choice A represents the inspiratory reserve volume, which is the volume that can be inspired after inspiration of the tidal volume.

Answer B is incorrect. Choice B represents the tidal volume, which is the volume inspired or expired with each normal breath.

Answer C is incorrect. Choice C represents the expiratory reserve volume, which is the volume that can be expired after the expiration of the tidal volume.

Answer E is incorrect. Choice E represents the inspiratory capacity, which is the sum of tidal volume and inspiratory reserve volume.

Answer F is incorrect. Choice F represents the functional reserve capacity. It is the sum of the expiratory reserve volume and the residual volume, and it is the volume that remains in the lungs after a tidal volume is expired.

Answer G is incorrect. Choice G represents vital capacity, which is the sum of tidal volume, inspiratory reserve volume, and expiratory reserve volume. Vital capacity (also called forced vital capacity) is the volume of air that can be forcibly expired after a maximal inspiration.

42. The correct answer is B. Hyaline membrane disease (neonatal respiratory distress syndrome) is the most common cause of death in premature infants. It is associated with prematurity, gestational diabetes, and cesarean section delivery.

Answer A is incorrect. Diffuse alveolar damage is caused by a wide variety of mechanisms and toxic agents. The formation of intra-alveolar hyaline membranes leads to impaired gas exchange.

Answer C is incorrect. Hypersensitivity pneumonitis is an immunologically induced, non-IgE-mediated inflammatory lung disease resulting from the sensitization and subsequent recurrent exposure to any of a wide variety of inhaled organic dusts.

Answer D is incorrect. Intra-alveolar exudative consolidation is typically seen in lobar pneumonia caused most frequently by *Streptococcus pneumoniae*(pneumococcus). There is no association with diabetic mothers.

Answer E is incorrect. Multiple noncaseating granulomas are seen in sarcoidosis, a disease of unknown etiology (i.e., it is not caused by early delivery) that affects multiple organ systems.

Answer F is incorrect. Panacinar emphysema is caused by α_1-antitrypsin deficiency, which is a genetically inherited condition affecting the lungs and liver.

Answer G is incorrect. Neither gestational diabetes nor prematurity are associated with an increased risk of patent foramen ovale.

43. The correct answer is D. The medical student should be very familiar with both the anatomy and the physiology of the sucking chest wound, as described in this patient. A penetrating wound to the chest can puncture the pleura, making an opening for air to be sucked into the pleural space. With inspiration, the diaphragm descends, lowering the intrapleural pressure. If there is a communication directly between the pleural space and the outside world, air is sucked into this negative pressure space and collapses the lung. Air in the pleural space is known as a pneumothorax and is seen on chest x-ray as a collapsed lung.

Answer A is incorrect. It is possible to have a hemopneumothorax, but this vignette describes a pneumothorax injury. One may also see blood in the dependent portions of the thorax. However, a hemothorax may not be present in this case, while a pneumothorax definitely will be present.

Answer B is incorrect. There may be rib fractures on x-ray of the chest, but the stab wound is above the nipple, which is about the level of the fourth and fifth ribs, superior to the ninth and tenth ribs.

Answer C is incorrect. A pleural effusion is seen on x-ray as a fluid collection in the dependent portions of the thorax. The injury above describes the chest wall around the wound moving with respirations. This is from air moving in and out of the pleural space. Fluid would fill the gravity-dependent portions of the lung and not move with respirations.

Answer E is incorrect. Right upper lobe consolidation would be consistent with right upper lobe pneumonia, which is not described in this vignette.

44. **The correct answer is A.** The patient described has typical community-acquired pneumonia, which is characterized by high-grade fever, productive cough, and acute onset. Common bacteria causing lobar pneumonia include *Streptococcus pneumoniae*, *Staphylococcus aureus*, and *Haemophilus influenzae*, which would be covered with ceftriaxone, a broad-spectrum third-generation cephalosporin.

Answer B is incorrect. Clindamycin is used to treat anaerobic infections. It can be used with an aminoglycoside for penetrating wound infections of the abdomen. It is also commonly used to treat female genital tract infections.

Answer C is incorrect. Doxycycline is a tetracycline analog that can be used in patients with renal failure. Its mechanism of action is binding to the 30S subunit and preventing attachment of aminoacyl-tRNAs. It can be used to treat causes of atypical pneumonia such as *Chlamydia* and *Mycoplasma* species infection. Side effects include gastrointestinal distress, photosensitivity, and rash.

Answer D is incorrect. Erythromycin is a macrolide antibiotic used to treat *Legionella*, *Chlamydia*, *Mycoplasma*, and *Neisseria* species infection. It is typically used to treat atypical pneumonias and upper respiratory infections. Erythromycin toxicity causes gastrointestinal discomfort, acute cholestatic hepatitis, eosinophilia, and skin rash.

Answer E is incorrect. Trimethoprim-sulfamethoxazole is used to treat a variety of infections, but is not first-line therapy for community-acquired pneumonias. Generally, in pulmonary infections, trimethoprim-sulfamethoxazole is first-line therapy for *Pneumocystis jiroveci* pneumonia.

45. **The correct answer is B.** The patient is suffering from TB, with the causative organism (*Mycobacterium tuberculosis*) seen as the red organism on acid-fast stain. His treatment regimen will include isoniazid. One of the adverse effects of isoniazid therapy is peripheral neuropathy, which can be prevented by coadministration of vitamin B_6.

Answer A is incorrect. There is no role for the administration of vitamin B_1 in the treatment of TB. Vitamin B_1 is used to treat alcoholics to prevent Wernicke-Korsakoff syndrome.

Answer C is incorrect. There is no role for the administration of vitamin B_{12} in the treatment of TB. Vitamin B_{12} is used to treat patients with vitamin B_{12} deficiency who are showing neurological symptoms and macrocytic anemia.

Answer D is incorrect. There is no role for the administration of vitamin C in the treatment of TB. Vitamin C is used to treat scurvy.

Answer E is incorrect. There is no role for the administration of vitamin E in the treatment of TB.

46. **The correct answer is A.** β-Agonists such as albuterol may cause potassium to shift into cells, resulting in hypokalemia. This may lead to ECG abnormalities due to destabilization of cardiac cell membranes, the classic examples of which are U waves. Short-acting β-agonists such as albuterol are used in the treatment of acute asthma exacerbations because of their relaxing effects on bronchial smooth muscle. Long-acting β-agonists such as salmeterol are used for prophylaxis of bronchospasm.

Answer B is incorrect. Ipratropium is an antimuscarinic agent that is used for both asthma and chronic obstructive pulmonary disease. Common adverse effects include cough, nausea, and dizziness. It is not known to cause hypokalemia.

Chapter 17: Respiratory • Answers   441

Answer C is incorrect. Theophylline most likely causes bronchodilation by increasing levels of cAMP. It does this by inhibiting phosphodiesterase, an enzyme that hydrolyses cAMP to AMP. Theophylline has a narrow therapeutic window and may cause cardiotoxicity (and neurotoxicity) but does not result in hypokalemia.

Answer D is incorrect. Zileuton is an asthma medication that blocks the production of leukotrienes. Serious adverse reactions include hepatotoxicity and neutropenia. It is not known to cause hypokalemia.

47. **The correct answer is B.** This histology shows noncaseating granulomas, characteristic of sarcoidosis. Sarcoidosis is a multiorgan inflammatory disorder of unknown etiology. It is thought to be immune mediated. The lung is the most frequently involved organ, but other commonly affected organs are lymph nodes, skin, eyes, kidneys, the heart, and the central nervous system. Findings that might be expected in a patient with sarcoidosis would include γ-**G**lobulinemia, **R**heumatoid arthritis, elevated **A**ngiotensin-converting enzyme levels, **I**nterstitial fibrosis, and **N**oncaseating granulomas (remember the mnemonic **GRAIN**).

Answer A is incorrect. Goodpasture's syndrome is caused by anti-basement membrane antibodies. It is not associated with noncaseating granulomas.

Answer C is incorrect. Small cell lung cancer is not associated with granulomas and is recognized by numerous small blue neoplastic cells.

Answer D is incorrect. Systemic lupus erythematosus can be associated with pleuritis, but it is not associated with noncaseating granulomas.

Answer E is incorrect. TB is characterized by caseating granulomas, which can be recognized by the necrotic, cheeselike center in the granuloma.

48. **The correct answer is A.** *Bacillus anthracis* can cause cutaneous anthrax, inhalation anthrax, and gastrointestinal anthrax. This patient had inhalation anthrax (also known as "woolsorter's disease"), which usually has two phases: the initial phase characterized by malaise, dry cough, and chest pressure that resolve in a few days; and the second phase in which patients suddenly develop acute respiratory distress and hypoxemia followed by hemorrhagic mediastinitis and bloody pleural effusions. If a patient is not rapidly treated with penicillin, doxycycline, ciprofloxacin, or levofloxacin, systemic infection can cause septic shock (due to exotoxins produced by the bacteria) and death within 24 hours.

Answer B is incorrect. *Brucella abortus* is transmitted from cattle to humans who have contact with infected animal meat, milk products, or aborted animal placentas. *Brucella* penetrates multiple organs, including the lungs, skin, conjunctiva, and gastrointestinal tract. Patients with brucellosis have systemic symptoms such as fever (undulant fever that is worse in the evening), chills, loss of appetite, and lymphadenopathy. Brucellosis is rarely fatal, and its symptoms can last from months to years.

Answer C is incorrect. *Francisella tularensis* causes tularemia, characterized by abrupt onset of fever, chills, malaise, and fatigue. Six clinical forms of tularemia exist: ulceroglandular, glandular, oculoglandular, oropharyngeal, pneumonic, and typhoidal (septicemic). Pulmonic tularemia is very similar to inhalational anthrax; however, hemorrhagic mediastinitis is not seen in tularemia, and death does not occur within 24 hours. Tularemia is also associated with rabbit, tick, or deerfly contact.

Answer D is incorrect. *Legionella* is a cause of severe pneumonia, particularly in cigarette smokers and immunocompromised individuals. It is associated with environmental water sources. It does not cause mediastinitis or hemorrhagic pleural effusions.

Answer E is incorrect. *Nocardia asteroides* is an acid-fast aerobe found in soil. This organism causes pulmonary infections primarily in immunocompromised individuals.

49. **The correct answer is D.** In the tissues, more CO_2 is being produced and entering the RBCs.

It is combined with H_2O by carbonic anhydrase to form H_2CO_3, which then becomes H^+ and HCO_3^-. The HCO_3^- leaves the RBCs while Cl^- enters.

Answer A is incorrect. Dissolved CO_2 that remains in the plasma accounts for about 5% of transport. In addition, bicarbonate does not bind to hemoglobin, H^+ does.

Answer B is incorrect. Bicarbonate travels in the plasma, not the RBCs. When it gets to the lung, it enters the RBCs, gets transformed back to H_2O and CO_2, and the CO_2 is exhaled.

Answer C is incorrect. The primary transport of CO_2 in the blood is via HCO_3^- (90%). Carbaminohemoglobin only accounts for about 5%.

Answer E is incorrect. The lungs do not have an acidic environment, the peripheral tissues do. The oxygenation of hemoglobin in the lungs promotes the dissociation of CO_2 (the Haldane effect).

50. **The correct answer is D.** The formula for calculating physiologic dead space (V_D) is: tidal volume × ([arterial carbon dioxide pressure – expired air carbon dioxide pressure] divided by the arterial carbon dioxide pressure); or $V_D = V_T \times ([Paco_2 - Peco_2] / Paco_2)$. Plugging, in the numbers given in the stem, the answer is 0.5 L.

Answer A is incorrect. See calculation.

Answer B is incorrect. See calculation.

Answer C is incorrect. See calculation.

Answer E is incorrect. See calculation.

Answer F is incorrect. See calculation.

SECTION III

Full-Length Examinations

Test Block 1

1. A new patient presents to a clinic in Denver, Colorado with complaints of dyspnea and fatigue on exertion. On history, the patient informs the doctor that she just moved from the California coastline less than 1 week ago, and has been attempting to do her 3-mile run every morning. The patient is told to limit her running until her body adjusts to the new altitude. Which of the following will occur in this woman's body in response to the high altitude?

(A) An increased partial oxygen pressure at 50% saturation on the hemoglobin-oxygen dissociation curve
(B) Decreased pulmonary vascular resistance
(C) Decreased RBC 2,3-diphosphoglycerate concentration
(D) Increased arterial partial oxygen pressure
(E) Right ventricular atrophy

2. A 32-year-old woman with pheochromocytoma is being treated with phenoxybenzamine. After surgical excision of the tumor, the patient has an episode of hypotension requiring 30 seconds of cardiopulmonary resuscitation and subsequent treatment in the intensive care unit. The attending physician asks his intern what physiologic responses he would expect to see if the patient had been given epinephrine during resuscitation. What would have been observed following administration of epinephrine?

(A) Decrease in blood pressure
(B) Decrease in heart rate
(C) Increase in blood pressure
(D) Increase in respiratory rate
(E) No changes in vital signs

3. A 35-year-old man with no significant past medical history presents to his primary care physician complaining of shortness of breath on exertion for the past several months. The patient acknowledges recent heart palpitations, but denies chest pain, cough, lower extremity edema, paroxysmal nocturnal dyspnea, or weakness. He further denies any recent illness, and he states that he does not smoke. Cardiac examination shows an irregularly irregular rhythm, a widely split fixed S_2, and a midsystolic ejection murmur over the left upper sternal border. ECG reveals that the patient is in atrial fibrillation. Based on these findings, the physician concludes that these symptoms are due to pathology of which of the following fetal structures?

(A) Aorticopulmonary septum
(B) Ductus arteriosus
(C) Ductus venosus
(D) Foramen ovale
(E) Interventricular septum

4. A 10-year-old boy is referred to the neurologist with intellectual deterioration, personality changes, generalized seizures, and visual disturbances that have worsened over the last few months. The patient's cerebrospinal fluid culture shows no bacterial growth. Further analysis shows normal glucose levels and normal protein. The patient is afebrile and reports no headache. The child's parents say that he has not received any vaccinations since arriving in the United States last year. They also say that he has had only one major illness prior to this. The child was approximately 2 years old when he developed a high fever, cough, and runny nose. Soon after the onset of these symptoms, he developed a red maculopapular rash that spread downward from his head. Antibodies against which of the following are likely to be found in this patient's cerebrospinal fluid?

(A) Herpes simplex virus type 2
(B) Measles virus
(C) Mumps virus
(D) *Neisseria meningitidis*
(E) Rubella virus
(F) *Treponema pallidum*

5. A 34-year-old man comes to the clinic because his gums have become swollen and have exhibited a tendency to bleed. He states that he has been brushing his teeth at least twice a day. On examination, he is found to have several bruises on his legs in different stages of heal-

ing. The patient adds that his bruises have been taking longer than usual to heal. His complete blood cell count and coagulation panel are within normal limits. What is the likely cause of this patient's symptoms?

(A) Decreased platelet count
(B) Decreased von Willebrand factor
(C) Defect in hydroxylation of collagen residues
(D) Mutation of dystrophin gene
(E) Mutation of spectrin

6. A 21-year-old woman with no family or personal history of breast cancer presents with a small, firm mass in the lower inner quadrant of her right breast that seems mobile when palpated. It is nontender. There are no overlying skin changes or nipple discharge. Which of the following would most likely be found on biopsy of this mass?

(A) Blue dome cysts and some atypical epithelial hyperplasia
(B) Cells in a single file formation
(C) Fibrosing stroma around normal-looking glands
(D) Large cells with clear "halos"
(E) Multicentric lobes with lymphocytic infiltrate

7. A 50-year-old woman who works as a secretary comes to the physician because of numbness and tingling in her hands. On examination, the patient is found to have decreased sensation in all of her fingers except her fifth digit. Which of the following muscles is most commonly weakened in patients with this condition?

(A) Adductor pollicis
(B) Dorsal interossei
(C) Lumbricals (3 and 4)
(D) Opponens digiti minimi
(E) Opponens pollicis

8. A 19-year-old man presents to the emergency department complaining of fatigue, lethargy, and a history of a recent upper respiratory infection. His temperature is 37° C (98.6° F) and his physical examination shows jaundice and prominent splenomegaly. Blood counts show decreased hemoglobin (9 g/dL), elevated mean cell hemoglobin concentration, and increased reticulocyte count. A peripheral blood smear is shown in the image. Which of the following is the definitive choice of therapy for this condition?

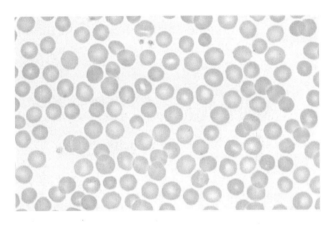

Reproduced, with permission, from Lichtman MA, Beutler E, Kipps TJ, Seligsohn U, Kaushansky K, Prchal JF. *Williams Hematology*, 7th ed. New York: McGraw-Hill, 2006: Color Plate III-7.

(A) Blood transfusion
(B) Chemotherapy
(C) Folic acid supplementation
(D) Iron chelation therapy
(E) Iron supplementation
(F) Splenectomy

9. A 22-year-old woman presents to her family physician because of increasing fatigue and because she looks "pale" despite spending many hours outside as a camp counselor. She also states that her urine looks "cola-colored" when she first goes to the bathroom in the morning. The patient feels well otherwise. Blood analysis shows a low platelet count, a low RBC count, and a low WBC count. The patient's RBCs are mixed with acidified normal serum and compared to normal RBCs at room temperature and at 37° C (98.6° F); both temperatures cause the patient's, but not the normal, RBCs to lyse. Based on this clinical picture and the laboratory tests, this patient most likely has which of the following disorders?

(A) Alkaptonuria
(B) Cystinuria
(C) Hemophilia A
(D) Maple syrup urine disease
(E) Paroxysmal nocturnal hemoglobinuria

10. A 34-year-old man presents to the emergency department complaining of a 2-day history of fatigue and double vision. Physical examination shows a right nystagmus. A detailed history reveals that he recently began treatment for recurrent tonic-clonic seizures. Laboratory studies show:

Na^+: 143 mEq/L
K^+: 4.5 mEq/L
Cl^-: 103 mEq/L
HCO_3^-: 26 mEq/L
Blood urea nitrogen: 45 mg/dL
Creatinine: 4.3 mg/dL

Which of the following agents is most likely responsible for this patient's condition?

(A) Clozapine
(B) Imipramine
(C) Lithium
(D) Phenytoin
(E) Sumatriptan
(F) Valproic acid

11. A 4-year-old boy has a sublingual mass. A scan using ^{99m}Tc pertechnetate, which behaves as iodine and approximates iodine uptake, shows significant uptake in this region with little activity lower in the neck. Which of the following is the embryologic explanation for this mass?

(A) The third and fourth branchial (pharyngeal) arches have hypertrophied
(B) The thymus has developed ectopically
(C) The thymus has hypertrophied
(D) The thyroid has failed to migrate caudally
(E) The thyroid has migrated too far rostrally

12. A 27-year-old healthy man presents because he and his wife have been repeatedly unsuccessful in conceiving a child. His wife has been tested and determined to be fertile. Upon questioning, the patient denies coronary or lipid abnormalities but admits to having multiple sinus infections and a chronic productive cough. Further analysis of his semen shows a normal number of sperm. Which of the following is the most likely etiology for the patient's infertility?

(A) Age-related increase in estradiol with possible prostate dihydrotestosterone sensitization
(B) Autosomal recessive dysfunction of a chloride ion channel
(C) Failure of testicles to descend into the scrotum
(D) Familial disease causing early atherosclerosis leading to erectile dysfunction
(E) Lack of dynein ATPase arms in microtubules of cilia

13. An anxious young woman presents to the emergency department with an acute onset of severe abdominal pain. She states that she "partied a little bit last night" and consumed approximately 8 or 9 alcoholic drinks. She also admits to using diuretics to "lose water weight." Her stool is guaiac-negative, but she has periumbilical tenderness to palpation. An arterial blood gas study shows that her pH is 7.55 and her bicarbonate level is 21 mEq/L, with a partial pressure of carbon dioxide of 25 mm Hg. Her serum shows normal sodium chloride levels. Which of the following is the origin of her acid-base disturbance?

(A) A build-up of unmeasured anions due to hepatic metabolism of alcohol
(B) Electrolyte imbalance due to diuretic use
(C) Hyperventilation secondary to pain and anxiety
(D) Hypoventilation due to the respiratory depression caused by alcohol ingestion
(E) Vomiting due to alcohol toxicity

14. A 38-year-old white woman presents to the physician with a 2-week history of aching pain in her left calf that is made worse by dorsiflexion of her foot. On physical examination, her left calf is found to be erythematous, warm, and swollen. Which of the following measures should she take to decrease similar problems in the future?

(A) Begin taking a bile acid resin
(B) Begin taking a statin
(C) Begin taking low-dose oral contraceptives
(D) Exercise 30 minutes three times per week
(E) Quit smoking
(F) Reduce alcohol consumption to one or two glasses of red wine per week

15. An 18-year-old woman presents to her physician's office with symptoms of nausea and vomiting as well as jaundice. She is taking oral contraceptives, but also reports consistent condom use. She denies illicit drug use. On physical examination the patient shows no hepatomegaly or right upper quadrant tenderness to deep palpation. Laboratory studies show a total bilirubin level of 4 mg/dL, direct bilirubin level of 1 mg/dL, and indirect bilirubin level of 3 mg/dL. Liver enzyme levels are within normal limits. A direct Coombs' test is negative. Which of the following is the most likely diagnosis?

(A) Autoimmune hemolytic anemia
(B) Crigler-Najjar syndrome type I
(C) Gilbert's disease
(D) Hepatitis C
(E) Oral contraceptive-associated cholestasis

16. A 74-year-old man is brought to the emergency department after he became combative and was screaming that "the little people" were after him. The staff is unable to obtain a history or physical examination because of his agitation, although the triage nurse is able to obtain his vital signs, which are significant for a temperature of 40° C (104° F) and a blood pressure of 90/50 mm Hg. His family reports that he was fine earlier in the day except for an occasional cough, and that he has never had any psychiatric issues before. By the time the psychiatrist arrives, the patient is somnolent and somewhat confused. Which of the following will confirm this patient's most likely diagnosis?

(A) Blood alcohol level
(B) Blood, urine, and sputum cultures
(C) CT of the head
(D) Electroencephalography
(E) Urine toxicology screen

17. A 34-year-old woman who is at 26 weeks of gestation and who has a history of multiple spontaneous abortions presents with severe abdominal pain, jaundice, ascites, and mental status change. Ultrasonography reveals an obscure hepatic venous connection to the inferior vena cava and absence of any waveform in the hepatic veins. She has a positive serum antiphospholipid antibody titer. Which of the following is the most likely diagnosis?

(A) Budd-Chiari syndrome
(B) Congestive heart failure
(C) Polymyalgia rheumatica
(D) Portal vein thrombosis
(E) Veno-occlusive disease

18. A 5-year-old girl is brought to the pediatrician by her mother for evaluation of readiness to enter school. The mother is worried because the child had to be withdrawn from preschool last year because of an inability to cope with the other children. She reports that the child becomes very upset if her daily routine is interrupted. The child's birth history and past medical history are unremarkable. She reached all of her neurodevelopmental milestones, including speech development, on schedule. Which of the following is the most likely diagnosis?

   (A) Asperger's syndrome
   (B) Autistic disorder
   (C) Childhood disintegrative disorder
   (D) Expressive language disorder
   (E) Rett's disorder

19. A 4-year-old boy with a history of mental retardation and seizures is brought to the physician with a 3-month history of worsening shortness of breath. During physical examination, the physician notices numerous acnelike papules on the patient's face. Echocardiography shows significant left ventricular outflow obstruction. Which of the following is the most likely diagnosis for this patient's heart condition?

   (A) Coronary artery disease
   (B) Dilated cardiomyopathy
   (C) Myxoma
   (D) Rhabdomyoma
   (E) Transposition of the great vessels

20. A 28-year-old male physician is seeing a new patient, who is a 25-year-old woman. At the beginning of the encounter he recognizes her as someone he met at a bar several weeks ago. He was highly attracted to her at that time, but she left the bar before he could invite her on a date. What is the physician's best course of action during this visit?

   (A) Ask her on a date
   (B) Continue the visit as normal
   (C) Refer her to another doctor
   (D) Refer her to another doctor, then ask her on a date
   (E) Return to the room with a chaperon and conduct the visit as normal

21. A 45-year-old man visited his primary care physician 1 month ago because of chest pain that he had experienced four times in the past 4 months. The onset of the pain is sudden and radiates to his left jaw. He usually feels the pain when he is watching television but has never felt it during exertion. During last month's visit, the physician prescribed sublingual nitroglycerin, and the patient reports that this has shortened the duration of his episodes. Last month's ECG is shown in the image. Which of the following is the most likely cause of this patient's chest pain?

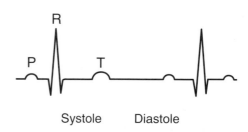

Reproduced, with permission, from USMLERx.com.

   (A) Myocardial infarction
   (B) Pericarditis
   (C) Prinzmetal's angina
   (D) Stable angina
   (E) Unstable angina

22. A clinical study is performed on young male subjects who have deafness, ocular abnormalities, and a nephritic syndrome. Kidney biopsies of these subjects reveal no pathology under immunofluorescence or light microscopy. Which of the following is the most common glomerular pathological characteristic likely to be seen under electron microscopy?

   (A) Diffuse epithelial foot process fusion
   (B) Immune complex deposits
   (C) Split basement membrane
   (D) Wire-loop appearance

23. A researcher is designing an in vitro experimental system to study the kinetics of GLUT4-mediated glucose transport into mammalian cells. The system will measure radiolabeled glucose concentrations in cell culture media

both before and at intervals following the addition of insulin. Which of the following cell types is the best choice for use in this experimental system?

(A) Adipocytes
(B) Cortical neurons
(C) Erythrocytes
(D) Hepatocytes
(E) Pancreatic β cells

24. Myasthenia gravis is an autoimmune disorder that affects approximately 3 in 100,000 people. Individuals with mysasthenia gravis classically present with complaints of muscle weakness and fatigue secondary to the formation of autoantibodies directed against the acetylcholine receptors at neuromuscular junctions. The most accurate method of diagnosis involves the detection of these autoantibodies. On average, this test is approximately 80% sensitive and 90% specific. If an individual has a positive test for autoantibodies against the acetylcholine receptor, what is the approximate post-test probability of having this disease, assuming a pre-test probability of 50%?

(A) 80%
(B) 85%
(C) 89%
(D) 90%
(E) 95%
(F) 99%

25. An 85-year-old man is rushed to the emergency department from his primary care physician's office after his physician palpates a pulsating mass in his abdomen. The patient is diagnosed with an abdominal aortic aneurysm. Instead of repairing the aneurysm by surgically opening the abdomen, the surgeon decides to perform endovascular stenting and grafting. The stent is inserted into the femoral artery and threaded up toward the aortic defect. To access the femoral artery the surgeon must open the femoral sheath and expose its contents. Which of the following structures is enclosed inside the femoral sheath?

(A) Cooper's ligament
(B) Femoral canal

(C) Femoral nerve
(D) Obturator nerve
(E) Tunica vaginalis

26. A 6-year-old girl is found to be nearsighted during a vision screening at school, and the school nurse tells the parents the child should be fitted for corrective lenses. Her mother is upset because her daughter is already much taller than her classmates, has an awkward gait, and was recently diagnosed with scoliosis. She is afraid that the glasses will only add to her daughter's problems at school, where her classmates frequently tease her. When the ophthalmologist observes that the patient's right lens is dislocated, he suspects that her symptoms are in fact related to an enzyme deficiency. As a result of this deficiency, which of the following amino acids is essential in this patient's diet?

(A) Cysteine
(B) Lysine
(C) Methionine
(D) Tryptophan
(E) Tyrosine

27. A 57-year-old man presents to his primary care physician with complaints of fatigue and nausea over the past month. On physical examination, the patient is found to have a low-grade fever, scattered lymphadenopathy including two firm 2-cm lymph nodes in the left axilla, and an enlarged spleen. Biopsy of the lymph nodes yields a diagnosis of diffuse large cell lymphoma. Upon consultation with an oncologist, the patient begins a multidrug regimen that includes cyclophosphamide. Although generally safe, cyclophosphamide treatment can produce severe adverse effects in some patients. Which of the following drug-symptom combinations correctly states the treatment strategy for a common adverse event associated with this medication?

(A) Acrolein for hemorrhagic cystitis
(B) Acrolein for myelosuppression
(C) Acrolein for nausea and vomiting
(D) N-acetylcysteine for hemorrhagic cystitis
(E) N-acetylcysteine for myelosuppression
(F) N-acetylcysteine for nausea and vomiting

28. An obese 46-year-old, multiparous woman presents to the physician with nonradiating right upper quadrant pain and fever that was preceded by nausea and vomiting. Ultrasonography shows hyperechogenic structures in the right upper quadrant. Laboratory testing reveals a WBC count of 14,500/mm^3, an erythrocyte sedimentation rate of 40 mm/hr, and a serum amylase level of 70 U/L. Which of the following is the most likely diagnosis in this patient?

(A) Acute acalculous cholecystitis
(B) Acute calculous cholecystitis
(C) Acute pancreatitis
(D) Carcinoma of the pancreas
(E) Cholesterolosis

29. A 60-year-old woman with a 25-year history of type 2 diabetes mellitus presents with pruritus, diffuse bone pain, and proximal muscle weakness. Laboratory studies show a serum Ca^{2+} level of 6.5 mg/dL, a serum phosphate level of 6.0 mg/dL, a serum creatinine level of 2.7 mg/dL, and an intact parathyroid hormone level of 300 pg/mL. The laboratory findings in this patient are most likely due to which of the following conditions?

(A) Parathyroid adenoma
(B) Parathyroid insufficiency
(C) Renal failure
(D) Underlying malignancy
(E) Vitamin D intoxication

30. A 73-year-old man who has atrial fibrillation has been treated pharmacologically for 10 years. He presents to his primary care physician complaining of generalized dyspnea. Pulmonary function tests show forced expiratory volume in 1 second (FEV_1) and forced vital capacity (FVC) are both less than 70% of the predicted value, with a ratio of FEV_1 to FVC of 81%. The flow-volume curve is shown in the image. Which of the following is a possible etiology of this presentation?

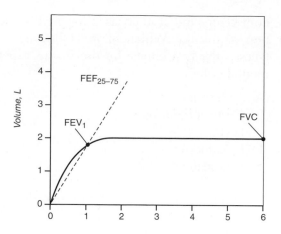

Reproduced, with permission, from USMLERx.com.

(A) Adult-onset asthma
(B) Amiodarone
(C) Diltiazem
(D) Sotalol
(E) Tobacco

31. A 23-year-old man comes to the emergency department complaining of bloody diarrhea and a fever. Laboratory tests of blood and stool cultures show an oxidase-negative, motile, gram-negative bacillus that grows as clear colonies on MacConkey agar. Which of the following is the most likely causative organism?

(A) *Escherichia coli*
(B) *Pseudomonas aeruginosa*
(C) *Salmonella* species
(D) *Shigella* species
(E) *Vibrio cholerae*

32. A 35-year-old man is brought to the emergency department by ambulance after having a tonic-clonic seizure at work. The patient reports that he has always been healthy and has never had a seizure before. On further questioning, the patient reports that he has been having intermittent bloody stools for the past 4 months. CT of the head reveals an irregular 3-cm × 4-cm mass extending from the right to the left hemisphere. CT of the abdomen shows multiple polypoid masses in the sigmoid colon. Which of the following is the most likely diagnosis?

(A) Familial adenomatous polyposis
(B) Gardner syndrome
(C) Hereditary nonpolyposis colorectal carcinoma
(D) Tuberous sclerosis
(E) Turcot syndrome

33. A patient's serum is placed on a plate that is pre-coated with a specific antigen. The plate is then washed free of non-antigen-binding antibodies. Anti-immunoglobulin antibodies coupled to an enzyme are then added to the mixture. Excess anti-immunoglobulin antibodies are washed free, and a substrate that changes color when cleaved by the enzyme is added to the plate. Which of the following laboratory techniques does this describe?

(A) Allele-specific oligonucleotide probe
(B) Enzyme-linked immunosorbent assay
(C) Northern blot
(D) Polymerase chain reaction
(E) Sequencing
(F) Southern blot
(G) Western blot

34. A 3-year-old boy comes to the physician because of fever and erythema in his conjunctivae, oral mucosa, palms, and soles for the past week. Physical examination is significant for fever, enlarged cervical lymph nodes, and edema of the hands and feet. Although the precise cause of the patient's disease is unknown, it is speculated that autoantibodies may play a role. Based on the known structure that is primarily affected in the patient's disease, what autoantibodies are suspected to be associated with this condition?

(A) Anticentromere antibodies
(B) Anti-endothelial cell antibodies
(C) Antihistone antibodies
(D) Anti-IgG antibodies
(E) Antinuclear antibodies

35. A 6-year-old boy arrives at the emergency department breathing rapidly and complaining of tinnitus and nausea. His parents explain that he swallowed half a bottle of aspirin that they had accidentally left out. The physician decides to administer a medication that alters the pH of the boy's urine in order to improve excretion of the drug. How does altering the pH of the urine improve the excretion of aspirin?

(A) Acidification of the urine traps ionized molecules in the tubule
(B) Acidification of the urine traps nonionized molecules in the tubule
(C) Acidification of urine will increase the glomerular filtration rate
(D) Alkalinization of the urine traps ionized molecules in the tubule
(E) Alkalinization of the urine traps nonionized molecules in the tubule
(F) Alkalinization of urine will increase the glomerular filtration rate

36. A 61-year-old man with a past medical history of cancer presents with a 2-week history of constant and severe headaches. He also notes changes in his vision associated with the headaches. Physical examination shows a healing ecchymotic lesion on the right forearm, papilledema in the left eye, a right-sided pronator drift, and weakness of the right arm. The diagnosis of an intracranial hemorrhage is confirmed with CT of the head. Which of the following cancers is most likely to have resulted in this patient's presentation?

(A) Angiosarcoma
(B) Basal cell carcinoma
(C) Colorectal carcinoma
(D) Melanoma
(E) Prostate cancer

37. A 7-year-old boy presents to the physician with acute-onset edema and facial swelling. Dipstick urinalysis reveals 4+ proteinuria. Renal biopsy shows no appreciable changes under light and fluorescence microscopy, but electron microscopy demonstrates glomerular epithelial cell foot process effacement. A diagnosis of minimal change disease is made. How does this disease affect the pressures governing the flow of fluid across the glomeruli?

(A) Bowman's space hydrostatic pressure will be decreased
(B) Bowman's space hydrostatic pressure will be increased
(C) Bowman's space oncotic pressure will be decreased
(D) Glomerular capillary hydrostatic pressure will be increased
(E) Glomerular capillary oncotic pressure will be decreased

38. A 15-year-old boy is riding his skateboard down a rail when the board slips and he falls, straddling the rail. He comes to the emergency department in extreme pain. On physical examination, he is found to be febrile and tachycardic. His genital examination is notable for ecchymosis and swelling of the scrotum and perineal region due to urinary leakage. Which of the following is the source of this urinary leakage?

(A) Anterior bladder wall rupture
(B) Penile urethra rupture
(C) Superior bladder wall rupture
(D) Urethral rupture above the urogenital diaphragm
(E) Urethral rupture below the urogenital diaphragm

39. A gram-positive organism is isolated and cultured. Analyses show the organism is catalase-negative with no hemolysis, and is resistant to optochin and penicillin. The organism is able to grow in 40% bile salts and in 6.5% sodium chloride solution. Which of the following organisms has been isolated?

(A) *Enterococcus faecalis*
(B) *Staphylococcus epidermidis*
(C) *Streptococcus agalactiae*
(D) *Streptococcus pneumoniae*
(E) *Streptococcus sanguis*

40. The mother of a 16-month-old girl is concerned because she noticed that her daughter became lethargic and irritable 2 days after an ear infection. The mother recalls periodically noticing sweet-smelling urine in her child's diaper but that otherwise her development has been normal. An inability to metabolize which of the following would explain these symptoms?

(A) Glucosylceramide
(B) Histidine
(C) Phenylalanine
(D) Sphingomyelin
(E) Tyrosine
(F) Valine

41. A 35-year-old man presents to the physician with a 2-month history of non-bloody, non-mucoid, non-oily watery diarrhea. He has a diastolic murmur that gets louder with inspiration and is best heard over the left lower sternal border. His face is warm and appears to be engorged with blood for several minutes during the examination. Laboratory studies show:

Vanillylmandelic acid: 5 mg/day (normal 0–7 mg/day)
Metanephrine, urine: 250 μg/g of creatinine (normal 0–300 μg/g)
Homovanillic acid, urine: 14 mg/day (normal 0–15 mg/day)
5-HIAA: 28 mg/day (normal 0–9 mg/day)

Gastrointestinal endoscopy is most likely to show a lesion located near which of the following?

(A) Gastroesophageal junction
(B) Ligament of Treitz
(C) Pancreaticoduodenal junction
(D) Rectosigmoid junction
(E) Splenic flexure

42. A 57-year-old woman presents with violet discoloration of her upper eyelids, periorbital edema, and erythematous patches over her knuckles, elbows, and knees for the past several months. She also complains of bilateral muscle weakness that causes difficulty swallowing and trouble getting up from a chair. Which additional disease process is this patient most likely to have?

(A) Cancer of a visceral organ
(B) Osteoarthritis
(C) Psoriasis
(D) Secondary syphilis
(E) Zenker's diverticulum

43. A 20-year-old man presents to the emergency department with a 3-day history of worsening fever and swelling and redness over his left leg. On physical examination, the patient has erythema and edema of his left leg that is exquisitely tender. The patient is admitted to the hospital and given intravenous antibiotics. The erythema and swelling decrease over the next 3 weeks. During the fourth week, the patient develops new onset of weakness, fatigue, fever, and a maculopapular rash. Significant laboratory findings include a blood urea nitrogen level of 45 mg/dL and creatinine level of 2.8 mg/dL. Blood studies show increased WBCs and eosinophils. Urinalysis shows hematuria, mild proteinuria, and increased WBCs, with a high number of eosinophils. Which of the following is the most likely cause of this patient's new onset of symptoms?

(A) IgA nephropathy
(B) Interstitial nephritis due to medications
(C) Poststreptococcal glomerulonephritis
(D) Rapidly progressive glomerulonephritis
(E) Systemic lupus erythematosus

44. A 10-year-old boy is brought to the emergency department after becoming less responsive following several bouts of nausea and vomiting. The patient is tachycardic and is breathing deeply and slowly. Laboratory studies are remarkable for a serum pH of 7.21, a serum glucose level of 700 mg/dL, a serum bicarbonate level of 16 mEq/L, and a serum anion gap of 22 (normal 7–16). Intravenous fluids and insulin are administered. Measurement and management of which of the following electrolytes are most critical in this patient?

(A) Bicarbonate
(B) Calcium
(C) Chloride
(D) Potassium
(E) Sodium

45. A 51-year-old man presents to the emergency department 30 minutes after his wife noticed drooping of the left side of his face and difficulty speaking. The patient is alert and oriented to person and place. His wife states that he has a history of benign prostatic hypertrophy, peptic ulcer disease, and high blood pressure. According to the wife, the patient has never experienced symptoms like this before and has never had surgery of any type. The physicians determine that the patient is hemodynamically stable and they obtain the CT scan shown in the image. Which of the following is the best next step in management?

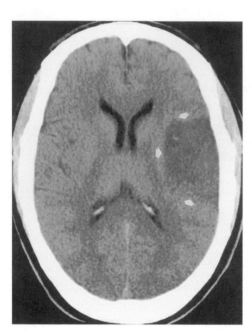

Reproduced, with permission, from Chen MYM, Pope TL, Ott DJ. *Basic Radiology.* New York: McGraw-Hill, 2004: Figure 12-20.

(A) Echocardiogram
(B) Hemicraniectomy
(C) Heparin
(D) Insulin
(E) Tissue plasminogen activator

46. A 3-year-old girl is brought to the emergency department because she is feeling sick and has had a temperature of 38.9° C (102° F) for 3 days.

The intern notices a shallow, healing laceration on the girl's right calf with an erythematous papule in the same area. On questioning, her brother states that a cat may have scratched the toddler because he "saw her playing with a stray." Which of the following organisms is the most likely cause of this illness?

(A) *Bartonella henselae*
(B) *Borrelia burgdorferi*
(C) *Eikenella corrodens*
(D) *Francisella tularensis*
(E) *Pasteurella multocida*

47. A 35-year-old man presents comes to his primary care physician with a chief complaint of palpitations and occasional chest pain. Further questioning reveals a recent history of weight loss, diarrhea, and heat intolerance. Laboratory evaluation shows anti-thyroid-stimulating hormone (TSH) receptor antibodies in the patient's serum. Which of the following best describes this patient's TSH and thyroid hormone levels relative to normal baseline values?

Choice	Thyroid-Stimulating Hormone	Total Thyroxine	Free Thyroxine
A	↑	↑	↑
B	↑	↓	↑
C	↑	↓	↓
D	↓	↑	↑
E	↓	↓	↓

(A) A
(B) B
(C) C
(D) D
(E) E

48. A 35-year-old woman presents to her primary care physician with a fever of 38.3° C (101° F), night sweats, and fatigue. The patient says that she has lost about 6.7 kg (15 lb) over the past year. A CT scan demonstrates mediastinal lymphadenopathy. Biopsy of the nodes shows a small number of large cells with "owl-eye" nucleoli, multiple nuclei, and an abundance of pale cytoplasm on a background of many reactive lymphocytes, macrophages, and granulocytes. Which of the following drugs could be used to treat this condition?

(A) Azathioprine
(B) Cisplatin
(C) Doxorubicin
(D) Paclitaxel
(E) β-Interferon

1. **The correct answer is A.** In response to high altitude, the hemoglobin-oxygen curve shifts right (to release oxygen more easily at the tissues). The P_{50} (the partial oxygen pressure) at 50% saturation of hemoglobin) will increase.

Answer B is incorrect. Pulmonary vasoconstriction (hypoxic vasoconstriction) is a result of hypoxemia (decreased arterial partial oxygen pressure), thus increasing pulmonary arterial pressure (i.e., pulmonary vascular resistance).

Answer C is incorrect. 2,3-Diphosphoglycerate (2,3-DPG) binds to the β chains of deoxyhemoglobin, decreasing the affinity of hemoglobin for oxygen. An increase in 2,3-DPG shifts the hemoglobin-oxygen dissociation curve to the right, which is what happens in response to high altitudes.

Answer D is incorrect. At increased altitudes, barometric pressure decreases, which decreases alveolar partial oxygen pressure. As a result, arterial partial oxygen pressure is decreased (hypoxemia).

Answer E is incorrect. As a result of increased pulmonary vascular resistance, there is increased work on the right side of the heart, resulting in hypertrophy of the right ventricle to counteract the increased afterload.

2. **The correct answer is A.** Phenoxybenzamine is a nonselective α-antagonist that will block both $α_1$- and $α_2$-receptors. In this patient, the administration of high-dose epinephrine (which is both an α- and a β-agonist) would result in unopposed $β_1$- (increased heart rate, increased contractility) and $β_2$- (vasodilation, bronchodilation) agonist effects because the α-effects of epinephrine are blocked by prior phenoxybenzamine administration. The net effect will be β-agonist effects, including an increase in heart rate and a decrease in blood pressure.

Answer B is incorrect. Unopposed β-agonist effects will cause an increase in heart rate because $β_1$-agonists result in increased heart rate.

Answer C is incorrect. Unopposed β-agonist effects will cause a decrease in blood pressure because $β_2$-agonists result in vasodilation.

Answer D is incorrect. Unopposed β-agonist effects do not have a significant effect on respiratory rate.

Answer E is incorrect. Unopposed β-agonist effects will cause changes in both blood pressure and heart rate.

3. **The correct answer is D.** The clinical picture is consistent with a patent foramen ovale (PFO), in which the foramen ovale fails to fully close at birth. A small PFO may go undetected well into adulthood, and it is the most commonly found congenital heart disease in adults. Atrial fibrillation, characterized by an irregularly irregular pulse and the sensation of palpitations, commonly accompanies PFO. A stroke in a young patient is another possible manifestation of PFO, as venous thrombi are able to bypass the pulmonary circulation via the PFO and lodge in the cerebral vasculature as "paradoxical emboli."

Answer A is incorrect. The aorticopulmonary septum forms the division between the pulmonary trunk and the aorta, which are both derived from the truncus arteriosus. Pathology of this septum is associated with transposition of the great vessels and tetralogy of Fallot. Both of these conditions cause early cyanosis and are present in infancy.

Answer B is incorrect. When the ductus arteriosus fails to close at birth, this produces a patent ductus arteriosus (PDA). While this can cause exertional dyspnea, it is typically discovered much earlier in life and produces a continuous "machine-like" murmur, not a purely systolic murmur. PDA is associated with maternal rubella infection during pregnancy and with premature birth. There is no association with atrial fibrillation.

Answer C is incorrect. The ductus venosus shunts blood from the portal vein to the inferior vena cava and thus is not associated with cardiac pathology.

Answer E is incorrect. The interventricular septum divides the fetal primitive ventricle into right and left ventricles. Pathology of this structure produces a membranous ventricular septal defect (VSD). A VSD produces exertional dyspnea and is usually discovered during infancy. VSD is characterized by a harsh pansystolic murmur heard best over the left lower sternal border.

4. **The correct answer is B.** This patient is most likely suffering from subacute sclerosing panencephalitis. This is a rare progressive demyelinating disease associated with chronic central nervous system infection with measles virus. There is often a history of primary measles infection at an early age (approximately 2 years) followed by a latent interval of 6–8 years. Initial manifestations include poor school performance and mood and personality changes. Fever and headache do not occur. As the disease progresses, patients develop progressive intellectual deterioration, focal and/or generalized seizures, myoclonus, ataxia, and visual disturbances. The cerebrospinal fluid (CSF) is acellular with normal or mildly elevated protein and markedly elevated gamma globulin (>20% of total CSF protein). CSF anti-measles antibodies are elevated. CT and MRI show evidence of multifocal white matter lesions, cortical atrophy, and ventricular enlargement.

Answer A is incorrect. Herpes simplex virus 2 (HSV-2) can cause a recurrent meningitis. As with the other examples, one would expect to see signs of meningeal irritation as well as an increase in lymphocytes. Infection with HSV-2 is often associated with genital lesions.

Answer C is incorrect. The patient has no evidence of current mumps infection. Mumps virus can cause acute viral meningitis, but one would expect to see classic signs of meningitis as well as an increase in lymphocytes in the cerebrospinal fluid.

Answer D is incorrect. *Neisseria meningitidis* can cause bacterial meningitis. These organisms would likely be discovered on culture of the CSF. Bacterial meningitis would also manifest in a high fever with meningeal signs (headache, nuchal rigidity) as well as decreased CSF glucose, increased CSF protein, and mononuclear and/or polymorphonuclear cells.

Answer E is incorrect. Rubella virus causes German measles, which is generally characterized by fever and upper respiratory symptoms that resolve with subsequent rash. The maculopapular rash usually starts with the face and descends to the extremities, lasting only several days.

Answer F is incorrect. Infection with *Treponema pallidum* can eventually lead to neurosyphilis, which can include some of the symptoms described in this case. The patient has neither elevated CSF protein nor the presence of mononuclear cells. There is also little evidence in the history of prior or current infection with *T. pallidum*.

5. **The correct answer is C.** A defect in the hydroxylation of proline and lysine residues of collagen is a result of vitamin C deficiency and is associated with scurvy. Patients with scurvy can present with swollen gums and poor wound healing.

Answer A is incorrect. Thrombocytopenia, or decreased platelet counts, may account for easy bleeding. Thrombocytopenia may be a result of many factors, including decreased platelet production (secondary to viral infections or to chemotherapy or radiation), increased platelet destruction (which may be idiopathic or secondary to disseminated intravascular coagulation, thrombotic thrombocytopenic purpura, or hemolytic uremic syndrome), or distribution (splenomegaly). The characteristic symptom of thrombocytopenia is mucosal or cutaneous bleeding. However, this diagnosis is ruled out by a normal platelet count.

Answer B is incorrect. Von Willebrand's factor (vWF) plays an important role in primary hemostasis by binding to both platelets and endothelial components, forming an adhesive bridge between platelets and vascular subendothelial structures as well as between adjacent platelets at sites of endothelial injury. It also contributes to fibrin clot formation by acting as a carrier protein for factor VIII, which has a greatly shortened half-life and abnormally low concentration unless it is bound to vWF. Von Willebrand's disease is characterized by mutations that lead to impairment in the synthesis or function of vWF. Patients with von Willebrand's disease have a tendency to bleed, as the disease is associated with an increased partial thromboplastin time and bleeding time, both of which are normal in this patient.

Answer D is incorrect. Dystrophin is a protein that is located on the cytoplasmic face of the plasma membrane of muscle fibers. It functions as a component of a large, tightly associated glycoprotein complex and shields the complex from degradation. Mutations in the dystrophin gene lead to digestion of the glycoprotein complex by proteases. Loss of these membrane proteins may initiate the degradation of muscle fibers, resulting in muscle weakness characteristic of Duchenne's muscular dystrophy.

Answer E is incorrect. Spectrin is a protein that ties the skeleton of an RBC to its outer lipid bilayer. Mutations of spectrin can lead to a disease called hereditary spherocytosis. Patients with this RBC membrane defect typically present with hemolytic anemia, jaundice, and splenomegaly.

6. **The correct answer is C.** Fibroadenomas are the most common tumor in young women, presenting as small, firm, mobile masses. They are not associated with malignancy. On histology, fibrosing stroma is seen around normal duct and gland structures.

Answer A is incorrect. Blue dome cysts are seen in fibrocystic diseases of the breast. These lesions have associated risks of carcinoma with the presence of atypia.

Answer B is incorrect. Infiltrating lobular carcinomas are often multilocular and bilateral. These cells are found in clusters or in a linear formation.

Answer D is incorrect. Paget's disease presents with eczematous skin findings with underlying ductal carcinomas. Paget's cells are large cells with halo-like clearings.

Answer E is incorrect. Any lymphocytic infiltrate suggests inflammatory carcinoma with a poor prognosis.

7. **The correct answer is E.** This woman has carpal tunnel syndrome, which occurs in individuals whose work involves repetitive hand motions. The median nerve is compressed in the carpal tunnel, leading to decreased sensation on the first three and one-half digits and loss of strength of the thumb due to weakness of the abductor pollicis brevis and opponens pollicis. The opponens pollicis is supplied by the median nerve and functions to aid in opposition.

Answer A is incorrect. The adductor pollicis is innervated by a branch of the ulnar nerve and thus would not be affected by carpal tunnel syndrome. It functions to adduct the thumb toward the middle digits.

Answer B is incorrect. Dorsal interossei muscles are innervated by a branch of the ulnar nerve, which functions to abduct the digits.

Answer C is incorrect. The third and fourth lumbricals are innervated by a branch of the ulnar nerve.

Answer D is incorrect. The opponens digiti minimi muscle is innervated by a branch of the ulnar nerve and brings the fifth digit in opposition with the thumb.

8. **The correct answer is F.** The most likely diagnosis in this patient is hereditary spherocytosis (HS) caused by a defect in cytoskeletal proteins in RBCs, such as spectrin and ankyrin. HS is most commonly inherited as an autosomal-dominant disorder and presents with a triad of anemia, jaundice, and splenomegaly. Anemia may be intermittent and can be aggravated by infection or bone marrow suppression. Laboratory indices that are supportive of HS include evidence of hemolytic anemia (elevated reticulocyte count and low hemoglobin), elevated mean cell hemoglobin concentration due to loss of membrane stability, and increased osmotic fragility. HS is most characteristically de-

fined on peripheral blood smear by the presence of spherocytic RBCs. Spherocytes are formed by the activity of splenic reticuloendothelial cells, which remove portions of abnormal membrane from the cytoskeletal defects found on these RBCs. Symptomatic treatment for anemic crises includes folic acid and blood transfusions. In more severe cases, the only treatment for HS anemia is splenectomy. Even following splenectomy, however, spherocytes will still be observed due to the underlying defect in the RBC membrane.

Answer A is incorrect. Both folic acid supplements and blood transfusion are important in treating the symptoms of anemia in hereditary spherocytosis, but they are not curative measures.

Answer B is incorrect. Chemotherapy is not appropriate and would induce a state of aplastic anemia.

Answer C is incorrect. Both folic acid supplements and blood transfusion are important in treating the symptoms of anemia in hereditary spherocytosis, but they are not curative measures.

Answer D is incorrect. Iron chelation therapy would be appropriate in iron-overloaded states, such as in thalassemic patients requiring many transfusions or in hemochromatosis.

Answer E is incorrect. Iron supplementation would be appropriate in iron deficiency anemia.

9. **The correct answer is E.** Paroxysmal nocturnal hemoglobinuria (PNH) is caused by a defect in synthesis of the cellular anchor used to hold surface proteins to the cell membranes of RBCs, WBCs, and platelets. This defect leads to the clinical manifestations of the disorder: anemia caused by intravascular hemolysis (leading to hemoglobinuria and the darkened urine), thromboses in unusual veins, and hematopoietic deficiencies leading to pancytopenia. The hemolysis occurs all day, but the concentrated urine formed overnight shows an obvious color change. The Ham test (mixing the patient's RBCs with acidified serum) is used to diagnose PNH. Lysis of the patient's RBCs indicates PNH.

Answer A is incorrect. Alkaptonuria presents with urine that darkens after exposure to air as a result of alkapton bodies (accumulations of homogentisic acid), as well as darkening of connective tissues. Patients may also have arthralgias.

Answer B is incorrect. Cystinuria is due to a defect in the tubular amino acid transporter in the kidneys. Patients can form cystine kidney stones due to excess cystine in the urine.

Answer C is incorrect. Hemophilia A is an X-linked disease characterized (in moderate to severe deficiency) by spontaneous bleeding, easy bruising into soft tissues, and hemarthrosis into weight-bearing joints (hip, knee, and ankle).

Answer D is incorrect. Maple syrup urine disease is caused by a deficiency of α-ketoacid dehydrogenase. Patients present with lethargy, seizures, failure to thrive, mental retardation, and urine that smells like maple syrup.

10. **The correct answer is D.** Phenytoin toxicity, as with toxicity of many antiepileptic medications, can lead to nystagmus, diplopia, lethargy, and ataxia. It can also lead to tubulointerstitial nephritis, which can cause a sharp increase in creatinine levels.

Answer A is incorrect. Clozapine is an antipsychotic that possesses extrapyramidal and anticholinergic adverse effects.

Answer B is incorrect. Imipramine is a tricyclic antidepressant that can lead to the "3 C's": Convulsion, Coma, and Cardiotoxicity.

Answer C is incorrect. Lithium toxicity presents with tremor, polyuria, slurred speech, and poor coordination.

Answer E is incorrect. Sumatriptan is a 5-HT$_1$ agonist used to treat migraines. Sumatriptan toxicity can present with chest discomfort and tingling.

Answer F is incorrect. Valproate, an antiepileptic that works primarily by increasing GABA in the central nervous system, can cause nystagmus. Although it does not cause nephritis, valproate has been known to disrupt the urea cycle, leading to hyperammonemia and cerebral edema. Other adverse effects include rare but severe hepatotoxicity, thrombocytopenia, and alopecia. Valproate can increase phenytoin levels by inhibiting CYP450 metabolism.

11. **The correct answer is D.** The uptake of ^{99m}Tc pertechnetate (which is captured by thyroid tissue just as iodine is) in this mass and its sublingual position strongly suggest that it is composed of ectopic thyroid tissue. Normally, the thyroid diverticulum develops from the floor of the primitive pharynx and descends from there into the neck. Therefore, finding thyroid tissue still attached to the tongue implies that it has failed to migrate caudally. The tongue is the most common site of ectopic thyroid tissue for this reason.

Answer A is incorrect. The third and fourth branchial (pharyngeal) arches form the posterior third of the tongue. However, the ^{99m}Tc pertechnetate uptake in this mass indicates that it is composed of thyroid, and not lingual, tissue.

Answer B is incorrect. The thymus is located in the anterior mediastinum, deep to the sternum. There would be no embryologic explanation for finding thymic tissue in the upper neck. Furthermore, the uptake of ^{99m}Tc pertechnetate implies that this mass is composed of thyroid, and not thymus, tissue.

Answer C is incorrect. The thymus is not normally found in the neck; it is instead located in the anterior mediastinum. Thymic hypertrophy would not explain this location. Furthermore, the uptake of ^{99m}Tc pertechnetate indicates that this mass is composed of thyroid, and not thymus, tissue.

Answer E is incorrect. The thyroid does not migrate rostrally during development. Instead, it develops near the tongue and migrates caudally (descends) to its normal position in the lower neck.

12. **The correct answer is E.** This patient has Kartagener's syndrome, which is caused by a lack of dynein arms in microtubules in cilia, rendering them immotile. It results in infertility due to immotile sperm, as well as recurrent sinusitis due to deficient removal of bacteria and other infectious particles. It is also associated with situs invertus, in which the major organs are reversed or mirrored from their original locations.

Answer A is incorrect. Benign prostatic hypertrophy could cause impairment of ejaculation by not allowing semen to be expelled from the body. Because the patient is without an enlarged prostate and is only 27 years old, this diagnosis is highly unlikely.

Answer B is incorrect. Cystic fibrosis does cause infertility, but usually because of bilateral absence of the vas deferens, which would lead to lack of sperm in semen.

Answer C is incorrect. Undescended testicles are associated with infertility and an increased risk of testicular cancer. It is usually found at a very young age and resolves by itself or is surgically corrected before serious complications occur.

Answer D is incorrect. Familial hypercholesterolemia can cause atherosclerosis of the vessels of the male genitalia, causing erectile dysfunction. Without a history of erectile dysfunction or elevated lipid levels, this diagnosis is highly unlikely.

13. **The correct answer is C.** According to her lab data, this young woman has an acute respiratory alkalosis. Respiratory alkalosis is caused by a loss of CO_2, which is balanced by an increased excretion of HCO_3^-. Hence, a low CO_2 and low HCO_3^- level indicate respiratory alkalosis. The key to this question is to recognize that respiratory alkalosis can be caused only by an increase in ventilation, which can be caused by low oxygen (in high altitudes) or by sympathetic stimulation such as anxiety, panic attack, or pain. In this case, the patient is described as anxious and presents with severe

abdominal pain, which is most likely the result of acute alcohol-induced pancreatitis. Both the anxiety and the pain could be causing her to hyperventilate.

Answer A is incorrect. An increase in anions would be consistent with anion-gap metabolic acidosis. Metabolic acidosis is indicated by the presence of a low pH with a low plasma HCO_3^- and a low CO_2, and an increased anion gap, measured by ($[Na^+] - [Cl^-] - [HCO_3^-]$), which is normally between 10 and 16 mEq/L.

Answer B is incorrect. Diuretic use can cause metabolic alkalosis by volume contraction. This causes the kidney to compensate by reabsorbing sodium and excreting hydrogen ions. A metabolic alkalosis would present with elevated pH, elevated CO_2, and elevated HCO_3^-.

Answer D is incorrect. Hypoventilation causes a reduction in pH due to CO_2 retention. This will lead to a respiratory acidosis with a low pH, a high CO_2, and a high HCO_3^-. The compensatory mechanism for respiratory acidosis is an increase in HCO_3^- retention by the kidneys to normalize the pH.

Answer E is incorrect. Vomiting causes a metabolic alkalosis secondary to the loss of acid and chloride from the stomach. If this were the cause, this patient's lab results would show a high pH, a high HCO_3^-, and (with respiratory compensation) a high CO_2. The causes of metabolic alkalosis include vomiting, diuretic therapy, and chloride restriction. The compensation for metabolic alkalosis is hypoventilation.

14. **The correct answer is E.** This patient presents with deep venous thrombosis (DVT). Erythematous, warm, and tender unilateral calf swelling is classic for DVT. Risk factors for DVT and subsequent pulmonary thromboembolism include Virchow's triad, which consists of stasis (eg., immobility, obesity, congestive heart failure), endothelial injury (e.g., trauma, surgery, previous DVT), and hypercoagulable state (e.g., pregnancy, oral contraceptive use, coagulation disorders, malignancies, smoking). This patient also has a positive Homans' sign (calf pain on forced dorsiflexion), which fur-

ther supports the diagnosis. Not only should this patient be anticoagulated with heparin or warfarin upon presentation, but she should quit smoking to decrease her clotting tendencies.

Answer A is incorrect. Bile acid resins such as cholestyramine and colestipol decrease serum triglycerides and cholesterol, which may indirectly, although not directly, improve vascular health.

Answer B is incorrect. Statins decrease LDL cholesterol but do not affect the rate of DVT formation.

Answer C is incorrect. Oral contraceptives are associated with hypercoagulable state, so they would make DVT more likely.

Answer D is incorrect. Moderate exercise has been linked to improved cardiovascular health and a decreased incidence of acute coronary syndromes, although it is not specifically linked to DVT. Stasis, however, can make DVT thrombosis more likely.

Answer F is incorrect. Modest alcohol consumption has been associated with improved cardiovascular health, although no specific link to DVT has been proven.

15. **The correct answer is E.** This patient has an increase in both direct and indirect bilirubin levels. Oral contraceptives can cause jaundice, which is very similar to intrahepatic cholestasis. This condition would lead to increased direct and indirect bilirubin levels. This condition is reversible when the medication is discontinued.

Answer A is incorrect. Autoimmune hemolytic anemia is a type of hemolytic anemia in which the body's immune system attacks its own RBCs. The antibodies involved in this reaction can be detected with the direct Coombs' test. Patients may present with a conjugated or unconjugated hyperbilirubinemia and right upper quadrant tenderness.

Answer B is incorrect. Crigler-Najjar syndrome type I is an indirect bilirubinemia that is caused by a complete absence of glucuronosyltransferase. It presents in infancy with high unconjugated bilirubin.

Answer C is incorrect. Gilbert's disease is an indirect bilirubinemia that typically presents in the second decade of life in response to a stressor (infection, surgery, excessive alcohol consumption, exertion, or fasting). These patients typically present with normal liver function tests, high serum bilirubin, and low/normal direct bilirubin levels.

Answer D is incorrect. Patients with hepatitis typically present with increased levels of both indirect and direct bilirubin. This patient also denies two of the common risk factors for hepatitis, unprotected intercourse and drug use.

16. **The correct answer is B.** This patient is experiencing delirium, which is characterized by a decreased attention span and level of arousal, disorganized thinking, hallucinations, illusions, misperceptions, disturbance in sleep-wake cycle, fluctuating levels of consciousness, and cognitive dysfunction. Delirium is the most common psychiatric diagnosis on medical and surgical floors, particularly among elderly patients. Delirium may be caused by infection, metabolic disturbances, electrolyte abnormalities, hypoperfusion, drug intoxication, alcohol intoxication or withdrawal, and adverse effects due to medication. In this patient, the combination of a high fever and hypotension suggests an infectious etiology. The causative agent is likely to be identified through blood, urine, and sputum cultures.

Answer A is incorrect. A blood alcohol level will give the physician insight into the presence of alcohol intoxication or withdrawal, both of which can cause delirium. In this patient, however, infection is the more likely cause given his fever.

Answer C is incorrect. CT of the head can detect the presence of structural brain abnormalities, hematomas, hemorrhages, infarcts, and masses. Although these processes can certainly lead to changes in mental status, this patient is presenting with clear signs of delirium most likely related to an infection. CT of the head is unlikely to be useful in this setting.

Answer D is incorrect. An electroencephalogram is useful in documenting a seizure or the postictal state following a seizure. While complex partial seizures can be associated with hostile, aggressive behavior, they are also typically associated with automatisms such as lip-smacking and grimacing, which this patient is not experiencing.

Answer E is incorrect. A urine toxicology screen will detect the presence of metabolites of recently ingested drugs. While drug intoxication is a well-established cause of delirium, infection is the more likely cause in this patient given his high fever. However, in delirious patients in whom the cause is not obvious, it is crucial to perform toxicology screens of the urine and blood.

17. **The correct answer is A.** Budd–Chiari syndrome (BCS) is a nearly complete obstruction to blood flow by an acute clot in the hepatic veins or in the inferior vena cava. This sudden event is followed by the onset of hepatomegaly, pain, ascites, and jaundice. The patient has classical hypercoagulable risk factors for developing BCS, including pregnancy and antiphospholipid antibody syndrome (positive antiphospholipid antibody titer, seizures, and multiple abortions). In addition to the clinical presentation and risk factors, imaging study further supports the diagnosis by suggesting hepatic venous occlusion.

Answer B is incorrect. Although pregnancy increases the patient's risk for congestive heart failure (CHF), this patient's clinical presentation, combined with the ultrasound findings, is unlikely to result from CHF.

Answer C is incorrect. Polymyalgia rheumatica is a rheumatologic disorder characterized by pain in several muscle groups with an increased erythrocyte sedimentation rate. It does not involve the liver or related vasculature.

Answer D is incorrect. Unlike BCS, the presenting symptom of portal vein thrombosis is almost always variceal hemorrhage with melena. In contrast to BCS, ultrasound testing reveals an echogenic thrombus in the portal vein.

Answer E is incorrect. Veno-occlusive disease is characterized by occlusion of terminal hepatic venules and hepatic sinusoids. It can clinically resemble BCS; however, the risk factors for developing this disorder are different. They include bone marrow transplantation, chemotherapy, hepatic irradiation, and Jamaican bush tea. Hypercoagulable states such as pregnancy and antiphospholipid syndrome are not risk factors for the disorder. Hence, the most likely diagnosis is not veno-occlusive disease.

18. **The correct answer is A.** Asperger's syndrome is now considered to be an autistic spectrum disorder. These children have normal intelligence but are unable to show emotion or attachment to other people. They exhibit some characteristics of autism, including repetitive behaviors and relationship problems, but what distinguishes Asperger's from autism is the lack of delay in language acquisition. This condition is associated with poor visuospatial skills, difficulty with subtle aspects of social interactions, and clumsiness. Many of the difficulties evident in patients with Asperger's syndrome are closely associated with right hemisphere dysfunction.

Answer B is incorrect. Children with autistic disorder exhibit pervasive cognitive and behavioral deficits. They display impaired social interaction and formation of peer relationships, delay in speech, and stereotyped patterns. Their intelligence is generally below normal. This child does not exhibit such a severe disability.

Answer C is incorrect. Children with childhood disintegrative disorder develop normally and reach developmental milestones until about 2 years of age, after which they show loss of abilities. Areas of loss include language ability, social skills, bowel/bladder control, play, or motor skills. Eventually these children become severely mentally retarded.

Answer D is incorrect. Expressive language disorder is a disorder of communication. These children are not mentally retarded and exhibit no difficulties other than with speech.

Answer E is incorrect. Rett's disorder is an X-linked condition that is seen only in girls (affected boys die at birth). Most of the classic signs and symptoms, including neurodevelopmental regression and mental retardation, are first noticed after the age of 4 years. Specifically, these children will display stereotypic hand movements, seizures, ataxia, and dementia.

19. **The correct answer is D.** Tuberous sclerosis is a genetic condition (autosomal dominant) characterized by nodular proliferation of multinucleated atypical astrocytes. These form tubers, which are found throughout the cerebral cortex and periventricular areas. The classic triad, which is manifest in only the most severe of cases, consists of seizures, mental retardation, and facial angiofibromas (also known as adenoma sebaceum). Half of patients with tuberous sclerosis develop rhabdomyomas, primary tumors of cardiac muscle that, although benign, may compromise cardiac function, especially of the atrioventricular valves. Tuberous sclerosis is also notable for a link to angiomyolipomas of the kidney.

Answer A is incorrect. Coronary artery disease (CAD) can cause progressive shortness of breath, but in conjunction with the facial lesions, the outflow obstruction on echo, and the patient's age, CAD is an unlikely diagnosis.

Answer B is incorrect. Dilated cardiomyopathy is often idiopathic. It involves four-chamber hypertrophy and dilation, and eventually heart failure. This condition is not associated with tuberous sclerosis. Note that hypertrophic cardiomyopathy also causes ventricular outflow obstruction and is often responsible for sudden death in young athletes.

Answer C is incorrect. Myxomas, like rhabdomyomas, are capable of obstruction. However, these are seen in adults and are often located in the atria.

Answer E is incorrect. Transposition of the great vessels is a situation in which the pulmonary trunk arises from the left ventricle and the aorta arises from the right ventricle. This arrangement is incompatible with life, and a compensatory anomaly such as a patent ductus arteriosus is necessary.

20. **The correct answer is B.** Personal (especially sexual) relationships with patients are inappropriate and should not be actively sought by either party of an existing physician-patient relationship. The doctor's best course of action here is to continue the interview and examination, while making no mention of his feelings for the woman, who is now his patient. If the physician had a prior or previously existing relationship with the patient, he could refuse to see her on that basis because the personal relationship preceded any would-be physician-patient relationship.

    Answer A is incorrect. The physician should not actively seek romantic (or other personal) liaisons with patients.

    Answer C is incorrect. Generally, referring the patient to another physician will be an incorrect answer to physician-patient encounter questions, unless the referring physician seeks the particular medical training, expertise, or knowledge of another doctor that is pertinent to the patient. Furthermore, differences in religious or moral beliefs about health care choices do not alone constitute a reason to refer because the patient should always be counseled about alternatives and provide informed consent. In these cases, referral should occur only if the patient's health care choice lends itself to better (i.e., more expert) care from another provider.

    Answer D is incorrect. This physician should not refer the patient in order to escape from the physician-patient relationship. The woman is now this physician's patient unless a proper hand-off is made.

    Answer E is incorrect. Chaperons are typically helpful in cases in which a patient makes inappropriate seductive gestures or remarks directed at the health care provider. The chaperon thus neutralizes the environment during an interview and physical examination, allowing the physician to comfortably serve the patient. Here, the female patient has not indicated any interest in the male physician, so he

should not behave any differently than normal during this visit.

21. **The correct answer is C.** This patient has classic symptoms of cardiac ischemia: chest pain with sudden onset that radiates to his left shoulder or jaw and is relieved by sublingual nitroglycerin. However, the patient is young, and the pain is not prompted by activity but occurs at rest. Additionally, his ECG is normal, showing no evidence of infarct or ischemia. As a result, he probably suffers from coronary vasospasm, also known as Prinzmetal's angina

    Answer A is incorrect. If myocardial infarctions were the etiology of the four episodes of chest pain in the past 4 months, his ECG would show evidence of infarct (T-wave inversion, pathologic Q waves, etc.).

    Answer B is incorrect. Pericarditis can cause sudden onset of chest pain without exertion, but the pain would be not relieved with nitroglycerin. Typically, an ECG would also show diffuse ST-segment elevations.

    Answer D is incorrect. Although the patient's clinical symptoms are of cardiac ischemia, they are not induced by a specific amount of exercise, which is the classic definition of stable angina.

    Answer E is incorrect. Because the patient's symptoms are not prompted by a light amount of exercise or strain, it is unlikely that they are due to unstable angina.

22. **The correct answer is C.** Alport's syndrome is a heterogeneous (although most commonly X-linked) genetic disorder with absent or mutated type IV collagen. It is characterized by renal disease, nerve disorders (deafness), and ocular disorders. There is no evidence of disease under low-power light or immunofluorescence microscopy, as it is not an immune-mediated disease. However, under electron microscopy, there is evidence of a split basement membrane due to the collagen IV mutation.

    Answer A is incorrect. Minimal change disease, the most common cause of nephrotic syndrome in children, includes a histopathologic finding of diffuse epithelial foot process fusion on electron microscopy.

Answer B is incorrect. Alport's syndrome is genetic, not immune-mediated. Therefore, there will be no immune complex deposits visible under electron microscopy.

Answer D is incorrect. A wire-loop appearance under electron microscopy is peculiar to systemic lupus erythematosus (SLE), which is accompanied by subendothelial basement membrane deposits. SLE is a chronic autoimmune disease that affects multiple organ systems, including the kidney. SLE affects young adults (women more than men) and usually presents with a combined nephritic and nephrotic picture.

23. **The correct answer is A.** Adipocytes are the cells that comprise adipose tissue. GLUT4-mediated glucose transport occurs in only two tissue types: adipose (fat) and skeletal muscle. This is the only choice among those listed that could be used in the hypothetical experimental system described.

Answer B is incorrect. Cortical neurons are derived from the brain, where glucose transport occurs independent of insulin stimulation. Thus, these cells could not be used in this hypothetical system.

Answer C is incorrect. Insulin has no effect on glucose uptake in erythrocytes, so this cell type could not be used in this hypothetical system.

Answer D is incorrect. Insulin has no effect on glucose uptake in hepatocytes, so this cell type could not be used in this hypothetical system.

Answer E is incorrect. Pancreatic β cells express GLUT2 transporters, which serve as glucose sensors. These cells do not express GLUT4 transporters and would not be appropriate for use in this hypothetical system.

24. **The correct answer is C.** The positive predictive value (PPV) of the test can be calculated with the following formula, where TP is true-positive results and FP is false-positive results: TP / (TP + FP). Given the pretest probability of 50%, we need to set up a hypothetical 2 × 2

table in which the number of subjects with the disease is equal to the number not having the disease (or to be said differently, the pretest probability becomes the prevalence). If we set the number of those with the disease as 10, then TP = 8 and FP = 1, given the sensitivity of 80% and specificity of 90%. Therefore, the PPV would be calculated as 8 / (8 + 1) = 89%, or about 90%. The same answer can also be obtained by converting the pretest probability to an odds ratio (1:1) and multiplying it by the test's positive likelihood ratio (LR+), which can be calculated using the formula LR+ = sensitivity / (1 - specificity) = 0.80 / (1 - 0.90) = 8. Therefore, the posttest odds of having the disease is 8:1 or 8/9 = 89% once the figure is converted back into a probability.

Answer A is incorrect. This value is too low to be the correct answer.

Answer B is incorrect. This value is too low to be the correct answer.

Answer D is incorrect. This value is too high to be the correct answer.

Answer E is incorrect. This value is too high to be the correct answer.

Answer F is incorrect. This value is too high to be the correct answer.

25. **The correct answer is B.** The femoral canal contains the deep inguinal lymph nodes and is enclosed inside the femoral sheath with the femoral artery and vein. In a femoral hernia, this is the potential space into which abdominal contents herniate. A mnemonic for the contents of the femoral triangle is "N(AVEL)" (laterally to medially) for Nerve, Artery, Vein, Empty space, Lymphatics.

Answer A is incorrect. Cooper's ligament (lacunar ligament) is an extension of the inguinal ligament and forms the medial border of the femoral ring.

Answer C is incorrect. The femoral nerve is found outside of the femoral sheath.

Answer D is incorrect. The obturator nerve runs along the medial edge of the psoas muscle and is posterior to the femoral triangle.

Answer E is incorrect. The tunica vaginalis is the reflection of the peritoneal membrane that invests the testis and spermatic cord. It is formed when the testis descends from the abdomen into the outpouching of peritoneum known as the processus vaginalis. The processus vaginalis normally closes but can remain patent in up to 20% of men. A patent processus vaginalis can lead to hydroceles or indirect hernias, but this structure is not found in the femoral triangle.

26. **The correct answer is A.** Homocystinuria is an inborn error of metabolism caused by a defect in cystathionine synthase, the enzyme that converts homocysteine to cystathionine. Cystathionine is later converted to cysteine, so patients with this enzyme deficiency are required to supplement their diets with exogenous cysteine. In addition to marfanlike features and subluxation of the lens, these patients are at increased risk of a variety of cardiovascular derangements, including premature vascular disease and early death.

Answer B is incorrect. Lysine is another of the essential amino acids (recall the mnemonic **PVT TIM HALL** used to remember the 10 essential amino acids: Phenylalanine, Valine, Tryptophan, Threonine, Isoleucine, Methionine, Histidine, Arginine, Lysine, and Leucine). It is not related to homocystinuria.

Answer C is incorrect. Homocystinuria is a disorder of methionine metabolism; this patient would actually have an excess of methionine as opposed to a deficiency.

Answer D is incorrect. Tryptophan is an amino acid often confused with tyrosine. It is already an essential amino acid and does not have any relationship to homocystinuria.

Answer E is incorrect. Tyrosine is the amino acid affected in phenylketonuria (PKU), a deficiency of phenylalanine hydroxylase. This enzyme deficiency results in an inability to convert phenylalanine to tyrosine, making the latter an essential amino acid in patients with PKU. However, it has no role in homocystinuria.

27. **The correct answer is D.** The adverse effects of cyclophosphamide include nausea, vomiting, myelosuppression, and hemorrhagic cystitis. During its metabolism, cyclophosphamide is converted to its active form by the hepatic cytochrome P-450 enzymes. The final step in the production of the active form is nonenzymatic and produces phosphoramide mustard, the desired cytotoxic agent, and acrolein, an unwanted cytotoxic compound that is directly responsible for hemorrhagic cystitis. This dreaded adverse effect is ameliorated by increasing fluid intake and administering N-acetylcysteine, a sulfhydryl donor. N-acetylcysteine has little impact on the other adverse effects. Mesna is another thiol compound commonly used to prevent cyclophosphamide-induced hemorrhagic cystitis.

Answer A is incorrect. Acrolein is an unwanted cytotoxic compound and is not a treatment.

Answer B is incorrect. Acrolein is an unwanted cytotoxic compound and is not a treatment.

Answer C is incorrect. Acrolein is an unwanted cytotoxic compound and is not a treatment.

Answer E is incorrect. N-acetylcysteine has little impact on myelosuppression.

Answer F is incorrect. N-acetylcysteine has little impact on nausea and vomiting.

28. **The correct answer is B.** Right upper quadrant pain in an obese, middle-aged, multiparous woman with ultrasonographic findings consistent with gallstones is a classic presentation of acute calculous cholecystitis. Acute calculous cholecystitis is an acute mechanical inflammation of the gallbladder commonly resulting from a gallbladder stone obstructing the gallbladder neck or cystic duct, chemical inflammation, and/or bacterial inflammation. Risk factors are the "4F's": Female, "Fat," Fertile, and Forty. Definitive treatment is cholecystectomy.

Answer A is incorrect. Acute acalculous cholecystitis, in contrast to acute calculous cholecystitis, occurs in the absence of gallstones, generally in a severely ill patient.

Answer C is incorrect. Acute pancreatitis usually presents with radiating epigastric pain and increased serum amylase levels. This is in contrast to the nonradiating right upper quadrant abdominal pain and normal amylase levels seen in this patient.

Answer D is incorrect. Carcinoma of the pancreas often presents with jaundice and abdominal pain radiating to the back. It may also present with migratory thrombophlebitis (Trousseau's sign). This presentation differs significantly from the one described in the question.

Answer E is incorrect. Cholesterolosis, or strawberry gallbladder, is characterized by yellow cholesterol-containing flecks in the mucosal surface. In contrast to this patient's diagnosis, it is not associated with inflammatory changes (normal erythrocyte sedimentation rate and WBC count) and has no special association with cholelithiasis.

29. **The correct answer is C.** This patient has secondary hyperparathyroidism due to chronic renal insufficiency or renal osteodystrophy. There are numerous etiologies of chronic renal failure; the most common cause in the U.S. is diabetic nephropathy secondary to diabetes mellitus. The central problems in secondary hyperparathyroidism are impaired Ca^{2+} reabsorption and phosphate excretion from the kidneys due to nephron loss. The resulting hypocalcemia stimulates increased secretion of parathyroid hormone (secondary hyperparathyroidism), causing increased bone turnover and contributing to the hyperphosphatemia. Moreover, nephron loss results in impaired conversion of 25-OH vitamin D to 1,25-dihydroxy vitamin D, reducing Ca^{2+} absorption from the intestines and thus exacerbating hypocalcemia in this syndrome.

Answer A is incorrect. Parathyroid adenoma would cause increased secretion of parathyroid hormone, resulting in hypercalcemia and hypophosphatemia rather than hypocalcemia and hyperphosphatemia.

Answer B is incorrect. Parathyroid insufficiency would result in hypocalcemia but cannot account for the hyperphosphatemia presented in this case.

Answer D is incorrect. Malignancy usually results in hypercalcemia either due to lytic metastases to bone (with increased serum alkaline phosphatase activity and hyperphosphatemia) or due to production of parathyroid hormone-related peptide (with hypophosphatemia).

Answer E is incorrect. Vitamin D intoxication results in hypercalcemia and hyperphosphatemia and thus would be inconsistent with the low calcium value presented in the vignette. However, vitamin D intoxication may indeed present with the clinical findings stated above, including pruritis, bone pain, weakness, and renal dysfunction.

30. **The correct answer is B.** This is a clinical picture of restrictive lung disease; the FEV_1:FVC ratio is approximately normal, but both are dramatically reduced. Amiodarone is an antiarrhythmic that can cause pulmonary fibrosis, a restrictive lung disease.

Answer A is incorrect. Asthma is a cause of chronic obstructive pulmonary disease.

Answer C is incorrect. Diltiazem is an antiarrhythmic that is sometimes used in intravenous form to treat atrial fibrillation. It infrequently causes hypotension or bradyarrhythmias, but is not known to cause pulmonary fibrosis.

Answer D is incorrect. Sotalol has both β-blocking and action potential-prolonging activity. It is used for treatment of ventricular and supraventricular arrhythmias in children and for life-threatening ventricular arrhythmias in adults. It can sometimes cause torsades de pointes when taken at higher doses. However, sotalol does not cause pulmonary fibrosis.

Answer E is incorrect. Tobacco is a known risk factor for chronic obstructive pulmonary disease (COPD). COPD presents with an FEV_1:FVC ratio of <80% and a sloping flow-volume curve.

31. **The correct answer is C.** Bloody diarrhea and fever can have a number of bacterial causes, including *Escherichia coli* (O157:H7), *Salmonella*, and *Shigella* species. Other bacterial

causes include *Campylobacter jejuni* and *Yersinia enterocolitica*. Both *Salmonella* and *Shigella* species are gram-negative rods that do not ferment lactose and are oxidase-negative. *Salmonella*, however, is motile, while *Shigella* is not. When a bacterium that ferments lactose is plated on MacConkey agar, the colonies are pink/red. If the plated bacteria do not ferment lactose, the colonies are clear.

Answer A is incorrect. Certain strains of *E. coli* (O157:H7) can cause bloody diarrhea. However, *E. coli* does ferment lactose, which would result in the growth of pink colonies on MacConkey agar.

Answer B is incorrect. *Pseudomonas aeruginosa* is a frequent cause of nosocomial pulmonary infection in intubated patients and those with cystic fibrosis. It does not cause bloody diarrhea, and although it is a non-lactose-fermenting, gram-negative bacillus, it is oxidase-positive.

Answer D is incorrect. Enteric shigellosis can present similarly to *Salmonella* species infection. They also are oxidase-negative, non-lactose-fermenting, gram-negative rods. However, *Shigella* species are nonmotile, while *Salmonella* species are motile.

Answer E is incorrect. *Vibrio* species are curved, motile, gram-negative rods. However, *Vibrio cholerae* causes rice-water stools, not bloody diarrhea.

32. **The correct answer is E.** This patient has Turcot syndrome, an autosomal dominant disease. All familial polyposis syndromes, with the exception of Peutz-Jeghers syndrome, predispose to colorectal cancer. Turcot syndrome is associated with two separate dominant mutations. The first is a mutation of the *APC* gene leading to polyposis and medulloblastoma, and the second is associated with the *hMLH1* DNA mismatch repair gene leading to polyposis and glioblastoma multiforme.

Answer A is incorrect. Familial adenomatous polyposis is associated with hundreds of colorectal polyps, and nearly all affected patients will develop colorectal cancer.

Answer B is incorrect. Gardner syndrome is characterized by colorectal polyposis and osteomas or other bone and soft tissue tumors.

Answer C is incorrect. Hereditary nonpolyposis colorectal carcinoma is associated with dozens of colorectal polyps, and a majority of affected patients will develop colorectal cancer.

Answer D is incorrect. Tuberous sclerosis is an autosomal dominant condition characterized by mental retardation, seizures, tuberous central nervous system tumors, angiomyolipomas of the kidneys, leptomeningeal tumors, and skin lesions such as ash-leaf spots and shagreen patches.

33. **The correct answer is B.** This question describes enzyme-linked immunosorbent assay (ELISA). ELISA is an immunologic technique used in laboratories to determine whether a particular antibody is present in a patient's blood. Labeled antibodies are used to detect whether the serum contains antibodies against a specific antigen precoated on an ELISA plate. The patient's serum can also be challenged with a specific antibody to determine whether the corresponding antigen is present in the patient's blood.

Answer A is incorrect. Allele-specific oligonucleotide probes are short labeled DNA sequences complementary to an allele of interest. These probes can be used to detect the presence of disease-causing mutations.

Answer C is incorrect. Northern blots are similar to Southern blots except that in Northern blotting, mRNA is separated by electrophoresis instead of DNA. This is not the technique described above.

Answer D is incorrect. Polymerase chain reaction is a laboratory technique used to produce many copies of a segment of DNA. In the procedure, DNA is mixed with two specific primers, deoxynucleotides and a heat-stable polymerase. The solution is heated to denature the DNA and is then cooled to allow synthesis. Twenty cycles of heating and cooling amplify the DNA over a million times. This is not the procedure described above.

Answer E is incorrect. Sequencing is a laboratory technique that utilizes dideoxynucleotides to randomly terminate growing strands of DNA. Gel electrophoresis is used to separate the varying lengths of DNA. The DNA sequence can then be read based on the position of the bands on the gel. This is not the technique described above.

Answer F is incorrect. In a Southern blot procedure, DNA is separated with electrophoresis, denatured, transferred to a filter, and hybridized with a labeled DNA probe. Regions on the filter that base-pair with the labeled DNA probes can be identified when the filter is exposed to film that is sensitive to the radiolabeled probe. This is not the technique described above.

Answer G is incorrect. In a Western blot procedure, protein is separated by electrophoresis and labeled antibodies are used as a probe. This technique can be used to detect the existence of an antibody to a particular protein.

34. **The correct answer is B.** To answer this question, one must know that Kawasaki's syndrome (also referred to as mucocutaneous lymph node syndrome) is an arteritis that primarily affects medium- and small-sized arteries. Hence, it makes sense that there is evidence suggesting the formation of anti-endothelial cell (and anti–smooth muscle cell) autoantibodies in patients with this disease. The clinical manifestations of this disease include fever for more than 5 days, cervical lymphadenopathy, a skin rash (which often has desquamation, or shedding of the skin), and erythema of the conjunctivae, oral mucosa, palms, and soles. Eighty percent of patients are under the age of 4 years. Twenty percent of patients develop cardiovascular disease, including coronary artery vasculitis and coronary artery aneurysm.

Answer A is incorrect. Anticentromere antibodies, which are found in 90% of patients with the CREST variant of scleroderma, are not particularly associated with Kawasaki's syndrome.

Answer C is incorrect. Antihistone antibodies, which are found in over 95% of patients with drug-induced lupus erythematosus, are not particularly associated with Kawasaki's syndrome.

Answer D is incorrect. Anti-IgG (rheumatoid factor) is not particularly associated with Kawasaki's syndrome. Elevated levels of serum rheumatoid factor are present in 80% of patients with rheumatoid arthritis.

Answer E is incorrect. Antinuclear antibodies, which are present in over 95% of patients with systemic lupus erythematosus, are not particularly associated with Kawasaki's syndrome.

35. **The correct answer is D.** Because aspirin is a weak acid with a pK_a near 3.5, it can interconvert between neutral and negatively charged forms depending on the pH. Increasing the pH of tubular fluid shifts the equilibrium toward the deprotonated charged state of the molecule. Thus, neutral molecules diffusing into the tubule will become ionized. Once in the charged state, molecules cannot diffuse back across tubular epithelial membranes to the bloodstream. Thus the clearance of aspirin is greatly increased when urine pH is alkalinized.

Answer A is incorrect. Acidification of the urine would lower the pH and shift the equilibrium toward the protonated neutral form of aspirin. These nonionized molecules could then move back into the bloodstream and clearance of aspirin would be decreased.

Answer B is incorrect. Acidification of the urine would lower the pH and shift the equilibrium toward the protonated neutral form of aspirin, but these molecules can diffuse across cell membranes back into the bloodstream and would not be excreted.

Answer C is incorrect. Acidification of the urine has no effect on the glomerular filtration rate (GFR). GFR is affected by the difference in pressures across the glomerulus and glomerular permeability.

Answer E is incorrect. Alkalinization of urine promotes ionization of aspirin in the urine; the concentration of nonionized molecules of aspirin in the tubule would decrease as the urine is alkalinized.

Answer F is incorrect. Alkalinization of the urine has no effect on the GFR. GFR is affected by the difference in pressures across the glomerulus and glomerular permeability.

36. **The correct answer is D.** Intracranial metastases represent nearly half of all brain tumors, yet only 15% of tumors metastasize to the brain. Intracranial hemorrhages are a recognized but relatively uncommon complication of brain tumors and can result in intraparenchymal, subarachnoid, subdural, and epidural hematomas. Focal neurologic signs are frequently evident and are due to pressure exerted on the brain parenchyma. Renal cell carcinomas, choriocarcinomas, melanomas, retinoblastomas, and lung and breast cancers can result in hemorrhagic brain metastases. Since melanoma is a relatively frequent source of metastatic lesions to the brain (although less common than breast or lung carcinoma) and demonstrates a tendency to hemorrhage, melanoma is the correct answer in this case.

Answer A is incorrect. Angiosarcomas are malignant endothelial neoplasms that resemble hemangiomas. Although these tumors may bleed, angiosarcomas rarely metastasize, and only a few case reports exist of hemorrhage of cerebral metastasis from angiosarcoma.

Answer B is incorrect. Some cancers rarely metastasize to the brain; these include carcinomas of the oropharynx, esophagus, and prostate, as well as nonmelanoma skin cancers.

Answer C is incorrect. Colorectal carcinoma does metastasize to the brain (though less frequently than melanoma) but does not typically result in intracranial hemorrhage. Since colorectal carcinoma is less likely than melanoma to result in brain metastases and is not as likely to hemorrhage, melanoma is a better answer.

Answer E is incorrect. Carcinoma of the prostate almost never results in metastatic brain disease and therefore represents an extremely unlikely etiology for this patient's disease.

37. **The correct answer is E.** Minimal change disease results in nephrotic syndrome, which is primarily manifested in the loss of significant protein in the urine. As a result of this protein loss, the plasma protein concentration will go down, thus decreasing the oncotic pressure in the glomerular capillary. According to the Starling equation ($GFR = K_f [(P_{GC} - P_{BS}) - (p_{GC} - p_{BS})]$), this change will lead to a higher GFR by decreasing the oncotic forces that normally oppose ultrafiltration.

Answer A is incorrect. Tubular hydrostatic pressures are not affected by nephrotic syndrome. The Bowman's space hydrostatic pressure generally does not decrease.

Answer B is incorrect. Tubular hydrostatic pressures are not affected by nephrotic syndrome. The Bowman's space hydrostatic pressure could be increased in a patient with an obstruction to urine flow.

Answer C is incorrect. Bowman's space oncotic pressure will increase, not decrease, as protein is filtered into Bowman's space and thus increases the protein concentration there.

Answer D is incorrect. Hydrostatic pressures are not affected in minimal change disease. The glomerular capillary hydrostatic pressure could be increased with constriction of the efferent arteriole, for example.

38. **The correct answer is E.** The male urethra is made up of three parts. The prostatic urethra runs through the prostate. The membranous urethra runs through the urogenital diaphragm, and the penile urethra runs through the penis. Rupture of the urethra below the urogenital diaphragm (at the junction between the membranous and the penile urethra) from a so-called "straddle injury" causes urine to flow into the scrotum and the perineal region.

Answer A is incorrect. Anterior bladder wall rupture is caused by a fractured pelvis. In this kind of injury, urine will flow into the retropubic space.

Answer B is incorrect. Penile urethra rupture occurs following a crush injury. Urine will flow into the deep fascia of Buck within the penis.

Answer C is incorrect. Superior bladder wall rupture, also called dome rupture, is caused by forceful compression of a full bladder. This form of bladder rupture causes urine to flow into the peritoneal cavity.

Answer D is incorrect. Urethral rupture above the urogenital diaphragm (at the junction of the prostatic and membranous urethra) due to a fractured pelvis or improper catheter insertion causes urine to flow into the retropubic space.

39. **The correct answer is A.** *Enterococcus faecalis* and *E. faecium* (Lancefield group D streptococci) are normal flora of the intestine and can cause both urinary tract infection and infectious endocarditis. They are very hardy organisms that are able to grow in salt and bile solutions. They can be γ- or α-hemolytic and are optochin- and penicillin-resistant. Recently, strains of enterococcus have become resistant to vancomycin. Vancomycin-resistant enterococci can cause a life-threatening nosocomial infection.

Answer B is incorrect. *Staphylococcus epidermidis* is a catalase-positive, coagulase-negative, novobiocin-sensitive organism. It is the cause of infection in many patients with artificial prosthetic devices such as catheters, heart valves, and vascular shunts.

Answer C is incorrect. *Streptococcus agalactiae* is a bacitracin-resistant, β-hemolytic group B streptococcus. It is the leading cause of neonatal meningitis but does not usually cause symptomatic infection in adults. *S. agalactiae* is usually penicillin-sensitive.

Answer D is incorrect. *Streptococcus pneumoniae* is a significant cause of many different types of infections, including pneumonia. *S. pneumoniae* is an α-hemolytic, optochin-sensitive organism. The majority of *S. pneumoniae* strains are still sensitive to penicillin and do not grow in bile.

Answer E is incorrect. *Streptococcus sanguis* is similar to *E. faecalis* in that it is optochin-resistant and bile-tolerant. Although resistance to penicillin among the viridans group of streptococci (which includes *S. sanguis*) is increasing, most strains are still susceptible. The viri-

dans streptococci are α-hemolytic, while the enterococci can be either α- or γ-hemolytic.

40. **The correct answer is F.** This child has intermittent maple syrup urine disease (MSUD). MSUD is caused by an inability to degrade the carbon skeleton of the three branched chain amino acids valine, leucine, and isoleucine. MSUD has many subtypes; the two most common are classical and intermittent. Classical MSUD presents with ketonuria 48 hours to 1 week after birth. The intermittent form presents during times of catabolism such as after infections. If left untreated, MSUD can lead to seizure, coma, and death. Dietary restriction of branched-chained amino acids is the mainstay of treatment.

Answer A is incorrect. Gaucher's disease results from an accumulation of glucosylceramide in macrophages of bone marrow, spleen, and liver due to deficiency of glucocerebrosidase. Patients may present with bone pain and fractures, thrombocytopenia, and hepatosplenomegaly.

Answer B is incorrect. Histidine breakdown is impaired in histidase deficiency, which can lead to histidinemia. Mental retardation is common but not always present in this disease. It is 20 times more common than MSUD.

Answer C is incorrect. Phenylalanine degradation deficiencies are characteristic of PKU. This is screened for at birth and the main symptom is mental retardation.

Answer D is incorrect. Deficiency of sphingomyelinase can lead to Niemann–Pick disease, an autosomal recessive disorder characterized by hepatosplenomegaly, macular cherry-red spot, and loss of motor skills and neurologic function.

Answer E is incorrect. Phenylalanine is converted to tyrosine, which is degraded by homogentisate oxidase. Deficiency of this enzyme leads to a buildup of phenylalanine and tyrosine. This disorder is known as alkaptonuria, which results in black-appearing urine when left untreated.

41. **The correct answer is B.** This patient presents with chronic diarrhea, intermittent facial flushing, and a murmur consistent with tricuspid stenosis, a triad of findings classic for carcinoid syndrome. One-third of carcinoid tumors of the gastrointestinal tract occur in the midgut-derived small bowel, which begins at the ligament of Treitz and ends at the mid transverse colon. While adenocarcinoma is the most common type of small bowel tumor, carcinoid tumors are most likely to occur in the small bowel. Carcinoid tumors of the small intestine secrete serotonin, which is usually metabolized by the liver and doesn't cause the symptoms of the carcinoid syndrome. However, when metastases to the liver are present, the bioactive amines can no longer be metabolized and enter the systemic circulation causing diarrhea, abdominal cramps, gastrointestinal bleeding, malabsorption, flushing, bronchospasm, and right heart valvular disease from serotonin-mediated fibroelastosis. Electron microscopy reveals "salt and pepper" granulation of cells, consistent with their neuroendocrine origin. An elevated urinary 5-HIAA level is diagnostic of carcinoid syndrome.

Answer A is incorrect. The gastroesophageal junction is affected by gastroesophageal reflux disease, not carcinoid tumors.

Answer C is incorrect. The pancreaticoduodenal junction is the site where pancreatic endocrine and exocrine secretions empty into the small bowel to aid in digestion. It is part of the foregut-derived intestine, and it is a rare site for carcinoid tumors.

Answer D is incorrect. The rectosigmoid junction is not a common location for carcinoid tumors.

Answer E is incorrect. The splenic flexure is a watershed area that is susceptible to ischemic damage if cardiac output becomes low. It is not, however, a common site for carcinoid tumors.

42. **The correct answer is A.** The clinical vignette gives a description of dermatomyositis, an im-mune-mediated disorder that involves the skin and skeletal muscles. The distinctive rash of this disease is characterized by a violet discoloration of the upper eyelids together with periorbital edema. Patients often develop a gradual symmetric muscle weakness of the proximal muscles, which may manifest as difficulty getting up from chairs; one-third of patients develop muscle weakness that causes dysphagia. The disease often also presents with Gottron's lesions, which are erythematous patches over the knuckles, elbows, and knees. Between 6% and 45% of patients with dermatomyositis have an underlying visceral cancer.

Answer B is incorrect. Osteoarthritis is a degenerative joint disease characterized by joint inflammation and destruction secondary to wear and tear. It is not notably associated with dermatomyositis.

Answer C is incorrect. The diagnosis of psoriasis is characterized by nonpruritic scaly/silvery erythematous plaques with well-defined borders. Nevertheless, psoriasis is not notably associated with dermatomyositis.

Answer D is incorrect. Secondary syphilis often develops 6 weeks after an untreated primary chancre of syphilis has healed. It is characterized by fever, lymphadenopathy, skin rashes (widespread small, flat lesions that particularly involve the palms, soles, and oral mucosa), and condylomata lata (painless wartlike lesions that present in the vulva, the scrotum, or other warm, moist areas of the body). This disease is not notably associated with dermatomyositis.

Answer E is incorrect. Zenker's diverticulum, also known as pharyngoesophageal diverticulum, is an outpouching of the esophageal wall above the level of the upper esophageal sphincter that results from herniation of mucosa through a defective muscular layer. While this disease may cause dysphagia, it is not notably associated with dermatomyositis.

43. **The correct answer is B.** Allergic interstitial nephritis is an intrarenal cause of acute renal failure. The cause of interstitial nephritis is usually medications, but infections and immu-

nologic disorders occasionally precipitate the disorder. Medications that cause interstitial nephritis include penicillins (particularly methicillin and nafcillin), cephalosporins, sulfonamides, and nonsteroidal anti-inflammatory drugs. Clinical findings include fever, rash, and peripheral eosinophilia. Eosinophilia is also seen on urinalysis, along with RBCs and proteinuria.

Answer A is incorrect. IgA nephropathy (Berger's disease) is a primary renal disease with deposition of IgA in the glomerulus. Patients usually present with gross hematuria of little clinical significance following an infection. Unlike postinfectious glomerulonephritis, no latent period exists between infection and renal symptoms. Eosinophilia is not present.

Answer C is incorrect. Poststreptococcal glomerulonephritis is a type of immune complex glomerulonephritis that causes enlargement of glomeruli with infiltration of neutrophils and mesangial cell proliferation. This condition usually presents in children about 2 weeks after skin or throat infection with *Streptococcus pyogenes*. Most patients have antistreptolysin O, which can be helpful in making the diagnosis. The classic presentation is oliguric renal failure with nephritic syndrome. It is not associated with eosinophilia.

Answer D is incorrect. In rapidly progressive glomerulonephritis (RPGN), patients develop renal failure over a period of weeks to months. They present with renal failure and nephritic syndrome. Pathologically, RPGN is characterized by crescent formation involving most glomeruli. There are many etiologies for nephritic syndrome/RPGN. One would not expect to see eosinophils

Answer E is incorrect. SLE is an inflammatory autoimmune disorder that affects multiple organ systems. SLE frequently causes renal damage that can present as either nephrotic or nephritic syndrome or be asymptomatic. Urinalysis typically shows microscopic hematuria and proteinuria but not eosinophilia. End-stage renal disease is a common cause of death in SLE.

44. **The correct answer is D.** This patient is in diabetic ketoacidosis (DKA), which is often the presenting syndrome in type 1 diabetes mellitus. The initial management of this condition requires aggressive fluid resuscitation and correction of hyperglycemia with insulin. Insulin stimulates the shift of potassium from the extracellular compartment to the intracellular compartment, causing a decrease in serum potassium levels and possible cardiac conduction abnormalities. In addition, the rise in serum pH (as a result of correcting the ketoacidosis with insulin) will cause hydrogen ions to come out of the cells, and their positive charge will be replaced by potassium ions moving intracellularly, leading to further hypokalemia. Thus, patients with a low serum potassium level before administering insulin should be considered to have a potentially life-threatening low total body potassium level. Hence, after the administration of insulin, judicious administration of potassium is the most important step in the treatment of DKA. In addition, calcium gluconate should be administered to protect cardiac myocytes and prevent arrhythmias.

Answer A is incorrect. Bicarbonate does not undergo insulin-mediated transcellular shifts as is the case with potassium. Bicarbonate levels often normalize with the correction of hyperglycemia and fluid administration with diuresis of serum ketoacids. Bicarbonate should be administered only when serum levels are <15 mEq/L.

Answer B is incorrect. Calcium does not undergo insulin-mediated transcellular shifts, as is the case with potassium; hence, serum levels of calcium do not fluctuate to the same extent with DKA and insulin administration. Calcium gluconate is generally administered to protect cardiomyocytes against arrhythmias that may result from abnormal serum potassium levels; serum calcium levels per se are usually not the concern in patients with DKA.

Answer C is incorrect. Chloride does not undergo insulin-mediated transcellular shifts, as is the case with potassium; hence, serum levels of chloride do not fluctuate to the same extent with DKA and insulin administration. Appropriate fluid resuscitation is generally sufficient to manage serum chloride levels in patients who may be dehydrated.

Answer E is incorrect. Sodium does not undergo insulin-mediated transcellular shifts, as is the case with potassium. Serum sodium levels therefore do not fluctuate to the same extent with DKA and insulin administration. Fluid resuscitation is generally sufficient to manage serum sodium levels in patients who may be dehydrated.

45. **The correct answer is E.** The history and physical examination suggest a possible cerebrovascular accident. Before any therapeutic intervention is done, an emergent CT scan must be performed to rule out hemorrhage. In the emergent setting, CT scans are favored over MRI. The CT scan shown does not demonstrate any signs of intracranial hemorrhage. Given the high clinical suspicion for stroke, your attention should focus on the likely possibility of an ischemic etiology. It is important to remember, however, that an ischemic infarct will often not be visible on the initial scan, especially if the scan is done within a few hours of symptom onset. Tissue plasminogen activator (t-PA), a thrombolytic agent, is the best next step in management given that the patient does not have any obvious contraindications to thrombolytic therapy. Treatment with t-PA has been shown to be very effective in the management of acute ischemic stroke, especially if administered within 3 hours of symptom onset. This form of treatment does, however, carry a risk of hemorrhage.

Answer A is incorrect. Once a hemorrhagic stroke has been ruled out by CT scan, the possibility of a cardioembolic source should be investigated with an echocardiogram. Patients with a history of atrial fibrillation are at significantly increased risk of thromboembolism. Thrombolysis/anticoagulation, however, helps restore perfusion to the brain and therefore should be done first.

Answer B is incorrect. Some strokes, particularly those involving the middle cerebral artery,

are associated with significant parenchymal edema and subsequent mass effect, with possible sequelae including herniation and death. Hemicraniectomy is a rather novel therapeutic intervention that involves temporarily removing half of the skull over the edematous area with the goal of relieving pressure and reducing the chance of herniation. This intervention is not widely used and is not considered the standard of care in the management of acute stroke.

Answer C is incorrect. Heparin therapy is the next step in management for patients who have contraindications to thrombolytic therapy. Such contraindications include past history of hemorrhagic stroke, active internal bleed, history of surgery within the past 3 weeks, and any form of coagulopathy. As with tissue plasminogen activator, it is imperative to rule out the presence of intracranial hemorrhage with a CT scan before initiating therapy.

Answer D is incorrect. Hyperglycemia worsens functional outcomes in cases of ischemic stroke. It has been hypothesized that hyperglycemia may increase local tissue acidosis and blood-brain barrier permeability. While glucose control with insulin would help minimize the harmful effects of hyperglycemia, it is not the next step in management.

46. **The correct answer is A.** *Bartonella henselae* is a gram-negative bacillus that is the cause of cat-scratch disease. Typically (in 60% of cases), a child is scratched by a bacteremic young cat, and a papule or pustule develops in the area 3–5 days later. Tender regional lymphadenopathy develops in 1–2 weeks. Most patients present with systemic symptoms such as anorexia, fever, and malaise.

Answer B is incorrect. The spirochete *Borrelia burgdorferi* is the cause of Lyme disease. The spirochete is carried by the *Ixodes* tick, which is most common in the northeastern United States. It initially presents with an expanding ring-shaped lesion known as erythema migrans, which begins at the site of the tick bite.

Answer C is incorrect. *Eikenella corrodens* is a gram-negative organism that is part of the normal flora of the mouth and nasopharynx. It is associated with infections resulting from human bites.

Answer D is incorrect. *Francisella tularensis* is the cause of tularemia. This disease is carried by wild rabbits and ticks in the southeastern United States. It often presents with lymphadenopathy and an ulcer at the site of entry as well as with fever.

Answer E is incorrect. *Pasteurella multocida* is caused by cat bites and dog bites. This infection causes a rapid inflammation (often within hours) and is accompanied by purulent drainage.

47. **The correct answer is D.** The vignette describes a classic history of an autoimmune hyperthyroidism, Graves' disease. In this disorder, thyroid follicular cells are stimulated to synthesized and secrete thyroid hormone by anti-TSH receptor antibodies, leading to increased levels of thyroxine (T_4) and triiodothyronine (T_3) in the blood, which results in negative feedback on the anterior pituitary and suppression of TSH secretion. Thus, both free T_4 and total T_4, which includes free T_4 and T_4 bound to proteins in the blood (e.g., albumin and thyroxine-binding globulin) will be increased, while blood TSH levels will be low relative to the normal baseline.

Answer A is incorrect. An elevated TSH level is not characteristic of Graves' disease, and elevated T_4 levels should result in a lower TSH level due to negative feedback on the anterior pituitary.

Answer B is incorrect. An elevated TSH level is not characteristic of Graves' disease, and an elevated T_4 level should result in a lower TSH level due to negative feedback on the anterior pituitary. Furthermore, thyroid hormone binding to proteins in the blood should not be decreased but instead should be increased in the setting of increased free T_4. Therefore, the total T_4 level should be elevated rather than low.

Answer C is incorrect. Graves' disease is characterized by a low TSH due to the circulating thyroid-stimulating immunoglobulins which elevate the T_3 and T_4 levels and, via negative feedback, downregulate the level of TSH. In this answer choice, the level of TSH is elevated, which would lead to elevated, not diminished, levels of T_3 and T_4.

Answer E is incorrect. Total and free T_4 levels are expected to be low in the setting of low TSH levels. However, in Graves' disease, stimulation of TSH receptors on the thyroid follicular cells by anti-TSH receptor antibodies stimulates the secretion of thyroid hormones and results in increased total and free T_4 levels in the setting of normal or even low TSH levels. The resulting negative feedback loop to the anterior pituitary leads to reduced TSH levels.

48. **The correct answer is C.** The classic symptoms of Hodgkin's disease include nonspecific constitutional symptoms such as night sweats, fatigue, fever, and weight loss. Additionally, mediastinal lymphadenopathy is common, and biopsy of affected nodes will show Reed-Sternberg cells on a background of reactive inflammatory cells, just as described in the question stem. A variety of chemotherapeutic agents can be used for treatment of Hodgkin's disease, including doxorubicin.

Answer A is incorrect. Azathioprine is used as an immunosuppressant in kidney transplant patients and those with autoimmune disorders.

Answer B is incorrect. Cisplatin (as well as other platinum-based chemotherapeutics) is used in the treatment of testicular, ovarian, and lung cancers.

Answer D is incorrect. Paclitaxel (Taxol) is used for treatment of ovarian and breast cancers.

Answer E is incorrect. β-Interferon is used in treatment of multiple sclerosis.

Test Block 2

1. An oncologist recently discovered that certain cancerous cells secrete a protein named ca-1panc. Using this protein, he developed a new blood test to detect this type of cancer. He performed the blood test on 1,000 patients. One hundred of these patients had the cancer, and the test came back positive for 60 of them, while for the remaining 40 patients the test was negative. Nine hundred of the patients did not have the cancer; however, the test was positive for 100 of them. In the remaining 800, the test came back negative. Which of the following numbers represents how well the test identified those who had the cancer?

(A) 10.0%
(B) 37.5%
(C) 60.0%
(D) 88.8%
(E) 90.0%
(F) 95.2%

2. A 27-year-old woman who is pregnant at 32 weeks' gestation presents to the emergency department following a motor vehicle accident. Results of fetal heart monitoring are reassuring, and there is no evidence of rupture of membranes. Radiologic studies show a fractured femur. The patient is admitted to the hospital for expectant management and is placed on strict bed rest with delivery planned at 37 weeks' gestation. Which of the following medications would be most appropriate for preventing deep venous thrombosis in this patient?

(A) Heparin
(B) Indomethacin
(C) Prostaglandin E_2
(D) Streptokinase
(E) Warfarin

3. A 38-year-old woman with a history of type 2 diabetes mellitus gives birth to a term male infant. Immediately after birth, the infant is noted to be cyanotic and tachypneic. His hypoxemia quickly worsens over minutes, and he is taken to cardiac catheterization, where a balloon is guided to perforate the atrial septum.

He is also given an infusion of prostaglandin E_1. The infant's hypoxia stabilizes, and he is later taken for definitive, corrective surgery. Which of the following is the underlying pathophysiology of this infant's hypoxemia?

(A) Coarctation of the aorta
(B) Concomitant ventricular septal defect
(C) Delayed closure of the ductus arteriosus
(D) Failure of the aorticopulmonary septum to spiral
(E) Overriding aorta

4. A 34-year-old man presents to his primary care physician with night sweats, a fever of 38° C (100.2° F), and weight loss of 5 kg (12 lb) over the last 3 months. A CT scan demonstrates mediastinal lymphadenopathy, and results of a biopsy of the node are shown in the image. Which of the following drugs is part of the multidrug regimen that would be used to manage this patient's disease?

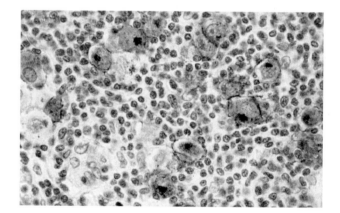

Reproduced, with permission, from Lichtman MA, Beutler E, Kipps TJ, Seligsohn U, Kaushansky K, Prchal JF. *Williams Hematology*, 7th ed. New York: McGraw-Hill, 2006: Color Plate XXII-34.

(A) Cyclosporine
(B) Hydroxyurea
(C) Imatinib
(D) Isoniazid
(E) Vinblastine

5. A 14-year-old high school freshman presents to her family doctor for a sports physical. She has not played organized sports in the past but is in good physical shape. She mentions that she experienced severe leg cramps after trying out for the soccer team last week. The night after the tryouts, she noticed that her urine had a reddish tinge. She has no other medical complaints. Her physician orders an ischemic forearm exercise test, which reveals no increase in venous lactate. Which of the following enzymes is most likely deficient in this patient?

(A) Cystathionine synthase
(B) Glucose-6-phosphatase
(C) α-1,6-Glucosidase
(D) Glycogen phosphorylase
(E) Lysosomal α–1,4-glucosidase

6. A 35-year-old man comes to the physician because he has been experiencing bone pain, in addition to confusion, lethargy, recurrent renal stones, duodenal ulcer, and a small nodule on the anterior neck. Laboratory tests show:

Calcium: 17 mg/dL
Phosphate: 1.0 mg/dL
Alkaline phosphatase: 500 U/L
Parathyroid hormone: 900 pg/mL

Which of the following is most likely to be seen in this patient's bones?

(A) Hypertrophic osteoarthropathy
(B) Osteitis fibrosa cystica
(C) Osteopetrosis
(D) Osteoporosis
(E) Paget's disease of the bone

7. A 45-year-old man comes to the physician with a 3-day history of a temperature of 39° C (102.2° F). He also complains of headache, neck stiffness, and a maculopapular rash on his trunk. A diagnosis of meningitis is made, and a smear and culture of his cerebrospinal fluid identify *Neisseria meningitidis* as the causative agent. In the most severe form of meningococcemia, which of the following symptoms is most likely to develop?

(A) Acute renal failure and thrombocytopenia with hemolytic anemia

(B) Fever, migratory polyarthritis, and carditis
(C) Fever, new murmur, small erythematous lesions on the palms, and splinter hemorrhages on the nail bed
(D) Shock, widespread purpura, disseminated intravascular coagulation, and adrenal insufficiency
(E) Symmetric ascending muscle weakness beginning in the distal lower extremities

8. Cyclooxygenase-2 (COX-2) inhibitors, unlike similar nonselective nonsteroidal anti-inflammatory drugs, may be associated with cardiovascular events, including myocardial infarction. Which of the following proposals might explain why selective COX-2 inhibitors may cause more cardiovascular events than does aspirin? (PGI_2 = prostaglandin I_2, TxA_2 = thromboxane A_2)

	CHOICE	PGI_2	TxA_2
A	COX-2 inhibitor	↑	—
	Aspirin	↓	↓
B	COX-2 inhibitor	—	↑
	Aspirin	↓	↓
C	COX-2 inhibitor	↓	↓
	Aspirin	↓	↓
D	COX-2 inhibitor	↓	—
	Aspirin	↑	↑
E	COX-2 inhibitor	↓	—
	Aspirin	↓	↓

(A) A
(B) B
(C) C
(D) D
(E) E

9. A 30-year-old woman with systemic lupus erythematosus treated with high-dose prednisone comes to her physician with symptoms of anemia. The patient's blood studies show a low hemoglobin level (10 g/dL), a low serum iron level, an elevated ferritin level, and a low total iron-binding capacity with normocytic RBCs on blood smear. Which of the following is the most appropriate treatment for this patient's anemia?

(A) Erythropoietin
(B) Ferrous sulfate
(C) Folate
(D) Parenteral vitamin B$_{12}$
(E) Phlebotomy

10. A 7-year-old girl is brought to the emergency department by her parents because of concerns that she is not growing and not developing appropriately. The parents say that the patient has cold intolerance, easy fatigability, and polyuria. A physical examination is notable for short stature and bilateral papilledema. Thyroid function tests are notable for low levels of triiodothyronine, thyroxine, and thyroid-stimulating hormone (TSH). An MRI shows an enhancing multilobulated suprasellar mass with ring calcification in the region of the sella turcica. If the lesion represents a primary intracranial neoplasm, which of the following is the most likely diagnosis?

(A) Craniopharyngioma
(B) Ependymoma
(C) Hemangioblastoma
(D) Prolactinoma
(E) Thyrotropinoma

11. An obese 56-year-old African-American man with a 25-pack-year history of smoking experiences chest pain associated with an apparent heart attack. The pain radiates to the man's left shoulder and down his left arm. What is the reason for referred pain to this region?

(A) Lymphatic drainage of mediators of inflammation and pain
(B) Proximity of sensory nerve fiber tracts in the anterior horn of the spinal cord
(C) Proximity of sensory nerve fiber tracts in the posterior horn of the spinal cord
(D) Shared parasympathetic pathways
(E) Shared sympathetic pathways

12. A 57-year-old man who is HIV-positive presents to his physician with headache, nausea and vomiting, and a change in mental status. No nuchal rigidity is noted. A lumbar puncture is performed and shows a high opening pressure. A preparation of his bronchoalveolar lavage fluid with India ink stain is shown in the image. Intravenous treatment is started for the acute condition. Which of the following adverse effects would most likely occur with this patient's initial treatment?

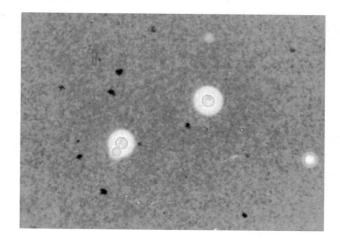

Reproduced, with permission, from Brooks GF, Carroll KA, Butel JS, Morse SA. *Jawetz, Melnick, & Adelberg's Medical Microbiology*, 24th ed. New York: McGraw-Hill, 2007: Figure 45-21.

(A) Arrhythmia
(B) Bone marrow suppression
(C) Gynecomastia
(D) Flushing
(E) Nausea and vomiting

13. A 21-year-old sexually active college student presents to the clinic complaining of odorous green vaginal discharge and itchiness. Multiple oval flagellated motile organisms are seen on wet mount. She is prescribed an antibiotic treatment. While on therapy she goes to a party, where on consumption of one alcoholic beverage she experiences flushing, tachycardia, headaches, and vomiting. The same effects could be observed when alcohol is mixed with which drug?

(A) Ampicillin
(B) Erythromycin
(C) Glipizide
(D) Imipenem
(E) Tolbutamide

14. A woman with a 2-year-old son comes to her physician because she has been unable to conceive a second child for more than a year. The woman is currently breastfeeding her son. Which of the following explains how lactation suppresses ovulation?

(A) Lactation antagonizes estrogen action
(B) Lactation decreases secretion of prolactin
(C) Lactation inhibits secretion of gonadotropin-releasing hormone
(D) Lactation increases secretion of follicle-stimulating hormone
(E) Lactation increases secretion of sterility hormones

15. A 5-day-old normally developed boy presents to the emergency department with vomiting and constipation. The mother states that the child has not passed stool since birth but only recently began vomiting. The vomitus has a greenish coloration. On examination, the abdomen is markedly distended and is dull to percussion. Digital rectal examination shows an empty rectum, but stool is passed explosively following the examination. A sweat chloride test is negative. The disorder in this infant arises from cells derived from which of the following embryologic cell populations?

(A) Endoderm
(B) Mesoderm
(C) Neural crest
(D) Neuroectoderm
(E) Surface ectoderm

16. A woman strikes her head in a car crash and is admitted to the hospital, where she begins urinating up to 1 L every few hours and complaining of constant thirst. Which of the following is the most appropriate treatment?

(A) Demeclocycline
(B) Desmopressin
(C) Furosemide
(D) Insulin
(E) Mannitol

17. A 65-year-old man presents to his family doctor for a regularly scheduled check-up. He is recently widowed and appears unkempt at this visit. His past medical history is significant for alcoholism, hypertension, and type 2 diabetes mellitus. His current medications are hydrochlorothiazide, metformin, and clonidine. On physical examination, his blood pressure is 158/90 mm Hg. His body mass index is 33 kg/m^2, and he reports a 4.5-kg (10-lb) weight loss over the past 3 months. On further questioning the patient admits to owning a gun and states that he has thought repeatedly of shooting himself in the head. Which of the following actions is most appropriate in the care of this patient?

(A) Hospitalize voluntarily or involuntarily
(B) Prescribe an antidepressant
(C) Refer to a psychiatrist
(D) Schedule for a regular visit
(E) Tell the patient's children so that they can intervene

18. A 5-year-old girl is brought to the emergency department with acute onset of projectile vomiting and severe headache. Her parents report that over the past couple of months her gait has become increasingly unstable. Her medical history is negative for seizures and signs of meningitis. Physical examination is notable for truncal ataxia and papilledema. CT reveals a mass at the cerebellar vermis. Which of the following is most likely to be seen on histological examination of tissue from this mass?

(A) Cells with round, regular, centrally located nuclei surrounded by a perinuclear halo
(B) Prolific vasculature and receding rows of nuclei
(C) Rod-shaped perinuclear inclusions
(D) Round calcifications
(E) Small cells with high nuclear:cytoplasmic ratios surrounding the vasculature

19. A patient presents to the emergency department with a crushing injury to her right ankle. A medical student working there is told to evaluate the vascular integrity of the patient's right lower extremity. She feels for femoral, dorsalis pedis, and posterior tibial pulses and finds that they are intact and symmetric bilaterally. In which of the following locations did the student palpate the posterior tibial pulse?

(A) Between the two heads of the gastrocnemius muscle
(B) Deep in the popliteal fossa
(C) Immediately anterior to the medial malleolus
(D) Immediately posterior to the lateral malleolus
(E) Immediately posterior to the medial malleolus
(F) On the dorsal surface of the foot

20. A 53-year-old man with a long-standing history of allergic rhinitis and asthma presents with uveitis, mild hearing loss, numbness and tingling in his right hand, and diffuse joint pain for the past 10 days. Physical examination shows weak to absent left knee patellar reflexes (right knee reflex strong and intact). Laboratory studies show a markedly elevated eosinophil count. A diagnosis is made, and the patient is treated with cyclophosphamide. Further laboratory studies show elevated serum levels of the most common autoantibody associated with this condition. What structure is primarily targeted by the autoantibodies that are most likely elevated in this patient's serum?

(A) Acetylcholine receptors
(B) Neutrophils
(C) Oligodendrocytes
(D) RBCs
(E) TSH receptors

21. A 32-year-old HIV-positive man with a recent CD4+ cell count of 84/mm³ and a 3-week history of worsening headaches is brought to the emergency department by ambulance because of acute mental status changes. Upon arrival he is noted to have papilledema, a third cranial nerve palsy, and a rigid neck that cannot be flexed or extended. He subsequently dies from an overwhelming infection involving his nervous system. An autopsy specimen of the patient's brain is shown in the image. What is the underlying cause of this patient's symptoms?

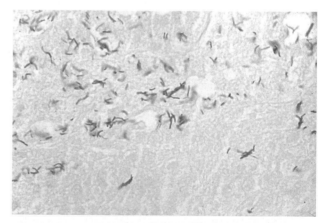

Reproduced, with permission, from PEIR Digital Library (http://peir.net).

(A) Bacterial meningitis
(B) Fungal meningitis
(C) Herpes encephalitis
(D) Mycobacterial meningitis
(E) Viral meningitis

22. A 32-year-old female dialysis patient visits her general internist for a health maintenance visit. She subsequently has a dual-energy x-ray absorption examination, which demonstrates significant osteoporosis. What is the most likely etiology of this patient's osteoporosis?

(A) Chronic metabolic alkalosis
(B) 1,25-Dihydroxycholecalciferol excess
(C) Hypercalcemia
(D) Hypophosphatemia
(E) Secondary hyperparathyroidism

23. A 62-year old man arrives at his doctor's office complaining of recent onset dull pain in his left flank region. He is a retired steel plant worker with a long history of excessive smoking, hypertension, and obesity. He does not recall any history of similar illness in his family. On physical examination a firm, homogeneous, nontender movable mass is palpated deep in the left umbilical region near the lower pole of the kidney. Laboratory tests show hypercalcemia, hypophosphatemia, and moderate polycythemia. Urinalysis reveals the presence of hematuria. Which of the following is the most likely diagnosis?

(A) Adult polycystic kidney disease
(B) Angiomyolipoma
(C) Pheochromocytoma
(D) Renal cell carcinoma
(E) Wilms' tumor

24. A 55-year-old woman presents to her primary care physician with complaints of nausea, fatigue, early satiety, and abdominal distension. Physical examination reveals the presence of ascites as well as significant pelvic discomfort. CT scanning reveals the presence of multiple masses spread diffusely throughout the abdomen. The patient is subsequently taken to surgery to reduce her tumor burden and to confirm a diagnosis of metastatic ovarian cancer.

Her oncologist then places her on a treatment regimen that includes paclitaxel. Which of the following characterizes the mechanism of this chemotherapy agent?

(A) Alkylating agent that covalently links DNA
(B) Binds tubulin and hyperstabilizes polymerized microtubules
(C) Depolymerizes microtubules
(D) Inhibits DNA polymerase
(E) Inhibits topoisomerase II

25. A 7-year-old girl has numerous vesicles on her face, particularly around her mouth. Over a few days, the vesicles turn into pustules and crust over, becoming flaky and light yellow in color. Which of the following statements about the organism most likely responsible for this girl's infection is correct?

(A) Sabouraud's agar is required to culture this bacterium
(B) The bacterium is a facultative intracellular organism
(C) The bacterium is a group B β-hemolytic organism
(D) The bacterium is bacitracin-sensitive
(E) The bacterium is protected from host defenses by protein M

26. An 18-year-old man has a history of a pancreatic cyst and multiple hemangioblastomas. Which of the following tumors is he at an increased risk of developing?

(A) Acute lymphocytic leukemia
(B) Colon cancer
(C) Pheochromocytoma
(D) Renal cell carcinoma
(E) Testicular seminoma

27. A 42-year-old woman comes to the physician with severe itching for the past 4 days. Her physical examination is significant for hepatomegaly and three xanthomas on her right lower extremity. Laboratory studies reveal a normal total bilirubin level and elevated serum cholesterol and alkaline phosphatase levels. A liver biopsy shows granulomatous destruction of medium-sized intrahepatic bile ducts. Which of the following autoantibodies is most likely to be significantly elevated in this patient?

(A) Anticentromere antibodies
(B) Antihistone antibodies
(C) Antimitochondrial antibodies
(D) Antinuclear antibodies
(E) Rheumatoid factor

28. A 25-year-old woman comes to her family physician for a routine check-up. Her physical examination shows a mildly overweight woman but is otherwise unremarkable. A fasting lipid panel, however, shows an LDL cholesterol level of 310 mg/dL, HDL cholesterol level of 42 mg/dL, triglyceride level of 150 mg/dL, and total cholesterol level of 382 mg/dL. Because a diagnosis of familial hypercholesterolemia is suspected, the doctor initiates treatment of her condition. Soon after starting treatment, however, she presents with myalgias. Laboratory values show elevated levels of aspartate aminotransferase, alanine aminotransferase, and creatinine kinase. Which of the following interventions is most likely responsible for the patient's myalgias?

(A) B complex vitamins
(B) Hormone replacement therapy
(C) LDL apheresis
(D) Liver transplant
(E) Statin medications

29. Informed consent is the legal demonstration of a patient's understanding of risks, benefits, and outcomes of treatments and alternatives. Which of the following circumstances represents an exception for obtaining informed consent?

(A) A competent patient whose son wishes to waive his father's right

(B) A mentally retarded patient who is legally competent
(C) A nursing volunteer has already obtained informed consent
(D) A paralyzed patient who cannot speak but can nod his head for consent
(E) A physician agrees that informing the patient will be detrimental to the patient's health

30. A 43-year-old man presents to the emergency department with the sudden onset of a headache, sweating, and palpitations. On physical examination, he appears anxious and his face is flushed. His blood pressure is 150/95 mm Hg. Urinalysis reveals high levels of vanillylmandelic acid. Which of the following is the most appropriate pharmacologic treatment for this patient's condition?

(A) Phenelzine
(B) Phenoxybenzamine
(C) Phenylephrine
(D) Propranolol

31. A 78-year-old man comes to the physician for evaluation after falling five times in 2 months. An x-ray skeletal survey reveals no fractures, but the patient admits to worsening urinary incontinence over the previous 4 months. His wife states that his memory and concentration have deteriorated recently. The patient's vital signs are normal, and his physical examination is notable for a wide-based gait with short steps. A Mini-Mental State Examination results in a score of 26/30. His funduscopic examination is normal, and his neurologic examination is notable for slight bradykinesia without tremor. Laboratory tests, including serum vitamin B_{12}, folate, and TSH, are normal. What is the most likely etiology of this patient's recent decline?

(A) Alzheimer's disease
(B) Hypothyroidism
(C) Multi-infarct dementia
(D) Normal pressure hydrocephalus
(E) Parkinson's disease

32. An 8-month-old girl is brought to the emergency department by her parents because she appears swollen. The parents weaned the child from formula 3 weeks ago. They have been giving her rice milk for 1 month. On examination the child has a protuberant belly and 2+ pitting edema in her wrists and shins. This type of malnutrition is caused by a deficiency of what type of nutrient?

(A) Calorie
(B) Carbohydrate
(C) Electrolyte
(D) Fat
(E) Protein

33. A 19-year-old man who recently immigrated from Asia comes to the emergency department because of blood in his sputum. On history, the patient mentions he has had weight loss and night sweats. On examination, the patient has a fever and bronchial breath sounds with crepitant rales. Laboratory tests show lymphocytosis and an increased erythrocyte sedimentation rate. X-ray film of the chest shows a calcified lung lesion and hilar lymphadenopathy. Which of the following is the stain used to identify the most likely infectious organism?

(A) Congo red
(B) Giemsa's
(C) India ink
(D) Periodic acid-Schiff
(E) Ziehl-Neelsen

34. A 65-year-old postmenopausal woman presents with progressive constipation and frequent, excessive urination. She mentions she has been smoking 1 pack per day since she was 19 years old. On further questioning she states she is having palpitations constantly. On physical examination, there are respiratory findings, which prompt an x-ray film of the chest. A circular, perihilar lesion in the lung is found. Laboratory testing shows a decreased phosphorus level. Which of the following is the most likely cause of this patient's symptoms?

(A) Central bronchogenic carcinoma
(B) Cervical sympathetic chain compression
(C) Chronic silica exposure

(D) Congenital chloride channel dysfunction
(E) Dynein arm defect in cilia
(F) Ectopic antidiuretic hormone production
(G) Solitary parathyroid adenoma

35. The image shows a specialized epithelium that overlies a type of peripheral lymphoid tissue. What is the main class of antibodies associated with this lymphoid tissue?

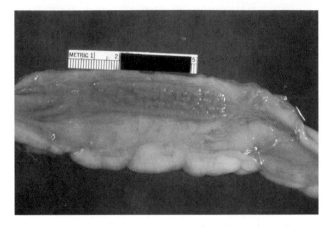

Reproduced, with permission, from PEIR Digital Library (http://peir.net).

(A) IgA
(B) IgD
(C) IgE
(D) IgG
(E) IgM

36. A 45-year-old man with essential hypertension presents to the emergency department with muscle weakness and palpitations. Peaked T waves and prolonged PR intervals are noted on ECG. Which of the following medications could be the underlying cause of the changes noted on this patient's ECG?

(A) Acetazolamide
(B) Furosemide
(C) Hydrochlorothiazide
(D) Mannitol
(E) Spironolactone

37. A physician is caring for a hospitalized 31-year-old man with long-standing, poorly controlled type 1 diabetes mellitus. He is blind and has peripheral neuropathy with sensory loss in both feet, and his most recent hemoglobin A1c level was 13.9%. He recently presented with altered mental status, polyuria, and polydipsia. At that time, his serum glucose level was 475 mg/dL, arterial blood pH was 6.96, and his anion gap was 27. Since then his acidosis has resolved with appropriate treatment, and fingerstick blood glucose levels have normalized. However, he has persistent nasal discharge; paranasal sinus tenderness; and new onset of periorbital edema, proptosis, facial numbness, and obtundation. Fungal stain of fluid obtained from urgent surgical sinus drainage would most likely reveal which of the following?

(A) Broad-based budding dimorphic fungi
(B) 45-degree angle branching, septate hyphae with rare fruiting bodies
(C) Irregular, broad, nonseptate hyphae with 90-degree branching
(D) Pseudohyphae with budding yeasts
(E) 5- to 10-μm yeasts with wide capsular halo on India ink stain

38. A 64-year-old woman presents to her primary care physician with fatigue, weakness, and a weight loss of 4.5 kg (10 lb) in the past 4 months. Additionally, she notes that her vision has deteriorated over that time, and has had several severe nosebleeds. Physical examination demonstrates hepatosplenomegaly, and laboratory tests show an increased total protein level. Serum protein electrophoresis reveals a large spike in the gamma region. A skeletal survey is negative. Which of the following is the most likely diagnosis?

(A) Chronic lymphocytic leukemia
(B) Diabetes mellitus
(C) Monoclonal gammopathy of undetermined significance
(D) Multiple myeloma
(E) Waldenström's macroglobulinemia

39. A pharmaceutical company has created a new drug that, when taken daily, is thought to be highly effective at preventing the onset of migraines. The company would like to market the drug and is conducting a study to look at its benefits and possible risks. In coordination with a physician at a local hospital, it enrolls 800 people for the study. The physician places 100 patients with the worst and most frequent migraines in the medication group, as he thinks that they are in most need of the drug's benefit. Which of the following best explains why the drug may not perform up to expectations?

(A) Differences in group size
(B) Late-look bias
(C) Recall bias
(D) Sampling bias
(E) Selection bias

40. The human papillomavirus promotes neoplasia through production of the viral proteins E6 and E7, which interfere with the normal function of *Rb* and *p53*. What general function is common to both *Rb* and *p53*?

(A) Cell cycle regulation
(B) Cellular adhesion
(C) Direct transcriptional control
(D) DNA repair
(E) Inhibition of signal transduction

41. A 95-year-old woman is transferred to the intensive care unit after a 3-day history of cough and declining mental status. Her blood pressure is 85/50 mm Hg, pulse is 124/min, temperature is 39.8° C (103.6° F), and respiratory rate is 27/min. Crackles are heard at the left lower lung base, and the patient is suffering from rigors intermittently. Blood and sputum cultures drawn at the onset of symptoms grow strains of *Klebsiella pneumoniae* resistant to all antibiotics except polymyxin B. Which of the following is a serious adverse reaction of polymyxin B?

(A) Granulocytopenia
(B) Hearing loss
(C) Hemolysis in patients with glucose 6-phosphate dehydrogenase deficiency
(D) Numbness of the extremities
(E) Severe vomiting

42. A 20-year-old woman presents to the physician with a history of bloody diarrhea and abdominal pain. She states that she has not traveled recently or changed her eating habits. A stool culture is negative for any known infectious cause of diarrhea. A flexible sigmoidoscopy is performed and shows numerous lesions in the descending colon interrupted by normal-appearing mucosa. Which of the following features would most likely be present on a tissue biopsy of the affected region?

(A) Cells with loss of mucin and hyperchromatic nuclei
(B) Hyperplastic goblet cells
(C) Mucus-filled cells in crypts
(D) Noncaseating granulomas
(E) Ulcerated mucosa only

43. A 38-year-old man from rural Guatemala dies in the emergency department due to heart failure. Autopsy reveals an enlarged and flaccid heart. Microscopy of a blood sample taken before the man's death shows flagellated parasites. A histologic section of the heart shows amastigotes. Which of the following parasites did this man most likely harbor?

(A) *Cryptosporidium* species
(B) *Entamoeba histolytica*
(C) *Giardia lamblia*
(D) *Toxoplasma gondii*
(E) *Trypanosoma cruzi*

44. A 27-year-old man presents to the emergency department with a cough productive of blood-tinged sputum. He also complains that in the past couple weeks he has noticed increased fatigue and some blood in his urine. A renal biopsy is performed that, upon immunofluorescence, shows a linear pattern of IgG deposition along the basement membrane. Which of the following is most likely responsible for this patient's disease?

(A) Antineutrophil cytoplasmic antibodies
(B) Anti-type III collagen antibodies
(C) Anti-type IV collagen antibodies
(D) Immune complexes
(E) T lymphocytes

45. A 36-year-old man who completed a marathon 6 hours earlier presents to the emergency department with severe muscle pain and swelling and complaints of red urine. Laboratory tests show a creatine kinase level of 6800 U/L but no RBCs on urinalysis. Which of the following symptoms would most likely also be present?

(A) Arrhythmia
(B) Hepatomegaly
(C) Inflammation of the metacarpophalangeal joints
(D) Pain in a dermatomal distribution
(E) Shuffling gait

46. Albinism is an autosomal recessive disorder in which a deficiency in tyrosinase activity leads to a lack of pigmentation in the hair, skin, and eyes. The cells most involved in this condition are derived from which of the following germ cell layers?

(A) Ectoderm
(B) Endoderm
(C) Mesoderm
(D) Neuroectoderm, neural crest cells
(E) Neuroectoderm, non-neural crest cells

47. The father of a 7-year-old boy is contacted by his child's schoolteacher because she is concerned about his inattentiveness during class. The teacher states that the boy appears to be daydreaming multiple times each day, during which time he blinks his eyes repeatedly. She reports that the boy's daydreaming episodes are brief and he is able to refocus shortly following the daydream. What is the most appropriate therapy for the child's underlying condition?

(A) Carbamazepine
(B) Clonazepam
(C) Ethosuximide
(D) Gabapentin
(E) Methylphenidate
(F) Tiagabine

48. A 53-year-old man presents to his physician with complaints of chest pain that worsens on exertion and at times of stress. An angiogram reveals fibrous plaques in the intima of the proximal portions of his coronary arteries. Fibrous plaques are indicative of which of the following pathologic processes?

(A) Arteriosclerosis
(B) Atherosclerosis
(C) Medial calcific sclerosis
(D) Mönckeberg's arteriosclerosis
(E) Takayasu's arteritis

1. The correct answer is C. It is important to understand that the question is asking for the sensitivity, the proportion of people who have the disease and test positive out of all the people who have the disease. It is calculated by TP / (TP + FN), where TP means true-positive and FN means false-negative. The true-positives in the vignette represent those with the cancer who correctly tested positive with this new test (n = 60). False-negatives are those with the cancer who tested negative with the new test (n = 40); thus, 60 / (60 + 40) = 60%. Screening tests theoretically would aim to identify all those with the disease, and therefore high sensitivities are desired. In this case 60% represents a low number, and the ca-1panc blood test would not be a good screening test for the cancer.

Answer A is incorrect. The 10.0% figure represents the prevalence of the disease, calculated as total cancer/total people (100/1,000).

Answer B is incorrect. The 37.5% figure is the positive predictive value, or the probability that someone with a positive test (ca-1panc) truly does have the cancer. The predictive values vary with how prevalent a disease is in the population. It is calculated as TP / (TP + FP) (where TP means true-positive and FP means false-positive) or 60 / (60 + 100) = 37.5%.

Answer D is incorrect. The 88.8% figure represents the specificity of the blood test, which measures the proportion of the people who don't have the disease and test negative out of all the people who don't have the disease. It is important to correctly detect those without the disease in order to prevent them from undergoing unnecessary treatment or studies that could be painful or harmful to the patient. It is calculated as TN / (TN + FP) (where TN means true-negative and FP means false-positive), or 800 / (800 + 100) = 88.8%.

Answer E is incorrect. The 90.0% figure simply represents the percentage of people without the cancer, 900/1000.

Answer F is incorrect. The 95.2% figure is the negative predictive value, or the probability that the person with a negative test really does not have the cancer. It is calculated as TN / (TN + FN) (where TN means true-negative and FN means false-negative), or 800 / (800 + 40) = 95.2%.

2. The correct answer is A. Pregnancy is considered to be a state of hypercoagulability with an increased risk for deep venous thrombosis (DVT) and pulmonary embolus. A major concern is that a DVT can lodge within the pulmonary arterial system. This, in turn, can result in pulmonary hypertension, hypoxia, and, in the worst case, right-sided heart failure and death. Pregnant women who have an indication for anticoagulation therapy (in this case, both stasis and endothelial injury secondary to her trauma) should be treated with an anticoagulant. Heparin is the preferred anticoagulant because it does not cross the placenta.

Answer B is incorrect. Indomethacin is a nonsteroidal anti-inflammatory agent and is contraindicated in the third trimester of pregnancy because it will close the ductus arteriosus prematurely. Indomethacin is also used as a tocolytic in preterm labor.

Answer C is incorrect. Prostaglandin E_2 can be applied topically to ripen the cervix and promote induction of labor; however, in this patient, immediate induction of labor is not desired.

Answer D is incorrect. Streptokinase is a thrombolytic agent used in the treatment of early myocardial infarction.

Answer E is incorrect. Warfarin cannot be used because it can cross the placenta and has been implicated in nasal hypoplasia and skeletal abnormalities in the fetus in the first trimester. It also causes diffuse central nervous system abnormalities, particularly optic atrophy during pregnancy.

3. The correct answer is D. The neonate suffers from transposition of the great vessels, in which the aorta rises from the right ventricle and the pulmonary artery from the left ventricle. It is a common congenital heart defect in the children of mothers with diabetes. Without a shunt, transposition is incompatible with life. If the infant is born without the shunt, an artificial shunt can be created by balloon atrial septostomy, and prostaglandin E_1 can be given to salvage whatever patent ductus arteriosus might remain. Once stabilized, the infant can then be taken for corrective surgery. Transposition is also associated with maternal diabetes.

Answer A is incorrect. Coarctation of the aorta would not cause early cyanosis and is not associated with transposition of the great vessels.

Answer B is incorrect. A concomitant ventricular septal defect (VSD), while sometimes present in patients with transposition of the great vessels, is not the underlying pathophysiology of this infant's cyanosis. Additionally, if this patient had a VSD, there would have been little reason to create an additional shunt in the atria.

Answer C is incorrect. A prostaglandin E_1 infusion delays the closure of the patent ductus arteriosus; however, this confers a protective advantage in patients with transposition of the great vessels, as it allows for mixing of blood. It is not the underlying pathophysiology of transposition of the great vessels.

Answer E is incorrect. An overriding aorta is one component of tetralogy of Fallot in addition to ventricular septal defect, right ventricular outflow tract obstruction, and right ventricular hypertrophy. Although tetralogy of Fallot is a cause of early cyanosis, an isolated overriding aorta would not cause the emergent hypoxia seen in this infant.

4. The correct answer is E. The patient presents with the classic signs of Hodgkin's lymphoma, and the biopsy demonstrates the presence of Reed–Sternberg cells with reactive lymphocytes. Reed–Sternberg cells are large with lobed nuclei that look like "owl's eyes" and appear to be two halves mirroring each other. Vinblastine is part of the **ABVD** regimen (**A**driamycin, **B**leomycin, **V**inblastine, **D**acarbazine) regimen used to treat Hodgkin's lymphoma. Vinblastine works by inhibiting microtubule formation necessary to build the mitotic spindle, so that cells in mitosis get stuck in metaphase. It is used to treat many solid tumors as well as Hodgkin's and non-Hodgkin's lymphoma. Adverse effects include alopecia, constipation, myelosuppression, and (rarely) neurotoxicity.

Answer A is incorrect. Cyclosporine is an immunosuppressant used in transplant patients and autoimmune disorders, but would not be appropriate for a patient with Hodgkin's lymphoma. It works by inhibiting the production and release of interleukin-2, which is necessary to induce cytotoxic T lymphocytes. Adverse effects include gastrointestinal upset, headache, and tremor but amazingly little myelosuppression.

Answer B is incorrect. Hydroxyurea is used for treatment of sickle cell anemia and to suppress high WBC counts in acute leukemia and chronic myelogenous leukemia. It would not be helpful in this patient, who is presenting with Hodgkin's lymphoma. Hydroxyurea is an antimetabolite, and although its exact mechanism is unknown, it is believed to work in the synthesis (S) phase of the cell cycle. The major adverse effect to remember is myelosuppression.

Answer C is incorrect. Imatinib is used to treat chronic myeloid leukemia (CML; a patient would present with increased neutrophils and metamyelocytes) and gastrointestinal stromal tumors, and would not be helpful in a patient with Hodgkin's lymphoma. Imatinib is a tyrosine kinase inhibitor that specifically inhibits *brl-abl* in CML, promoting apoptosis in these cells. Adverse effects include weight gain, gastrointestinal distress, musculoskeletal pain, and myelosuppression.

Answer D is incorrect. Isoniazid is one of the drugs used to treat tuberculosis (other drugs include rifampin, pyrazinamide, streptomycin, or ethambutol). Although the patient presents with some symptoms that would be expected with tuberculosis, such as night sweats, fever, and weight loss, the biopsy results clearly show the Reed–Sternberg cells of Hodgkin's lymphoma. Isoniazid works by inhibiting mycolic acid synthesis and therefore disrupting the cell wall. Adverse effects include hepatotoxicity, neuropathy, and potentially psychiatric symptoms.

5. **The correct answer is D.** This patient suffers from McArdle's disease, a glycogen storage disorder in which glycogen phosphorylase is deficient in muscle. The enzyme is responsible for liberating individual units of glucose-1-phosphate from branches of a glycogen molecule. Onset of the disease typically occurs in adolescence or early adulthood and is characterized by muscle cramping, rapid fatigue, and poor endurance during exertion. Severe myoglobinuria is also observed in some patients.

Answer A is incorrect. Homocystinuria is an inborn error of metabolism caused by a defect in cystathionine synthase, the enzyme that converts homocysteine to cystathionine. In addition to Marfan-like features, these patients are at increased risk for a variety of cardiovascular derangements due to increased atherosclerosis, including premature vascular disease and early death.

Answer B is incorrect. Glucose-6-phosphatase is the enzyme responsible for converting glucose-6-phosphate to glucose. It is a component of gluconeogenesis. A deficiency of this enzyme causes Von Gierke's disease, characterized by a severe fasting hypoglycemia, increased glycogen in the liver, hepatomegaly, and increased blood lactate. These findings are inconsistent with the symptoms observed in this patient.

Answer C is incorrect. α-1,6-Glucosidase is the enzyme responsible for the debranching of glycogen. It is implicated in Cori's disease, which is a mild form of Von Gierke's disease with normal blood lactate levels. It is not implicated in McArdle's disease as it wouldn't cause the muscle cramping.

Answer E is incorrect. Lysosomal α-1,4-glucosidase is the defective enzyme in Pompe's disease, another glycogen storage disorder. The findings in Pompe's disease typically manifest in early childhood and include respiratory difficulties (due to diaphragmatic weakness), cardiomegaly, and progressive loss of muscle tone leading to early death.

6. **The correct answer is B.** This patient is likely suffering from hyperparathyroidism due to a parathyroid adenoma. Primary hyperparathyroidism causes hypercalcemia, hypophosphatemia, increased alkaline phosphatase activity, and an increase in serum parathyroid hormone (PTH). Hypercalcemia can cause metastatic calcification, including nephrocalcinosis, and development of renal stones and peptic duodenal ulcer disease. Furthermore, PTH elevation can lead to a variety of bone abnormalities, including osteitis fibrosa cystica, a condition that results from excessive bone resorption and fibrous replacement of the marrow, leading to cystic spaces and areas of hemorrhage, or "brown tumors." Clinically, patients may present with bone pain and fractures.

Answer A is incorrect. Hypertrophic osteoarthropathy is seen in patients with a variety of illnesses, including lung cancer, sepsis, endocarditis, and inflammatory bowel disease. Patients frequently present with digital clubbing and painful swelling of wrists, fingers, elbows, and other joints. New bone formation is present at the ends of these bones.

Answer C is incorrect. Osteopetrosis is characterized by brittle, dense, thickened bones that fracture easily. The disease has an autosomal dominant and recessive mode of inheritance

Answer D is incorrect. Osteoporosis, which is characterized by decreased bone mass, pain, and fractures, is most commonly seen in postmenopausal women and the elderly. Osteoporosis is associated with normal calcium, phosphorus, and alkaline phosphatase levels.

Answer E is incorrect. Paget's disease of the bone, like osteitis fibrosa cystica, is a result of excessive bone resorption. In Paget's disease, the resorbed bone is replaced by a soft, disorganized bone matrix with a mosaic, rather than trabecular, pattern. Alkaline phosphatase activity is increased. Patients can present with bone pain, fractures, deformity, and sensory deficits due to nerve impingement.

7. **The correct answer is D.** Waterhouse-Friderichsen syndrome is a possible complication of meningococcemia. In this disorder, bilateral hemorrhage into the adrenal gland causes adrenal insufficiency. This results in hypotension, tachycardia, a rapidly enlarging petechial skin lesion, disseminated intravascular coagulation, and coma.

Answer A is incorrect. Hemolytic-uremic syndrome (HUS) is characterized by acute renal failure and thrombocytopenia with hemolytic anemia. HUS can be a complication of infection caused by *E. coli* O157:H7 and not *Neisseria meningitidis.*

Answer B is incorrect. Rheumatic fever is characterized by fever, migratory polyarthritis, and carditis. It may follow group A streptococcal pharyngitis.

Answer C is incorrect. Fever, a new murmur, Janeway lesions, and nail-bed hemorrhages are all signs of bacterial endocarditis. Acute endocarditis is caused by *Staphylococcus aureus* and subacute infection can be caused by *Streptococcus viridans.*

Answer E is incorrect. Guillain–Barré syndrome is characterized by rapidly progressing ascending paralysis. It is thought to follow a variety of infectious diseases, such as cytomegalovirus, Epstein-Barr virus, HIV, and gastroenteritis caused by *Campylobacter jejuni.*

8. **The correct answer is E.** PGI_2 inhibits platelet aggregation and therefore is an antithrombotic agent. On the other hand, TxA_2 increases platelet aggregation and is a prothrombotic agent. COX-2 inhibitors selectively decrease PGI_2, leaving the action of TxA_2 unopposed. This could well result in increased cerebrovascular and cardiovascular events due to the tonic, unopposed prothrombotic action of TxA_2.

Answer A is incorrect. COX-2 inhibitors do not increase PGI_2. They are thought to spare the gastric mucosa because they selectively block the synthesis of other prostaglandins, not because they increase the production of PGI_2.

Answer B is incorrect. COX-2 inhibitors do not increase TxA_2. COX-2 inhibitors in general do not increase PGI_2 and TxA_2, which are downstream products.

Answer C is incorrect. COX-2 inhibitors and aspirin do not have the same actions.

Answer D is incorrect. COX-2 inhibitors do decrease PGI_2, but aspirin does not increase PGI_2 and TxA_2. Aspirin is a nonselective COX inhibitor that decreases both PGI_2 and TxA_2.

9. **The correct answer is A.** This patient's clinical presentation is consistent with anemia of chronic disease (ACD) in the setting of systemic lupus erythematosus. ACD presents with low serum iron levels, elevated ferritin levels, decreased total iron-binding capacity, and microcytic/normocytic RBCs on blood smear. ACD resolves if the underlying condition is corrected, but in the absence of a successful primary treatment, erythropoietin can be effective in treating the anemia. Iron therapy is not effective in treating this disorder.

Answer B is incorrect. Iron therapy is inappropriate in treating anemia of chronic disease, since iron stores are not low.

Answer C is incorrect. Folate supplementation would be appropriate in macrocytic anemia caused by folate deficiency.

Answer D is incorrect. Parenteral vitamin B_{12} therapy is appropriate for pernicious anemia caused by lack of intrinsic factor, which is necessary for vitamin B_{12} absorption.

Answer E is incorrect. Phlebotomy is appropriate in treating cases of iron overload, as seen in patients with chronic transfusion therapy and hemochromatosis.

10. **The correct answer is A.** Craniopharyngiomas account for 80%–90% of neoplasms arising in the pituitary region and are the most common supratentorial tumor of childhood. They originate from squamous rest cells in the remnant of Rathke's pouch between the adenohypophysis and neurohypophysis. Eighty percent of patients have evidence of endocrine dysfunction

at diagnosis; growth hormone deficiency is the most common (75%), followed by gonadotropin deficiency (40%), and ACTH or TSH deficiency (25%). Even though these masses are frequently large at presentation, it is rare for the pituitary stalk to be disrupted; only 20% of patients have prolactinemia, and 10%–15% have diabetes insipidus (DI) secondary to pituitary stalk dysfunction. This patient has symptoms of growth hormone deficiency (short stature), biochemically documented hypothyroidism, DI (polyuria), and increased intracranial pressure as suggested by bilateral papilledema (nonspecific for craniopharyngioma). Imaging in craniopharyngioma may reveal calcification within the tumor.

Answer B is incorrect. Ependymomas are most commonly found in the fourth ventricle and can result in hydrocephalus; however, it is very rare for ependymomas to cause the hormonal changes evident in this patient.

Answer C is incorrect. Hemangioblastomas are associated with von Hippel–Lindau syndrome when found with retinoblastomas. Such a tumor would not affect hormonal release.

Answer D is incorrect. While a prolactinoma can cause many of the same symptoms (pubertal delay/failure) and may present with symptoms similar to those of a craniopharyngioma, it represents a far less likely diagnosis (accounting for 2.7% of childhood tumors) than craniopharyngioma.

Answer E is incorrect. Thyrotropinomas present with hyperthyroidism without TSH suppression, goiter, visual symptoms, and headache. It would be uncommon for them to suppress growth hormone release, and they are very rare in childhood.

11. **The correct answer is C.** Afferent pain fibers of the heart enter the posterior horn of the spinal cord at the same level as the brachial plexus, thus leading to pain that is perceived as being located in the neck and shoulder region.

Answer A is incorrect. Lymphatic drainage does occur in the left upper quadrant, but it plays no role in the model of referred myocardial pain.

Answer B is incorrect. Sensory neurons have their origin in the dorsal root ganglion and send their axons to the posterior horn of the spinal cord instead of the anterior horn, which is where efferent neurons arise.

Answer D is incorrect. The heart and the neck and shoulder region do not share similar parasympathetic innervation patterns.

Answer E is incorrect. The heart and the neck and shoulder region do not share similar sympathetic innervation patterns.

12. **The correct answer is A.** Patients with AIDS are susceptible to a variety of infections that are unusual in the immunocompetent population. Among diseases that cause fever and headache in these patients are *Cryptococcus*, toxoplasmosis, and central nervous system lymphoma. An encapsulated yeast that stains with India ink is a pathognomonic description of *Cryptococcus neoformans*, which is a yeast found in pigeon droppings. Infection occurs when patients inhale fungus particles, which can lead to pneumonia. Initial treatment of *C. neoformans* is intravenous amphotericin B, followed by fluconazole once the patient's condition is stable. Amphotericin toxicity can cause fever and chills, hypotension, nephrotoxicity, and arrhythmias. The arrhythmias are due to QT prolongation, which is exacerbated by changes in potassium and magnesium levels.

Answer B is incorrect. Bone marrow suppression is seen with a number of drugs, including flucytosine.

Answer C is incorrect. Gynecomastia is an adverse effect of fluconazole treatment. The -azole antifungals inhibit ergosterol synthesis. They are used to treat systemic mycoses but are less effective than amphotericin B. Other adverse effects include liver dysfunction and fever.

Answer D is incorrect. Flushing can be caused by caspofungin, an antifungal medication used to treat aspergillosis infection. Caspofungin inhibits synthesis of an essential component of the fungal cell wall. Other adverse effects include gastrointestinal upset.

Answer E is incorrect. Nausea and vomiting are seen with flucytosine, which is used to treat systemic fungal infections. Flucytosine inhibits DNA synthesis because it is converted to fluorouracil in vivo.

13. **The correct answer is E.** The patient consumed alcohol while taking metronidazole for her trichomoniasis. Metronidazole and tolbutamide both have disulfiram-like adverse effects when combined with alcohol use. These effects include flushing, tachycardia, headaches, and vomiting. Tolbutamide is a first-generation sulfonylurea that can also produce these effects.

Answer A is incorrect. Ampicillin is a penicillin family antibiotic often used to treat gram-positive infections or *Listeria* infections. It does not have disulfiram-like adverse effects.

Answer B is incorrect. Erythromycin is a macrolide antibiotic and is not commonly used to treat trichomoniasis. It does not have disulfiram-like adverse effects.

Answer C is incorrect. Glipizide is a second-generation sulfonylurea that does not have the disulfiram-like adverse effects of first-generation sulfonylureas.

Answer D is incorrect. Imipenem is a carbapenem-type antibiotic with a very broad spectrum of action. The main adverse effect is that it can cause seizures in rare cases. It does not have disulfiram-like adverse effects.

14. **The correct answer is C.** Lactation is maintained by prolactin secretion from the anterior pituitary. Prolactin prevents ovulation by several mechanisms. It inhibits the secretion of gonadotropin-releasing hormone (GnRH) from the hypothalamus and inhibits the action of GnRH at the anterior pituitary, thus decreasing the secretion of luteinizing hormone (LH) and follicle-stimulating hormone (FSH). Finally, it

inhibits the actions of LH and FSH on the ovaries. This woman might have a better chance of becoming pregnant if she were to stop breastfeeding her son.

Answer A is incorrect. Lactation and the resulting high levels of prolactin do not affect estrogen's action on the ovary.

Answer B is incorrect. Lactation is maintained by prolactin. It does not decrease its secretion.

Answer D is incorrect. Lactation results in decreased secretion of FSH.

Answer E is incorrect. Lactation does not cause sterility.

15. **The correct answer is C.** The disorder described in the question is Hirschsprung's disease, a disorder of neural crest cells. Specifically, neural crest cells fail to migrate to distal portions of the colon, leading to a congenital lack of parasympathetic ganglion cells. This produces a functional obstruction of the colon, as peristalsis cannot take place. As a result, the abdomen becomes distended and bilious vomiting eventually results, while the rectum is empty on digital examination. Pathologic exam will reveal a lack of ganglia in Meissner's and Auerbach's plexuses and nerve fiber hypertrophy in Meissner's plexus.

Answer A is incorrect. The endoderm gives rise to the epithelial lining of much of the gastrointestinal tract, but this is not a disorder of the epithelium.

Answer B is incorrect. The mesoderm gives rise to smooth muscle, but this patient has Hirschsprung's disease, a disorder of colonic ganglion cells, not smooth muscle.

Answer D is incorrect. The neuroectoderm gives rise to most components of the nervous system but not to the ganglia.

Answer E is incorrect. The surface ectoderm gives rise to the epithelial lining of the lower anal canal, but this patient has Hirschsprung's disease, which is not a disorder of the epithelium.

16. **The correct answer is B.** Desmopressin (dDAVP) is 1-deamino-8-D-arginine vasopressin, an analog of ADH. This woman has central DI caused by trauma to the posterior pituitary. This inhibits secretion of ADH. Repleting her ADH is the most appropriate therapy of the options given. If dDAVP is chosen, the patient's sodium and fluid status should be carefully monitored, because acute trauma to the posterior pituitary can lead to a triphasic response. In phase 1, the injured pituitary ceases secretion of ADH, resulting in the clinical picture presented in the question stem. In phase 2, the death of pituitary tissue causes the release of ADH stores, leading to fluid retention and hyponatremia consistent with the syndrome of inappropriate ADH secretion. Phase 3 arises from permanent damage to the posterior pituitary, resulting in persistent central diabetes insipidus.

Answer A is incorrect. Demeclocycline is used to treat the syndrome of inappropriate ADH secretion. This compound acts to inhibit ADH action and would exacerbate her condition.

Answer C is incorrect. Furosemide is a loop diuretic and is likely to exacerbate her condition.

Answer D is incorrect. Insulin is an inappropriate treatment. Central DI shares only the symptoms of polydipsia and polyuria with diabetes mellitus. The treatments and causes are completely different.

Answer E is incorrect. Mannitol is an osmotic diuretic that would exacerbate her condition.

17. **The correct answer is A.** This patient has a number of risk factors for suicide, including an organized plan, male gender, older age, depression, ethanol abuse, and single status. Other risk factors include loss of rational thinking, lack of social support, and chronic illness. If a patient has suicidal ideation and is deemed at high risk to himself, hospitalization is an appropriate intervention.

Answer B is incorrect. This patient may be given an antidepressant while in the hospital, but a prescription alone is insufficient care for this patient. In addition, antidepressants may take up to 1 month to have a therapeutic effect.

Answer C is incorrect. While the patient will certainly benefit from referral to a psychiatrist, he should be hospitalized because he represents an imminent threat to himself.

Answer D is incorrect. Scheduling this patient for a regular visit will ignore his symptoms of major depressive disorder and place him at risk for harming himself.

Answer E is incorrect. The patient has not been declared incompetent; it is therefore a breach of confidentiality to tell his children without his consent.

18. **The correct answer is E.** Gait disturbances and ataxia are results of the tumor impinging on the cerebellar vermis. Some of the symptoms arise from obstructive hydrocephalus. Medulloblastomas, ependymomas, and hemangioblastomas are childhood primary brain tumors that can result in hydrocephalus by obstruction of the fourth ventricle. However, the patient's gait disturbances and truncal ataxia indicate medulloblastoma, the most common pediatric brain tumor, as the most likely cause. Medulloblastomas are a form of primitive neuroectodermal tumor and appear as small blue cells arranged in perivascular rosettes. They are most often found at the cerebellar vermis.

Answer A is incorrect. "Fried egg" cells have round, regular nuclei with a perinuclear halo and are typical of oligodendrogliomas, which are more common in adults.

Answer B is incorrect. Pseudopalisading tumor cells and microvascular proliferation indicate glioblastoma multiforme, which is more common in adults.

Answer C is incorrect. Rod-shaped blepharoblasts (basal ciliary bodies) are typical of ependymomas.

Answer D is incorrect. Psammoma bodies, which are round, extracellular concretions of calcium, are typical of meningiomas, which are not likely to cause the symptoms listed. In addition, meningiomas are more common in adults.

19. **The correct answer is E.** Recall that blood supply to the entire leg comes from the femoral artery. The femoral artery runs anteriorly on the thigh until reaching the adductor hiatus, where it dives deep and becomes the popliteal artery. The posterior tibial artery branches from the popliteal artery and runs deep in the calf until the ankle, where it lies in the superficial fossa immediately posterior to the medial malleolus. When there is a penetrating or crushing injury to the leg, it is important to palpate this artery and assess for symmetry.

Answer A is incorrect. The posterior tibial artery does run between the heads of the gastrocnemius muscle, but it is deep in the leg and is not easily palpable. You should remember from anatomy that the palpable pulses in the leg are the femoral artery in the groin, the popliteal artery in the popliteal fossa on the posterior aspect of the knee, the posterior tibial posterior to the medial malleolus, and the dorsalis pedis in the first interosseous space on the dorsum of the foot.

Answer B is incorrect. The popliteal artery is found in the popliteal fossa on the posterior aspect of the knee.

Answer C is incorrect. There is no palpable artery anterior to the medial malleolus.

Answer D is incorrect. The popliteal artery gives off three branches in the lower leg, one for each compartment: the posterior tibial, the fibular, and the anterior tibial artery. To assess the anterior tibial artery, one can palpate the dorsalis pedis pulse on the dorsal surface of the foot. The branches of the anterior tibial artery that supply the lateral ankle are too small to palpate.

Answer F is incorrect. The dorsalis pedis artery runs along the dorsal surface of the foot and is a continuation of the anterior tibial artery.

20. **The correct answer is B.** This patient has Churg–Strauss syndrome (also known as allergic granulomatosis and angiitis), which is one of a trio of diseases (Wegener's granulomatosis and microscopic polyangiitis being the others) that are commonly referred to as the ANCA (antineutrophil cytoplasmic antibody)-associated vasculitides (i.e., diseases causing inflammation of blood or lymphatic vessels). Fifty to seventy percent of patients have elevated levels of ANCA, usually the perinuclear pattern of staining type. Patients often have preexisting asthma and allergic rhinitis, and they often present with markedly elevated eosinophil counts and mononeuritis multiplex (simultaneous deficits of two or several peripheral nerves in different areas of the body). Other symptoms include uveitis, conductive hearing loss, and muscle/joint pain. An eosinophilic gastroenteritis may precede the onset of the other symptoms.

Answer A is incorrect. Autoantibodies to acetylcholine receptors are not particularly associated with Churg–Strauss syndrome. Myasthenia gravis is characterized by an autoimmune attack on the acetylcholine receptors of the neuromuscular junction between motor neurons and skeletal muscle fibers.

Answer C is incorrect. Autoantibodies to oligodendrocytes are not particularly associated with Churg–Strauss syndrome. There is evidence suggesting that multiple sclerosis may be partially caused by autoimmune antibody attack on central nervous system myelin-secreting oligodendrocytes.

Answer D is incorrect. Autoantibodies to RBCs, which may be found in certain cases of immune hemolytic anemia, are not particularly associated with Churg–Strauss syndrome.

Answer E is incorrect. Autoantibodies to TSH receptors are not particularly associated with Churg–Strauss syndrome. Graves' disease is a disorder resulting from IgG-type autoantibodies to the TSH receptor.

21. **The correct answer is D.** This patient suffered from tuberculous meningitis, which is demonstrated by the characteristic acid-fast bacilli present in the patient's brain tissue. Immunocompromised patients are at risk for developing tuberculous meningitis, which occurs after the central nervous system (CNS) is seeded with mycobacteria that subsequently produce a thick, gelatinous exudate. This exudate typically collects in the basilar region of the CNS and can cause cranial nerve dysfunction (com-

monly cranial nerves III, VI, and VII) as well as obstruction of the basilar cisterns, resulting in obstructive hydrocephalus. The presence of cranial nerve involvement and/or obstructive hydrocephalus portends a poor prognosis.

Answer A is incorrect. Although bacterial meningitis may occur in immunocompromised patients, this tissue section is not consistent with a bacterial infection. *Streptococcus pneumoniae* and *Neisseria meningitidis*, the two most common causes of bacterial meningitis, are cocci-shaped organisms.

Answer B is incorrect. Although fungal meningitis may occur in immunocompromised patients, this tissue section is not consistent with a fungal infection.

Answer C is incorrect. Although herpes encephalitis may occur in immunocompromised patients, this tissue section is not consistent with a viral herpetic infection.

Answer E is incorrect. Although viral meningitis may occur in immunocompromised patients, this tissue section is not consistent with a viral infection.

22. **The correct answer is E.** Patients with significant renal disease are at particularly high risk for developing skeletal complications, generally known as renal osteodystrophy. Renal failure produces numerous downstream consequences that affect bone health, including increased phosphate retention (resulting in calcium phosphate deposition leading to hypocalcemia and secondary hyperparathyroidism), decreased renal conversion of 25-hydroxcholecalciferol to 1,25-dihydroxycholecalciferol (resulting in decreased intestinal calcium absorption and decreased suppression of parathyroid hormone production), and chronic metabolic acidosis (resulting in increased bone reabsorption). The resulting secondary hyperparathyroidism increases osteoclast activity and the reabsorption of bone.

Answer A is incorrect. Patients with renal failure have a chronic metabolic acidosis due to decreased renal handling of acid anions. Metabolic alkalosis does not result in osteoporosis.

Answer B is incorrect. Patients with renal failure have decreased levels of 1,25-dihydroxycholecalciferol because of decreased renal conversion of 25-hydroxycholecalciferol to 1,25-dihydroxycholecalciferol. 1,25-Dihydroxycholecalciferol excess does not result in osteoporosis.

Answer C is incorrect. Patients with renal failure have hypocalcemia as a result of decreased intestinal absorption of calcium and increased calcium phosphate deposition in tissues. Hypercalcemia is not associated with renal failure and does not result in osteoporosis.

Answer D is incorrect. Patients with renal failure have hyperphosphatemia due to decreased renal excretion of phosphorous. Hypophosphatemia does not result in osteoporosis.

23. **The correct answer is D.** This patient most likely suffers from renal cell carcinoma (RCC). RCC is characterized by the triad of flank pain, hematuria, and abdominal mass, although <10% of patients have all three symptoms. It occurs most commonly in men and is associated with risk factors such as obesity, hypertension, smoking, and environmental toxin exposure (this patient was a worker in a steel plant). Importantly, the major distinguishing feature of RCC is its association with paraneoplastic syndromes due to the ectopic production of hormones such as parathyroid hormone-related protein (hypercalcemia, hypophosphatemia), erythropoietin (polycythemia), and ACTH. RCC is also associated with hereditary conditions such as von Hippel–Lindau (VHL) syndrome. In VHL-related RCC, patients usually present with bilateral tumors. RCC has a relatively poor prognosis because most tumors are asymptomatic until they have undergone metastasis.

Answer A is incorrect. Adult polycystic kidney disease (APKD) is usually an autosomal dominant genetic disease that causes rapid cystic enlargement of the kidneys, leading to renal failure. It usually manifests with hypertension, pain, and hematuria. Patients with APKD do have occasional palpable masses, but renal masses are usually bilateral.

Answer B is incorrect. Angiomyolipomas are relatively rare, benign vascular tumors that occur in the kidney. Renal angiomyolipomas, however, have a more insidious course of progression than RCC, are more common in women, and do not cause paraneoplastic syndromes. Nevertheless, the triad of flank pain, hematuria, and palpable abdominal mass can also occur with angiomyolipomas.

Answer C is incorrect. Pheochromocytoma is a rare tumor derived of catecholamine-producing chromaffin cells of the adrenal glands. Major clinical findings usually result from the ectopic production of catecholamines, including episodic headache, palpitations, and sweating with severe hypertension. It can also be associated with café-au-lait spots and neurofibromas. These clinical features predominate in the presentation of the pheochromocytoma-affected patient, rather than the triad of flank pain, hematuria, and palpable mass and the electrolyte abnormalities seen in this patient.

Answer E is incorrect. Wilms' tumor is a common pediatric malignancy and is not found in adult patients. It can be sporadic or familial. In almost all cases, Wilms' tumor is caused by mutations in the *WT1* gene. In familial Wilms' tumor the disease can be associated with numerous congenital abnormalities, including single, horseshoe, or ectopic kidney; hypospadias; cryptorchidism; and aniridia.

24. **The correct answer is B.** Paclitaxel (Taxol) binds tubulin and hyperstabilizes polymerized microtubules, thus preventing anaphase. It is derived from the pacific yew tree *(Taxus brevifolia)*, and is currently used with carboplatin as first-line therapy for metastatic ovarian carcinoma. It is also used to treat metastatic adenocarcinoma of the breast.

Answer A is incorrect. Cyclophosphamide and ifosfamide are alkylating agents that covalently link DNA and are useful in the treatment of non-Hodgkin's lymphoma and breast and ovarian carcinomas. Cisplatin and carboplatin are platinum-derived compounds that are also thought to act like alkylating agents; they are used with paclitaxel for primary chemotherapy for ovarian cancer, and are also effective for treatment of testicular, bladder, and lung carcinomas.

Answer C is incorrect. Colchicine depolymerizes microtubules and is derived from the autumn crocus *(Colchicum autumnale)*. It is used in the treatment of acute gout attacks.

Answer D is incorrect. Cytarabine inhibits DNA polymerase and is useful in the treatment of acute myelogenous leukemia.

Answer E is incorrect. Etoposide inhibits topoisomerase II and is derived from a springtime herb *(Podophyllum peltatum)*. It is used in the treatment of oat cell and testicular carcinomas.

25. **The correct answer is D.** This girl has impetigo, caused by *Streptococcus pyogenes*, a gram-positive group A β-hemolytic organism that is bacitracin-sensitive. This infection is characterized by an eruption of vesicles on the face. These vesicles later turn into pustules with a characteristic honey-colored crust. A distinctly *bullous* form of impetigo is caused by S. *aureus*.

Answer A is incorrect. Sabouraud's agar is required to culture fungi, not *Streptococcus pyogenes*.

Answer B is incorrect. *Mycobacterium, Brucella, Francisella, Listeria, Yersinia, Legionella,* and *Salmonella* are facultative intracellular organisms, but *Streptococcus pyogenes* is not.

Answer C is incorrect. The bacterium is a group A β-hemolytic organism. *Streptococcus agalactiae* is a group B β-hemolytic organism.

Answer E is incorrect. Protein M protects the bacterium from phagocytosis, but it makes the bacterium more sensitive to host defenses due to antibody production against protein M.

26. **The correct answer is D.** Patients with VHL disease have hemangioblastomas, or cavernous hemangiomas of the retina, cerebellum, and medulla. They can also present with adenomas and cysts of the liver, kidneys, and pancreas. Patients with VHL disease are also at increased risk of developing renal cell carcinoma.

Answer A is incorrect. Patients with Down's syndrome, or trisomy 21, are at increased risk of developing acute lymphocytic leukemia.

Answer B is incorrect. Patients with familial adenomatous polyposis develop colon cancer if the polyps are not resected.

Answer C is incorrect. Patients with neurofibromatosis type 1 are at increased risk of developing pheochromocytoma and malignancies such as Wilms' tumor, rhabdomyosarcoma, and leukemia.

Answer E is incorrect. Patients with androgen insensitivity are normal-appearing females but can have undescended (inguinal) testicles. If these are not excised, the risk of malignancy, including testicular seminoma, is greatly increased.

27. **The correct answer is C.** This patient most likely has primary biliary cirrhosis, which is a chronic autoimmune liver disorder that may initially present with severe itching, hepatomegaly, and xanthomas (yellow nodules/plaques filled with lipid-laden histiocytes, often a sign of hypercholesterolemia). Jaundice develops later in the disease, as hyperbilirubinemia does not occur until there is marked liver damage. The pathologic hallmark is described by the liver biopsy results in the question stem. Over 90% of patients have elevated levels of antimitochondrial antibodies.

Answer A is incorrect. While patients with primary biliary cirrhosis may also have other autoimmune disorders, the association with anticentromere antibodies is not as strong as the association with antimitochondrial antibodies. It is worth noting that the presence of elevated levels of anticentromere antibodies is often associated with the CREST variant of scleroderma.

Answer B is incorrect. While patients with primary biliary cirrhosis may also have other autoimmune disorders, the association with antihistone antibodies is not as strong as the association with antimitochondrial antibodies. It is worth noting that the presence of antihistone antibodies is often associated with drug-induced lupus syndromes.

Answer D is incorrect. While patients with primary biliary cirrhosis may also have other autoimmune disorders, the association with antinuclear antibodies is not as strong as the association with antimitochondrial antibodies.

Answer E is incorrect. While patients with primary biliary cirrhosis may also have other autoimmune disorders, the association with rheumatoid factor is not as strong as the association with antimitochondrial antibodies. It is worth noting that the presence of elevated levels of rheumatoid factor is often associated with rheumatoid arthritis.

28. **The correct answer is E.** Dietary modification (drastically limiting saturated and trans fats and cholesterol), weight loss, and aerobic exercise are the first-line treatment options for any patient with elevated cholesterol levels, and these lifestyle modifications should be attempted by this patient but will likely have only a minimal effect in a patient with familial hypercholesterolemia. Statin medications are 3-hydroxy-3-methylglutaryl coenzyme A reductase inhibitors. By blocking the rate-limiting step in cholesterol synthesis, they can lower cholesterol levels. High-dose therapy with a statin such as atorvastatin, or combined therapy with one of the fibrate drugs, is usually initiated. In terms of toxicity, statins can potentially cause myositis, which is causing this patient's symptoms as well as her elevated creatinine kinase levels. Rarely, patients can develop rhabdomyolysis with renal failure. Elevated liver enzyme levels can also be observed with statin treatment, although this is usually reversible.

Answer A is incorrect. Niacin (vitamin B_3) can lower LDL and increase HDL levels. However, statin medications are first-line therapy for this disorder. Niacin can be added to the regimen as a third drug (with a fibrate) or can be used in patients who are refractory to statin treatment. Its use is often limited by tolerability (it causes flushing in the majority of patients).

Answer B is incorrect. Hormone replacement therapy is contraindicated in patients with high cholesterol due to the increased risk of heart attack and stroke. Also, hormone replacement therapy is not necessary for a woman in her 20s.

Answer C is incorrect. LDL apheresis is a method for selectively removing LDL molecules from the blood using immunoadsorption columns. This process takes at least 3 hours and is done every 1–2 weeks. It is very expensive and not readily available.

Answer D is incorrect. Liver transplantation can dramatically lower LDL levels in patients with familial hypercholesterolemia by providing them with normal LDL receptors. However, the risks associated with transplantation make this option a last resort.

29. **The correct answer is E.** The therapeutic privilege is a rare case of an appropriate exception to informed consent. The principle is that informing the patient will not be medically sound for the patient. In general, a physician should consult another physician not involved in the patient's care, a psychiatrist, and/or an ethics committee when invoking this principle. It does not refer to withholding information a physician believes will make a patient less likely to have a procedure performed.

Answer A is incorrect. Only a patient can waive their own right to informed consent.

Answer B is incorrect. Any competent adult can make informed consent.

Answer C is incorrect. Usually, physicians must obtain informed consent. In some instances, a qualified nurse or other medical professional may obtain informed consent; however a nursing volunteer can certainly not.

Answer D is incorrect. A competent patient may acknowledge informed consent by any means.

30. **The correct answer is B.** This patient has the classic presentation of pheochromocytoma, a tumor of the adrenal medulla that causes hypersecretion of catecholamines. Patients tend to experience sudden "spells" of elevated blood pressure, palpitations, headache, diaphoresis, and anxiety. Diagnosis of this disorder is made by demonstration of elevated urinary excretion of catecholamines or their metabolites, metanephrines and vanillylmandelic acid. Pharmacologically, this disorder is managed with nonselective α-antagonists (phenoxybenzamine and phentolamine). It is also useful to keep in mind that pheochromocytoma is a part of multiple endocrine neoplasma (MEN) type II (medullary carcinoma of the thyroid, pheochromocytoma, and parathyroid tumor) and MEN type III (medullary carcinoma of the thyroid, pheochromocytoma, and mucosal neuromas).

Answer A is incorrect. Phenelzine, a monoamine oxidase inhibitor, is used to treat depression is in fact contraindicated in patients with pheochromocytoma because it can exacerbate hypertension.

Answer C is incorrect. Phenylephrine, an α-agonist, would not be appropriate for the treatment of pheochromocytoma because it would worsen the patient's hypertension via its vasoconstrictive effect at α_1-receptors.

Answer D is incorrect. Propranolol, a nonselective β-blocker, is not indicated for the treatment of pheochromocytoma because its actions are limited to β receptors. Thus, it would have little effect in antagonizing the α_1-agonist actions of norepinephrine that are of concern in these tumors.

31. **The correct answer is D.** This patient has a potentially reversible case of dementia: normal pressure hydrocephalus (NPH), with the classic triad of incontinence, gait difficulty, and mental decline ("wet, wobbly, and wacky"). Patients with NPH often demonstrate mild bradykinesia and their gait has been described as "magnetic" because their feet seemingly cling to the floor. The score of 26/30 on the Mini-Mental State Examination indicates only that some mild abnormality is present. Regardless, the patient should undergo magnetic resonance imaging to rule out a mass lesion that could cause similar symptoms. The pathophysiology of NPH is not well understood, but it is

thought that neurons are stretched secondary to ventricular dilation caused by excessive cerebrospinal fluid production, decreased absorption, or both. It is imperative to identify these patients because timely intervention with a ventriculoperitoneal shunt can reverse the dementia and decline.

Answer A is incorrect. Alzheimer's disease can present with some of the symptoms in this case. However, significant physical impairment tends to occur later in the Alzheimer's disease process and would thus correlate with a much lower score on the Mini-Mental State Examination. The time course and the relatively rapid progression in symptoms are not consistent with this diagnosis.

Answer B is incorrect. Hypothyroidism, another potential cause of reversible dementia in the elderly, should be ruled out early in the work-up. This patient's TSH level is normal, indicating euthyroidism.

Answer C is incorrect. Multi-infarct dementia is the most common cause of cognitive decline with a stepwise drop in function in the setting of prior cerebrovascular disease and stroke. In this case, the decline has been steadily progressive in a patient with no history of vascular disease.

Answer E is incorrect. Parkinson's disease classically presents with bradykinesia, masklike facies, shuffling gait, tremor, and rigidity. This patient has mild bradykinesia and no rigidity or tremor, so this diagnosis is a less likely possibility.

32. **The correct answer is E.** Protein malnutrition, or kwashiorkor, is characterized by an inadequate intake of protein but adequate intake of calories. Edema is the most common presenting symptom, but depigmented hair, anorexia, fatty liver changes, and skin lesions are also seen. Edema is caused by low levels of protein that decrease the plasma oncotic pressure and result in a loss of fluid into interstitial spaces. This patient's history and presentation are consistent with a low-protein, normal-calorie diet.

Answer A is incorrect. Marasmus describes caloric deficiency that can occur even with an adequate protein intake. Like kwashiorkor, marasmus is seen in infants at times of diet change such as weaning from breast milk in areas of the world where food can be scarce. However, marasmus is a generalized starvation with loss of body fat and protein. The symptoms of marasmus are muscle wasting, weakness, arrested growth, and anemia.

Answer B is incorrect. When the intake of carbohydrates is low, amino acids are deaminated to provide carbon skeletons for gluconeogeneis. However, this will not produce edema as seen in kwashiorkor.

Answer C is incorrect. Electrolyte deficiencies have various effects, but some are clinically difficult to recognize in an 8-month-old infant. For example, hyponatremia can manifest with confusion, muscle cramps, anorexia, nausea, seizures, and coma; hypokalemia can manifest with nausea, vomiting, muscle weakness or paralysis, rhabdomyolysis, and cardiac arrhythmias. However, overt edema from solely an electrolyte deficiency is a highly unlikely presentation.

Answer D is incorrect. Fat malnutrition would be unlikely in this child based on the presentation. Rice milk has about one-fourth the amount of fat in cow's milk or soy milk. Fats, especially the essential fatty acids linoleic acid and linolenic acid, are largely obtained in the diet. They are required for the development of cell membranes and nerve cell sheaths. Deficiency in fat causes developmental delays but not edema. In addition, with adequate calories the body can generate most fatty acids.

33. **The correct answer is E.** This patient most likely has *Mycobacterium tuberculosis* infection. *M. tuberculosis* is an acid-fast bacillus, and Ziehl–Neelsen stain is used to reveal acid-fast bacteria. Characteristics favoring a diagnosis of tuberculosis include immigrant status, night sweats, weight loss, and chest x-ray findings. Primary tuberculosis is known to result in

Ghon complexes, which show up as calcifications on x-ray imaging. Ghon complexes are a combination of parenchymal lesions and involved hilar and/or mediastinal lymph nodes. The lesions are calcified because of the caseating granuloma formation. Secondary tuberculosis presents with cavitary lesions and is seen more in immunocompromised patients. Other pathologies that can present with hilar/mediastinal nodes are lymphoma and sarcoidosis, making the Gram stain important in diagnosis. *M. tuberculosis* is aerobic and gram positive.

Answer A is incorrect. Congo red is used to visualize amyloid, showing apple-green birefringence in polarized light.

Answer B is incorrect. Giemsa's stain is useful for *Borrelia*, *Plasmodium*, trypanosomes, and *Chlamydia*.

Answer C is incorrect. India ink is the stain of choice for *Cryptococcus neoformans*.

Answer D is incorrect. Periodic acid-Schiff stains glycogen, and thus it can be used to visualize mucopolysaccharides. In addition, is used to diagnose Whipple's disease.

34. **The correct answer is A.** The patient has symptoms of hypercalcemia. With a history of smoking and "coin" lesion in the lung, one should suspect a lung tumor that produces parathyroid hormone-related peptide. Squamous cell carcinoma is a centrally located bronchogenic carcinoma.

Answer B is incorrect. Horner's syndrome is characterized by ptosis, miosis, and anhidrosis. It is a complication of lung cancer at the apex, referred to as a Pancoast tumor.

Answer C is incorrect. Chronic silica exposure is associated with increased tuberculosis susceptibility. Tuberculosis usually presents with chronic cough, hemoptysis, fevers, chills, and weight loss.

Answer D is incorrect. Cystic fibrosis causes respiratory, reproductive, and gastrointestinal symptoms.

Answer E is incorrect. Kartagener's syndrome is associated with sinusitis, bronchiectasis, and infertility.

Answer F is incorrect. ADH, which one could see with small-cell carcinoma, would cause water retention (oliguria) and fatigue.

Answer G is incorrect. Solitary parathyroid adenoma can present with hypercalcemia and low phosphorus levels. However, the patient's smoking history and new findings on chest imaging cannot be ignored.

35. **The correct answer is A.** The image depicts the epithelium that lies above the Peyer's patches, lymphoid tissues found within the ileum. This gut-associated lymphoid tissue is a vital collection of peripheral lymphoid tissue. Note that on a microscopic image of Peyer's patches, this epithelium has several M cells, specialized cells that function to endocytose and phagocytose particles in the lumen of the gut. Thus, they serve as immune surveillance in the intestines. In adults, B lymphocytes predominate in Peyer's patches and secrete IgA, the main antibody present within the mucosal lining of the gut. It is synthesized by plasma cells that reside within the lamina propria. Of note is the fact that several gut pathogens express virulence factors, known as IgA proteases, which cleave and therefore deactivates the dimeric IgA antibodies.

Answer B is incorrect. IgD is found only on the surface of B lymphocytes; its function is not known.

Answer C is incorrect. IgE orchestrates the type I hypersensitivity response.

Answer D is incorrect. IgG is the main antibody produced during a secondary immune response and also the most abundant.

Answer E is incorrect. While IgM can be found within the gut lumen, IgA predominates.

36. **The correct answer is E.** Peaked T waves and prolonged PR intervals are evident on ECG in

cases of hyperkalemia. Spironolactone is a potassium-sparing diuretic that inhibits K⁺ secretion at the cortical collecting duct; therefore, an important side effect of spironolactone use is hyperkalemia.

Answer A is incorrect. Acetazolamide inhibits carbonic anhydrase at the proximal convoluted tubule to cause increased excretion of HCO_3^-. It has no effect on potassium concentrations and thus would not result in hyperkalemia.

Answer B is incorrect. As a loop diuretic, furosemide inhibits the Na^+-K^+-$2Cl^-$ cotransporter in the thick ascending loop of Henle and causes secretion of potassium from the kidney. Hypokalemia can result.

Answer C is incorrect. Thiazide diuretics inhibit an Na^+-Cl^- cotransporter in the distal tubule. Increased distal nephron filtrate flow and activation of the renin-angiotensin-aldosterone axis cooperate to encourage potassium loss during thiazide diuresis. Thus, hypokalemia is an adverse effect of excess hydrochlorothiazide.

Answer D is incorrect. Mannitol is an osmotic diuretic that increases urine output by drawing fluid into the filtrate. It has no effect on ion transport proteins and thus does not change potassium excretion.

37. **The correct answer is C.** A feared infectious complication seen in patients with long-standing diabetic ketoacidosis is invasive rhinocerebral mucormycosis. As in this case, this infection leads to persistent sinusitis with inevitable invasion into adjacent neural structures such as the trigeminal nerve and the frontal lobe. *Rhizopus* organisms thrive in serum containing high glucose levels and low pH. Other conditions predisposing patients to this aggressive infection include iron overload/chelator treatment, AIDS, immunosuppression due to prolonged steroid use, and hematologic malignancies. Under the microscope, *Mucor* species appear as irregular, broad, nonseptate hyphae with 90-degree branching. Both *Mucor* and *Rhizopus* species can cause this condition.

Answer A is incorrect. *Blastomycetes* species appear as broad-based, budding, dimorphic fungi. Blastomycosis is mainly a pulmonary infection, endemic to states east of the Mississippi River and Central America. Infection of the lung leads to polygranulomatous infection with frequent hematogenous dissemination. These fungal species are cultured on Sabouraud's agar.

Answer B is incorrect. *Aspergillus* species appear microscopically as 45-degree angle branching, septate hyphae with rare fruiting bodies. Invasive *Aspergillus* infection occurs mainly after prolonged profound immunosuppression (as in patients with AIDS or cancer or in individuals with chronic granulomatous disease) and typically leads to bronchopulmonary aspergillosis with cavitary lesions in the lung.

Answer D is incorrect. Candidal species appear microscopically as pseudohyphae with budding yeasts. Candidal infections are more common in patients with poorly controlled diabetes, but they rarely cause invasive rhinocerebral infections as described in this patient. Rather, candidal infection may cause vulvovaginosis, chronic mucocutaneous infections, or disseminated candidiasis in advanced cases.

Answer E is incorrect. *Cryptococcus* species appear as 5- to 10-μm yeasts with a wide capsular halo. These infections represent an important opportunistic infection in patients with AIDS, causing cryptococcal meningitis. Cryptococcal infections are extremely rare in patients with normal CD4⁺ T-lymphocyte counts.

38. **The correct answer is E.** The disease that is described is Waldenström's macroglobulinemia, which is characterized by weakness, weight loss, a monoclonal M spike on serum protein electrophoresis (seen as a large spike in the gamma region), and a hyperviscosity syndrome (manifesting as nosebleeds, headaches, and vision disturbances). Hyperviscosity is caused by the large amount of IgM protein in the blood produced by a B-cell neoplasm. These large proteins interfere with microvascular and cellular processes, causing blood vessel

damage, which results in headaches due to impaired cranial blood flow and in disturbances in vision due to poor ocular blood flow. Additionally, circulating IgM proteins can bind to clotting factors and inhibit them, causing increased bleeding.

Answer A is incorrect. Chronic lymphocytic leukemia (CLL) typically presents with lymphadenopathy, hepatosplenomegaly, a warm antibody autoimmune hemolytic anemia, and smudge cells in the peripheral blood. The hyperviscosity syndrome is not present in CLL.

Answer B is incorrect. Diabetes presents with nocturia, polyuria, and polydipsia. Blood tests would demonstrate increased glucose. Superficial resemblances between the hyperviscosity syndromes and diabetic retinopathy, and diabetic kidney disease with the renal insufficiency of multiple myeloma, may be misleading. However, bleeding complications due to diabetes alone would be rare.

Answer C is incorrect. Monoclonal gammopathy of undetermined significance (MGUS) is similar to the condition described above in that it, too, has a monoclonal spike. An important difference is that MGUS is asymptomatic due to a lower level of protein. Some patients may experience mild polyneuropathy, but they will not have the bone pain, renal failure, and anemia of multiple myeloma or the hyperviscosity of Waldenström's macroglobulinemia. Nonetheless, MGUS may be a premalignant lesion that can progress to multiple myeloma.

Answer D is incorrect. Multiple myeloma is similar to the condition described above and it also involves abnormal plasma cells overproducing immunoglobulin, seen as a monoclonal M spike (critical for diagnosis). However, instead of a hyperviscosity syndrome, multiple myeloma typically presents with a collection of other characteristic symptoms. These symptoms include with lytic bone lesions causing bone pain and hypercalcemia, renal insufficiency and azotemia, increased susceptibility to infection, and anemia. Additionally, one may find Bence Jones protein (Ig light chains)

in the urine and a rouleaux formation of RBCs on peripheral blood smear.

39. **The correct answer is E.** Selection bias is being displayed in this scenario. The physician is selecting his more serious cases for the treatment group (i.e., those who are in most need of the benefit). The placebo group contains patients who are healthier, less symptomatic, and more likely to have a better outcome. Therefore, when it comes time for collecting data, the drug's beneficial effect compared to placebo may be blunted.

Answer A is incorrect. Studies can still be valid if there are differences in group size. There is no evidence that there is a difference in group size in this scenario.

Answer B is incorrect. Late-look bias occurs when information or results are gathered at an inappropriate time. Late-look bias is not displayed in this scenario.

Answer C is incorrect. Recall bias occurs when knowledge of the presence of a disorder alters the way a subject remembers his or her history. For example, a patient may over- or underestimate his or her consumption of a certain drug upon learning of its detrimental effect to the body. Recall bias is not displayed in this scenario.

Answer D is incorrect. Sampling bias occurs when those in the trial are not truly representative of the general population. Therefore, the results (both positive and negative) of the study cannot be truly applied to the general population. There is no evidence of sampling bias in this scenario.

40. **The correct answer is A.** This question addresses mechanisms of neoplastic transformation via loss of tumor suppressors. Each of the choices is a valid tumor suppressor function which, if lost, promotes malignancy. *Rb* and *p53* act as red flags that halt the cell cycle if, for example, DNA is damaged.

Answer B is incorrect. E-cadherin is a tumor suppressor that is involved in cellular adhesion.

Some breast and stomach cancers are associated with mutations in e-cadherin.

Answer C is incorrect. WT-1, a nuclear transcription factor, is mutated in Wilms' tumor. *p53* is a transcription factor, but *Rb* interacts only with transcription factors, thereby indirectly affecting gene expression.

Answer D is incorrect. The breast cancer-associated genes *BRCA1* and *BRCA2* are involved in DNA repair.

Answer E is incorrect. Tumor suppressors such as *APC* (gastrointestinal cancers and melanoma) and *NF1* (neurofibromatosis type 1) inhibit signal transduction.

41. **The correct answer is D.** Polymyxins bind to gram-negative bacterial cell membrane phospholipids and destroy the membrane by acting like a detergent. They have no activity against gram-positive organisms or fungi. Polymyxins are predominantly used to treat severe gram-negative infections that are resistant to less toxic antimicrobials. Polymyxins are rarely used owing to their association with nephrotoxicity and neurotoxicity. Numbness of the extremities is one manifestation of neurotoxicity, but dizziness, drowsiness, confusion, nystagmus, and blurred vision are also possible.

Answer A is incorrect. Granulocytopenia refers to a low number of granulocytes (neutrophils, eosinophils, and basophils). Certain medications can cause granulocytopenia, most commonly clozapine, ticlopidine, sulfasalazine, and antithyroid drugs. Among antibiotics, trimethoprim and dapsone are most commonly implicated.

Answer B is incorrect. Ototoxicity is a common adverse effect of aminoglycosides and vancomycin, particularly when the two agents are used in combination. It is not an adverse effect of polymyxins.

Answer C is incorrect. Patients with glucose 6-phosphate dehydrogenase deficiency are predisposed to hemolysis, and drugs with a high redox potential can precipitate rapid destruction of RBCs. In particular, primaquine and sulfonamides can precipitate a severe anemia characterized by sudden onset of jaundice, pallor, and dark urine with back pain.

Answer E is incorrect. Vomiting is an adverse effect of many antibiotics, but it is not an adverse effect of polymyxins.

42. **The correct answer is D.** Inflammatory bowel disease (IBD) typically presents during late adolescence to early adulthood with symptoms of abdominal pain and frequent bouts of diarrhea. Types of IBD are differentiated and diagnosed on the basis of their clinical picture, their appearance on endoscopy and biopsy, and the exclusion of other intestinal infectious etiologies. In this patient, the areas of normal-appearing mucosa should immediately point to the diagnosis of Crohn's disease as opposed to ulcerative colitis. Ulcerative colitis is characterized by mucosal inflammation that is limited to the colon and frequently involves the rectum. Crypt abscesses and ulceration of the mucosa are classically seen on biopsy. Crohn's disease, however, shows transmural inflammation interspersed with normal mucosa (skip lesions), as seen in this patient. It can affect any part of the gastrointestinal tract but usually spares the rectum. Noncascating granulomas may be found in Crohn's disease but are not found in ulcerative colitis.

Answer A is incorrect. Cells with loss of mucin and hyperchromatic nuclei are present in colon cancer, which is more commonly associated with ulcerative colitis.

Answer B is incorrect. Hyperplasia of goblet cells is the central feature of hyperplastic polyps, the most common type of non-neoplastic polyp. Although usually asymptomatic, they may cause bleeding, abdominal pain, and, rarely, obstruction.

Answer C is incorrect. Mucus-filled cells in crypts are part of normal colonic mucosa.

Answer E is incorrect. Ulceration limited to the mucosa is a feature of ulcerative colitis. In Crohn's disease, the inflammation is often transmural and interspersed with areas of normal-appearing tissue, as described in this vignette.

43. **The correct answer is E.** *Trypanosoma cruzi* infection can cause aganglionic megacolon and Chagas' disease, a condition in which the heart is enlarged and flaccid. *T. cruzi* is transmitted via the reduviid bug. Microscopic examination reveals flagellated trypomastigotes in the blood and nonflagellated amastigotes in cardiac muscle. *T. cruzi* infection is treated with nifurtimox. The fact that this man is from Central America is a second clue to his illness; epidemiologically, *T. cruzi* infections are most common among the poor in rural Central and South America.

Answer A is incorrect. *Cryptosporidium* infection presents with severe diarrhea in HIV-positive patients and mild watery diarrhea in HIV-negative patients. *Cryptosporidium* is transmitted via cysts in water (fecal-oral transmission). Microscopically, acid-fast staining cysts are found. Unfortunately, there is no treatment available for *Cryptosporidium* infection; however, in healthy patients, cryptosporidiosis is self-resolving.

Answer B is incorrect. *Entamoeba histolytica* infection presents with bloody diarrhea (dysentery), abdominal cramps with tenesmus, and pus in the stool. It can also cause liver abscesses accompanied by right upper quadrant pain. *E. histolytica* is transmitted via cysts in water (fecal-oral transmission). On microscopy one observes amebas with ingested RBCs. Treatment for *E. histolytica* infection includes metronidazole and iodoquinol.

Answer C is incorrect. *Giardia lamblia* infection presents with bloating, flatulence, foul-smelling diarrhea, and light-colored fatty stools. *G. lamblia* is transmitted via cysts in water (fecal-oral transmission). On microscopy, one observes teardrop-shaped trophozoites with a ventral sucking disc or cysts. Metronidazole is used to treat *G. lamblia* infection.

Answer D is incorrect. *Toxoplasma gondii* infection presents with brain abscesses in HIV-positive patients and with birth defects if infection occurs during pregnancy (toxoplasmosis is one of the ToRCHeS organisms). *T. gondii* is transmitted via cysts in raw meat or cat feces.

The definitive stage (sexual stage) occurs in cats. The diagnosis is most often made serologically. Sulfadiazine and pyrimethamine are used to treat toxoplasmosis.

44. **The correct answer is C.** A young man presenting with hemoptysis should raise a high index of suspicion for Goodpasture's syndrome. This diagnosis is supported by his fatigue and hematuria (although typically renal symptoms follow pulmonary symptoms by weeks to months). As the disease progresses, one would expect a nephritic picture with hematuria, hypertension, and oliguria. The diagnosis of Goodpasture's syndrome is confirmed by the renal biopsy, which on immunofluorescence staining shows a linear pattern of IgG deposition along the basement membrane. These anti–glomerular basement membrane (GBM) antibodies are specific to the α3 chain of type IV collagen, and cause injury to both the glomerular and alveolar basement membranes.

Answer A is incorrect. ANCAs are found in certain pauci-immune glomerulonephritides such as Wegener's granulomatosis. This could account for a nephritic picture, but immunofluorescence would show an absence of any immune deposition. Furthermore, if the patient had Wegener's granulomatosis, one would expect to see a specific pattern of symptoms involving the sinuses, lungs, and kidneys.

Answer B is incorrect. Goodpasture's syndrome is caused by anti-GBM antibodies specific to the α3 chain of type IV collagen. Type III collagen is found in skin, blood vessels, and other organs and is not affected by anti–GBM antibodies. The most common pathology involving type III collagen is Ehlers–Danlos syndrome, a connective tissue disorder in which patients bleed very easily and have hyperelastic skin.

Answer D is incorrect. Immune complex deposition causes damage to the glomerulus in many diseases such as poststreptococcal glomerulonephritis and systemic lupus erythematosus. The cause can be idiopathic, due to an antigenic stimulus, or due to a systemic immune complex disorder. On immunofluorescence one would see a less even distribution of staining, with lumpy or granular deposition of immune complexes in the glomerulus.

Answer E is incorrect. The patient's presentation is characteristic of Goodpasture's syndrome, which is caused by antibodies specific to type IV collagen. Immune-related injury to the glomerulus can be separated into three categories: immune-complex glomerulonephritis, anti–GBM, and pauci-immune glomerulonephritis (no antibodies, complement, or immune deposition). It has been proposed that pauci-immune glomerulonephritis is mediated by T lymphocytes, which release cytokines and thereby recruit inflammatory cells.

45. **The correct answer is A.** The patient has experienced rhabdomyolysis secondary to extreme muscle strain. Rhabdomyolysis causes the release of muscle cell contents into the bloodstream, leading to an elevated creatine kinase level and myoglobinuria (red urine characterized by a urine dipstick test that is positive for blood but shows no RBCs on urinalysis). Release of intracellular potassium may lead to the development of significant arrhythmias and possibly death.

Answer B is incorrect. Hepatomegaly is a nonspecific sign of many medical conditions but is not a typical consequence of rhabdomyolysis.

Answer C is incorrect. Inflammation of the metacarpophalangeal joints is characteristic of rheumatoid arthritis and is unrelated to rhabdomyolysis.

Answer D is incorrect. Pain in a dermatomal distribution is characteristic of shingles and is unrelated to rhabdomyolysis.

Answer E is incorrect. A shuffling gait may be seen in Parkinson's disease and is unrelated to rhabdomyolysis.

46. **The correct answer is D.** The lack of pigmentation in the hair, skin, and eyes that is seen in albinism results from a lack of tyrosinase activity in melanocytes. Without tyrosinase, these cells are unable to convert tyrosine to melanin, putting the affected person at an increased risk of squamous and basal cell carcinoma (BCC) and malignant melanoma. Melanocytes, odontoblasts, pia and arachnoid mater, Schwann cells, cells of the ganglia, parafollicular C cells of the thyroid, chromaffin cells, the aorticopulmonary septum, pharyngeal arch skeletal components, and the neurocranium are all derived from neural crest cells, a specific portion of the neuroectoderm.

Answer A is incorrect. Although the ectoderm does give rise to the epidermis and the hair (as well as many other structures), it does not produce melanocytes.

Answer B is incorrect. The endoderm is responsible for the epithelial lining of many internal organs as well as other structures, but plays no role in albinism.

Answer C is incorrect. The mesoderm produces many structures, including the dermis, but does not produce melanocytes.

Answer E is incorrect. The neuroectoderm cells outside of the neural crest are the source of the iris (as well as several other optic and non-optic structures) but do not give rise to melanocytes.

47. **The correct answer is C.** The boy has a history consistent with absence seizures. On clinical examination, typical absence seizures appear as brief staring spells with no warning or postictal phase. Children are not responsive during the seizure and are amnestic of what happened during the attack. In fact, patients are generally unaware that a seizure has occurred. Classically, a regular and symmetric 3-Hz spike is found on electroencephalography. Ethosuximide is the primary treatment option in cases of absence (petit mal) seizures.

Answer A is incorrect. Carbamazepine has been associated with the exacerbation of absence seizures.

Answer B is incorrect. Clonazepam and the ketogenic or medium-chain triglyceride diet have been attempted to reduce seizure frequency.

These adjunctive therapies, however, have limited efficacy.

Answer D is incorrect. Gabapentin has been associated with the exacerbation of absence seizures.

Answer E is incorrect. The teacher's concerns regarding the boy are quite common in the case of absence seizures. Often such concerns will be incorrectly attributed to inattentiveness and may even lead to a misdiagnosis of attention deficit/hyperactivity disorder (ADHD). Methylphenidate, a central nervous system stimulant, is the cornerstone of therapy in ADHD.

Answer F is incorrect. Tiagabine has been associated with the exacerbation of absence seizures.

48. **The correct answer is B.** Atherosclerosis begins with the formation of a fatty streak, which is caused by the deposition of cholesterol and cholesterol esters, lipid-laden macrophages (foam cells), calcium, and necrotic debris in the intima of the coronary arteries. Over time, the fatty streak becomes a proliferative plaque and then a complex atheroma under the influence of specific risk factors such as smoking, hypertension, diabetes, hyperlipidemia, and family history. The most common arteries affected are the abdominal aorta, coronary, popliteal, carotid, renal, and mesenteric arteries.

Answer A is incorrect. Arteriosclerosis is a general term for vascular disease characterized by rigidity caused by calcification and often thickening of blood vessels. The most common places for arteriosclerosis are the radial and ulnar arteries.

Answer C is incorrect. Medial calcific sclerosis, also known as Mönckeberg's arteriosclerosis, involves the media of medium-sized muscular arteries.

Answer D is incorrect. Mönckeberg's arteriosclerosis is characterized by ringlike calcifications that do not cause obstruction to arterial flow because the intima is not involved.

Answer E is incorrect. Takayasu's arteritis is also known as "pulseless disease" because of thickening of the aortic arch or proximal great vessels, which leads to weak pulses in the upper extremities and ocular disturbances.

Test Block 3

1. An 18-month-old child is brought to the physician by her parents because of a sore throat, difficulty breathing, and a barking cough for the past day. On physical examination the toddler is found to have some respiratory stridor and a runny nose but is not in acute distress. The rest of the examination is unremarkable. Which of the following is the most appropriate treatment?

(A) Amantadine
(B) Bronchoalveolar lavage
(C) emergency department admittance
(D) Penicillin
(E) Supportive therapy

2. A 64-year-old man with a history of coronary artery disease and high cholesterol presents to the physician with increasing lower extremity edema. His blood pressure is 190/110 mm Hg, and laboratory studies show hypernatremia and hypokalemia. Imaging shows no abnormalities except an area of right renal artery vessel constriction. Which of the following are the likely aldosterone and renin levels, respectively, in this patient?

(A) Decreased/decreased
(B) Decreased/elevated
(C) Elevated/decreased
(D) Elevated/elevated
(E) No change/no change

3. A 41-year-old man is admitted to the hospital for progressive obtundation. On admission the patient's serum sodium level is 114 mEq/L. Treatment is initiated, and 7 hours later the patient's serum sodium level is 134 mEq/L. Over the next 4 days the patient's condition worsens with the development of dysarthria, dysphagia, and paraparesis. What pathologic process is most likely responsible for this patient's new symptoms?

(A) Cerebral edema
(B) Diffuse axonal injury
(C) Intracerebral hemorrhage

(D) Osmotic demyelination
(E) Uncal herniation

4. When a particular ligand binds to its receptor, there is an increase in the cleavage of phosphatidylinositol biphosphate into inositol triphosphate and diacylglycerol. Both of these substances have actions within the cell. Which of the following would be an example of a receptor that functions in this manner?

(A) γ-Aminobutyric acid receptor
(B) Dopamine receptor
(C) Insulin receptor
(D) Muscarinic acetylcholine receptor
(E) Serotonin receptor

5. A 59-year-old man presents to his primary care physician with a 2-year history of increasing lethargy, weakness, bone pain, a pathologic hip fracture 1 year ago, and polyuria. X-rays show lytic bone lesions in the hip and spine. Total serum protein is elevated, and serum protein electrophoresis shows an M spike in the gamma immunoglobulin region. Bence Jones proteins are seen in the urine. If a kidney biopsy were taken, which of the following would most likely be found in this patient?

(A) Destruction of glomeruli with crescents of proliferating cells adherent to Bowman's capsule
(B) Fibrillary deposits in the mesangium and subendothelium that stain positive with Congo red
(C) Focal lesions involving collapse of the basement membrane, increase in matrix, and deposition of hyaline masses with detachment of the epithelial cells from the basement membrane
(D) Normal appearance under light microscopy but with foot process effacement observed under electron microscopy
(E) Ovoid hyaline masses located in the periphery of the glomerulus, with prominent wire looping

6. A 5-year-old boy is brought to the emergency department with a 2-day history of abdominal pain, vomiting, and a rash. His mother reports that he had a runny nose and mild cough about a week ago. On examination there is diffuse abdominal tenderness and a rash over the buttocks and the legs. His complete blood cell count is within normal limits and urinalysis shows 12 RBCs/mm³, 2 WBCs/mm³, no protein, and no glucose. A photograph of the rash is shown in the image. What is the most likely etiology of this patient's symptoms?

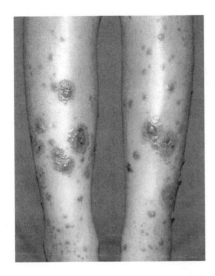

Reproduced, with permission, from Lichtman MA, Beutler E, Kipps TJ, Seligsohn U, Kaushansky K, Prchal JF. *Williams Hematology*, 7th ed. New York: McGraw-Hill, 2006: Color Plate XXV-15.

(A) Deficiency of von Willebrand factor-cleaving metalloproteinases
(B) IgA antibody deposition in the mesangium
(C) IgA immune complexes deposited in small vessels
(D) IgG antibodies against platelets
(E) IgG antibodies deposited in the glomerular basement membrane

7. A 70-year-old man is brought to the emergency department after a 2-day history of altered mental status. His past medical history is significant for alcoholism with hepatic cirrhosis, but he has no history of dementia. His current medications are hydrochlorothiazide, ranitidine, metoprolol, metformin, and testosterone. Laboratory tests show:

Na⁺: 137 mEq/L
K⁺: 3.1 mEq/L
Cl⁻: 101 mEq/L
HCO₃⁻: 18 mEq/L
Blood urea nitrogen: 15 mg/dL
Creatinine: 1.1 mg/dL
Glucose: 83 mg/dL

Which of his medications is most likely to have caused his delirium?

(A) Hydrochlorothiazide
(B) Metformin
(C) Metoprolol
(D) Ranitidine
(E) Testosterone

8. An 8-year-old boy comes to the physician with a fever of 39.4° C (103° F), cough, chills, and dyspnea. His mother reports that he has had numerous respiratory infections over the past 3 years and has a history of foul-smelling, fatty stools. Physical examination is significant for crackles, decreased breath sounds, dullness to percussion in the lower left lung, and clubbing of the digits. The patient's work-up reveals colonization by a non-lactose-fermenting, oxidase-positive organism that produces procyanin. What is the virulence factor used by the organism that is most likely responsible for this patient's current illness?

(A) Cord factor
(B) F protein
(C) Polysaccharide capsule
(D) Protein P1 adhesin factor

9. Referring to the image, where A = afferent arteriole and B = efferent arteriole, which of the following most accurately reflects the actions of angiotensin II and prostaglandins on the glomerular filtration rate (GFR) and renal plasma flow (RPF) in a dehydrated patient?

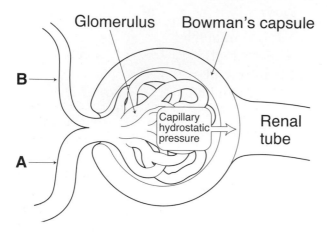

Reproduced, with permission, from USMLERx.com.

(A) Angiotensin II vasoconstricts A; prostaglandins vasodilate B; there is an overall decrease in GFR and increase in RPF
(B) Angiotensin II vasoconstricts A; prostaglandins vasodilate B; there is an overall increase in GFR and decrease in RPF
(C) Angiotensin II vasoconstricts B; prostaglandins vasodilate A; there is an overall decrease in GFR and increase in RPF
(D) Angiotensin II vasoconstricts B; prostaglandins vasodilate A; there is an overall increase in GFR and decrease in RPF
(E) Angiotensin II vasodilates B; prostaglandins vasoconstrict A; there is an overall decrease in GFR and increase in RPF

10. A 24-year-old man presents to the emergency department with hypertension, tachycardia, an elevated body temperature, diaphoresis, mydriasis, and severe agitation. When asked, his mother states that her son and his friends "probably used some drugs they got in the neighborhood." Which of the following is the most appropriate therapy for this patient?

(A) Atropine
(B) Flumazenil

(C) Fluoxetine
(D) Labetalol
(E) Naloxone
(F) Physostigmine

11. A 39-year-old woman presents to the physician with complaints of itchy skin and diarrhea. On examination, the patient appears slightly confused and is having trouble remembering what she did earlier in the day. A physical examination shows that the patient has a large, deeply pigmented tongue with thickened papillae. On further questioning, it is discovered that the patient has been taking isoniazid for suspected tuberculosis infection. Which of the following supplements should this patient take?

(A) Ascorbic acid
(B) Biotin
(C) Folic acid
(D) Niacin
(E) Riboflavin
(F) Thiamine
(G) Vitamin D

12. Acute allograft rejection is mediated by cytotoxic T lymphocytes that recognize and are activated by the major histocompatibility complex proteins expressed by the donated organ. A depleting monoclonal antibody to which of the following cell surface molecules would be most useful in reducing this immune-mediated graft rejection?

(A) CD3
(B) CD4
(C) CD14
(D) CD16
(E) CD19

13. Routine blood studies for a 73-year-old man show an elevated serum alkaline phosphatase level. The physician subsequently checks the patient's prostate-specific antigen level, which is elevated. A fine-needle biopsy of the prostate is done, revealing adenocarcinoma. Which of the following might also be expected in this patient?

(A) Hepatitis
(B) Hypercalcemia

(C) Hyperuricemia

(D) Paraneoplastic syndrome

(E) Severe anaplasia

14. A 28-year-old woman with a past medical history significant for pelvic inflammatory disease presents to the emergency department with right lower quadrant abdominal pain. The pain began 2 hours ago, has been consistently localized to the right lower quadrant without migration, and has been associated with nausea and vomiting. Although her periods are usually regular, her last menstruation was approximately 6 weeks ago. On examination, she is found to be afebrile with a blood pressure of 90/60 mm Hg, a pulse of 110/min, and a respiratory rate of 26/min. Abdominal examination shows localized tenderness with guarding in the right lower quadrant. Pelvic examination is deferred due to excessive pain, but vaginal bleeding is noted. Laboratory studies show a hematocrit of 29.8% and an elevated human chorionic gonadotropin (hCG) level. Which of the following is the most likely etiology of this patient's illness?

(A) A blastocyst has implanted in the ampulla, leading to uterine tube rupture

(B) A blastocyst has implanted in the posterior superior uterine wall, leading to rupture of the uterine wall

(C) A fecalith has obstructed the appendiceal lumen, leading to rupture of the appendix

(D) Ectopic endometrial tissue has implanted on the ovary

(E) Two spermatozoa have fertilized a single ovum

15. On the same day one pediatrician sees two children with a hereditary defect in fructose metabolism. The physician reminds the parents of the first child to maintain the child on a low-fructose, low-sucrose diet. However, he tells the parents of the second child that their child is unlikely ever to experience any symptoms of the disorder despite the fact that fructose was detected in her blood and urine. Which of the following actions describes the function of the enzyme deficient in the second child?

(A) Converts fructose to fructose-1-phosphate

(B) Converts fructose-1-phosphate to dihydroxyacetone-phosphate

(C) Converts fructose-1-phosphate to glyceraldehydes

(D) Converts glyceraldehyde to glyceraldehyde-3-phosphate

(E) Converts glyceraldehyde-3-phosphate to 1,3-bisphosphoglycerate

16. Calcium channel blockers are commonly used cardiovascular drugs that are effective antihypertensives, antianginals, and antiarrhythmics. Diltiazem is more effective than nifedipine for cardiac indications because diltiazem slows the recovery of the slow calcium channel while also reducing the influx of calcium into the myocyte. Which of the following is an effect of diltiazem?

(A) Increase in cardiac chronotropy

(B) Increase in cardiac inotropy

(C) Increase in conduction velocity

(D) Increase vascular smooth muscle tone

(E) Prolongation of the PR interval

17. A 68-year-old woman presents to the emergency department with altered mental status. Her temperature is 38.8° C (101.8° F,) heart rate is 116/min, respiratory rate is 23/min, and blood pressure is 132/87 mm Hg. Arterial blood gas shows a pH of 7.28, partial pressure of carbon dioxide of 15 mm Hg, and a bicarbonate level of 7 mEq/L. Which of the following is the most accurate description of the patient's acid-base status?

(A) Metabolic acidosis

(B) Metabolic acidosis with respiratory alkalosis

(C) Metabolic acidosis with respiratory compensation

(D) Metabolic alkalosis with respiratory acidosis

(E) Respiratory alkalosis

18. A 69-year-old smoker presents with "double vision," lower extremity muscle weakness with exertion, and diminished deep tendon reflexes. Results of neurologic, cardiovascular, and ophthalmologic examinations are negative. X-ray of the chest reveals a small circular lesion in the right lung hilum. A full cancer work-up reveals metastases throughout the body. A biopsy report from the pathologist gives the diagnosis of oat cell carcinoma. Which of the following is the most likely cause for this man's diplopia and weakness?

(A) Antibodies against presynaptic calcium channels at the neuromuscular junction
(B) Autoantibodies to acetylcholine receptors at the neuromuscular junction
(C) Autoimmune disease with anti-double-stranded DNA, anti-DNA, and anti-Smith antibodies
(D) Inflammatory disorder of synovial joints with pannus formation
(E) Reactivation of a peripheral subpleural parenchymal lesion and hilar lymph nodes

19. A 33-year-old man from Connecticut comes to his physician because he began experiencing flulike symptoms and an expanding rash on his leg following a camping trip 1 week ago. The physician diagnoses him with Lyme disease and prescribes tetracycline. The man finds some tetracycline in his bathroom from about 6 years ago and decides to use this instead of buying a new bottle. One week later, the man presents to the emergency department and is diagnosed with which of the following renal conditions?

(A) Acute tubular necrosis
(B) Glomerulonephritis
(C) Kidney stones
(D) Renal papillary necrosis
(E) Renal tubular dysfunction

20. A 26-year-old woman presents to her physician because of difficulty swallowing for the past 2 weeks. Her physical examination is unremarkable. For the past 4 years, this patient has presented to her doctor with complaints of episodic nausea, vomiting, and diarrhea as well as dyspareunia, low back pain, and menorrhagia.

She had a negative ultrasound of the gallbladder after complaining of severe right upper quadrant pain. She also had a normal colonoscopy with biopsies after complaining of rectal pain and the passage of blood and mucus in her stool. In the absence of organic pathology, what is this patient's most likely diagnosis?

(A) Body dysmorphic disorder
(B) Conversion disorder
(C) Hypochondriasis
(D) Pain disorder
(E) Somatization disorder

21. A 68-year-old farmer presents to his physician for evaluation of a "bump" on his ear. Detailed physical examination reveals three pearly, flesh-colored lesions on the ear (see image), left forearm, and right lower leg. On questioning, the patient reports that his father, also a farmer, developed similar lesions as an elderly man. Which of the following best describes the normal function of the cell type responsible for this patient's disease process?

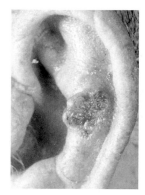

Reproduced, with permission, from Fauci AS, Braunwald E, Kasper DL, Hauser SL, Longo DL, Jameson JL, and Loscalzo J, eds. *Harrison's Principles of Internal Medicine*, 17th ed. New York: McGraw-Hill, 2008: Figure 83-2.

(A) Antigen presentation
(B) Regeneration of new skin cells
(C) Secretion of sweat
(D) Skin pigmentation and ultraviolet protection
(E) Waterproofing

22. A 2-year-old boy presents to his pediatrician with hepatosplenomegaly, failure to thrive, and progressive central nervous system deterioration. Liver biopsy shows that hepatocytes and Kupffer cells have a foamy, vacuolated appearance. The pediatrician suspects that the boy will die by 3 years of age. Which of the following is the function of the metabolic enzyme deficient in this patient?

(A) Converts ceramide trihexoside to lactosyl cerebroside
(B) Converts galactocerebroside to cerebroside
(C) Converts ganglioside M_2 to ganglioside M_3
(D) Converts glucocerebroside to cerebroside
(E) Converts sphingomyelin to cerebroside

23. A 60-year-old man with Wolff-Parkinson-White syndrome currently receiving pharmacologic treatment presents to the clinic with fatigue and a 2.3-kg (5-lb) weight gain over the past 3 months. Physical examination results are normal. Laboratory tests show:

Na^+: 136 mEq/L
K^+: 3.8 mEq/L
Cl^-: 100 mEq/L
HCO_3^-: 24 mEq/L
Blood urea nitrogen: 12 mg/dL
Creatinine: 1.1 mg/dL
WBC: 7,000/mm^3
Platelet count: 270,000/mm^3
Hematocrit: 44%
Hemoglobin: 15.6 g/dL
Thyroid-stimulating hormone: 23 U/mL
Thyroxine: 2.0 µg/dL
Prothrombin time: 12 sec
Activated partial thromboplastin time: 30 sec

The patient did not bring a list of his current medications. Which medication is most likely the cause of his condition?

(A) Amiodarone
(B) Enoxaparin
(C) Metoprolol
(D) Quinidine
(E) Warfarin

24. A patient with major depression that is resistant to treatment with selective serotonin receptor inhibitors and therapy is tapered off of his existing antidepressant medications and subsequently given a monoamine oxidase inhibitor by a physician who has been treating him for 3 years. The patient develops the serotonin syndrome, which results in her death. Considering the defining characteristics of malpractice, which of the following best describes the actions of the physician?

(A) Not malpractice because no harm was caused directly from the treatment
(B) Not malpractice because the patient was not harmed at all by this physician
(C) Not malpractice because the physician did not neglect her duties
(D) Not malpractice because the physician had no obligation to treat this patient
(E) This is an instance of malpractice

25. A 36-year-old woman comes to the physician because of dysphagia. Physical examination shows clawlike hands secondary to "tightened" skin; small, flat red skin marks around the upper extremities; and three small (<2.5 cm) subcutaneous nodules in her right forearm. Her hands are very sensitive to cold weather, and she wears winter gloves in air-conditioned stores to prevent her hands from cramping up and getting pale. Which of the following would most likely be abnormally elevated on further evaluation?

(A) Anticentromere antibody
(B) anti-Smith antibodies
(C) IgM anti-IgG
(D) Lower esophageal sphincter tone
(E) P-ANCA

26. A clinical laboratory technician is processing serum samples for HIV diagnostics. In order to confirm a positive enzyme-linked immunosorbent assay result, the technician performs a Western blot, assaying for the presence of antibodies to three different HIV proteins in the patient's serum. The image shows the results; tube 1 is the control for positives, tube 2 is the control for negatives, and tube 3 is the patient's sample. Which of the following is the most correct interpretation of the Western blot shown in the image?

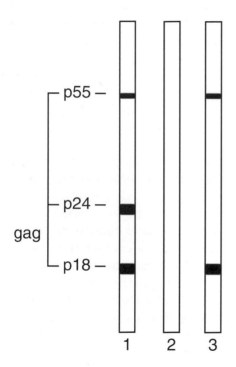

Reproduced, with permission, from USMLERx.com.

(A) The patient does not have HIV
(B) The patient's sample was most likely contaminated with positive control antibodies
(C) The positive control did not work; the blot must be redone
(D) The Western blot confirms a diagnosis of HIV
(E) The Western blot reveals that there are no antibodies to the HIV proteins in the patient's serum

27. A 24-year-old man presents to his physician for a routine physical examination before begin-

ning a new job. During testicular examination, the physician notes a nodule on the left testicle. The patient is subsequently diagnosed with a seminoma and is treated by an oncologist. Soon after beginning chemotherapy, the patient returns to his physician with complaints of a 1-week history of cough and shortness of breath. His physician orders an x-ray film of the chest that shows bilateral interstitial infiltrates. What is the mechanism of the chemotherapeutic agents this patient is most likely using to treat his seminoma?

(A) Alkylation of DNA
(B) Formation of superoxide or hydroxide radicals
(C) Inhibition of microtubule polymerization
(D) Intercalation into DNA
(E) Stabilization of microtubules against depolymerization

28. After a very difficult delivery 2 months ago, a new mother presents with complaints of amenorrhea, hair loss, weight gain, cold intolerance, constipation, puffy eyes, and flaky skin. Her blood pressure is 118/60 mm Hg, and her laboratory studies show a sodium level of 133 mEq/L, potassium of 5.1 mEq/L, and thyroid-stimulating hormone (TSH) of 1.5 μU/mL. Physical examination is otherwise unremarkable. Which of the following is the most likely cause of her symptoms?

(A) Antimicrosomal antibodies
(B) Ectopic TSH secretion
(C) Hemorrhage and shock
(D) Subacute thyroiditis
(E) Thyroid stimulating antibodies

29. Cells of the immune system are often difficult to distinguish from each other by light microscopy, even when they have very different functions. Surface marker proteins, which are often functionally important, are used to classify immune cells into one lineage or another. These marker proteins are traditionally named by the "cluster of differentiation" (or "CD") numerical system. Which of the following cell surface receptors is correctly paired with the immune cell that expresses it?

(A) B lymphocytes: CD3
(B) Cytotoxic T lymphocytes: CD19
(C) Dendritic cells: CD28
(D) Helper T lymphocytes: CD8
(E) Natural killer cells: CD16

(A) A
(B) B
(C) C
(D) D
(E) E

30. A 3-year-old boy is brought to the pediatrician because of decreased vision and pain in his right eye. Past medical history is significant for the diagnosis of glaucoma shortly after birth that has been refractory to standard medical therapies. Focused physical examination reveals iris hamartomas. Which of the following additional signs is most likely on physical examination?

(A) Bilateral acoustic neuromas
(B) Bilateral renal cell carcinomas
(C) Cystic medial necrosis of the aorta
(D) Leptomeningeal angioma
(E) Scoliosis

31. A 10-year-old boy is brought to the emergency department after falling from his bicycle. He presents with a large, painfully swollen knee; aspiration shows gross hemarthrosis. On further questioning, the patient's parents say that he bruises easily and that he had an episode of prolonged bleeding after losing a tooth 1 month ago. His maternal uncle had similar bleeding difficulties. After further testing, the patient is diagnosed with an X-linked recessive disorder. Which of the following laboratory test results corresponds to the patient's disorder?

Choice	Platelet Count	Bleeding Time	Prothrombin Time	Partial Thromboplastin Time
A	Normal	Normal	Normal	↑
B	Normal	↑	Normal	Normal
C	Normal	↑	Normal	↑
D	↓	↑	Normal	Normal
E	↓	↑	↑	↑

32. A 35-year-old man comes to the physician because of a fever, headache, malaise, and a cough and sore throat. The causative virus is established and the patient is given zanamivir. Which of the following is the mechanism of action of zanamivir?

(A) Blocks viral penetration and uncoating
(B) Inhibits the activity of a viral surface protein that binds to the cell surface receptor and initiates infection
(C) Inhibits the activity of an enzyme that allows budding virions to be released from the host cell membrane
(D) Inhibits viral DNA polymerase, preventing viral replication
(E) It is a nucleoside analog that causes inhibition of guanine nucleotide synthesis, preventing viral protein synthesis

33. A 32-year-old woman presents to the emergency department with a temperature of 38.7° C (101.7° F), petechiae covering her abdomen, and mental status changes. On questioning, her husband states that "she had been fine 3 weeks ago but got sick real fast." Physical examination shows severe weakness, petechiae and ecchymoses on the abdomen and back, and pale conjunctiva. A laboratory study shows severe anemia and thrombocytopenia with leukocytosis. The peripheral blood smear demonstrates the presence of abundant myeloblasts. Which of the following chromosomal translocations is most likely involved in this disorder?

(A) t(8:14) c-myc activation
(B) t(9:22), bcr-abl
(C) t(11:14), BCL1/PRAD1
(D) t(11:22), EWS gene
(E) t(15:17), PML-RAR-α

34. A 17-year-old girl who is 6 weeks pregnant presents to the emergency department with abdominal pain and vaginal bleeding. Ultrasound shows no fetal heartbeat and incomplete fetal development, and the pregnancy is terminated by aspiration to remove the fetal tissue. On questioning, the patient reports that she has been taking high doses of her mother's ulcer medication for her own heartburn. Which of the following medications did this patient most likely take?

(A) Cimetidine
(B) Magnesium hydroxide
(C) Misoprostol
(D) Omeprazole
(E) Sucralfate

35. A 43-year-old man with a history of hypercalcemia and bitemporal hemianopsia presents to the emergency department with muscle weakness, lethargy, and watery diarrhea. He reports brief episodes of complete paralysis in his lower extremities. The pH of the patient's nasogastric suction fluid is increased. An abdominal mass is noted on CT scan. The patient's family history is positive for numerous endocrine organ abnormalities. Which of the following is the most likely cause of this patient's symptoms?

(A) Gastrinoma
(B) Insulinoma
(C) Medullary thyroid carcinoma
(D) Pancreatic adenocarcinoma
(E) VIPoma

36. A 74-year-old man presents to his physician complaining of a 2-month history of left hip pain, intermittent headaches, and right-sided hearing loss. Laboratory studies show:

WBC: 5000/mm³
Hemoglobin: 14.2 g/dL
Platelet count: 390,000/mm³
Na⁺: 141 mEq/L
K⁺: 4.3 mEq/L
HCO₃⁻: 24 mEq/L
Ca²⁺: 8.6 mg/dL

Phosphate: 3.2 mg/dL
Alkaline phosphatase: 770 U/L
Creatinine: 0.8 mg/dL

X-ray of the pelvis is shown in the image. Which of the following is the most likely diagnosis?

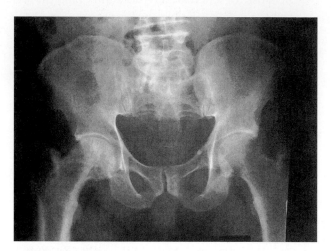

Reproduced, with permission, from Fauci AS, Braunwald E, Kasper DL, Hauser SL, Longo DL, Jameson JL, and Loscalzo J, eds. *Harrison's Principles of Internal Medicine*, 17th ed. New York: McGraw-Hill, 2008: Figure 349-3.

(A) Metastatic cancer
(B) Multiple myeloma
(C) Osteitis fibrosa cystica
(D) Osteoporosis
(E) Paget's disease

37. A 60-year-old Scandinavian woman presents to her doctor with a 2-month history of progressive fatigue. She also says that she has been feeling tingling and numbness in her lower extremities bilaterally and that she has felt "wobbly" lately. She does not have any significant past medical history. Her pulse is 101/min, and she has decreased lower extremity vibratory sensation as well as decreased sensation to light touch. Her laboratory studies show a hemoglobin level of 9 g/dL and a mean corpuscular volume of 110 mm³. Her peripheral blood smear is shown in the image. The pathogenesis of this patient's nutrient deficiency results from which of the following factors?

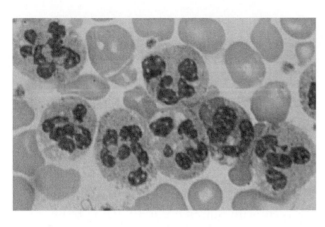

Reproduced, with permission, from Lichtman MA, Beutler E, Kipps TJ, Seligsohn U, Kaushansky K, Prchal JF. *Williams Hematology*, 7th ed. New York: McGraw-Hill, 2006: Color Plate VI-8.

(A) Abnormal neural crest cell migration
(B) Antibodies against parietal cells
(C) Bacterial overgrowth of colon
(D) Diet deficient in leafy vegetables
(E) Embolus to the superior mesenteric artery

38. A 37-year-old man with end-stage liver disease secondary to hepatitis C presents to the emergency department confused and lethargic. He has ascites, spider angiomata, and asterixis. Bowel sounds are normal. Laboratory studies show the following results:

Aspartate aminotransferase: 46 U/L
Alanine aminotransferase: 55 U/L
Alkaline phosphatase: 100 U/L
Bilirubin, total serum: 1.4 mg/dL
Prothrombin time: 38 sec
Albumin: 2.0 g/dL

Which of the following is the most appropriate acute treatment of this patient's condition?

(A) Lactulose
(B) Liver transplantation
(C) Lorazepam
(D) Neomycin
(E) Restricted protein diet

39. A 13-day-old child is brought to the pediatrician because of a purulent yellow discharge oozing from his eyes. He was born in Central America, where prophylactic erythromycin eye drops are not given to newborns at birth. On physical examination both eyelids are swollen, and the conjunctivae appear inflamed. Under microscopic view, scrapings from the conjunctival surface show epithelial cells with basophilic inclusions in the cytoplasm. Which of the following organisms is most likely responsible for this infant's conjunctivitis?

(A) *Chlamydia pneumoniae*
(B) *Chlamydia psittaci*
(C) *Chlamydia trachomatis*
(D) *Neisseria gonorrhoeae*
(E) *Ureaplasma urealyticum*

40. A 7-year-old girl comes to the dermatologist for the removal of a malignant melanoma. Her face, legs, and arms are covered with freckles. She also suffers from severe persistent sunburns. Which of the following is the most likely cause of these findings?

(A) A defect in nucleotide excision repair
(B) A defect in mismatch repair
(C) A defect in proofreading enzymes
(D) Exposure to ionizing radiation

41. A researcher at a pharmaceutical company develops an assay that can detect and quantify very low levels of hCG in the blood by binding with high affinity to the α subunit. Which of the following hormones may interfere with the ability of this assay to achieve an accurate measure of hCG levels in the blood?

(A) ACTH
(B) Gonadotropin-releasing hormone
(C) Growth hormone
(D) Melanocyte-stimulating hormone
(E) Thyroid-stimulating hormone

42. A 3-month-old boy who was born at full term presents to the pediatrician for evaluation of his congenital heart condition. His 39-year-old mother is healthy. She states that the pregnancy was notable for a decreased level of α–fetoprotein. The boy has flat facies, prominent epicanthal folds, and a simian crease on each hand. This child most likely has a heart condition that involves tissue derived from which of the following structures?

   (A) Bulbus cordis
   (B) Neural crest cells
   (C) Primitive atrium
   (D) Primitive ventricle
   (E) Truncus arteriosus

43. A 27-year-old man walks into the emergency department in an agitated state. He complains of severe abdominal pain and eventually becomes combative, requiring five-point restraint. His vital signs show elevated blood pressure and tachycardia. When a straight catheter is inserted, reddish urine enters the Foley bag. The urine is negative for RBCs, and a toxicity screen is negative. His doctor suspects a porphyria; laboratory tests for urine porphobilinogen are positive. Which of the following enzyme deficiencies is responsible for this patient's disorder?

   (A) Aminolevulinate dehydratase
   (B) Aminolevulinate synthase
   (C) Ferrochelatase
   (D) Heme oxygenase
   (E) Porphobilinogen deaminase
   (F) Uroporphyrinogen decarboxylase
   (G) Uroporphyrinogen III cosynthase

44. A patient with adult T-lymphocyte leukemia receives a bone marrow transplant from an unrelated donor. Despite an immunosuppressive post-transplant treatment regimen, over the course of several weeks the patient develops a severe cutaneous rash and intractable diarrhea. Blood tests were normal except for alanine aminotransferase (1032 U/L), aspartate aminotransferase (829 U/L), lactate dehydrogenase (634 U/L), and alkaline phosphatase (446 U/L). Which of the following is the most likely etiology of the patient's current symptoms?

   (A) Acute graft rejection
   (B) Graft-versus-host disease mediated by alloreactive donor T lymphocytes
   (C) Graft-versus-host disease mediated by alloreactive recipient T lymphocytes
   (D) Hyperacute graft rejection
   (E) Recurrence of leukemia

45. A 59-year-old man with a history of obesity, myocardial infarction, retinal detachment, and foot ulcers presents to the emergency department with numbness and tingling in his lower extremities. He has been receiving dialysis for the past 2 years. His hemoglobin A_{1c} level is increased. Which of the following describes the glomerular pathology most likely seen on light microscopy of this patient's kidneys?

   (A) Diffuse capillary and basement membrane thickening
   (B) Enlarged hypercellular glomeruli with neutrophils
   (C) Nodular glomerulosclerosis with thickened basement membrane
   (D) Segmental sclerosis with hyalinosis
   (E) Wire-loop appearance with subendothelial basement membrane deposits

46. A full-term newborn girl is noted to be hypotensive at birth. Despite intravenous fluid support, the baby remains hypotensive. During the medical work-up, the following data are obtained:

   Na^+: 127 mEq/L
   K^+: 5.5 mEq/L
   Cl^-: 92 mEq/L
   HCO_3^-: 18 mEq/L
   17-Hydroxyprogesterone: 74 nmol/L (normal 7–45 nmol/L)

   Which of the following is most likely to be found on further examination and work-up?

   (A) Biopsy of the gonads reveals the presence of testicular tissue
   (B) Chromosome analysis shows a 47,XXX karyotype
   (C) Endocrinology tests reveal a 5α-reductase deficiency

(D) Physical examination reveals an enlarged clitoris and partially fused labioscrotal folds

(E) Radiographic examination shows evidence of ovarian dysgenesis

47. A healthy woman presents to the physician for a checkup. Her physical examination is unremarkable, and laboratory studies are all within normal limits. She expresses concern about "inheriting" breast cancer because she had an aunt who recently died of the disease. The gene that would most likely indicate an inheritable form of breast cancer in this patient is located on which of the following chromosomes?

(A) 3
(B) 5
(C) 11
(D) 17
(E) 18
(F) 22

48. A 39-year-old woman presents to her physician with sporadic shooting pains across the left side of her face. She has no history of migraine headaches. On further questioning she says that 3 years ago she experienced several weeks of tingling in her right lower extremity, and as recently as 1 year ago was unable to drive her car because of bilateral arm weakness. The physician proceeds with a full neurologic workup, including MRI of the head (see image). Given the patient's likely diagnosis, what is the best long-term therapy?

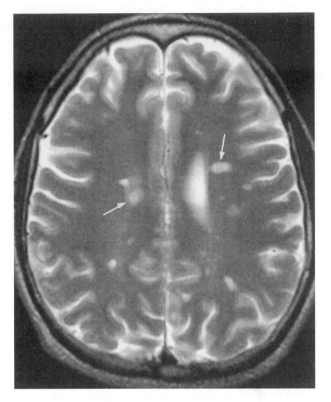

Reproduced, with permission, from Chen MYM, Pope TL, Ott DJ. *Basic Radiology.* New York: McGraw-Hill, 2004: Figure 12-36.

(A) Acetaminophen
(B) Corticosteroids
(C) Heparin
(D) Interferon
(E) Sumatriptan

1. **The correct answer is E.** The most likely diagnosis is croup, which is most commonly caused by parainfluenza virus. Croup is an infection of the upper airway causing narrowing that leads to inspiratory wheezing and a barking cough. Most cases of croup require only supportive therapy as treatment. Severe cases may require supplemental oxygen, corticosteroids, and epinephrine. While parainfluenza is the most common agent responsible for croup, it can also be caused by influenza, respiratory syncytial virus, and measles.

   Answer A is incorrect. Amantadine is an antiviral that has a narrow spectrum and is used to treat influenza type A. While influenza can cause croup, it is not the most common cause of this disease.

   Answer B is incorrect. Bronchoalveolar lavage is used to sample the lower respiratory tract in severe pneumonia, in the diagnosis of a lung tumor, and in the assessment of fibrosing alveolitis, among other indications.

   Answer C is incorrect. Admission to the emergency department may be called for if the child is in acute respiratory distress.

   Answer D is incorrect. Penicillin can be used to treat streptococcal pharyngitis, which presents with red, swollen tonsils and pharynx and a high fever.

2. **The correct answer is D.** The patient has renal artery stenosis leading to secondary hyperaldosteronism. The constriction in the right renal artery is causing hypoperfusion of the right kidney leading to an increase in renin production. The increased renin production is causing an increase in aldosterone levels, resulting in high blood pressure, hypernatremia, and hypokalemia. Thus, levels of both aldosterone and renin would be increased in this patient.

   Answer A is incorrect. Decreased levels of aldosterone and renin would be an unlikely combination in a patient unless both renin-angiotensin system dysfunction and adrenal dysfunction are present.

   Answer B is incorrect. A decreased aldosterone and an increased renin level is seen in patients with primary adrenal hypofunction, such as occurs in patients with Addison's disease. The renin-angiotensin system kicks into overdrive in these patients as a response to the low aldosterone levels.

   Answer C is incorrect. An increased aldosterone level paired with a decreased renin level would be seen in a patient with primary hyperaldosteronism, such as in a patient with an aldosterone-secreting adenoma or adrenal hyperplasia. These patients have a decreased level of renin due to the negative feedback effect of increased aldosterone levels on the renin-angiotensin system.

   Answer E is incorrect. Changes in aldosterone and renin levels would be expected in this patient.

3. **The correct answer is D.** Osmotic demyelination, also known as central pontine myelinolysis, can result from overaggressive treatment of hyponatremia. As hyponatremia develops, the brain prevents cerebral edema by gradually reducing its own osmolarity, thus reducing the osmotic gradient that would otherwise force water intracellularly. The brain can gradually replace these lost osmoles as the serum osmolarity is corrected, but correction of the serum sodium level at a rate faster than about 1 mEq/L/hr outpaces the brain's ability to compensate, resulting in neuronal shrinkage and death. The clinical manifestations occur several days later and include dysarthria, dysphagia, and flaccid quadriparesis that can become spastic and may progress to a "locked-in" syndrome, in which the patient retains full awareness but can move only the extraocular muscles.

   Answer A is incorrect. Cerebral edema occurs with acute hyponatremia as water flows freely across both the blood-brain barrier and cell membranes and into brain cells to compensate for the drop in serum sodium. However, cerebral edema does not typically accompany overly aggressive treatment of hyponatremia with hypertonic saline, but rather the opposite, as cell shrinkage and death occur as a result of water leaving the cells.

Answer B is incorrect. Diffuse axonal injury occurs in the setting of central nervous system trauma or angular acceleration or both and results in disruption of the axon at the nodes of Ranvier. Diffuse axonal injury does not occur with electrolyte abnormalities.

Answer C is incorrect. Intracerebral hemorrhage can occur as a result of hypertension, arteriovenous malformations, anticoagulation, thrombolysis, or amyloid angiopathy; however, it does not occur as a result of hyponatremia or the associated treatment.

Answer E is incorrect. Uncal herniation can result only from focal processes within the cranial vault, such as intracranial hemorrhage, but does not occur with diffuse processes associated with electrolyte abnormalities.

4. **The correct answer is D.** The muscarinic acetylcholine receptor, as well as the α_1-adrenergic and histamine$_1$ receptors, activates phospholipase C to cleave phosphatidylinositol biphosphate. Inositol triphosphate increases calcium ions for use in calmodulin activity, and diacylglycerol (DAG) activates protein kinase C. This is done through the G_q receptor.

Answer A is incorrect. The γ-aminobutyric acid receptor is a neurotransmitter-activated ion-channel-linked receptor.

Answer B is incorrect. The dopamine$_1$ receptor is a G_s receptor and functions to increase adenyl cyclase activity. The dopamine$_2$ receptor is a G_i receptor and inhibits adenyl cyclase activity.

Answer C is incorrect. The insulin receptor is an enzyme-linked receptor.

Answer E is incorrect. The serotonin receptor, like the γ-aminobutyric acid receptor, is an ion-linked receptor.

5. **The correct answer is B.** The patient has multiple myeloma. The big clues to the diagnosis are pathologic fractures, lytic lesions on X-ray, Bence Jones protein in the urine, and an M spike on serum protein electrophoresis. One possible consequence of multiple myeloma is systemic amyloidosis, as the plasma cells secrete misfolded aggregates of amyloid secondary to immunoglobulin light chain overproduction. These are deposited in the kidney and, in early stages, in the mesangium and subendothelial space; they stain positive with Congo red, with apple green birefringence in polarized light. Later in the course of the disease, they obliterate the glomerulus. These patients present with heavy proteinuria that progresses to renal insufficiency and uremia.

Answer A is incorrect. This describes rapidly progressive glomerulonephritis, which is caused by a variety of conditions, including Goodpasture's syndrome.

Answer C is incorrect. This is the description of focal segmental glomerulosclerosis, which occurs in HIV infection, heroin addiction, and sickle cell disease or in response to other events that cause scarring in the kidney (such as IgA nephropathy).

Answer D is incorrect. Minimal change disease (lipoid nephrosis) is characterized by normal-appearing glomeruli under light microscopy but foot process effacement under the electron microscope. It is common in children and presents with nephrotic syndrome. It is highly responsive to treatment with steroids.

Answer E is incorrect. The description of ovoid hyaline masses is characteristic of the Kimmelstiel-Wilson nodules seen in advanced diabetic glomerulosclerosis.

6. **The correct answer is C.** Henoch-Schönlein purpura (HSP) is a systemic vasculitis caused by the deposition of IgA immune complexes. It often follows a respiratory infection, and is characterized by the triad of purpura, abdominal pain, and glomerulonephritis. Some children also present with arthritis in major joints. The rash of HSP is usually described as palpable purpura on the buttocks and legs. It is the

most common small-vessel vasculitis in children, and rarely affects adults. The disease is self limiting and treatment is supportive. An older adult presenting with the same symptomatology is more likely to have a vasculitis associated with antineutrophil cytoplasmic antibodies.

Answer A is incorrect. The metalloproteinase ADAMTS-13 normally cleaves von Willebrand factor (vWF) multidimers, which then enter the circulation and rest on the surface of endothelial cells. In thrombotic thrombocytopenic purpura (TTP), deficiency of ADAMTS-13 leads to large von Willebrand factor (vWF) multidimers in the circulation, where they bind platelets causing the formation of platelet thrombi. TTP is characterized by fever, thrombocytopenia, hemolytic anemia, and renal and neurologic impairment.

Answer B is incorrect. IgA antibody deposition in the mesangium is the characteristic pattern of nephropathy associated with Berger's disease, which presents with hematuria and low-grade proteinuria during or a few days after an infection.

Answer D is incorrect. IgG antibodies against platelets is the pathophysiology of idiopathic thrombocytopenic purpura, which is characterized by thrombocytopenia leading to mucosal or skin bleeding, purpura or petechiae, and epistaxis. In children it has an acute onset after a viral infection, whereas in adults it has a gradual onset and often follows a viral infection or the administration of a new drug (e.g., sulfa drugs).

Answer E is incorrect. IgG antibodies deposited in the glomerular basement membrane is the etiology of Goodpasture's syndrome, which is a type II hypersensitivity reaction and presents with glomerulonephritis and pneumonitis.

7. **The correct answer is A.** Patients with cirrhosis are at risk for hepatic encephalopathy, which in chronic liver disease is frequently a reversible delirious state. Hepatic encephalopathy can be precipitated by several different factors, including hypokalemia, azotemia, alkalosis,

and hypovolemia, all of which can be induced by diuretics. Hydrochlorothiazide is especially known for causing hypokalemic metabolic alkalosis.

Answer B is incorrect. As with all medications used in hepatically impaired patients, metformin should be used with caution. The most grave adverse effect of metformin is lactic acidosis. However, hydrochlorothiazide is the most likely cause of this patient's delirium because he does not have a low blood glucose level.

Answer C is incorrect. As with all medications used in hepatically impaired patients, metoprolol should be used with caution. β-Blockers can produce adverse effects in the central nervous system (including sedation and sleep alterations), but exacerbation of asthma and other adverse cardiovascular effects are more common. Considering hydrochlorothiazide's association with hypokalemia, it is the most likely cause of this patient's delirium. It is worth noting that β-blockers are used in patients with chronic liver disease to treat portal hypertension.

Answer D is incorrect. As with all medications used in hepatically impaired patients, ranitidine should be used with caution. This is especially true in patients concomitantly using other medications that are metabolized hepatically due to ranitidine's inhibition of cytochrome P-450. The most likely adverse effects of ranitidine are antiandrogenic effects, but due to its hydrophobic nature, it can also cross the blood-brain barrier to cause confusion and dizziness. Still, hydrochlorothiazide is the most likely cause of this patient's delirium.

Answer E is incorrect. Testosterone should be used with caution in patients with impaired liver function, but in comparison to hydrochlorothiazide's association with hypokalemia, the diuretic is the most likely cause of this patient's delirium.

8. **The correct answer is C.** This patient has clinical and physical findings associated with a typical bacterial pneumonia caused by *Pseudomonas*

aeruginosa, an aerobic gram-negative bacteria. A major virulence factor of *Pseudomonas* is its alginate exopolysaccharide capsule, which forms a slime layer and mediates adherence. This patient also has signs and symptoms of cystic fibrosis: foul-smelling, fatty stools; frequent pneumonia; and digital clubbing (a sign of chronic hypoxia). Pulmonary infection by alginate-producing *P. aeruginosa* is the leading cause of death in patients with cystic fibrosis.

Answer A is incorrect. Cord factor is produced by *Mycobacterium tuberculosis*. It inhibits neutrophil migration, damages mitochondria, and leads to cachexia (weight loss). While pulmonary tuberculosis presents with coughing, fever, and night sweats, signs of lobar pneumonia are not commonly seen on physical exam. Tuberculosis is also not commonly associated with cystic fibrosis.

Answer B is incorrect. The F protein is released by the respiratory syncytial virus (RSV) and causes the formation of multinucleated giant cells (syncytial cells). RSV causes an atypical pneumonia and is not thought to be associated with cystic fibrosis.

Answer D is incorrect. Protein P1 adhesin virulence factor is used for attachment to respiratory cells by *Mycoplasma pneumoniae*, which causes atypical pneumonia, sometimes called walking pneumonia. Patients show few symptoms of infection with this type of infection (typically coughing with low-grade fever and some malaise). It is also not thought to be particularly associated with cystic fibrosis.

9. **The correct answer is D.** During hemorrhage, blood loss leads to an increase in the renin-angiotensin-aldosterone (RAA) system. Angiotensin II has the effect of preferentially constricting the efferent arteriole. Renal prostaglandins are produced in response to increased sympathetic activity and act to preferentially vasodilate afferent arterioles. The overall result is an increase in GFR and a decrease in RPF. It is notable that the reason angiotensin converting enzyme inhibitors are protective for the kidney is that they prevent vasoconstriction of the efferent arterioles and thereby prevent a decrease in RPF. The reason that drugs blocking the formation of prostaglandins (i.e., nonsteroidal anti-inflammatory drugs) are damaging to the kidney is that they block vasodilation at the afferent arterioles and thereby cause a decrease in both GFR and RPF.

Answer A is incorrect. Angiotensin II would cause vasoconstriction of B, while the prostaglandins would cause vasodilation of A. The overall result would be an increase in GFR and a decrease in RPF.

Answer B is incorrect. Angiotensin II would cause vasoconstriction of B, while the prostaglandins would cause vasodilation of A. The overall result would be an increase in GFR and a decrease in RPF.

Answer C is incorrect. Angiotensin II would cause vasoconstriction of B, while the prostaglandins would cause vasodilation of A. The overall result would be an increase in GFR and a decrease in RPF.

Answer E is incorrect. Angiotensin II would cause vasoconstriction of B, while the prostaglandins would cause vasodilation of A. The overall result would be an increase in GFR and a decrease in RPF.

10. **The correct answer is D.** The patient described above is probably under the influence of a central nervous system (CNS) stimulant such as methamphetamine. Labetalol is a nonselective α and β antagonist that would block many of the dangerous peripheral adverse effects of CNS stimulants, such as hypertension and cardiac stimulation. Other appropriate medications that could be administered under these conditions would be antipsychotic agents (to control the agitation and psychotic symptoms) and diazepam (to control possible seizures).

Answer A is incorrect. Atropine is a muscarinic antagonist that would be an appropriate therapy for an overdose by an acetylcholinesterase inhibitor. A patient presenting with an acetylcholinesterase inhibitor overdose would have miotic pupils and bradycardia.

Answer B is incorrect. Flumazenil is a benzodiazepine receptor antagonist. It is used in cases of benzodiazepine overdose. The clinical features of acute benzodiazepine intoxication include slurred speech, lack of coordination, unsteady gait, and impaired attention or memory. A severe overdose may lead to stupor or coma.

Answer C is incorrect. Fluoxetine is a selective serotonin reuptake inhibitor antidepressant. It would not be indicated in the case of CNS stimulant overdose.

Answer E is incorrect. Naloxone is an opioid-receptor antagonist that would be an appropriate therapy for an opiate overdose such as with heroin or morphine. A patient who presents with an opioid overdose would appear sleepy, lethargic, or comatose depending on the degree of overdose. Pupils would be miotic, not mydriatic. Blood pressure and heart rate would usually be decreased, and respiration would be depressed.

Answer F is incorrect. Physostigmine is an acetylcholinesterase inhibitor that might be used for an antimuscarinic drug overdose, such as with atropine, scopolamine, or Jimson weed. An antimuscarinic overdose can look similar to a CNS stimulant overdose, with at least one important exception. The hyperthermia seen with an antimuscarinic overdose is accompanied by hot and dry skin (because of blockade of the sympathetic cholinergics to the sweat glands). Stimulant overdose is often characterized by profuse sweating. Tachycardia, hypertension, hyperthermia, mental changes, and mydriasis are common to both.

11. **The correct answer is D.** This patient most likely has pellagra, caused by a niacin deficiency. Isoniazid impairs the conversion of tryptophan to niacin, and therefore its use can cause symptoms of niacin deficiency. Pellagra is characterized by the **3 D's: D**ermatitis, **D**iarrhea, and **D**ementia (and beefy glossitis, as described in the vignette). Isoniazid also produces pyrodixine (vitamin B_6) deficiency, which may manifest as convulsion, hyperirritability, and anemia.

Answer A is incorrect. A deficiency of ascorbic acid (vitamin C) would cause scurvy, which would present with swollen gums, bruising, anemia, and poor wound healing.

Answer B is incorrect. A deficiency of biotin would cause pruritic skin (dermatitis) and enteritis, but the above presentation, which includes beefy glossitis and dementia, is more characteristic of niacin deficiency.

Answer C is incorrect. A deficiency of folic acid would cause a macrocytic, megaloblastic anemia and would include symptoms such as fatigue. It would not result in this patient's presentation.

Answer E is incorrect. A deficiency of riboflavin (vitamin B_2) would cause angular stomatitis, cheilosis, and corneal vascularization.

Answer F is incorrect. A deficiency of thiamine (vitamin B_1) would cause beriberi and Wernicke–Korsakoff syndrome. Signs of beriberi include polyneuritis, cardiac pathology, and edema. Wernicke–Korsakoff syndrome is associated with dementia and a confabulating patient.

Answer G is incorrect. A deficiency of vitamin D would cause rickets in children and osteomalacia (soft bones) in adults, along with symptoms such as hypocalcemic tetany.

12. **The correct answer is A.** Anti-CD3 antibodies that bind to CD3 and trigger destruction of T lymphocytes (via phagocytes or complement-mediated lysis) would be most useful in this scenario, as CD8$^+$ T lymphocytes are the main effectors mediating acute allograft rejection. Note that monoclonal antibodies may be triggering, depleting, or blocking, and therefore it is absolutely necessary to characterize which of these effector functions they elicit, as those three scenarios would have three very different therapeutic applications.

Answer B is incorrect. Cytotoxic T lymphocytes express CD8, while helper T lymphocytes express CD4. While targeting CD4$^+$ T lymphocytes may be partially effective, it would be more useful to deplete all T lymphocytes with an anti-CD3 monoclonal antibody.

Answer C is incorrect. CD14 is a common macrophage cell surface marker.

Answer D is incorrect. CD16 is a common natural killer-cell surface marker.

Answer E is incorrect. CD19 is a common B-lymphocyte surface marker.

13. **The correct answer is B.** Prostatic carcinoma is the most common cancer in men. Metastasis can occur via hematogenous spread, often to the vertebral column, following the path of venous drainage of the prostate. An increased alkaline phosphatase level in the serum can be a sign of increased bone turnover caused by the metastatic tumor growth. Metastasis to bone is associated with loss of bone mineralization and matrix, as evidenced by hypercalcemia (>10.5 mg/dL) in some patients.

Answer A is incorrect. Hepatitis may increase alkaline phosphatase levels, as inflammation of the liver may obstruct parts of the biliary tree. However, hepatitis would not explain the increased prostate-specific antigen level.

Answer C is incorrect. Hyperuricemia (serum uric acid >7.4 mg/dL in males, >5.8 mg/dL in females) is a feature of myeloproliferative disorders in which tumor burden is high and there is rapid cell turnover. Hyperuricemia is also seen in gout, renal failure (whereby secretion of urate is defective), and certain metabolic conditions.

Answer D is incorrect. A paraneoplastic syndrome occurs when a tumor aberrantly produces a hormone; ADH production by small-cell lung carcinoma is one example. In this case, the alkaline phosphatase is not coming from the tumor itself, and no syndrome is described.

Answer E is incorrect. Although severe anaplasia may be present in the prostate biopsy, tumor grade and differentiation are not associated with elevated alkaline phosphatase levels unless bony metastasis has occurred.

14. **The correct answer is A.** This patient is presenting with a ruptured ectopic pregnancy, which occurs when a blastocyst implants in an inappropriate location, most commonly the ampulla of the uterine tube. This typically presents as described in the question stem and constitutes a medical emergency. The most common risk factors are pelvic inflammatory disease, or PID (usually gonorrheal), prior appendicitis or endometriosis, and previous abdominal surgery.

Answer B is incorrect. This describes appropriate implantation of a blastocyst in a normal pregnancy and is therefore not directly associated with pathology.

Answer C is incorrect. This describes the likely etiology of acute appendicitis. This will present with right lower quadrant (RLQ) abdominal pain but typically begins with diffuse periumbilical pain that later migrates to the RLQ. This condition is not associated with prior PID, a missed period, or elevated hCG level, and will typically produce a fever.

Answer D is incorrect. This describes endometriosis. Although this can be associated with irregular bleeding and abdominal/pelvic pain, it does not typically result in missed periods, shock-like signs, or elevated hCG level.

Answer E is incorrect. When two sperm fertilize a single ovum, a partial hydatidiform mole is formed. Like a ruptured ectopic pregnancy, this will produce vaginal bleeding and an elevated hCG level but will not cause acute shock-like signs and is not associated with prior PID. It will also cause a rapid increase in uterine size.

15. **The correct answer is A.** Fructokinase converts fructose to fructose-1-phosphate. This is the first step in fructose metabolism, and it is deficient in patients with essential fructosuria, also known as benign fructosuria. Patients with this condition are asymptomatic with the incidental finding of a reducing substance in the urine.

Answer B is incorrect. Aldolase B, also known as fructose-1,6-bisphosphate aldolase, converts fructose-1-phosphate to dihydroxyacetone-phosphate, the second step in fructose metabolism. This enzyme is deficient in patients with hereditary fructose intolerance, in which fructose-1-phosphate accumulates as a toxic metabolite. Patients will present with jaundice, hepatomegaly, vomiting, lethargy, convulsions, and hypoglycemia following ingestion of fructose. Chronic ingestion will lead to renal and liver failure. Treatment is avoidance of fructose. The first child in this vignette most likely has this condition.

Answer C is incorrect. Aldolase B converts fructose-1-phosphate to glyceraldehydes.

Answer D is incorrect. Triose kinase converts glyceraldehyde to glyceraldehyde-3-phosphate.

Answer E is incorrect. Glyceraldehyde-3-phosphate dehydrogenase converts glyceraldehyde-3-phosphate to 1,3-bisphosphoglycerate, one of the steps that fructose metabolites undergo in glycolysis.

16. **The correct answer is E.** By inhibiting the voltage-dependent calcium channels in cardiac pacemaker cells and slowing the rate of recovery, diltiazem will prolong phase 0 and phase 2 of the cardiac action potential. As a result, the PR interval will be prolonged, especially in the atrioventricular nodal cells, which is why this medication is indicated to prevent nodal arrhythmias.

Answer A is incorrect. Diltiazem decreases cardiac chronotropy because it slows the recovery of the slow calcium channels. Nifedipine does not have this effect.

Answer B is incorrect. Because it inhibits calcium ion influx, diltiazem reduces cardiac inotropy.

Answer C is incorrect. By the same mechanism of PR prolongation, diltiazem will decrease the conduction velocity of the action potential in the myocardial cells.

Answer D is incorrect. By inhibiting calcium influx in vascular smooth muscle cells, calcium channel blockers will decrease vascular tone, which is the source of their efficacy as antihypertensive medications. Nifedipine is the calcium channel blocker that is more effective on vessel receptors, whereas diltiazem and verapamil have more cardiac function.

17. **The correct answer is B.** This patient is acidemic, with a pH below the normal range of 7.35–7.45. Her bicarbonate level is low, so this is a metabolic acidosis. Next we look to see if she has appropriate respiratory compensation using Winter's formula: partial pressure of carbon dioxide = $1.5 (HCO_3^-) + 8 (\pm 2)$. The expected partial pressure of carbon dioxide would therefore be 16.5 mm Hg at the lowest, but the patient's level is 15 mm Hg, telling us that there is a simultaneous respiratory alkalosis. This picture of metabolic acidosis with respiratory alkalosis is seen with severe salicylate intoxication, which would explain the patient's altered mental status.

Answer A is incorrect. The patient is experiencing a metabolic acidosis, but there is also a simultaneous respiratory alkalosis.

Answer C is incorrect. If the patient were experiencing metabolic acidosis with respiratory compensation, given the bicarbonate level of 7 mEq/L, we would expect to see a partial pressure of carbon dioxide of 16.5 mm Hg. However, the patient's partial pressure of carbon dioxide is 15 mm Hg, suggesting that there is a simultaneous respiratory alkalosis that is more than compensatory.

Answer D is incorrect. This patient is acidemic, and her bicarbonate level is low, so we know this is a metabolic acidosis, not a respiratory acidosis or metabolic alkalosis.

Answer E is incorrect. The patient is experiencing a respiratory alkalosis, but there is also a simultaneous metabolic acidosis.

18. **The correct answer is A.** A paraneoplastic syndrome results from the production of a hormonally active substance that develops from what is usually a tumor focus and acts through hormonal action on distant areas of the body. Oat (small) cell carcinoma is an example of a cancer that frequently produces paraneoplastic

syndromes. One of these, Lambert–Eaton syndrome, involves the production of antibodies against presynaptic calcium channels at the neuromuscular junction. This produces proximal muscle weakness, decreased deep tendon reflexes, and, rarely, diplopia.

Answer B is incorrect. Myasthenia gravis is similar to Lambert–Eaton syndrome, but is not associated with oat cell carcinoma. It is occasionally seen with thymoma. Symptoms often include muscle weakness and diplopia. Repetitive nerve stimulation testing can be used to differentiate Lambert–Eaton from myasthenia gravis if the diagnosis is unclear. Repetitive nerve testing will show progressive increase in muscle action potential amplitude in Lambert–Eaton but no increase in myasthenia gravis.

Answer C is incorrect. Systemic lupus erythematosus is associated with multiple symptoms, including skin rash, hair loss, fever, and anorexia, and is usually seen in females 14-45 years old.

Answer D is incorrect. Rheumatoid arthritis is seen mostly in females, and presents with symmetric morning stiffness, joint inflammation, and systemic symptoms (fever and fatigue).

Answer E is incorrect. Secondary tuberculosis is uncommon except in immunocompromised patients. Because the biopsy came back as oat cell carcinoma, tuberculosis is highly unlikely.

19. **The correct answer is E.** Degraded tetracycline is associated with Fanconi's syndrome, a disorder of proximal tubule function that results in severe loss of protein, glucose, and essential minerals (e.g., calcium and magnesium). Tetracycline degrades over time to the toxic degradation product, anhydro-4-epitetracycline. Fanconi's syndrome is often caused by the accumulation of toxins in the proximal tubules.

Answer A is incorrect. Acute tubular necrosis is typically associated with hypoperfusion and is not associated with either Fanconi's syndrome or tetracycline.

Answer B is incorrect. Glomerulonephritis is most often caused by immune mechanisms and is not associated with either Fanconi's syndrome or tetracycline.

Answer C is incorrect. Kidney stones, commonly caused by hypercalciuria or infection, are not associated with either Fanconi's syndrome or tetracycline.

Answer D is incorrect. Renal papillary necrosis, often caused by diabetes or acute pyelonephritis, is not associated with either Fanconi's syndrome or tetracycline.

20. **The correct answer is E.** Patients with somatization disorder present with many physical complaints. To be diagnosed, they must have had at least eight symptoms, including at least two gastrointestinal symptoms, four pain symptoms, one sexual symptom, and one pseudoneurotic symptom. The patient finds the symptoms to be disabling out of proportion to the examination. These patients tend to be female with onset before the age of 30, and many patients also meet the criteria for a personality disorder.

Answer A is incorrect. Patients with body dysmorphic disorder have a severely distorted body image. All they see are imagined or minor physical flaws. They tend to obsess over their appearance, frequently look in mirrors, compare the flawed features with other people, and perform grooming rituals in order to hide the flaw. Onset tends to be in the late teens.

Answer B is incorrect. Patients with conversion disorder typically present with the sudden onset of loss of a single sensory or motor function, usually after a stressful life event. These patients tend to be adolescents or young adults, live in a rural area, lack education, and be of low socioeconomic status. The loss of function is not under voluntary control, and pain is not the predominant aspect of their complaint.

Answer C is incorrect. Patients with hypochondriasis misinterpret normal body symptoms and worry excessively about physical illness despite negative tests and positive reassurance. The diagnosis is made after their worries persist for more than 6 months. These patients tend to be middle-aged, and the incidence is roughly equal between men and women.

Answer D is incorrect. Patients with pain disorder complain of intense pain that is not explained by organic disease and lack symptoms other than pain. They tend to be in their 30s and 40s.

21. **The correct answer is B.** The lesion described is basal cell carcinoma (BCC). BCC most often occurs after chronic exposure to ultraviolet (UV) light and is therefore most common on sun-exposed regions of the body. The characteristic fleshy and pearly appearance of BCC helps distinguish it from squamous cell carcinoma (SCC), which is generally scaly in appearance. Basal cells comprise the deepest epidermal cell layer, the stratum basalis, and serve to divide and replenish skin cells normally lost through sloughing.

    Answer A is incorrect. Skin antigen presentation is carried out by Langerhans cells, which are specialized variants of dendritic cells. Langerhans cells are rarely involved in abnormal proliferations, termed histiocytosis X. However, in contrast to this case, histiocytosis X is almost always a pediatric disease and is characterized by numerous systemic complications.

    Answer C is incorrect. Sweat glands are composed of secretory cells and ducts that carry secreted substances to the skin surface. Importantly, both apocrine and eccrine sweat glands are present only in the dermis, not the epidermis. Tumors of sweat glands and sweat gland ducts are exceptionally rare.

    Answer D is incorrect. Skin pigmentation and UV protection depends on the synthesis and secretion of melanin by melanocytes. Melanocytes exocytose melanin, and it is subsequently taken up by neighboring cells where it remains. Most aberrant proliferations of melanocytes are benign nevi, or moles. However, malignant transformation of melanocytes secondary to UV exposure is a common cause of melanoma, but the lesion in the image can be distinguished from most melanomas by the absence of pigmentation and the presence of irregular borders.

    Answer E is incorrect. The waterproofing function of skin is carried out by keratinocytes of the stratified squamous epithelium. Carcinoma of these flattened cells occurs quite commonly and is termed SCC. SCC can be distinguished from BCC by gross morphology and by histopathologic examination.

22. **The correct answer is E.** Sphingomyelinase converts sphingomyelin to cerebroside. Deficiency of sphingomyelinase in Niemann–Pick disease causes accumulation of sphingomyelin and cholesterol in parenchymal and reticuloendothelial cells.

    Answer A is incorrect. α-Galactosidase A converts ceramide trihexoside to lactosyl cerebroside. This enzyme is deficient in Fabry's disease.

    Answer B is incorrect. β-Galactosidase converts galactocerebroside to cerebroside. This enzyme is deficient in Krabbe's disease.

    Answer C is incorrect. Hexosaminidase A converts ganglioside M_2 to ganglioside M_3. This enzyme is deficient in Tay–Sachs disease.

    Answer D is incorrect. β-Glucocerebrosidase converts glucocerebroside to cerebroside. This enzyme is deficient in Gaucher's disease.

23. **The correct answer is A.** Amiodarone is a class III antiarrhythmic that can be used as part of the pharmacologic treatment of Wolff–Parkinson–White syndrome. One of its potential adverse effects is hypothyroidism. However, it can also cause hyperthyroidism. This patient's elevated TSH and decreased thyroxine levels indicates a hypothyroid state. Other adverse effects of amiodarone include pulmonary fibrosis, hepatotoxicity, photodermatitis, and neurologic effects. You should always remember to check liver function tests, pulmonary function tests, and thyroid function tests in a patient taking amiodarone.

    Answer B is incorrect. Enoxaparin is a low-molecular-weight heparin that inhibits factor

Xa. It is used in patients with atrial fibrillation. It does not cause hypothyroidism.

Answer C is incorrect. Metoprolol is a β-blocker and a class II antiarrhythmic agent. Its adverse effects include dyslipidemia, fatigue, and sexual dysfunction. It does not cause hypothyroidism.

Answer D is incorrect. Quinidine is a class Ia antiarrhythmic agent. Its adverse effects include cinchonism (tinnitus, headaches, thrombocytopenia, and torsades des pointes). It is rarely used to treat Wolff–Parkinson–White syndrome.

Answer E is incorrect. Warfarin is an anticoagulant used in certain arrhythmias to prevent thrombus formation. It does not cause hypothyroidism.

24. **The correct answer is C.** Malpractice is civil litigation as a result of the "4 D's" on the part of the physician: **D**ereliction of **D**uty **D**irectly causing **D**amage to the patient. The physician in this case prescribed a treatment that was not a deviation from standard treatment. This was not negligence on the part of the physician.

Answer A is incorrect. This choice is not correct because the treatment did directly cause the death of this patient.

Answer B is incorrect. The patient was indeed harmed by the actions of this physician.

Answer D is incorrect. The patient had an established physician-patient relationship with the patient so he had an obligation to treat the patient; therefore this choice is not correct.

Answer E is incorrect. A skilled lawyer may produce a civil suit, but legally this is not a case of malpractice.

25. **The correct answer is A.** This patient has CREST syndrome. It is a variant of scleroderma (progressive systemic sclerosis), which is a disease characterized by extensive fibrosis throughout the body, most notably of the skin. **CREST** stands for **C**alcinosis (skin nodules formed from the deposition of calcium salts), **R**aynaud's phenomenon (intermittent ischemia, pallor, pain, or paresthesias of the fin-

gers, nose, ears, or toes brought on by cold or stress and alleviated by heat), **E**sophageal dysfunction, **S**clerodactyly, and **T**elangiectasias (small focal red skin marks from abnormally dilated blood vessels). Ninety-six percent of patients with anticentromere antibody have CREST syndrome.

Answer B is incorrect. While not all patients with lupus have anti-Smith antibodies, an elevation of these antibodies is highly specific for the disease. Systemic lupus erythematosus is diagnosed by the presence of four of the 11 symptoms summarized by the mnemonic "**BRAIN SOAP, MD**": **B**lood dyscrasias (such as hemolytic anemia or thrombocytopenia), **R**enal disorder, **A**rthritis, **I**mmunologic disorder (such as anti-DNA antibody and anti-Smith antibody), **N**eurologic disorder, **S**erositis (such as pleuritis or pericarditis), **O**ral ulcers, **A**ntinuclear antibody (elevated titers in the absence of drugs associated with drug-induced lupus syndrome), **P**hotosensitivity, **M**alar rash, and **D**iscoid rash.

Answer C is incorrect. Rheumatoid arthritis is an autoimmune disorder of synovial joints and often presents with morning joint stiffness, subcutaneous joint nodules (particularly in the proximal interphalangeal joints), and symmetric joint involvement. Eighty percent of patients test positive for rheumatoid factor, which is IgM anti-IgG antibodies, and the disease may include systemic symptoms such as fever, pleuritis, and pericarditis.

Answer D is incorrect. Achalasia is characterized by aperistalsis of the esophagus, incomplete relaxation of the lower esophageal sphincter with swallowing, and increased tone of the lower esophageal sphincter even in its resting state. While achalasia also presents with difficulty swallowing, this diagnosis does not subsume the other symptoms this patient presented with.

Answer E is incorrect. An elevated perinuclear anti-neutrophil cystoplasmic antibody (P-ANCA) level is not associated with "classic" polyarteritis nodosa, but is present in a form of the disease affecting smaller blood vessels known as microscopic polyangiitis or leukocytoclastic angiitis. Polyarteritis nodosa, a necrotizing immune complex vasculitis that usually affects small or medium-sized muscular arteries, commonly presents with fever, malaise, myalgias, and hypertension. Findings may include pericarditis, myocarditis, palpable purpura, and cotton-wool spots (white or grey opacities in the retina). While no single lab test is diagnostic, erythrocyte sedimentation rate and C-reactive protein levels are generally increased.

26. **The correct answer is D.** A positive enzyme-linked immunosorbent assay result must be confirmed by Western blot. The Western blot is a highly specific test with a very low false-positive rate, such that a positive reaction for two of the three commonly tested HIV antigens indicates disease. The Western blot technique is generally performed as follows: (1) Run three HIV antigens on a protein gel. (2) Transfer proteins to the nitrocellulose membrane. (3) Add the patient's serum. If the patient is infected, then antibodies to HIV antigens will be present and will bind to the HIV antigens on the membrane. (4) Add secondary enzyme-linked anti-Ig antibody. (5) Add substrate for enzyme and observe for product. As shown in the figure, it is wise to add a positive control lane where a known concentration of anti-HIV antigen antibodies are added; additionally, a negative control lane where antibodies that are known not to bind the HIV antigen is included. If the positive control demonstrates three bands, one can be assured that the assay was successful; if the negative control demonstrates no bands, cross-contamination is unlikely. The Western blot shown in this question demonstrates that the patient's serum contains antibodies that bind two of three HIV antigens. Thus, the patient would receive a diagnosis of HIV infection.

Answer A is incorrect. The Western blot is confirmatory for HIV.

Answer B is incorrect. There is no reason to believe contamination has occurred. In fact, if the positive control antibodies were mistakenly loaded in the patient's sample lane, one would expect that there would be three bands present in that lane.

Answer C is incorrect. Both the positive and negative control worked well, as three bands are clearly present in the positive control lane, and no bands are evident in the negative control lane.

Answer E is incorrect. The bands seen on the Western blot indicate that there are HIV-reactive antibodies in the patient's serum.

27. **The correct answer is B.** These symptoms of pulmonary toxicity and fibrosis are often associated with bleomycin, a chemotherapeutic agent used as first-line treatment for testicular tumors. Bleomycin is a mixture of glycopeptides that have the unique feature of forming complexes with Fe^{2+} while also bound to DNA. Oxidation of Fe^{2+} gives rise to superoxide and hydroxyl radicals that attack the DNA bonds, causing strand breakage. Although its main adverse effect is pulmonary toxicity, bleomycin can also cause skin changes and alopecia.

Answer A is incorrect. Mitomycin C is a broadly active antineoplastic agent that alkylates DNA. Although it can cause delayed bronchospasm 12–14 hours after dosing, it rarely produces a pulmonary fibrosis syndrome like that caused by bleomycin.

Answer C is incorrect. Vincristine binds to the tubulin dimer to disaggregate microtubules. It is used to treat acute lymphoblastic leukemia, Wilms' tumor, and lymphomas, not testicular carcinoma. Its adverse effects include cellulitis and peripheral neuropathies.

Answer D is incorrect. Doxorubicin is the most frequently used antineoplastic agent. It can intercalate into DNA to alter DNA structure, replication and topoisomerase function. Its adverse effects include myelosuppression, alopecia, nausea, and acute cardiotoxicity in the form of atrial and ventricular dysrhythmias.

Answer E is incorrect. Paclitaxel stabilizes microtubules against depolymerization, and these "stabilized" microtubules are not able to undergo the normal dynamic changes of microtubule function necessary for cell cycle completion. It is used to treat ovarian and breast cancers, not testicular cancer. Major adverse effects of paclitaxel include hypersensitivity and neutropenia.

28. **The correct answer is C.** Low thyroid (indicated by the constellation of signs and symptoms described in the vignette, or myxedema) and TSH levels indicate a secondary pituitary hypothyroidism. Sheehan's syndrome results from hemorrhage and shock of the pituitary gland after hypotension from postpartum hemorrhage. Gonadotropin levels decline first, followed by TSH and ACTH. This results in amenorrhea and myxedema, as well as in hypotension and electrolyte imbalances due to adrenocortical insufficiency.

Answer A is incorrect. Antimicrosomal antibodies are found in Hashimoto's hypothyroidism. This results in high compensatory TSH levels. Hashimoto's may or may not be associated with goiter but does not affect electrolyte levels.

Answer B is incorrect. Ectopic TSH secretion may arise exogenously or endogenously from malignancies such as struma ovarii, an ovarian monodermal germ cell tumor that secretes TSH. This condition would be associated with high TSH levels.

Answer D is incorrect. De Quervain's thyroiditis is a self-limiting subacute hypothyroidism that occurs following a flu-like viral illness. Patients present with a tender thyroid gland, jaw pain, and elevated TSH levels.

Answer E is incorrect. Thyroid-stimulating or TSH receptor antibodies are associated with Graves' disease, which may present during pregnancy or the postpartum period. This would result in hyperthyroidism, presenting as menorrhagia, weight loss, heat intolerance, sweats, diarrhea, and exophthalmos.

29. **The correct answer is E.** CD16 (also called Fc-g RIII) is an important cell surface receptor found on natural killer (NK) cells. As an Fc receptor, CD16 can bind to antibodies coating virally infected cells. CD16 recognizes the Fc portion of certain IgG subclasses, and once bound intracellular signaling results in the release of perforin and granzymes, thereby killing the virally infected cells. This mechanism of NK Fc receptor-mediated destruction is called antibody-dependent cell-mediated cytotoxicity.

Answer A is incorrect. CD3 is a key component of the T-lymphocyte receptor complex and is thus expressed by T lymphocytes.

Answer B is incorrect. Helper T lymphocytes express CD4; cytotoxic T lymphocytes express CD8.

Answer C is incorrect. CD28, found on T lymphocytes, receives a costimulatory signal that allows full activation of T lymphocytes by antigen presenting cells. The ligand for CD28, B7, is found on dendritic cells and macrophages.

Answer D is incorrect. Helper T lymphocytes express CD4; cytotoxic T lymphocytes express CD8.

30. **The correct answer is E.** This patient demonstrates several characteristics classic for neurofibromatosis type 1 (also known as von Recklinghausen's disease). Potential findings include café au lait spots, two or more neurofibromas, optic glioma, iris hamartomas (Lisch's nodules), a positive family history (autosomal dominant inheritance), and a distinctive bony lesion such as sphenoid dysplasia or scoliosis. Patients with this disease generally demonstrate 95% of the criteria by age 8 years and all of the criteria by age 20. These patients are also at increased risk for tumors. The gene is located on the long arm of chromosome 17.

Answer A is incorrect. Bilateral acoustic neuromas are characteristic of neurofibromatosis type 2. It is much less common than type 1 and typically manifests with multiple central nervous system tumors. The *NF2* gene is located on chromosome 22.

Answer B is incorrect. Bilateral renal cell carcinoma occurs in von Hippel–Lindau disease, an autosomal dominant disease that is characterized by hemangioblastomas of the retina, cerebellum, and medulla. About half of patients develop bilateral renal cell carcinomas. The disease is associated with the deletion of the *VHL* gene located on chromosome 3, which is a tumor suppressor gene.

Answer C is incorrect. Cystic medial necrosis of the aorta leading to aortic insufficiency and dissecting aortic aneurysm is associated with Marfan's syndrome, a connective tissue disorder caused by the autosomal dominant inheritance of a defective fibrillin gene.

Answer D is incorrect. Leptomeningeal angioma is associated with Sturge–Weber syndrome, which is a rare congenital vascular disorder of unknown etiology affecting capillary-sized blood vessels. Its characteristic features include angiomas and a facial port-wine stain. Only a small portion of patients with port-wine stains at birth have Sturge–Weber syndrome.

31. **The correct answer is A.** Hemophilia (types A and B) is an X-linked recessive disorder, with affected male individuals inheriting a defective copy of the X chromosome from heterozygous (asymptomatic) mothers. It is caused by a deficiency in factor VIII (hemophilia A) or factor IX (hemophilia B) of the clotting cascade. Platelet number and bleeding time are normal because there is no deficiency of platelet function. Prothrombin time measures activity of factors VII, X, V, prothrombin, and fibrinogen, thus it is also normal in hemophilia. Partial thromboplastin time (PTT) measures activity of factors VIII, IX, XI, and XII in addition to factors X, V, prothrombin and fibrinogen. PTT is therefore elevated in the case of factor VIII or IX deficiency.

Answer B is incorrect. This profile describes qualitative platelet defects such as Bernard–Soulier disease and Glanzmann's thrombasthenia. Since there is no clotting factor deficiency, prothrombin time and PTT are normal.

Answer C is incorrect. This profile describes von Willebrand's disease, an autosomal dominant disease. vWF promotes platelet adhesion to damaged endpothelium, therefore its deficiency prolongs bleeding time. It also serves as a carrier for factor VIII, so PTT is also prolonged in this disorder.

Answer D is incorrect. This profile describes thrombocytopenia. Since there is no clotting factor deficiency, prothrombin time and partial thromboplastin time are normal. Since platelets are low, bleeding time is prolonged.

Answer E is incorrect. This profile describes disseminated intravascular coagulation (DIC). In this disorder, widespread intravascular coagulation consumes platelets and clotting factors, resulting in lab findings indicative of a deficiency in all elements of the clotting machinery. In DIC one would also see an increase in fibrin split products and D-dimers.

32. **The correct answer is C.** Zanamivir is used in the treatment of both influenza A and influenza B. The mechanism of action is inhibition of the neuraminidase enzyme, which is critical to the influenza life cycle. First, hemagglutinin binds to neuraminic acid on host cells, allowing infection of the cell. After entering the cell, the virus replicates, and progeny viral assembly takes place in the cytoplasm. The virions bud from the cell membrane while bound to neuraminic acid. Neuraminidase cleaves the neuraminic acid, releasing the virions from the host. Zanamivir prevents the release of progeny virions by blocking neuraminidase.

Answer A is incorrect. Amantadine blocks viral penetration and uncoating. It is used to treat influenza A and rubella, as well as idiopathic Parkinson's disease.

Answer B is incorrect. Hemagglutinin binds to neuraminic acid, initiating infection.

Answer D is incorrect. Acyclovir inhibits viral DNA polymerase. It is used to treat herpes simplex virus, varicella-zoster virus, and Epstein-Barr virus.

Answer E is incorrect. Ribavirin is a guanine analog that blocks viral protein synthesis. It is used to treat respiratory syncytial virus.

33. **The correct answer is E.** The disease that is described in this patient is acute myelogenous leukemia (AML), which is characterized by acute onset of myelosuppression and the presence of increased myeloblasts in the peripheral smear and bone marrow. One subtype of AML is acute promyelocytic leukemia with abnormal presence of t(15:17), which encodes for a fusion protein of the retinoic acid receptor with the promyelocytic leukemia gene. This fusion protein renders these cancer cells sensitive to treatment with all-trans retinoic acid, causing differentiation of myeloblasts into mature granulocytes. Combination treatment with retinoic acid and chemotherapy leads to overall response rates of 70%–80% in this disease.

Answer A is incorrect. In general, chromosomal translocations involving chromosome 14 commonly occur in B- lymphocyte lymphomas, as the locus for immunoglobulin production is on chromosome 14. This translocation is associated with Burkitt's lymphoma and induces overproduction of the c-myc oncogene.

Answer B is incorrect. Translocation t(9:22), encoding bcr-abl, also known as the Philadelphia chromosome, is found in over 90% of chronic myelogenous leukemia (CML) and also in some acute leukemias, where it is associated with a poor prognosis. The bcr-abl fusion protein is a constitutively active tyrosine kinase that drives the cells to express a cancerous phenotype. Treatment of CML with imatinib mesylate, a specific bcr-abl kinase inhibitor, may control disease growth for several years without cytotoxic chemotherapy.

Answer C is incorrect. Translocation t(11:14) is associated with mantle cell lymphoma, a type of lymphoma with a very poor prognosis.

The translocation produces increased activity of cyclin D1, which causes rapid progression of the cell cycle.

Answer D is incorrect. Translocation t(11:22), found in Ewing's sarcoma, results in production of the Ewing's sarcoma transcription factor, which induces the overexpression of various oncogenes such as c-myc. Ewing's sarcoma is a bone tumor that presents as a rapidly enlarging mass in the diaphysis of long bones. It most commonly occurs in children.

34. **The correct answer is C.** Misoprostol is a prostaglandin E_1 analog that can be used to prevent nonsteroidal anti-inflammatory drug-induced peptic ulcers. It is also used as a medical abortifacient in many countries, particularly Latin American countries, and is therefore strictly contraindicated in pregnant women. Prostaglandins E_1 (misoprostol) and E_2 have been successfully used to induce labor, because prostaglandins activate dissolution of collagen bundles and increase the submucosal water content of the cervix. Prostaglandin E also has potentiating effects on endogenous oxytocin, the combination of which increases the probability of labor induction and abortion.

Answer A is incorrect. Cimetidine is an H_2 antagonist and is associated with inhibition of the cytochrome P450 system. It is not considered a teratogen and can be taken by pregnant women.

Answer B is incorrect. Magnesium hydroxide is an antacid and is associated with diarrhea. It is not considered a teratogen and can be taken by pregnant women.

Answer D is incorrect. Omeprazole is a proton pump inhibitor and is associated with atrophic gastritis due to hypergastrinemia and carcinoid tumors. It is not considered a teratogen and can be taken by pregnant women.

Answer E is incorrect. Sucralfate binds to ulcers, allowing a physical protective barrier, and has no known significant adverse effects. It is not considered a teratogen and can be taken by pregnant women.

35. **The correct answer is E.** This patient has clinical evidence of multiple endocrine neoplasia (MEN) type I, which can cause tumors in the "3 P's": the **P**ituitary gland, the **P**arathyroid gland, and the **P**ancreas. The MEN I syndrome follows an autosomal dominant pattern of inheritance, thus this patient's family history of multiple endocrine organ abnormalities further supports this diagnosis. In this patient, parathyroid involvement is suggested by hypercalcemia; and a pituitary adenoma is most likely causing his bitemporal hemianopsia. This patient has signs and symptoms consistent with elevated levels of vasoactive intestinal peptide (VIP). VIP acts on the gut mucosa to promote sodium secretion, causing a secretory diarrhea. VIP also stimulates potassium secretion in the colon, causing hypokalemia, which can lead to the muscle weakness, tetany, and even periodic paralysis seen in this patient. Finally, VIP inhibits gastric acid secretion, leading to hypochlorhydria, which can be tested by an elevated pH on nasogastric suction fluid. The majority of VIPomas arise within the pancreas and are one type of pancreatic tumor seen in MEN I.

Answer A is incorrect. Gastrinomas are non-β islet cell tumors that commonly arise from the pancreas and secrete gastrin, leading to hypersecretion of hydrochloric acid. Although gastrinomas do cause diarrhea and are associated with MEN I, the pH of the nasogastric suction fluid would be decreased, not increased, in a patient with a gastrinoma.

Answer B is incorrect. Insulinomas are islet cell tumors that secrete insulin. These tumors are associated with Whipple's triad: hypoglycemia, symptoms of hypoglycemia that include mental status changes, and relief of symptoms upon glucose administration.

Answer C is incorrect. Medullary thyroid carcinoma is associated with increased levels of calcitonin, which rarely causes hypocalcemia and muscle weakness in these patients. Medullary thyroid carcinoma is associated with MEN IIA and IIB but not with MEN I.

Answer D is incorrect. Although an abdominal mass noted on CT scan could be a pancreatic adenocarcinoma, the patient's symptoms point to the diagnosis of VIPoma.

36. **The correct answer is E.** Paget's disease is a metabolic bone disorder characterized by overactive osteoclastic bone resorption followed by a compensatory increase in osteoblastic new bone formation, creating widespread structurally disorganized bone. Patients are often asymptomatic, or may present with a variety of symptoms or complications including bone pain, pathologic fractures, and bowing deformities of the skeleton. Skull involvement may cause headaches, frontal bossing, increased head size, hearing loss, and other neurologic complications secondary to nerve compression due to increased bone remodeling and narrowed cranial foramina. Asymptomatic patients are often diagnosed incidentally by the discovery of an elevated alkaline phosphatase level in the setting of normal calcium and phosphate levels on routine blood testing, or from an abnormality on a skeletal radiograph obtained for another indication. Radiographic findings typical of Paget's disease include enlargement or expansion of an entire bone or area of a long bone, cortical thickening, coarsening of trabecular markings, and typical lytic and sclerotic changes like those seen in this patient's x-ray film.

Answer A is incorrect. Certain types of cancer, such as breast and lung carcinomas, can metastasize to bone and produce lytic lesions that may lead to pathologic fractures. However, Paget's disease is the most likely diagnosis for this patient.

Answer B is incorrect. Multiple myeloma is a malignancy of plasma cells characterized by bone destruction, bone marrow failure, and renal failure. This condition commonly results in lytic bone lesions with resulting hypercalcemia, hyperphosphatemia, elevated alkaline phosphatase levels, bone pain, and pathologic fractures; replacement of bone marrow by cancerous cells, leading to bone marrow failure and anemia; and renal failure secondary to hypercalcemia and excess light chain components secreted by the cancerous plasma cells.

Answer C is incorrect. Osteitis fibrosa cystica is a distinctive bone manifestation of hyperparathyroidism characterized histologically by a pathognomonic increase in giant multinucleated osteoclasts in scalloped areas on the surface of the bone and a replacement of the normal cellular and marrow elements by fibrous tissue. Radiographic changes include resorption of the phalangeal tufts and replacement of the usually sharp cortical outline of the bone in the digits by an irregular outline (subperiosteal resorption); lytic lesions are not typically seen in this condition. Routine laboratory tests in hyperparathyroidism reveal elevated calcium and low phosphate levels.

Answer D is incorrect. Osteoporosis is a common disease characterized by decreased bone mineral density leading to an increased susceptibility to fractures. Risk factors for osteoporosis include female gender, low estrogen levels (e.g., postmenopausal state), positive family history, white and Asian ethnicity, smoking, low body mass index, alcohol use, malnutrition, and insufficient physical activity. Osteoporosis usually presents with pathologic fractures (including vertebral compression fractures) in otherwise asymptomatic patients. Calcium, phosphate, and alkaline phosphatase levels are all normal in this condition.

37. **The correct answer is B.** This patient has neurological symptoms consistent with vitamin B_{12} (cobalamin) deficiency caused by demylination of the dorsal columns, spinocerebellar tract, and lateral corticospinal tract. Pernicious anemia is a vitamin B_{12} deficiency associated with chronic atrophic gastritis. Autoantibodies are directed against gastric parietal cells, leading to an intrinsic factor deficiency. Without intrinsic factor, vitamin B_{12} cannot be absorbed in the ileum. Patients may present with fatigue, dyspnea, and tachycardia. A peripheral blood smear will show macrocytic RBCs with hypersegmented polymorphonuclear leukocytes, consistent with megaloblastic anemia (as

seen in the image). Treatment includes vitamin B_{12} injections.

Answer A is incorrect. Abnormal neural crest cell migration leads to Hirschsprung's disease, which is a congenital aganglionic motility disorder affecting the large bowel. Patients present with obstructive symptoms such as megacolon and not with vitamin B_{12} deficiency.

Answer C is incorrect. The colon is not the site of vitamin B_{12} absorption, and bacterial overgrowth there, such as with *Clostridium difficile*, will produce symptoms such as diarrhea, flatulence, and weight loss.

Answer D is incorrect. Green leafy vegetables contain folate, not vitamin B_{12}. Folate is an essential cofactor in nucleic acid synthesis and its deficiency commonly leads to megaloblastic anemia as seen in the image. However, folate deficiency does not explain the neurologic symptoms experienced by this patient.

Answer E is incorrect. An embolus to the superior mesenteric artery can lead to an acute bowel infarction, a life-threatening problem. Patients typically present with abdominal pain, bloody stools, fever, and peritoneal signs, not with signs of vitamin B_{12} deficiency.

38. **The correct answer is A.** This patient has developed cirrhosis of the liver from chronic hepatitis C infection. In addition to the physical exam findings suggestive of cirrhosis (jaundice, spider angiomata, ascites), the patient has decreased liver synthetic function (elevated PTT, low albumin). This patient also manifests signs of hepatic encephalopathy, including asterixis (flapping tremor), confusion, and lethargy. The etiology of hepatic encephalopathy is not entirely understood, but it is thought that ammonia acts as a toxin to the CNS when it is not converted into urea by the cirrhotic liver. Lactulose, when digested by colonic bacteria, acidifies the colonic contents. This acidification then converts ammonia into a nonabsorbable protonated form. It also changes the bowel flora so that fewer ammonia-forming organisms are present.

Answer B is incorrect. Although this patient may benefit from liver transplantation, it is not an acute treatment strategy.

Answer C is incorrect. Lorazepam, as well as other benzodiazepines that are metabolically cleared by the liver, should not be used and can actually worsen the encephalopathy.

Answer D is incorrect. While neomycin can be used as an adjunct to decrease ammonia production by gut flora, it is not first-line therapy. Neomycin works by destroying the gut flora that normally produce ammonia.

Answer E is incorrect. While a restricted protein diet should be standard in all patients with end-stage liver disease, it will not acutely decrease ammonia concentrations.

39. **The correct answer is C.** Swollen eyelids, conjunctival inflammation, and yellow purulent discharge are symptoms of conjunctivitis. *Chlamydia trachomatis* is the most common sexually transmitted disease in the United States, and can cause conjunctivitis in newborns who are colonized by the bacteria (serotypes D through K, the same serotypes causing urogenital infections) during passage through the birth canal of an affected mother. It tends to develop a few days to several weeks after birth. The conjuctival epithelial cells will demonstrate basophilic cytoplasmic inclusions when viewed microscopically. These inclusions, in fact, are the causative bacteria existing in the reticulate/initial body phase of their life cycle. In the United States, all newborns receive erythromycin eye drops prophylactically. The fact that the child in the question stem was born outside of the country should raise suspicion that he did not receive this prophylaxis.

Answer A is incorrect. *Chlamydia pneumoniae* is another cause of atypical pneumonia worldwide. It is transmitted person-to-person.

Answer B is incorrect. *Chlamydia psittaci* causes psittacosis. This disease causes symptoms similar to atypical pneumonia. The bacteria are spread through poultry and birds.

Answer D is incorrect. *Neisseria gonorrhoeae* causes gonorrhea, and is also a cause of neonatal conjunctivitis acquired by passage through the birth canal. However, it typically appears one to two days after birth and would not be associated with cytoplasmic inclusions. The erythromycin eye drops administered to children at birth also act as prophylaxis against Neisseria conjunctivitis. Other treatments include silver nitrate 1% aqueous solution or tetracycline 1% ophthalmic ointment. One of these preparations should be applied into both eyes immediately after birth.

Answer E is incorrect. *Ureaplasma urealyticum* can produce nongonococcal urethritis. This organism has the ability to convert urea into ammonia and carbon dioxide.

40. **The correct answer is A.** This patient has xeroderma pigmentosum, a disease characterized by extreme sensitivity to sunlight, skin damage, and a predisposition to malignancies such as melanoma. The disease results from a defective excision repair mechanism for ultraviolet light-damaged DNA.

Answer B is incorrect. The mismatch repair mechanism replaces segments of DNA that include mismatched bases. Hereditary nonpolyposis colorectal cancer is caused by defects in mismatch repair.

Answer C is incorrect. A defect in proofreading enzymes would not cause xeroderma pigmentosum. It would affect DNA replication in all body tissues, not just those exposed to UV light.

Answer D is incorrect. Ionizing radiation, such as x-rays, removes electrons from atoms and molecules such as DNA. This causes chromosome breakage, translocations, and point mutations. Bloom's syndrome and ataxia-telangiectasia are rare autosomal recessive genetic disorders that are hypersensitive to ionizing radiation. Patients with xeroderma pigmentosum are hypersensitive to UV light.

41. **The correct answer is E.** TSH, hCG, luteinizing hormone (LH), and follicle-stimulating

hormone, are all composed of an identical α subunit paired with a β subunit that is unique to each of these hormones. Hence, any of these may interfere with the accurate detection and measurement of hCG by this hypothetical assay. TSH is the only hCG structural homologue listed among the answer choices.

Answer A is incorrect. ACTH is a melanocortin and does not share structural homology with hCG and should not interfere with the assay. It does, however, share homology with Melanocyte-stimulating hormone, as both are cleavage products of the same precursor, pro-opiomelanocortin.

Answer B is incorrect. Gonadotropin-releasing hormone does not share structural homology with hCG and should not interfere with the assay.

Answer C is incorrect. Growth hormone does not share structural homology with hCG and should not interfere with the assay.

Answer D is incorrect. Melanocyte-stimulating hormone is of the melanocortin group and does not share structural homology with hCG and should not interfere with the assay.

42. **The correct answer is C.** Based on the physical findings and the low α-fetoprotein during pregnancy, this child most likely has Down's syndrome caused by trisomy 21. Down's syndrome is associated with many defects of embryology; the most common cardiac abnormality is an atrial septal defect of the septum primum, present in 45% of patients. The atrial septum develops as an outgrowth of the wall of the primitive atrium. The primitive atrium also develops into the trabeculated part of both atria. The second most common heart defect in children with Down's syndrome is ventricular septal defect, appearing in 35% of patients.

Answer A is incorrect. The bulbus cordis gives rise to the smooth part of both ventricles. These are not commonly malformed in children with Down's syndrome.

Answer B is incorrect. The neural crest cells give rise to many structures, including the aorticopulmonary septum, which divides the truncus arteriosus into the aorta and pulmonary trunk. Several malformations related to this structure exist, including a persistent truncus arteriosus, transposition of the great vessels, and tetralogy of Fallot. However, the most likely cardiac defect in a patient with Down's syndrome is an atrial septal defect.

Answer D is incorrect. The primitive ventricle gives rise to the trabeculated part of both ventricles and the interventricular septum. Malformations of these structures are possible but are not the most likely cardiac defect in children with Down's syndrome.

Answer E is incorrect. The truncus arteriosus gives rise to the aorta and pulmonary trunk. Malformations of these structures are not common in children with Down's syndrome.

43. **The correct answer is E.** Acute intermittent porphyria (AIP) and porphyria cutanea tarda (PCT) are the two most common porphyrias seen clinically. AIP is a defect in the enzyme porphobilinogen (PBG) deaminase, also called uroporphyrinogen I synthase. Uroporphyrinogen I synthase is the third enzyme in the heme synthetic pathway and results in aberrant accumulation of aminolevulinate (ALA) and PBG. In contrast, PCT is a defect in the enzyme uroporphyrinogen decarboxylase, the fifth step in the heme pathway, which causes an accumulation of uroporphyrinogen but not ALA or PBG. In this case, the patient presents with symptoms most consistent with AIP, which is manifested by acute intermittent attacks between periods of disease remission. Symptoms during acute attacks are marked by neurovisceral symptoms (most commonly abdominal pain, muscle weakness, and psychiatric manifestations such as anxiety, paranoia, and depression) and by high PBG levels in urine, which in severe cases can present as red port wine-colored urine. No increased photosensitivity is seen with this disease.

Answer A is incorrect. ALA dehydratase deficiency is associated with ALA dehydratase porphyria, which resembles acute intermittent porphyria.

Answer B is incorrect. ALA synthase deficiency is associated with X-linked sideroblastic anemia.

Answer C is incorrect. Ferrochelatase deficiency results in anemia and porphyria.

Answer D is incorrect. Heme oxygenase catalyzes the oxidation of heme to biliverdin.

Answer F is incorrect. PCT is one of the most common porphyries seen clinically. Uroporphyrinogen decarboxylase deficiency is responsible for PCT. This deficiency may be inherited or acquired, due to the inactivation of uroporphyrinogen decarboxylase by iron, alcohol, estrogens, and infection with hepatitis C or HIV. In contrast to acute Intermittent porphyria, patients with PCT present with photosensitivity and chronic, blistering lesions of sun-exposed skin in the absence of neuropsychiatric signs.

Answer G is incorrect. Uroporphyrinogen III cosynthase deficiency is associated with congenital erythropoietic porphyria, which resembles porphyria cutanea tarda.

44. **The correct answer is B.** Graft-versus-host disease (GVHD) is an unwanted side effect of bone marrow transplantation whereby donor T lymphocytes recognize the recipient as foreign and mount an immune response. The organs most often affected are the gut, skin, and liver. Human leukocyte antigen matching of the donor and recipient can help reduce the severity of GVHD, but the disease may still occur due to a minor histocompatibility mismatch.

Answer A is incorrect. Acute graft rejection is a potential side effect of solid organ transplant and is mediated by the recipient's cytotoxic T lymphocytes. The recipient of a bone marrow transplant undergoes myeloablative therapy before transplant, and therefore it is not expected that the patient would have significant numbers of T lymphocytes.

Answer C is incorrect. Graft-versus-host disease is mediated by donor T lymphocytes; recipient T lymphocytes are ablated before transplant.

Answer D is incorrect. Hyperacute graft rejection is a potential side effect of solid organ transplant and is mediated by preformed recipient antibodies. It occurs within minutes to hours post-transplant.

Answer E is incorrect. The clinical scenario described is more suggestive of graft-versus-host disease than recurrence of leukemia.

45. **The correct answer is C.** This patient has symptoms consistent with type 2 diabetes mellitus. Long-term hyperglycemia in these patients, reflected by the increased hemoglobin A1c level, causes many health problems including diabetic nephropathy. The pathogenesis of diabetic nephropathy involves nonenzymatic glycosylation of the glomerular and tubule basement membranes, increasing vessel permeability to proteins (this is why microalbuminuria is the first sign of diabetic nephropathy). Glomerular hypertrophy also occurs due to cytokine release, leading to hemodynamic changes in the vessels of the kidneys. On light microscopy, early changes show diffuse mesangial expansion in the glomeruli, while more advanced diabetic nephropathy (as seen in this patient) demonstrates nodular glomerulosclerosis. Nodular glomerulosclerosis is characterized by increased cellularity and mesangial matrix deposition, as well as hyaline masses and thickening of the lamina densa. Diabetic nephropathy can present with either a nephrotic or a nephritic syndrome, although nephrotic is more common.

Answer A is incorrect. Diffuse capillary and basement membrane thickening is associated with membranous glomerulonephritis.

Answer B is incorrect. Enlarged hypercellular glomeruli with neutrophils can be found in acute poststreptococcal glomerulonephritis.

Answer D is incorrect. Segmental sclerosis with hyalinosis is seen in focal segmental glomerulosclerosis.

Answer E is incorrect. Glomeruli demonstrating a wire-loop appearance with subendothelial basement membrane deposits are seen in lupus nephropathy.

46. The correct answer is D. The baby suffers from 21-hydroxylase deficiency, the most common cause of congenital adrenal hyperplasia and the underlying cause of the girl's virilism. Without functioning 21-hydroxylase, the precursor molecule 17-hydroxyprogesterone accumulates. 21-Hydroxylase deficiency also causes salt wasting with hypotension, hyponatremia, and hyperkalemia. Congenital adrenal hyperplasia is a common cause of female pseudohermaphroditism, a condition in which patients may have ambiguous genitalia but have a 46,XX karyotype.

Answer A is incorrect. In true hermaphroditism, both ovarian and testicular tissue can be found within the gonads. However, in 21-α-hydroxylase deficiency, the ovaries develop normally; it is the adrenal glands that cause the male-looking genitalia.

Answer B is incorrect. A 47,XXX karyotype would not cause congenital adrenal hyperplasia, salt wasting, or pseudohermaphroditism. Most women with an extra X chromosome are asymptomatic; an extra Barr body can be seen microscopically.

Answer C is incorrect. A deficiency in 5α-reductase is a cause of male pseudohermaphroditism and is also known as testicular feminization syndrome. A lack of 5α-reductase means that testosterone cannot be converted to dihydrotestosterone, the necessary hormone in the masculinization of genitalia.

Answer E is incorrect. Ovarian dysgenesis, the "streak ovary," is found in Turner's syndrome (45,XO). It does not cause salt wasting or virilism. Patients with Turner's present with poorly developed secondary sexual characteristics and amenorrhea.

47. The correct answer is D. The *BRCA1* and *BRCA2* genes are strongly associated with breast cancer and are found on chromosomes 17 and 13, respectively. *BRCA* is an example of a tumor suppressor gene. A mutation results in loss of function, and thus both alleles must be lost for expression of the cancer.

Answer A is incorrect. The *VHL* gene results in von Hippel–Lindau syndrome and is found on chromosome 3. Patients with this condition often present with hemangioblastomas of the retina, cerebellum, and medulla as well as renal cell carcinomas. The gene responsible for achondroplasia is also found on chromosome 3.

Answer B is incorrect. The *APC* gene, which is responsible for causing familial adenomatous polyposis, is found on chromosome 5. Adenomatous polyps form after puberty.

Answer C is incorrect. The *WT1* gene, which causes Wilms' tumor, is found on chromosome 11. Children affected with this disease present with solid, palpable renal masses.

Answer E is incorrect. The genes *DCC* and *DPC*, responsible for colon and pancreatic cancers, respectively, are both found on chromosome 18.

Answer F is incorrect. The *NF2* gene, which causes neurofibromatosis type 2, is found on chromosome 22. These patients often have bilateral acoustic neuromas.

48. The correct answer is D. Multiple sclerosis (MS) is a chronic inflammatory demyelinating disease of unknown etiology. It typically has a relapsing-remitting course and is most commonly seen in female patients with peak age of onset between 20 and 40 years. MS usually presents with weakness and/or numbness in one or more extremities. Another common presentation is visual loss secondary to optic neuritis and unilateral shooting facial pain secondary to trigeminal neuralgia. MRI is the most sensitive radiographic technique for imaging MS, with sensitivity of nearly 85%. Classic findings on MRI are periventricular white matter lesions known as "Dawson's fingers," as seen in the image. Commonly, foci identified on MRI imaging are clinically silent. A combination of history, physical examination, laboratory tests such as cerebrospinal fluid oligoclonal banding, and imaging findings is used to diagnose MS. Interferon beta-1a is indicated for the long-term treatment of patients with relapsing forms of the disease to slow the accumulation of physical disability and decrease the frequency of clinical exacerbations. Patients with MS in whom interferon's efficacy has been demonstrated include patients who have experienced a first clinical episode and have MRI features consistent with MS.

Answer A is incorrect. The patient presents with trigeminal neuralgia in the setting of several other past neurologic complaints. While trigeminal neuralgia is characterized by unilateral shooting facial pains, it is important to distinguish this pain from that of a headache (e.g., migraine, cluster, or tension). Acetaminophen may be considered in the initial treatment of tension headache.

Answer B is incorrect. Short courses of intravenous corticosteroids are commonly used to treat acute MS flares associated with neurologic deficits. However, interferon or glatiramer, not corticosteroids, are appropriate for the long-term treatment of MS.

Answer C is incorrect. Heparin would be an appropriate therapeutic intervention in the case of an ischemic stroke. Given that the patient's neurologic signs and symptoms are separated both by time and space, a stroke is not likely. Moreover, the patient is quite young and an ischemic stroke in such a young patient would be exceedingly rare.

Answer E is incorrect. Unilateral facial pain is more characteristic of trigeminal neuralgia (a common feature of multiple sclerosis) than of migraine headache. Triptans are used as initial treatment in the case of cluster and migraine headache.

Test Block 4

1. A 2-year-old boy who started treatment for absence seizures 2 weeks ago presents to the physician with blistering around his nose and mouth. On examination it is noted that there is extensive shedding of the skin. Which first-line drug prescribed for absence seizures most likely caused this result?

(A) Carbamazepine
(B) Ethosuximide
(C) Lamotrigine
(D) Phenytoin
(E) Valproic acid

2. A 15-year-old girl presents to the physician with underdeveloped breasts and hirsutism. Her medical history includes early appearance of axillary and pubic hair and amenorrhea. On examination her blood pressure is 90/55 mm Hg. The enzyme deficient in this patient is needed for the production of which of the following hormones?

(A) Aldosterone
(B) Estradiol
(C) Estrone
(D) Progesterone
(E) Testosterone

3. A 4-year-old child whose family arrived in the United States from China last month is brought to the pediatrician for a checkup. On physical examination, the patient is found to be short, potbellied, and pale with a puffy face, a protruding umbilicus, and a protuberant tongue. The child shows clear signs of significant mental retardation. Upon questioning, the mother reveals that she did not suspect any abnormality because of many children in their village in China share the same appearance. The physician suspects thyroid abnormalities and orders a thyroid function test. Which of the following are the most likely results for this patient?

Choice	Thyroid-Stimulating Hormone	Triiodothyronine	Thromboplastin
A	↓	↓	↓
B	↓	↑	↓
C	↓	↑	↑
D	↑	↓	↓
E	↑	↑	↓

(A) A
(B) B
(C) C
(D) D
(E) E

4. A 59-year-old woman was recently admitted to the hospital because of oral ulcers and diffuse crusted, denuded, erythematous plaques on her torso and upper arms (see image). She has tested positive for anti-epithelial cell antibodies. Which of the following is the most likely diagnosis?

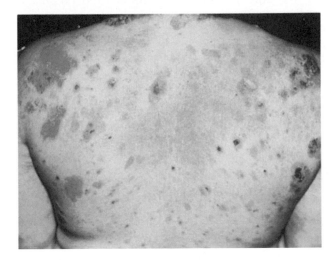

Reproduced, with permission, from Fauci AS, Braunwald E, Kasper DL, Hauser SL, Longo DL, Jameson JL, and Isselbacher KJ, eds. *Harrison's Principles of Internal Medicine*, 17th ed. New York: McGraw-Hill, 2008: Figure 55-1.

(A) Bullous pemphigoid
(B) Eczema
(C) Erythema multiforme
(D) Impetigo
(E) Pemphigus vulgaris

5. A 28-year-old woman has a 1-year history of recurrent abdominal pain relieved by defecation. She reports that her diarrhea has gotten worse in the last 2 weeks, since she started a new job. Her examination is unremarkable except for mild abdominal tenderness. Laboratory studies show:

Hemoglobin: 13.0 g/dL
Hematocrit: 39%
WBC count: 6000/mm³
Platelet count: 200,000/mm³
Erythrocyte sedimentation rate: 8 mm/h

Which of the following is most appropriate in the treatment of this patient's symptoms?

(A) Bactrim
(B) Bismuth
(C) Loperamide
(D) Metronidazole
(E) Octreotide
(F) Omeprazole

6. A 46-year-old man comes to the clinic with a cough that is occasionally productive of blood, diffuse muscle and joint pain in the upper extremities, and blood in his urine for the past several days. On further questioning, the patient reveals that he has had chronic sinusitis for the past several years. The patient has a low-grade fever and nasal ulcerations. Laboratory studies show a markedly elevated erythrocyte sedimentation rate, and staining for antibodies to cytoplasmic antigens of neutrophils is positive. Biopsy of a nasal ulceration reveals vasculitis and necrotizing granulomas. Which of the following is the most likely diagnosis?

(A) Alport's syndrome
(B) Giant cell (temporal) arteritis
(C) Goodpasture's syndrome
(D) Takayasu's arteritis
(E) Wegener's granulomatosis

7. A peripheral T-helper lymphocyte engages peptide-bound class II major histocompatibility complex molecules on the surface of an antigen-presenting cell (APC). No other contact is made between cell surface molecules present on the T lymphocyte and the APC. Which of the following can be correctly concluded about this peripheral T lymphocyte?

(A) The T lymphocyte will be activated and fully able to perform effector functions
(B) The T lymphocyte will be activated but unable to perform effector functions
(C) The T lymphocyte will cause the APC to undergo apoptosis
(D) The T lymphocyte will undergo anergy
(E) The T lymphocyte will undergo clonal expansion

8. A 54-year-old man is diagnosed with adenocarcinoma of the colon. Genetic analysis of the tumor reveals the presence of the *ras* oncogene, which is the most common abnormality in human cancer and is involved in approximately 30% of tumors. To which of the following families of molecules does *ras* belong?

   (A) Cyclin-dependent kinases
   (B) Epidermal growth factor receptor
   (C) Guanosine triphosphate-binding proteins
   (D) Non-receptor-associated tyrosine kinase
   (E) Transcriptional activators

9. A 22-year-old white man with metastatic testicular carcinoma is undergoing treatment with high doses of cisplatin. Which class of drugs is most likely to suppress his chemotherapy-related nausea?

   (A) 5-HT$_3$ antagonists
   (B) Benzodiazepines
   (C) Cholinergic antagonists
   (D) Histamine receptor antagonists

10. A 3-year-old girl is brought to her pediatrician because of a progressive loss of motor function and a decline in her cognitive abilities. On physical examination, it is noted that the patient has decreased deep tendon reflexes, truncal ataxia, and a decreased attention span in comparison to the child's last visit 6 months ago. The physician knows that her pathology is due to an abnormal accumulation of cerebroside sulfate in her brain, peripheral nerves, kidney, and liver. A deficiency of which of the following enzymes leads to this condition?

    (A) α-Galactosidase A
    (B) β-Galactosidase
    (C) Arylsulfatase A
    (D) Hexosaminidase A
    (E) Sphingomyelinase

11. A 35-year-old woman comes to the physician with right-handed paralysis, ataxia, and difficulty urinating for the past 36 hours. The patient states that she has had generalized right-sided weakness for years along with episodes of sensory numbness and/or motor paralysis. The

episodes normally last a few days, and the last episode occurred 18 months ago. Her left hand became so weak that she could not write with it. MRI of the brain is significant for periventricular white matter plaques. Which of the following signs and symptoms commonly occurs in patients with this disease?

   (A) Forceful, spastic involuntary movements of the limbs and/or facial muscles; onset is gradual, but spasms are permanent
   (B) Permanent bilateral resting tremor of the upper extremities
   (C) Permanent progressive paralysis of respiratory muscles
   (D) Spasm of digital arteries, causing blanching, numbness, and pain to the fingers whenever the patient is exposed to cold temperatures
   (E) Vision loss in one eye, usually lasting a few days

12. A researcher studying a pedigree of familial type 1 diabetes mellitus discovers a mutation in the potassium channel expressed in the cell membrane of pancreatic islet β cells. This mutation impairs closing of the potassium channel. The efficacy of which of the following agents would be most profoundly affected by this mutation?

    (A) Acarbose
    (B) Glargine
    (C) Glipizide
    (D) Metformin
    (E) Troglitazone

13. A 47-year-old woman presents to her family practitioner because of depression of 1 month's duration. Approximately 1.5 years ago her husband died of pancreatic cancer after a rapidly deteriorating course. She says she returned to work 2 weeks after his death and felt little emotional difficulty at that time. During the past month she has noted near constant sadness and frequent episodes of crying. She also notes new onset of frequent tension headaches, particularly during times of stress. She feels guilty that she is alive while he is dead. Her physical examination is unremarkable except that she

weighs about 1.3 kg (2.9 lb) less than she did 2 months previously. Which of the following is an indication of an abnormal grief reaction in this patient?

(A) Delayed grief
(B) Denied grief
(C) Feelings of guilt
(D) Headache in times of stress
(E) Weight loss

14. A 27-year-old woman is brought to the emergency department with an intense headache, left-sided weakness, and blurred vision that began after she was ejected from her vehicle in a motor vehicle accident. Paramedics report that she was ambulatory and cooperative at the scene of the crash but was unable to tell them what had happened. The patient had an episode of projectile vomiting while in the ambulance, and her mental status has deteriorated since then. A CT scan of the head shows extra-axial fluid collection on the right side and a temporal bone fracture on the same side. Injury to which of the following is the most likely cause of the patient's presentation?

(A) Inferior cerebral veins
(B) Middle meningeal artery
(C) Posterior ethmoidal artery
(D) Sigmoid sinus
(E) Superior sagittal sinus

15. An infant with severe jaundice that is not corrected by phototherapy is in danger of developing kernicterus. This can occur in infants with Crigler–Najjar syndrome, a genetic disorder in which there is a near-complete deficiency of glucuronyl transferase. Which of the following laboratory findings would be expected in blood tests in an infant with Crigler–Najjar syndrome?

(A) Decreased hematocrit
(B) Decreased indirect bilirubin
(C) Increased direct bilirubin
(D) Increased indirect bilirubin
(E) Increased reticulocyte count

16. A 72-year-old man who receives treatment for congestive heart failure (CHF) presents to the emergency department with vomiting, abdominal pain, and changes in his color vision. He is confused and does not remember the names of his medications. His heart rate is 36/min. Which of the following most likely caused this patient's symptoms?

(A) Recent decrease in his digoxin dosage
(B) Recent decrease in his verapamil dosage
(C) Recent increase in his enalapril dosage
(D) Recent increase in his furosemide dosage

17. A 78-year-old man has a 3-day history of diarrhea, left lower quadrant abdominal pain, and fever. His leukocyte count is slightly elevated, his hematocrit level reveals slight anemia, and his platelets are normal. A biopsy is obtained and shown in the image. Which of the following is the most likely anatomical location for this condition?

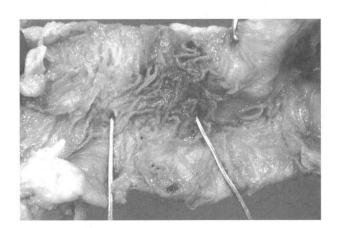

Reproduced, with permission, from PEIR Digital Library (http://peir.net).

(A) Appendix
(B) Ileum
(C) Rectum
(D) Sigmoid colon
(E) Transverse colon

18. A 36-year-old man who is HIV-positive presents to the physician with fever, cough, headaches, and myalgias. Questioning reveals that the man has just returned from a visit with his brother, who lives in Mississippi. No action is taken at the time, and the patient is sent home. A few weeks later, the patient returns to the hospital with an intracellular lung disease resembling tuberculosis (TB). Microscopic examination of the patient's sputum reveals a fungal infection. This patient is most likely infected with which of the following types of fungus?

(A) *Blastomyces*
(B) *Cryptococcus neoformans*
(C) *Histoplasma*
(D) *Mucor*
(E) *Tinea versicolor*

19. A 65-year-old obese man with a 60-pack-year smoking history presents with partial loss of vision after suffering a stroke. Physical examination reveals a bilateral defect in the upper left visual quadrants. Where is this patient's lesion most likely located?

(A) Dorsal optic radiation in the left parietal lobe
(B) Dorsal optic radiation in the right parietal lobe
(C) Left optic tract
(D) Loop of Meyer in the left temporal lobe
(E) Loop of Meyer in the right temporal lobe
(F) Right optic tract

20. A 44-year-old woman with end-stage renal disease on hemodialysis presents to the physician with abdominal pain. Laboratory tests are positive for HBsAg, anti-HBc, and HBeAg, but negative for anti-HBs and anti-HBe. Which of the following is the most appropriate treatment?

(A) Lamivudine and interferon-α
(B) Lamivudine and interferon-β
(C) Ribavirin and interferon-α
(D) Ribavirin and lamivudine
(E) Ribavirin and pegylated interferon-α

21. A 40-year-old woman presents to her physician with complaints of blood in her urine and decreased urine output for the past week. She had a sore throat 3 weeks ago, which has since resolved. Her temperature is 37° C (98.6° F), heart rate is 70/min, and blood pressure is 147/93 mm Hg. Physical examination reveals bilateral pedal edema to the mid-calf. In addition to several serologic tests, the patient undergoes renal biopsy (see image). Which of the following is the most accurate diagnosis?

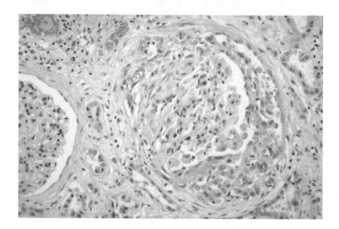

Reproduced, with permission, from PEIR Digital Library (http://peir.net).

(A) Diabetic nephropathy
(B) Goodpasture's syndrome
(C) IgA nephropathy
(D) Lupus nephritis
(E) Poststreptococcal glomerulonephritis
(F) Rapidly progressive glomerulonephritis
(G) Renal amyloidosis

22. A healthy 26-year-old woman delivers a single chorion and placenta but two amniotic sacs following a normal, full-term delivery. Which of the following is the most likely cause of these findings?

(A) Chorioamnionitis
(B) Complete hydatidiform mole
(C) Dizygotic twins
(D) Monozygotic twins
(E) Sheehan's syndrome

23. A 54-year-old alcoholic is brought to the emergency department by fire rescue after being found lying face down in the street. He is incoherent and is unable to walk in a straight line. His pulse is 110/min, his blood pressure is 135/80 mm Hg, and his respiration rate is 20/min. Physical examination reveals a diaphoretic man with generalized weakness passing in and out of consciousness. A glucose fingerstick test shows a glucose level of 45 g/dL. This patient's hypoglycemia most likely resulted from an elevated ratio of which of the following?

(A) NAD^+:NADH
(B) NADH:NAD^+
(C) NADP:NADPH
(D) NADPH:NADP
(E) Pyruvate:lactate

24. Eukaryotic genes can contain thousands of nucleotides that define the sequence. Not all the nucleotides are actually used to code for corresponding RNA molecules. Genes are divided into introns and exons based on whether or not a region of DNA within a gene is transcribed into messenger RNA. A mutation in a eukaryotic cell is shown below. The mutation is located at the 5′ end of an intron. This change is most likely to affect which of the following processes?

| Normal | 5′ TTCGUTCCGACT 3′ |
| Mutant | 5′ TTCAUTCCGACT 3′ |

(A) Capping
(B) Hybridization
(C) Polyadenylation
(D) Splicing
(E) Transcription

25. A 20-year-old college student complains to student health services of severe fatigue and lethargy. She reports a recent mononucleosis infection that has resolved. Physical examination shows scleral icteral jaundice, cervical lymphadenopathy, and splenomegaly. The tips of her fingers are purple. Laboratory testing shows a decreased hemoglobin level and appropriate reticulocytosis. A heterophile test is positive. Which of the following is the most likely diagnosis?

(A) Aplastic anemia
(B) Disseminated intravascular coagulation
(C) IgG-mediated (warm) hemolytic anemia
(D) IgM-mediated (cold) hemolytic anemia
(E) Paroxysmal nocturnal hemoglobinuria

26. A 37-year-old woman requests diagnostic testing before her frozen embryos are implanted. The physician requests a work-up for cystic fibrosis, as both the patient and her husband are carriers. The laboratory isolates some of the DNA from each 8- to 10-cell embryo prior to implantation and proceeds to run tests to determine the genotype of the embryos. Which of the following procedures is the first step performed in determining the genotype of the embryos?

(A) Enzyme-linked immunosorbent assay
(B) Ligase chain reaction
(C) Northern blot
(D) Polymerase chain reaction
(E) Southern blot

27. A 71-year-old Russian man comes to the physician complaining of a 4-month history of fatigue, low-grade fevers, night sweats, and cough. He became extremely worried yesterday when he noticed blood in his sputum. On physical examination, he is extremely thin, with enlarged, nontender left-sided cervical lymph nodes. His x-ray film of the chest is shown in the image. Which of the following organisms is the most likely cause of this patient's illness?

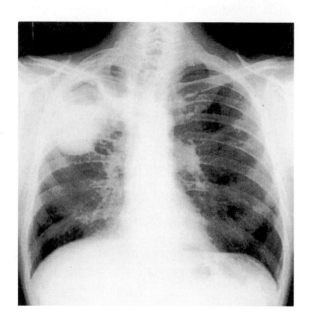

Reproduced, with permission, from Doherty GM, Way LW. *Current Surgical Diagnosis and Treatment*, 12th ed. New York: McGraw-Hill, 2006: Figure 18-19.

(A) *Legionella pneumophila*
(B) *Mycobacterium tuberculosis*
(C) *Mycoplasma pneumoniae*
(D) Respiratory syncytial virus
(E) *Streptococcus pneumoniae*

28. A 47-year-old woman presents to the physician with weight gain, fatigue, and lethargy. She says her appetite has decreased recently, and she has been constipated. A thyroid biopsy shows an enlarged, symmetric, and firm thyroid. Histological findings are significant for a lymphocytic and plasma cell infiltrate with occasional germinal center formation. Follicles contain little colloid, while the follicular epithelial lining shows enlarged epithelial cells containing acidophilic cytoplasm. Results of laboratory tests are pending. Which of the following antibodies would most likely be found in this patient?

(A) Anti-basement membrane antibodies
(B) Anti-epithelial cell antibodies
(C) Antimicrosomal antibodies
(D) Antimitochondrial antibodies
(E) Antineutrophil antibodies

29. A couple brings their 3-year-old daughter to her doctor because she has not behaved normally in the past month. The physician notes that the girl is quiet and less expressive than she was at her well-child visit several months ago. She was previously able to name four colors, but she now stutters and recalls only one. Furthermore, she responds to questions with one- or two-word sentences, which is uncharacteristic of her usually articulate personality. What other symptom might be expected in this patient?

(A) Hand wringing
(B) Hearing loss
(C) Hyperactivity
(D) Psychosis
(E) Repetitive behaviors
(F) Tics

30. A 64-year-old woman is brought to her primary care physician by her son because she has been progressively losing her vision. The patient emigrated from Southeast Asia 1 week ago. The son says that his mother's poor vision worsens at night, causing her to frequently run into the bedroom wall. Her nutrition was poor in Asia. On physical examination her conjunctivae are dry with a small build-up of keratin debris. The patient is diagnosed with a vitamin A deficiency. What other medical condition is the result of a fat-soluble vitamin deficiency?

(A) Iron deficiency anemia
(B) Megaloblastic anemia
(C) Osteomalacia
(D) Pellagra
(E) Wernicke-Korsakoff syndrome

31. A 62-year-old woman has sudden onset of stab-bing epigastric pain and hematemesis of bright red blood. She has a history of heartburn and has been taking over-the-counter antacids for most of her adult life. She has no history of liver disease. In the emergency department, she is stabilized with intravenous fluids and sent for esophagogastroduodenoscopy. A bleed-ing ulcer is visualized on the posterior duode-num approximately 2 cm from the pylorus. Which of the following vessels is the most likely source of the bleeding?

(A) Gastroduodenal artery
(B) Left gastric artery
(C) Left gastroepiploic artery
(D) Right gastric artery
(E) Right gastroepiploic artery

32. A 70-year-old woman is hospitalized for a change in mental status. During the course of her hospitalization, she develops a urinary tract infection and her urinary catheter is removed. Urine cultures show a gram-negative bacillus that is determined to be Enterobacter cloacae. Which of the following is the most appropriate therapy?

(A) Cephalosporin
(B) Gentamicin
(C) Imipenem
(D) Penicillin G
(E) Piperacillin-tazobactam

33. A 30-year-old African-American man comes to the physician with white macules on both his hands bilaterally. The patient is otherwise asymptomatic and states that he has had this condition for the past several years. Which of the following best describes the embryological origin of the affected cells in this patient?

(A) Endoderm
(B) Mesoderm
(C) Neural crest
(D) Neuroectoderm
(E) Surface ectoderm

34. A 3-month-old infant presents with failure to thrive, poor feeding, and lethargy. A physical examination reveals an enlarged liver and jaun-dice. Laboratory analysis reveals an elevated blood galactitol level and increased urinary re-ducing substance. Which of the following could correctly describe the levels of interme-diates of galactose metabolism in this patient?

(A) Decreased galactose
(B) Decreased uridine diphosphoglucose
(C) Elevated glucose-1-phosphate
(D) Increased galactose-1-phosphate
(E) Increased glycogen

35. A 25-year-old white woman of Ashkenazi Jewish descent presents to the physician with a 3-week history of lower abdominal cramps and intermittent bloody stools two times per day. She has not been febrile and reports no sick contacts, unusual food exposures, or travel history. She has an aunt with similar symptoms. Gross pathologic findings from a patient with similar symptoms are shown in the image. Laboratory tests show:

Hemoglobin: 13.0 g/dL
Hematocrit: 39%
WBC count: 6000/mm³
Platelet count: 200,000/mm³
Erythrocyte sedimentation rate: 35 mm/h

Which of the following is the most appropriate treatment?

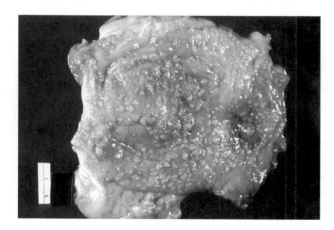

Reproduced, with permission, from the PEIR Digital Library (http://peir.net).

(A) Ciprofloxacin
(B) Emergent surgery
(C) Infliximab
(D) Loperamide
(E) Oral steroids
(F) Sulfasalazine

36. A 32-year-old man presents with progressive dementia and sudden, jerky, purposeless movements. On evaluation the patient is noted to be depressed. The patient states that his father, who died at age 50 years, had a similar condition as a young man. Which of the following is the most likely location of this man's brain lesion?

(A) Amygdala
(B) Caudate nucleus
(C) Lateral corticospinal tracts
(D) Mammillary bodies
(E) Nucleus basalis of Meynert
(F) Substantia nigra

37. A new genetic test for cystic fibrosis was developed and tested on 100 neonates known to have the disease. It returns a positive result in 98 of the neonates and a negative result in the other 2 neonates. Which of the following can be correctly concluded from these data?

(A) It has a negative predictive value of 98%
(B) It has a positive predictive value of 98%
(C) It has a prevalence of 98%
(D) It has a sensitivity of 98%
(E) It has a specificity of 98%
(F) It has an incidence of 98%

38. A 51-year-old man with HIV infection presents to the clinic with a 4-month history of increasing cognitive decline characterized by increasing apathy and mental slowing. His medical history is significant for several infections with *Pneumocystis jiroveci* (formerly *carinii*) pneumonia, and a recent CD4+ cell count was 112/mm³. Physical examination is notable for impaired saccadic eye movements, diffuse hyperreflexia, frontal release signs, and dysdiadochokinesia. Lumbar puncture reveals a total protein level of 72 mg/dL and an elevated IgG level. MRI of the brain shows global cerebral atrophy with multiple ill-defined areas of signal hyperintensity on T2-weighted images. Which of the following is the most likely cause of this patient's cognitive decline?

(A) Central nervous system lymphoma
(B) Cytomegalovirus encephalitis
(C) Disseminated *Mycobacterium avium* complex infection
(D) HIV-associated dementia
(E) Toxoplasmosis

39. A 62-year-old man presents to his physician complaining of a milky discharge from his nipples. The physician determines that the patient is suffering from a prolactinoma. What is the embryologic derivative of the region of the pituitary gland responsible for prolactin secretion?

(A) Endoderm
(B) Mesoderm
(C) Neural crest cells
(D) Neuroectoderm
(E) Oral ectoderm

40. A 34-year-old man with a history of Berger's disease who recently underwent renal transplantation following several years of glucocorticoid treatment and hemodialysis presents to the emergency department unable to walk properly. His mentation is normal, and he denies any chest pain or shortness of breath. During the interview, he says that he has recently been taking a pill for "a bug I had" and had recent severe pain around the back of his ankle. On physical examination, the patient is unable to plantar flex his right foot, and there is a large soft muscular mass high on his right calf. Which of the following medications has this patient most likely been taking?

(A) Amoxicillin
(B) Ceftriaxone
(C) Ciprofloxacin
(D) Erythromycin
(E) Metronidazole
(F) Penicillin G
(G) Vancomycin

41. A 35-year-old woman presents with a fever of 38.2° C (100.8° F), night sweats, fatigue, and a weight loss of 4.5 kg (10 lb) over the past 6 months. CT scan demonstrates mediastinal lymphadenopathy in multiple contiguous nodes. A photomicrograph of the biopsy specimen of the nodes is shown in the image. Which of the following is the most likely diagnosis?

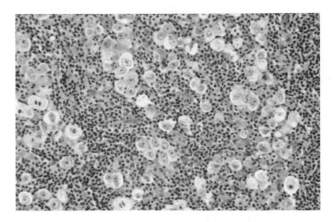

Reproduced, with permission, from Lichtman MA, Beutler E, Kipps EJ, Seligsohn U, Kaushansky K, and Prchal JT. *Williams Hematology*, 7th ed. New York: McGraw-Hill, 2006: Plate XXII-35.

(A) Acute myelogenous leukemia
(B) Burkitt's lymphoma
(C) Lymphocyte depletion Hodgkin's disease
(D) Mixed cellularity Hodgkin's disease
(E) Nodular sclerosing Hodgkin's disease

42. A second-year medical student is under a lot of stress due to her impending biochemistry examination. She knows that her psychological stress leads to the release of endogenous glucocorticoid, which increases the glucose levels in her body. To raise glucose levels, glucocorticoids act via the enzyme phosphoenolpyruvate carboxykinase to increase which of the following?

(A) Acetyl-CoA
(B) Malate
(C) Oxaloacetate
(D) Phosphoenolpyruvate
(E) Pyruvate

43. After 3 days of flulike symptoms, a patient is feeling unsteady on her feet and dizzy when she attempts to stand up. During her illness she has eaten very little and has had frequent emesis. Blood tests reveal an arterial pH of 7.5 and partial pressure of carbon dioxide of 53 mm Hg. What is the most likely etiology of this acid-base disturbance?

(A) Consumption of antacids
(B) Decreased hydrogen excretion in the distal tubule
(C) Increased bicarbonate reabsorption by the proximal tubule
(D) Production of ADH
(E) Volume depletion and increased hydrogen excretion in the distal tubule

44. If either the ulnar or radial arteries are occluded, which arteries ensure adequate collateral arterial flow in the hand?

(A) Anterior and posterior interosseous
(B) Arcuate
(C) Common and proper palmar digitals
(D) Deep and superficial dorsalis pedis
(E) Deep and superficial palmar arch

45. An obese 35-year-old woman presents to her physician with a 6-month history of amenorrhea. Her blood pressure is 128/88 mm Hg, and her laboratory studies show a luteinizing hormone (LH) level of 300 mIU/mL, a follicle-stimulating hormone (FSH) level of 5 mIU/mL, and a thyroid-stimulating hormone (TSH) level of 0.7 μU/mL. She also complains of increased hair growth. Physical examination reveals a normally developed woman, and a pelvic examination shows enlarged ovaries bilaterally. Her pregnancy test is negative. Which of the following additional findings is most commonly associated with her condition?

(A) Abdominal striae
(B) Exophthalmos
(C) Galactorrhea
(D) Hyperglycemia
(E) Weak pulses in the lower extremities

46. A 4-year-old girl is brought to the emergency department by ambulance late at night. Her caretaker reports that the child refuses to bear weight on her left leg and reports that she fell down the stairs this morning. X-ray of the leg shows a spiral fracture of her left femur. Which of the following is the most likely diagnosis?

(A) Child abuse
(B) Normal play injury
(C) Osteogenesis imperfecta
(D) Osteosarcoma
(E) Vitamin D deficiency

47. A 1-month-old boy presents to the pediatrician with bilious vomiting, an intolerance of feeding, and bloody diarrhea. X-ray of the abdomen is shown in the image. Which of the following is the anatomical cause of this patient's condition?

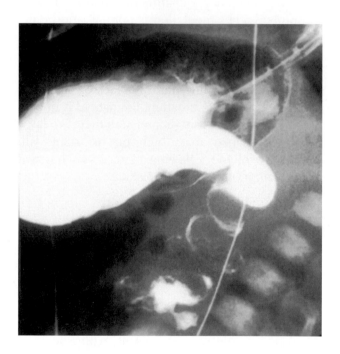

Reproduced, with permission, from PEIR Digital Library (http://peir.net).

(A) Failure of neural crest cell migration
(B) Incomplete rotation of the midgut during fetal development
(C) Intussusception of the small intestine
(D) Midgut loop remaining outside the abdominal cavity after umbilical hernia
(E) Persistent remnant of the vitelline duct

48. Antiviral agents used in the treatment of herpes virus infections are effective only during the acute phase of infection and are ineffective during the latent phase. Which of the following medications is a guanosine analog used in the treatment of active herpes virus infection?

(A) Acyclovir
(B) Didanosine
(C) Foscarnet
(D) Stavudine
(E) Zalcitabine

1. **The correct answer is B.** Ethosuximide is the only agent that is both used for absence seizures and associated with Stevens–Johnson syndrome. Ethosuximide is an antiepileptic indicated for absence seizures that works by blocking T-type calcium channels. A rare but severe adverse effect is drug-induced Stevens–Johnson syndrome. This is characterized by blistering of the nasal, oral, and genital mucosa as well as the conjunctivae. Erythema, palpable purpura, and epidermal necrolysis may also ensue.

Answer A is incorrect. Carbamazepine is used to treat partial and tonic-clonic seizures, but not absence seizures. It acts by increasing sodium channel inactivation. Carbamazepine can cause diplopia, induction of the cytochrome P450 system, blood dyscrasias, liver toxicity, and Stevens–Johnson syndrome.

Answer C is incorrect. Lamotrigine is used to treat partial and tonic-clonic seizures, but not absences seizures. It acts by blocking voltage-sensitive sodium channels. Lamotrigine can cause gastrointestinal upset, dizziness, diplopia, amnesia, and Stevens–Johnson syndrome.

Answer D is incorrect. Phenytoin is used to treat partial and tonic-clonic seizures, but not absence seizures. It acts by increasing sodium channel inactivation. Phenytoin toxicity causes nystagmus, diplopia, ataxia, gingival hyperplasia, hirsutism, and Stevens–Johnson syndrome.

Answer E is incorrect. Valproic acid is also indicated for absence seizures, and adverse effects include gastrointestinal distress and a rare, but fatal, hepatotoxicity. It acts by elevating concentrations of gamma-aminobutyric acid (GABA) in the brain. Valproic acid is not associated with Stevens–Johnson syndrome.

2. **The correct answer is A.** 21-Hydroxylase deficiency constitutes the most common form of congenital adrenal hyperplasia. It is marked by deficits in glucocorticoid and mineralocorticoid synthesis coupled with increased sex steroid production due to the increased flow of precursors, such as pregnenolone and progesterone, through androgen-yielding pathways. The resultant low serum cortisol and mineralocorticoid levels (aldosterone) and high sex steroid levels manifest clinically as hypotension, hyponatremia, hyperkalemia, volume depletion, masculinization, and female pseudohermaphroditism.

Answer B is incorrect. Estradiol is the most potent of the estrogens. It functions to stimulate ovarian follicle development, endometrial proliferation and myometrial excitability, development of female reproductive tract and secondary sexual characteristics, breast development, LH surge, feedback inhibition of FSH, and hepatic synthesis of transport proteins. 17α-Hydroxylase is necessary for the synthesis of estradiol, but 21-hydroxylase is not.

Answer C is incorrect. Estrone is one of the estrogens and is less potent than estradiol. Like the other estrogens, estrone stimulates ovarian follicle development, endometrial proliferation and myometrial excitability, development of female reproductive tract and secondary sexual characteristics, breast development, LH surge, feedback inhibition of FSH, and hepatic synthesis of transport proteins. 17α-Hydroxylase is necessary for the synthesis of estrone, but 21-hydroxylase is not.

Answer D is incorrect. Progesterone is produced by the corpus luteum, placenta, adrenal cortex, and testes. Elevation of progesterone is indicative of ovulation. The functions of progesterone include stimulation of endometrial glandular secretions, ovulation, spiral artery development, maintenance of pregnancy, decreased myometrial excitability, production of thick cervical mucus that inhibits sperm entry into the uterus, increased body temperature, inhibition of gonadotropins (LH, FSH); and uterine smooth muscle relaxation. 17α-Hydroxylase is necessary for the synthesis of progesterone, but 21-hydroxylase is not.

Answer E is incorrect. Testosterone is an androgen, the most potent of which is dihydrotestosterone. The androgens stimulate development of the male reproductive tract, male secondary sexual characteristics, and the pubertal growth spurt. They are responsible for increased anabolic effects, such as increased muscle mass and red blood cell production; they mediate normal spermatogenesis; and they increase libido. 17α-Hydroxylase is necessary for the synthesis of testosterone, but 21-hydroxylase is not.

3. **The correct answer is D.** This patient is likely suffering from endemic cretinism due to a deficiency in dietary iodine, a disorder that is still common in parts of the world, including parts of China. Lack of dietary iodine leads to deficient thyroid hormone production and thus hypothyroidism. Thyroid hormone is critical during development and thus children who grow up in iodine-deficient areas may manifest skeletal and central nervous system abnormalities, including short stature and mental retardation. Unfortunately for this child, once the syndrome is clinically apparent, it cannot be reversed. Thyroid function tests detect the presence of TSH secreted by the pituitary gland, as well as circulating levels of total serum triiodothyronine (T_3) and thyroxine (T_4). T_3 and T_4 levels usually fluctuate in the same direction in most abnormalities, whereas the balance between TSH and T_3/T_4 levels helps determine the cause of the thyroid abnormality. In primary hypothyroidism, T_3 and T_4 levels will both be low, and a compensatory increase in pituitary activity will increase TSH.

Answer A is incorrect. These findings suggest an abnormality in the pituitary that is accounting for the hypothyroidism (such as a pituitary adenoma), reducing TSH production. Reduced TSH production, in turn, reduces production of triiodothyronine and thyroxine from the thyroid.

Answer B is incorrect. This combination of findings would be not be normally seen in patients.

Answer C is incorrect. These findings will be seen in patients with primary hyperparathyroidism, such as thyroid carcinoma or Graves' disease. Due to autonomous production of triiodothyronine and thyroxine by the thyroid gland, there is a compensatory decrease in TSH production by the pituitary.

Answer E is incorrect. This combination of findings almost never occurs. It would theoretically suggest an abnormality in the terminal iodination step of thyroxine synthesis.

4. **The correct answer is E.** This patient has pemphigus vulgaris, a potentially fatal autoimmune disorder characterized by easily ruptured superficial vesicles that often crust and erode. It is thought to be due to IgG antibody against epidermal cell membrane. Lesions of the oral mucosa are characteristic of pemphigus vulgaris.

Answer A is incorrect. In bullous pemphigoid, patients have skin vesicles that are filled with a clear fluid; however, unlike pemphigus vulgaris, patients have IgG antibody against epidermal basement membrane. The bullae generally heal without scarring and do not rupture as easily as do the vesicles of pemphigus vulgaris. Oral mucosal lesions are found in 10%–40% of patients with bullous pemphigoid.

Answer B is incorrect. Eczema is characterized by itchy, red papulovesicular skin that, through excessive scratching, can become denuded and prone to bacterial superinfection.

Answer C is incorrect. Erythema multiforme is characterized by a combination of macules, papules, vesicles, bullae, and "target lesions" (spreading halos of erythema and central clearing) that often symmetrically affect the extremities.

Answer D is incorrect. Impetigo is a common skin infection caused by staphylococci or streptococci. It often presents as shallow skin erosions that have honey-crust-appearing edges.

5. **The correct answer is C.** This young woman has irritable bowel syndrome (IBS). IBS, a diagnosis of exclusion, is an idiopathic functional disorder characterized by abdominal pain and

changes in bowel habits that increase with stress (e.g., starting a new job) and are relieved with bowel movements. A normal complete blood count, erythrocyte sedimentation rate, and physical exam are consistent with this benign disease. Most people with this condition need reassurance from their physicians. However, pharmacologic treatment with antidiarrheals such as loperamide (an opioid) may be used in patients with diarrhea-predominant IBS.

Answer A is incorrect. Bactrim (trimethoprim-sulfamethoxazole) is an antibiotic used to treat conditions of infectious origin. Bactrim is not used for the treatment of IBS.

Answer B is incorrect. Bismuth is an agent used in peptic ulcers. This drug binds to the ulcer base, providing physical protection from acid. It has no clinical use in IBS.

Answer D is incorrect. Metronidazole is an antibiotic that is effective against anaerobes, protozoans, and gram-negative bacteria. It has no role in IBS treatment.

Answer E is incorrect. Octreotide, a somatostatin analog, may be useful in carcinoid syndrome and acromegaly. It has no known benefit in IBS treatment.

Answer F is incorrect. Omeprazole is a proton pump inhibitor that is useful in therapy for gastroesophageal reflux disease, gastritis, and peptic ulcer disease. It has no use in treatment of IBS.

6. **The correct answer is E.** This patient has Wegener's granulomatosis, a disease characterized by necrotizing, granulomatous vasculitis affecting several organs, most notably the upper respiratory tract, lung, and kidney. The hematuria is suggestive of glomerulitis. The presence of granulomas and the dramatic response to immunosuppressive therapy suggest that this disease process may be immunologic in origin. Elevated serum cytoplasmic antineutrophil cytoplasmic antibody is found in 90% of patients and is highly specific for the disease. Other clinical findings include skin rashes, muscle pains, and fever.

Answer A is incorrect. Patients with Alport's syndrome may have hematuria, but the hallmarks are ocular disorders and nerve deafness from defective synthesis of collagen type IV.

Answer B is incorrect. Giant cell (temporal) arteritis is a type of vasculitis that affects the arteries of the head (especially, of course, the temporal arteries). The highlights of this disease can be remembered by the mnemonic **JOE**, because patients get **J**aw pain and **O**cular disturbances from ischemia to the arteries supplying them. Patients also often have markedly elevated **E**rythrocyte sedimentation rates. The disease is often associated with the presence of polymyalgia rheumatica.

Answer C is incorrect. Goodpasture's syndrome is a type II hypersensitivity reaction against collagen type IV, found in the lungs and the kidneys. The disease commonly presents with concurrent hemoptysis and hematuria. Exposure to hydrocarbon solvents (such as those found in the dry-cleaning industry) and cigarette smoking have been associated with an increased risk of developing Goodpasture's syndrome.

Answer D is incorrect. Takayasu's arteritis is a vasculitis characterized by fibrotic thickening of the aortic arch (it also affects the pulmonary arteries, the branches of the aortic arch, and the rest of the aorta in up to one-third of patients). Clinically, patients often have lower blood pressure and weaker pulses in the upper extremities than in the lower extremities; some patients also have ocular disturbances as well.

7. **The correct answer is D.** This is a phenomenon known as peripheral tolerance. It is an important factor because deletion of self-reactive T lymphocytes within the thymus ("central tolerance") is not completely efficient at removing all self-reactive T lymphocytes. Thus, one mechanism of peripheral tolerance is that of anergy: When a T lymphocyte receives the first signal (peptide-major histocompatibility complex) but no second signal (costimulation, such as CD28-B7 ligation), that T lymphocyte undergoes a reprogramming known as anergy, wherein it is subsequently made refractory to any future stimulation.

Note that an anergic T lymphocyte cannot be activated later even if costimulation is present.

Answer A is incorrect. For a T lymphocyte to become activated and fully able to perform its effector functions, it must receive a second or costimulatory signal. Without a costimulatory signal, the T lymphocyte cannot be activated and instead becomes anergic.

Answer B is incorrect. A T lymphocyte that becomes anergic does not undergo activation.

Answer C is incorrect. Causing cells to undergo apoptosis is a function of an activated T-cytotoxic lympocyte.

Answer E is incorrect. The T lymphocyte will not clonally expand. Clonal expansion is more typical of B lymphocytes and requires a costimulatory signal to first activate the lymphocyte.

8. **The correct answer is C.** Ras is a G protein that cycles between two conformations: the activated ras-GTP and the inactivated ras-GDP. Mutation of the *ras* gene results in an aberrant protein with intact GTP binding but with a loss of GTPase activity, which prevents it from getting inactivated, resulting in a constitutively active G protein.

Answer A is incorrect. Cyclin-dependent kinases direct progression of cells through the cell cycle. They are activated by cyclins.

Answer B is incorrect. The oncogenes *erb* and *HER2* are examples of oncogenes that encode growth factor receptors.

Answer D is incorrect. *Abl* is an example of a proto-oncogene with tyrosine kinase activity. In chronic myeloid leukemia, *abl* on chromosome 9 is translocated to chromosome 22, fusing it with *bcr* and creating a hybrid tyrosine kinase with potent activity.

Answer E is incorrect. The myc protein is an example of a transcriptional activator that binds DNA, activating many growth-related genes.

9. **The correct answer is A.** The most effective drugs for the treatment of chemotherapy-induced nausea are the serotonin 5-HT$_3$ antagonists. This class includes ondansetron, dolasetron, and granisetron. These drugs can cause fatigue, headache, constipation, urinary retention, and dizziness; however, setrons are generally not very toxic.

Answer B is incorrect. Benzodiazepines include lorazepam and diazepam. They may be effective in treatment of the anticipatory nausea associated with chemotherapy, but they are not as effective as the 5-HT$_3$ antagonists.

Answer C is incorrect. Cholinergic antagonists include scopolamine. These drugs are not used for the treatment of chemotherapy-induced nausea. They are used for motion sickness.

Answer D is incorrect. Histamine receptor antagonists include diphenhydramine and promethazine. They are used for acid reflux and allergies.

10. **The correct answer is C.** Arylsulfatase A converts sulfatide to galactocerebroside. This enzyme is deficient in patients with metachromatic leukodystrophy, an autosomal recessive lysosomal storage disease in which patients cannot degrade sulfatides, leading to accumulation of cerebroside sulfate in both neuronal and nonneuronal tissues. There is abnormal myelination with widespread loss of myelination in the central nervous system (CNS) and peripheral nerves, leading to the clinical signs. Metachromatic granules can be seen on histologic examination.

Answer A is incorrect. α-Galactosidase A converts ceramide trihexoside to lactosyl cerebroside. This enzyme is deficient in Fabry's disease.

Answer B is incorrect. β-Galactosidase converts galactocerebroside to cerebroside. This enzyme is deficient in Krabbe's disease.

Answer D is incorrect. Hexosaminidase A converts ganglioside M$_2$ to ganglioside M$_3$. This enzyme is deficient in Tay–Sachs disease.

Answer E is incorrect. Sphingomyelinase converts sphingomyelin to cerebroside. This enzyme is deficient in Niemann–Pick disease.

11. **The correct answer is E.** This patient most likely has multiple sclerosis, a CNS demyelinating disorder characterized by neurologic lesions that produce signs and symptoms that are separated by both time (i.e., episodes greater than 1 month apart) and anatomic location within the white matter of the CNS. Patients typically also have difficulty in urination or incomplete voiding. By definition, multiple sclerosis (MS) episodes produce symptoms that last longer than 24 hours. The exact etiology is unknown, but there is evidence supporting a role of autoimmune antibodies that attach to CNS myelin-secreting oligodendrocytes. Episodes of optic neuritis (temporary unilateral vision loss) occur in 15%–20% of MS patients. Over 90% of patients have multiple periventricular plaques found on MRI of the brain.

   Answer A is incorrect. Chorea, the condition described in this answer, is not particularly associated with MS.

   Answer B is incorrect. Permanent bilateral resting tremors of the upper extremities are not particularly associated with MS. Intention tremors and ataxia (denoting cerebellar disease) are commonly associated with MS.

   Answer C is incorrect. Permanent progressive paralysis of the respiratory muscles is not particularly associated with MS.

   Answer D is incorrect. Raynaud's phenomenon, the condition described in this answer, is not particularly associated with MS.

12. **The correct answer is C.** Glipizide is a sulfonylurea that acts by stimulating the closing of potassium channels expressed in the cell membrane of pancreatic acinar β cells. It causes cellular depolarization and then calcium influx, which in turn triggers insulin release. Hence, a mutation that impairs closing of the β cell potassium channels would profoundly reduce the efficacy of the sulfonylureas.

   Answer A is incorrect. Acarbose is an α-glucosidase inhibitor that acts at the intestinal brush border to decrease the absorption of starches and other polysaccharides. This agent would be effective in maintaining glycemic control in someone with type 2 diabetes.

   Answer B is incorrect. Glargine is a long-acting synthetic insulin that provides a continuous baseline level of insulin in the blood. This agent would be appropriate for use in this patient in combination with a short- or intermediate-acting insulin to cover the glycemic loads associated with meals and snacks.

   Answer D is incorrect. Metformin is an oral hypoglycemic agent that is thought to inhibit gluconeogenesis and glycolysis, resulting in decreased blood glucose concentrations. This agent would be effective in helping to maintain glycemic control in someone with type 2 diabetes.

   Answer E is incorrect. Troglitazone is a thiazolidinone that acts to sensitize peripheral tissues to insulin and increase target cell response; it does not act on pancreatic acinar cells. This agent would be effective in helping to maintain glycemic control in someone with type 2 diabetes.

13. **The correct answer is A.** Pathologic grief includes excessive, intense, or prolonged grief as well as grief that is delayed, inhibited, or denied. The patient's quick return to work and lack of emotional impact at the time of death, combined with her grief symptoms 1.5 years after her husband's death, most likely reflect a delayed grief reaction. This patient is at higher risk for an abnormal grieving process given the rapid course of her husband's illness and death.

   Answer B is incorrect. Although denied grief is a pathologic entity, no symptoms of denial are elicited here.

   Answer C is incorrect. Guilty feelings are a normal part of the grieving process. They are abnormal if the feelings are intense and include feelings of worthlessness.

   Answer D is incorrect. Somatic symptoms such as headaches may be part of the normal bereavement process.

Answer E is incorrect. Weight loss of 1.3 kg (2.9 lb) or less is not worrisome. A weight loss of 3.6 kg (8.0 lb) or more would be worrisome for pathologic grief.

14. **The correct answer is B.** Such a presentation is consistent with a significant mechanism of injury such as ejection from a vehicle at a high rate of speed. The patient was able to talk with the police at the scene of the accident but was unable to recall how the accident occurred, which likely demonstrates an initial loss of consciousness followed by normal mentation and subsequent deterioration of consciousness. This lucid interval is classically seen with an epidural hematoma. An urgent neurosurgical consult is indicated for immediate evacuation of the clot to prevent herniation.

Answer A is incorrect. Injury to the inferior cerebral veins would result in subarachnoid bleeding. Bleeding from the inferior cerebral veins does not result from a fracture of the temporal bone and is unlikely to cause the rapid deterioration evident in this case because it has a slower rate of bleeding. However, subarachnoid bleeding is frequently seen in the setting of trauma and could be an associated finding with the epidural hematoma.

Answer C is incorrect. The posterior ethmoidal artery supplies the anterior superior nose and nasal septum with blood; its tearing would not result in an epidural hematoma secondary to a temporal bone fracture.

Answer D is incorrect. Injury to the sigmoid sinus would result in a subarachnoid hemorrhage. Thus such a finding is inconsistent with an injury to the temporal bone, the lucid interval in this patient's history, and the CT findings.

Answer E is incorrect. Injury to the superior sagittal sinus would also result in a subarachnoid hemorrhage, but this is a far less likely cause of this patient's deterioration than an epidural hematoma.

15. **The correct answer is D.** In Crigler–Najjar syndrome, the absence of glucuronyl trans-ferase results in an inability to conjugate bilirubin, leading to an unconjugated hyperbilirubinemia (high indirect bilirubin). The jaundice will become more severe as bilirubin accumulates, and at high levels will result in brain damage. Two entities have been identified: type 1 (autosomal recessive) and type 2 (autosomal dominant). A partial glucuronyl transferase deficiency is found in Gilbert's syndrome.

Answer A is incorrect. While the patient may have abnormalities in hematocrit, they would not be due to a glucuronyl transferase deficiency.

Answer B is incorrect. If an enzyme for conjugation is lacking, unconjugated (indirect) bilirubin will increase, not decrease.

Answer C is incorrect. Because the enzyme missing is used for conjugating bilirubin, direct bilirubin will decrease, not increase.

Answer E is incorrect. A hemolytic anemia would cause an increased reticulocyte count and also increase bilirubin level, which would result in jaundice. While this would further complicate the infant's condition, hemolytic anemia is not the cause of Crigler–Najjar syndrome, nor is it associated with that syndrome.

16. **The correct answer is D.** This patient presents with symptoms of digoxin toxicity. Severe bradycardia in a patient with complete heart block is a sign of severe digoxin toxicity. Digoxin toxicity is fairly common given the narrow therapeutic range of this medication, which is commonly prescribed for CHF. An increase in furosemide would result in increased potassium secretion in the nephron, which could cause hypokalemia, a state that potentiates the effects of digoxin and results in bradycardia.

Answer A is incorrect. A decrease in digoxin dosage would not cause an overdose of digoxin and would not cause any changes in the patient's ECG.

Answer B is incorrect. Verapamil, a calcium channel blocker, does not directly affect digoxin levels. However, increased levels of a calcium channel blocker will impair renal clearance in general and digoxin clearance specifically, thus resulting in digoxin toxicity. A reduced dosage of verapamil would not affect digoxin nor directly change the patient's ECG.

Answer C is incorrect. Enalapril, an angiotensin-converting enzyme inhibitor, has no direct or indirect effect on digoxin levels and would not produce any changes in the patient's ECG.

17. **The correct answer is D.** Diverticulitis is inflammation of diverticula, often in the sigmoid colon. It is related to retention of material within a diverticulum and fecalith formation. Diverticulitis typically manifests as left lower quadrant pain with fever, anorexia, and diarrhea and presents most commonly in older people. Diverticulitis should be distinguished from diverticulosis, which simply refers to the presence of diverticula. Diverticula occur when pressure causes herniation of the colonic wall through its own muscularis propria. A low-fiber diet is a known risk factor for diverticulosis. The sigmoid colon is the most common location affected by diverticulosis, likely due to the high pressure in this region. Occasionally, a diverticulum may cause rupture of a nutrient artery where it penetrates the muscularis propria; this results in bright red, painless bleeding from the rectum. However, only 20% of patients with diverticula experience hemorrhage. Thus, hemorrhage from diverticula is not always associated with diverticulitis, and diverticulitis may occur in the absence of bleeding.

Answer A is incorrect. The appendix contains similar layers to the colon with additional lymphoid tissue in the mucosa and submucosa. Acute appendicitis occurs more often in adolescents and young adults, and typically presents with right lower quadrant or periumbilical pain, nausea, and vomiting.

Answer B is incorrect. The ileum is not affected in diverticulosis.

Answer C is incorrect. Hemorrhoidal disease affects the rectum. The vasculature in this region normally protects the sphincter muscle, but prolonged straining and engorgement re-sults in prolapse into the anal canal. Symptoms include pain, bleeding, and protrusion of hemorrhoidal vessels.

Answer E is incorrect. The transverse colon is rarely affected in diverticulitis, and only 5% of patients have pancolonic diverticula.

18. **The correct answer is C.** Histoplasmosis does not typically lead to a symptomatic presentation. When symptoms are present, they usually manifest as a flu-like illness with fever, cough, headaches, and myalgias. Histoplasmosis can result in a lung disease resembling tuberculosis and widespread disseminated infection affecting the liver, spleen, adrenal glands, mucosal surfaces, and meninges. On light microscopy, histoplasmosis appears as small particles inside macrophages. Histoplasmosis occurs most commonly in the Mississippi and Ohio river valleys.

Answer A is incorrect. Blastomycosis can present with flu-like symptoms, fevers, chills, productive cough, myalgia, arthralgia, and pleuritic chest pain. Some patients will fail to recover from an acute infection and progress to develop chronic pulmonary infection or widespread disseminated infection. Fluconazole or ketoconazole is used for the treatment of local blastomycosis, and amphotericin B is used for the treatment of systemic infections.

Answer B is incorrect. *Cryptococcus neoformans* infection does not often present with any symptoms in an immunocompetent host. However, in an immunocompromised individual, it can present with meningoencephalitis. *Cryptococcus* is a heavily encapsulated yeast that is not dimorphic. The fungus is found in soil and pigeon droppings.

Answer D is incorrect. *Mucor* species is a mold with irregular nonseptate hyphae branching at wide angles (>90 degrees). Symptoms of *Mucor* infection include an allergic reaction and infarction of distal tissue due to fungal proliferation in the walls of blood vessels. The disease is mostly seen in patients with ketoacidotic diabetes and leukemia. High doses of amphotericin B are used to treat mucormycosis.

Answer E is incorrect. *Malassezia furfur* infection causes tinea versicolor. Symptoms of this infection include hypo- or hyperpigmented skin lesions that occur in hot and humid weather. Topical miconazole or selenium sulfides (Selsun) are used to treat *M. furfur*.

19. **The correct answer is E.** The loop of Meyer is located in the temporal lobe. It carries fibers from the inferior retina that are responsible for the contralateral upper quadrant of vision. The fibers first pass through the ipsilateral optic tract. Damage to the loop of Meyer on the right temporal lobe would result in bilateral left upper quadrant anopsia.

Answer A is incorrect. The dorsal optic radiation carries fibers from the superior retina that are responsible for the contralateral lower quadrant of vision. Damage to the left dorsal optic radiation causes bilateral right lower quadrant anopsia.

Answer B is incorrect. The dorsal optic radiation carries fibers from the superior retina that are responsible for the contralateral lower quadrant of vision. Damage to the right dorsal optic radiation causes bilateral left lower quadrant anopsia.

Answer C is incorrect. The optic tract carries fibers from the temporal retina of the ipsilateral eye and from the nasal retina of the contralateral eye. Damage to the left optic tract would cause right homonymous hemianopia.

Answer D is incorrect. Damage to the loop of Meyer in the left temporal lobe would result in bilateral right upper quadrant anopsia.

Answer F is incorrect. The optic tract carries fibers from the temporal retina of the ipsilateral eye and from the nasal retina of the contralateral eye. Damage to the right optic tract would cause left homonymous hemianopia.

20. **The correct answer is A.** This patient has recently acquired acute hepatitis B infection. Abdominal pain, positive hepatitis B surface antigen, and presence of IgM anti-HBc antibody are consistent with the diagnosis. Up to 15 weeks after exposure, patients with hepatitis B

infection are positive for HBV DNA, HBsAg, Anti-HBc, and HBeAg, but they are negative for anti-HBe and anti-HBs. The correct combination therapy for hepatitis B is lamivudine and interferon-α. Lamivudine is a reverse transcriptase inhibitor that blocks the action of an enzyme that is necessary in hepatitis replication. It is also used as an HIV medication. Interferon-α is thought to block viral replication and thereby inhibit hepatitis replication.

Answer B is incorrect. Interferon-β is not used in the treatment of hepatitis.

Answer C is incorrect. Ribavirin, in combination with pegylated interferon-α, is used in the treatment of hepatitis C. Lamivudine, in combination with interferon-α, is used in the treatment of hepatitis B.

Answer D is incorrect. Ribavirin, in combination with pegylated interferon-α, is used in the treatment of hepatitis C. Lamivudine, in combination with interferon-α, is used in the treatment of hepatitis B.

Answer E is incorrect. Ribavirin, in combination with pegylated interferon-α is used in the treatment of hepatitis C.

21. **The correct answer is F.** The image shows a crescent of epithelial cells and fibrin as well as a hypercellular glomerulus, which together are characteristic of rapidly progressive glomerulonephritis (RPGN). Furthermore, the clinical scenario demonstrates a nephritic syndrome, with hematuria, oliguria, and hypertension, which one would expect with RPGN. In about 50% of cases, RPGN is caused by deposition of immune complexes, but it can also be caused by pauci-immune glomerulonephritis and antiglomerular basement membrane (GBM) disease (called Goodpasture's syndrome when associated with pulmonary hemorrhage).

Answer A is incorrect. The most common cause of end-stage renal disease in the United States is diabetic nephropathy, which causes a nephrotic syndrome. A renal biopsy would show Kimmelstiel–Wilson lesions, which are nodules of mesangial matrix.

Answer B is incorrect. Patients with Goodpasture's syndrome present with pulmonary hemorrhage and glomerulonephritis. The syndrome is caused by anti-GBM antibodies. On immunofluorescence, renal biopsy would show a linear pattern tracing the basement membrane of the glomeruli. Anti-GBM antibodies are implicated in the pathogenesis of type 1 RPGN.

Answer C is incorrect. IgA nephropathy, or Berger's disease, often presents in children as hematuria following infection. Renal biopsy shows mesangial expansion due to deposition of IgA.

Answer D is incorrect. Lupus nephritis is the most serious symptom of systemic lupus erythematosus and often determines the prognosis of the disease. Additional symptoms of systemic lupus erythematosus included malar rash, discoid rash, photosensitivity, oral ulcers, arthritis, serositis, neurologic disorders, and immunologic disorders. Lupus nephritis causes a nephrotic syndrome with proteinuria, hypoalbuminemia, edema, and hyperlipidemia; many patients also develop hypertension. Renal biopsy is important to determine treatment, and histologic findings are classified in five patterns, including mesangial and subendothelial deposits (called "wire-loop" lesions).

Answer E is incorrect. Poststreptococcal glomerulonephritis is a common cause of nephritic syndrome that occurs about 10 days after pharyngitis. On light microscopy one would see diffuse proliferative glomerulonephritis without crescents. Electron microscopy would show subepithelial humps. Most cases are subclinical, and usually patients recover on their own, but some go on to develop RPGN, like the patient in this vignette.

Answer G is incorrect. Renal amyloidosis is associated with chronic inflammatory diseases and causes nephrotic syndrome. Glomerular amyloid deposits can be seen on renal biopsy by staining with Congo red and examining the specimen under polarized light.

22. **The correct answer is D.** This woman has had a normal delivery of monozygotic (identical) twins. Monozygotes may also develop separately, producing two amniotic sacs, two placentas, and two chorions, but this would not be distinguishable from dizygotic twins. In the case of a single chorion and placenta, the pregnancy must have developed from a single zygote, and in the womb the identical twins would appear within a single chorion with separate amniotic sacs.

Answer A is incorrect. Chorioamnionitis is typically caused by an infection ascending from the cervix or vagina following a premature membrane rupture. It requires early delivery and has a high risk of mortality for the fetus and would not, therefore, be considered a normal delivery.

Answer B is incorrect. A complete hydatidiform mole would not produce a normal delivery. Gross pathology shows a single enlarged placenta with edematous villi resembling grapes. Clinically, it produces a significant increase in human chorionic gonadotropin, vaginal bleeding, and fast uterine growth. It confers a 2%–3% risk of choriocarcinoma. Complete moles have no embryo present and are exclusively of paternal derivation.

Answer C is incorrect. Dizygotic twins would produce two chorions and two placentas, as well as two amniotic sacs.

Answer E is incorrect. Sheehan's syndrome is postpartum anterior pituitary necrosis resulting from hypotension and infarction following blood loss in pregnancy. It causes the gradual loss of anterior pituitary function. It has no relation to multiple amniotic sacs.

23. **The correct answer is B.** This patient is suffering from hypoglycemia related to his alcohol use. Ethanol is metabolized to acetaldehyde, which is then metabolized to acetate (acetaldehyde dehydrogenase). During both steps of ethanol metabolism, NADH is generated from NAD^+. With an elevated $NADH:NAD^+$ ratio in the liver, pyruvate is diverted to lactate,

while oxaloacetate is diverted to malate, thus inhibiting gluconeogenesis. The metabolism of ethanol is also responsible for the hepatic fatty changes seen in chronic alcoholics (increased fatty acid synthesis).

Answer A is incorrect. An elevated $NAD^+:NADH$ ratio does not result from alcohol metabolism. In any event, lactate would generate pyruvate, and gluconeogenesis would not be inhibited.

Answer C is incorrect. An elevated NADP:NADPH results from a faulty pentose shunt. NADPH is used for fatty acid synthesis and to reduce glutathione. The above presentation and decreased gluconeogenesis are consistent with an elevated $NADH/NAD^+$ ratio.

Answer D is incorrect. NADPH is produced by the pentose pathway. NADPH is used for fatty acid synthesis and to reduce glutathione. Glutathione helps prevent oxidative damage to cells by reducing hydrogen peroxide. An elevated NADPH:NADP ratio would not inhibit gluconeogenesis.

Answer E is incorrect. An elevated lactate: pyruvate ratio would be seen in alcohol intoxication rather than an elevated pyruvate:lactate ratio. During alcohol metabolism, the elevated $NADH:NAD^+$ ratio leads to diversion of pyruvate to lactate.

24. **The correct answer is D.** Introns are noncoding regions of RNA that are spliced out of mature mRNA. Almost all introns begin and end with 5′ GU———AG 3′. A mutation in one of those nucleotides affects splicing. This type of mutation is one of those found in thalassemia.

Answer A is incorrect. Capping of the mRNA occurs at the 5′ end as it is being transcribed. A mutation at the 5′ end of an intron would not affect capping.

Answer B is incorrect. Hybridization is a process in which single-stranded DNA base-pairs with a complementary sequence. A mutation at the 5′ end of an intron would not affect hybridization.

Answer C is incorrect. A poly(A) tail is added to the 3′ end of RNA after transcription. Poly(A) polymerase uses ATP as a precursor for adding adenosine one at a time. A mutation at the 5′ end of an intron would not affect polyadenylation.

Answer E is incorrect. Transcription of the DNA into RNA would not be affected by this mutation.

25. **The correct answer is D.** This patient's presentation is suggestive of IgM-mediated (cold) hemolytic anemia secondary to recent Epstein–Barr virus infection. Mononucleosis, which is caused by Epstein–Barr virus, is associated with IgM antibodies directed at the i antigen found on RBCs. In contrast, *Mycoplasma pneumoniae* infection typically yields a hemolytic anemia in which IgM antibodies are directed at the I antigen. IgM binds in the periphery at lower temperatures, binding complement, but IgM then falls off the RBCs as it returns to the central circulation. Agglutination of RBCs in the periphery can lead to the gray/purple discoloration seen in this patient's fingers.

Answer A is incorrect. Aplastic anemia results in pancytopenia, malaise, and severe infection. This disorder is a hypoproliferative anemia and would not have appropriate reticulocytosis as is seen in this patient.

Answer B is incorrect. Acute disseminated intravascular coagulation (DIC) results in bleeding and shock. Chronic DIC results in thrombosis and clotting. DIC is typically not associated with mononucleosis, but with gram-negative sepsis, acute myelogenous leukemia, and obstetric complications.

Answer C is incorrect. Coombs' test for IgG-mediated (warm) hemolytic anemia is positive for IgG. Warm hemolytic anemia is associated with autoimmune disease, lymphoproliferative disorders, and drug abuse.

Answer E is incorrect. Paroxysmal nocturnal hemoglobinuria is caused by a defect in the RBC's protection mechanism against complement-mediated lysis. Loss of the enzyme PIG-

A, which is required for glycosylphosphatidylinositol anchoring of decay-accelerating factor, results in episodic acute intravascular hemolysis and thrombosis.

26. **The correct answer is D.** Polymerase chain reaction is a laboratory procedure used to exponentially amplify DNA. Based on the primer sequences chosen, it results in the production of many copies of a desired fragment of DNA. These can then be used in a Southern blot.

    Answer A is incorrect. Enzyme-linked immunosorbent assay is a test of antigen-antibody hybridization used to detect an antigenic match in a patient's blood sample.

    Answer B is incorrect. Ligase chain reaction is a technique performed on mutant alleles for the purpose of detecting single-point mutations.

    Answer C is incorrect. A Northern blot is used to detect RNA through RNA-DNA hybridization.

    Answer E is incorrect. A Southern blot is used to detect DNA by DNA-DNA hybridization. It is performed after amplified DNA has been obtained.

27. **The correct answer is B.** The symptoms of fever, fatigue, night sweats, lymphadenopathy, and hemoptysis are consistent with the diagnosis of TB. The causative agent of TB is *Mycobacterium tuberculosis*. Primary tuberculosis infections are only rarely symptomatic in patients with normal immune function due to rapid containment by resident alveolar macrophages and infiltrating monocytes and lymphocytes. Symptomatic primary infection is mostly seen in the elderly, children, and immunocompromised individuals. Primary TB resembles an acute bacterial pneumonia, is typically located in the lower and middle lobes, and rarely causes cavitation. Secondary TB often localizes to the apex/upper lobes of the lungs, such shown in the x-ray film. A caseating granuloma is formed in which necrotic tissue and bacteria are surrounded by macrophages and giant cells.

Answer A is incorrect. *Legionella pneumophila* causes an atypical pneumonia and is associated with environmental water sources. It does not cause the symptoms described in the question. A chest film may demonstrate patchy interstitial infiltrates or nodular infiltrates.

Answer C is incorrect. *Mycoplasma pneumoniae* causes atypical pneumonia with cough and shortness of breath, and is visible as bilateral infiltrates on an x-ray film. The symptoms described in this patient are not consistent with this disease.

Answer D is incorrect. Respiratory syncytial virus is an etiologic agent of bronchiolitis in children, pneumonia in the elderly, and severe pneumonia culminating in respiratory failure in immunocompromised individuals. X-ray of the chest in patients with respiratory syncytial virus infection may demonstrate patchy infiltrate.

Answer E is incorrect. *Streptococcus pneumoniae* causes acute pneumonic symptoms reaching a crescendo within days, not weeks or months. Infection would not involve several months of fatigue, night sweats, and weight loss. A chest film in pneumonia caused by *S. pneumoniae* typically shows lobar consolidation.

28. **The correct answer is C.** The patient is suffering from Hashimoto's thyroiditis, an autoimmune disorder of the thyroid that is a common cause of hypothyroidism. Other classic signs and symptoms of this disorder include cold intolerance; hypoactivity; decreased appetite; weakness; decreased reflexes; dry, cool skin; and coarse, brittle hair. Laboratory values demonstrate an increased TSH level (the most sensitive test for primary hypothyroidism) and decreased total triiodothyronine and thyroxine levels. The thyroid gland is usually goitrous and firm, while histology reveals a significant lymphocyte and plasma cell infiltrate with germinal center formation, colloid-sparse follicles, and Hürthle cells (the acidophilic cells mentioned above). Like patients with Graves' disease, patients with Hashimoto's thyroiditis frequently have a history or family history of autoimmune disease. There is an increased incidence of Hashimoto's thyroiditis in HLA-

DR5 and -B5 individuals. Antimicrosomal antibodies, also called anti-thyroid peroxidase antibodies, are associated with Hashimoto's thyroiditis.

Answer A is incorrect. Anti-basement membrane antibodies are associated with Goodpasture's syndrome.

Answer B is incorrect. Anti-epithelial cell antibodies are associated with pemphigus vulgaris.

Answer D is incorrect. Antimitochondrial antibodies are associated with primary biliary cirrhosis.

Answer E is incorrect. Antineutrophil antibodies are associated with vasculitides such as Wegener's granulomatosis and polyarteritis nodosa.

29. **The correct answer is A.** This is a typical clinical picture of Rett's syndrome, a rare pervasive developmental disorder nearly always affecting girls 4 years old or younger. The hallmark features include decelerating social, cognitive, and verbal development that slowly progress to degeneration in these areas. Children become mentally retarded, expressionless, and nonverbal over the course of several years. Characteristic hand-wringing movements begin at about the same time as the developmental decline.

Answer B is incorrect. Although language and social degeneration occurs in patients with Rett's syndrome, gross hearing is unaffected.

Answer C is incorrect. Hyperactivity is not associated with Rett's syndrome; in fact, children with Rett's syndrome are typically withdrawn, apathetic, and solemn.

Answer D is incorrect. Psychosis is not a feature of Rett's syndrome.

Answer E is incorrect. Repetitive and compulsive behaviors such as self-injury and purposeless movements characterize autism and Asperger's disorder. They are not associated with Rett's syndrome.

Answer F is incorrect. Tics are characteristic of Tourette's syndrome, which typically begins in childhood. Loss of social and cognitive function is not associated with this disorder.

30. **The correct answer is C.** Vitamins A, D, K, and E are fat-soluble vitamins. They are released, absorbed, and transported with the fat from one's diet. Vitamin D deficiency reduces intestinal absorption of calcium and phosphate, leading to rickets in children and osteomalacia in adults. In oteomalacia there is demineralization of preexisting bone, leading to increased susceptibility to fracture. Patients with osteomalacia present with bone pain and muscle weakness with reduced bone density on radiographs. Hypophosphatemia, hypocalcemia, and elevated alkaline phosphatase levels are commonly seen. Treatment for osteomalacia depends on the underlying cause of the disease and includes pain control and orthopedic intervention when indicated. The patient should be given vitamin D supplementation and the low phosphate and calcium levels should be corrected.

Answer A is incorrect. Iron is an inorganic mineral, not a vitamin. A deficiency of iron causes a reduction in the rate of hemoglobin synthesis, resulting in iron deficiency anemia, the most common form of anemia in the United States. Iron deficiency occurs when loss of the iron component exceeds dietary intake of iron, such as occurs in gastrointestinal blood loss due to ulcer or menstrual blood loss. Like all anemia, iron deficiency anemia is characterized by fatigue and weakness, and includes additional epithelial changes such as brittle nails and atrophic tongue. Blood smear shows hypochromia and microcytosis. Lab tests show abnormally low levels of ferritin and low serum iron levels in association with an elevated total iron binding capacity.

Answer B is incorrect. Megaloblastic anemia is commonly caused by a deficiency of the water-soluble vitamins B_{12} or folate.

Answer D is incorrect. Pellagra is characterized by the "**3 D's**": **D**ermatitis, **D**iarrhea, and **D**ementia and, if untreated, **D**eath. It is a disease caused by niacin deficiency. Niacin is a water-soluble vitamin that form the biologically active coenzymes NAD^+ and its phosphorylated derivative, $NADP^+$. $NADP^+$ and NAD^+

serve as coenzymes in oxidation-reduction reactions, in which they are reduced to NADH and NADPH, respectively.

Answer E is incorrect. Thiamine (vitamin B$_1$) deficiency causes Wernicke–Korsakoff syndrome. Thiamine is a water-soluble vitamin and its deficiency is most commonly encountered in patients with chronic alcoholism. Wenicke–Korsakoff syndrome is characterized by a rapid onset of confusion, paralysis of extraocular muscles, and ataxia. If not treated promptly by administration of thiamine, a permanent memory deficit known as Korsakoff psychosis may result; this is characterized by an inability to form new memories or retrieve old ones, often accompanied by confabulation. The morphologic changes in Wernicke–Korsakoff syndrome are most evident in the mamillary bodies of the hypothalamus.

31. **The correct answer is A.** The gastroduodenal artery passes posterior to the duodenum. When an ulcer in the posterior duodenum erodes through the intestinal wall, it commonly erodes into this vessel. This requires urgent surgical repair, as an arterial bleed can rapidly lead to exsanguination and hemodynamic instability. Ulcers that occur in the anterior duodenum have a greater tendency to perforate than bleed.

Answer B is incorrect. The left gastric artery is a branch of the celiac trunk and supplies the superior lesser curvature of the stomach. It has anastomoses with the right gastric artery.

Answer C is incorrect. The left gastroepiploic artery supplies the greater curvature of the stomach and arises from the splenic artery, which arises from the celiac trunk.

Answer D is incorrect. The right gastric artery branches from the gastroduodenal artery proximal to the pylorus and supplies the lesser curvature of the stomach.

Answer E is incorrect. The right gastroepiploic artery branches from the gastroduodenal artery after it emerges inferior to the duodenum. It supplies the greater curvature of the stomach and has anastomoses with the left gastroepiploic artery.

32. **The correct answer is C.** *Enterobacter* species can cause pneumonia, and urinary tract and surgical site infections. Many strains have developed antibiotic resistance through the production of a β-lactamase that confers resistance to even the penicillin/penicillinase inhibitor combinations. However, coverage by the carbapenems (i.e., imipenem and meropenem) has been shown to be excellent.

Answer A is incorrect. In general, third-generation cephalosporins have good gram-negative rod coverage and can be used to treat pneumonia, sepsis, and urinary tract infection. However, when used against *E. cloacae*, there is a high risk of the development of resistance, making this a less good choice.

Answer B is incorrect. Gentamicin is an aminoglycoside antibiotic used to treat gram-negative bacilli. Adverse effects include nephrotoxicity and ototoxicity. Gentamicin is effective in treating *Enterobacter*, but it is not as efficacious as imipenem, and resistance is relatively common.

Answer D is incorrect. Penicillin G is not effective against *Enterobacter*. It is an intravenous β-lactam antibiotic useful in treating gram-positive bacteria as well as some gram-negative cocci and spirochetes. The most common adverse effect is a hypersensitivity reaction.

Answer E is incorrect. Piperacillin-tazobactam is a combination of an extended-spectrum penicillin with a penicillinase inhibitor. It is used to treat *Pseudomonas* infections as well as gram-negative rods. There is a risk of *E. cloacae* developing resistance to this drug during treatment, so it would not be used as first-line therapy.

33. **The correct answer is C.** This patient has vitiligo, a disorder characterized by partial or total absence of melanocytes within the epidermis. Studies have suggested an autoimmune connection to the disease process, citing associations to antibodies against tyrosinase, antigens that co-migrate with tyrosinase, or other antigens on melanocytes. Melanocytes produce skin pigment by synthesizing melanin from tyrosine and secreting it to keratinocytes. They

are derived from neural crest cells. Other neural crest derivatives include the adrenal medulla, Schwann cells, and sensory as well as autonomic ganglia.

Answer A is incorrect. Endoderm gives rise to the epithelial parts of the gastrointestinal tract, lungs, and urethra. It also gives rise to the parenchyma of organs such as the pancreas and liver. However, it does not give rise to melanocytes.

Answer B is incorrect. Mesoderm gives rise to muscle, connective tissues, bone and cartilage, blood and lymph, cardiovascular organs, the adrenal cortex, and reproductive organs as well as spleen and kidney. It does not give rise to melanocytes.

Answer D is incorrect. Neuroectoderm gives rise to the majority of the CNS as well as astrocytes, oligodendrocytes, and the pineal gland. It does not give rise to melanocytes.

Answer E is incorrect. While the surface ectoderm does give rise to the epidermis, hair, and nails, it does not give rise to melanocytes.

34. **The correct answer is D.** Elevated galactitol is the cause of clinical symptoms in patients with galactosemia. Galactose is utilized in glycolysis and gluconeogenesis by a two-step conversion to glucose-1-phosphate. The first step is catalyzed by the enzyme galactokinase, which phosphorylates galactose to galactose-1-phosphate. The second enzyme activity involves galactose-1-phosphate uridyl transferase (G1PUR), which converts galactose-1-phosphate to glucose-1-phosphate. A deficiency in G1PUR results in classic galactosemia (which is depicted in the case scenario). A deficiency in the other pathways of galactose metabolism leads to a much milder presentation (i.e., only infantile cataracts). Increased galactose-1-phosphate is the correct answer because the patient demonstrates classic galactosemia, and the damaging elevated galactitol that follows can occur in G1PUR deficiency. Although treatment is not available, prevention of progression involves avoidance of galactose from the diet (i.e., no breast milk or lactose formulas). This deficiency, which occurs between the conversion

of galactose to galactose 1-phosphate, would lead to relatively decreased galactose-1-phosphate. Galactose reduction by aldose reductase is then increased, forming galactitol.

Answer A is incorrect. Galactose would be elevated.

Answer B is incorrect. Classic galactosemia is caused by a deficiency of this uridyltransferase and would theoretically lead to a build up of galactose-1-phosphate, uridine diphosphoglucose, and galactose, and decreased glucose-1-phosphate.

Answer C is incorrect. Glucose-1-phosphate is the final product of galactose metabolism before glycolysis and would be decreased in all types of galactosemia.

Answer E is incorrect. Glucose-1-phosphate is an intermediate in glycogen pathways and the final product of galactose metabolism. However, galactosemia does not result in glycogen level fluctuations.

35. **The correct answer is F.** Based on the presenting symptoms of abdominal pain, bloody stools, Ashkenazi Jewish ancestry, and family history, this patient is suffering from inflammatory bowel disease, most likely ulcerative colitis. The image shows classical diffuse mucosal inflammation with pseudopolyps. Pseudopolyps are areas where mucosa has been eroded away such that only islands of intact mucosa remain; given their polypoid shape, these islands are referred to as pseudopolyps. However, they are actually the only "normal" parts of mucosa left, and the pathology is the ulcerative lesions all around these pseudopolyps. Infectious etiologies of diarrhea are less likely given the patient's absence of fever, left shift, sick contacts, and foreign travel. Increased erythrocyte sedimentation rate is also consistent with diagnosis of inflammatory bowel disease. Sulfasalazine is first-line therapy for ulcerative colitis. It is metabolized to 5-aminosalicylic acid in the digestive tract and decreases inflammation locally. Adverse effects include renal insufficiency and increased risk of bleeding.

Answer A is incorrect. Ciprofloxacin may be useful in the treatment of ulcerative colitis complicated by strictures and infections of the gastrointestinal tract; however, it is not first-line treatment for inflammatory bowel disease.

Answer B is incorrect. Surgery, specifically colectomy in the case of ulcerative colitis, should be reserved for patients who have failed medical therapy.

Answer C is incorrect. Infliximab, a monoclonal antibody against tumor necrosis factor-α, is used for the treatment of severe ulcerative colitis following failure of more conservative therapies.

Answer D is incorrect. Loperamide, an antidiarrheal, should be used only in mild ulcerative colitis. While it may be useful for treatment of mild symptoms, it is not first-line therapy. Caution for development of fulminant colitis and/or toxic megacolon should preclude the use of antidiarrheals in patients with severe disease.

Answer E is incorrect. Oral steroids are used for treatment of moderate-severity ulcerative colitis that is refractory to first-line therapy. This patient is suffering from mild disease and may benefit from the addition of oral steroids if sulfasalazine therapy fails.

36. **The correct answer is B.** Huntington's disease is inherited in an autosomal dominant manner. It is caused by the expansion of CAG repeats on chromosome 4, which is associated with the progressive degeneration of the caudate nucleus and subsequent loss of GABAergic neurons. A primary function of the caudate is to modulate motor action plans arising from the frontal cortex. Patients typically present in the third or fourth decades of life with symptoms of chorea, depression, and dementia.

Answer A is incorrect. Klüver–Bucy syndrome, clinically manifested by hyperorality, hypersexuality, and disinhibited behavior, is associated with bilateral obliteration of the amygdala.

Answer C is incorrect. Amyotrophic lateral sclerosis, more commonly known as Lou Gehrig's disease, is associated with degeneration of the lateral corticospinal tracts.

Answer D is incorrect. Wernicke's encephalopathy, which is most commonly seen in malnourished alcoholics, is associated with atrophy of the mammillary bodies.

Answer E is incorrect. Alzheimer's disease is marked by a decreased number of neurons in the nucleus basalis of Meynert.

Answer F is incorrect. Parkinson's disease is characterized histologically by neuronal depletion and depigmentation of cells in the substantia nigra.

37. **The correct answer is D.** Sensitivity is the probability that, given a disease, a test for that disease will correctly diagnose it. It is calculated by dividing the number of true positives (98) by the total number with the disease (100) = 98%.

Answer A is incorrect. Negative predictive value is the probability that, given a negative test result, the subject is actually free of the disease being tested. It is calculated by dividing the number of true negatives by the total number of subjects who tested negative. Since this experimental group included no healthy control subjects, one cannot determine the negative predictive value.

Answer B is incorrect. Positive predictive value is the probability that, given a positive test result, the patient actually has the disease. It is calculated by dividing the number of true positives by the total number of subjects who tested positive. Since this experimental group included no healthy control subjects, one cannot determine the positive predictive value.

Answer C is incorrect. Prevalence is the total number of disease cases in a population at a given time.

Answer E is incorrect. Given that the test was only performed on subjects known to have the disease, one cannot infer specificity from these data. Specificity is the probability that given a healthy subject, a given test returns a negative result. Thus, it is calculated by dividing the number of false-negatives by the total number of disease-free subjects on which the test was performed.

Answer F is incorrect. Incidence is the number of new cases of a disease in a population per unit time.

38. **The correct answer is D.** HIV-associated dementia (also known as AIDS dementia complex) presents with memory loss, gait disorder, and spasticity. It represents the most common direct CNS complication of HIV disease and generally occurs later in the course of illness. Early symptoms may be subtle and may include depressive symptoms and apathetic withdrawal; later symptoms include global dementia and motor deficits. As the dementia progresses, patients experience difficulty with smooth limb movement, dysdiadochokinesia (impairment in performing rapid, alternating movements), impaired saccadic eye movements, hyperreflexia, and frontal release signs. Imaging studies are imperative to rule out mass lesions; 20%–40% of patients will demonstrate nonenhancing, poorly demarcated areas of increased T2 signal intensity in the deep white matter. The symptoms must be distinguished from typical focal neurologic signs and symptoms that may be evident in patients with mass lesions. Elevated levels of protein and IgG on CSF examination are present in approximately 45% and 80% of cases, respectively.

    Answer A is incorrect. CNS lymphoma typically affects patients with AIDS whose CD4+ cell counts are <50/mm³ with one or more enhancing lesions on MRI (50% multiple; 50% single). It can present with many signs and symptoms that overlap with HIV-associated dementia, but it is less insidious and typically causes more focal signs earlier in the course of the illness. CNS lymphoma can present with a positive polymerase chain reaction for Epstein–Barr virus within the CSF.

    Answer B is incorrect. Cytomegalovirus encephalitis can mimic HIV-associated dementia, but is usually more rapidly progressive and is typically concurrent with more generalized cytomegalovirus infections. MRI typically demonstrates enhancing periventricular white matter lesions in cortical and subependymal regions.

    Answer C is incorrect. Disseminated *Mycobacterium avium* complex infection is a late-stage complication of acquired immunodeficiency syndrome and is associated with CD4+ cell counts <50/mm³. It typically presents with constitutional signs and symptoms that include fever, night sweats, lymphadenopathy, hepatosplenomegaly, weight loss, and pancytopenia. The symptoms are more generalized and severe than those in HIV-associated dementia.

    Answer E is incorrect. Space-occupying lesions secondary to toxoplasmosis infection begin to occur with CD4+ cell counts <100/mm³ and typically appear as enhancing central nervous system lesions (which may be multiple) on MRI, with positive serologies. Treatment is typically with sulfadiazine and pyrimethamine, with imaging studies repeated after a few weeks. If no regression has occurred, the diagnosis should be reconsidered, and central nervous system lymphoma should be considered the most likely diagnosis.

39. **The correct answer is E.** The hormone prolactin is secreted by the anterior pituitary. In contrast to the posterior pituitary, which is derived from neuroectoderm and considered an extension of the brain, the anterior pituitary is derived from oral ectoderm on the roof of the mouth.

    Answer A is incorrect. Neither the anterior nor the posterior pituitary is derived from endoderm. The patient's adenoma developed in the anterior pituitary, which is derived from oral ectoderm.

    Answer B is incorrect. Neither the anterior nor the posterior pituitary is derived from mesoderm. The patient's adenoma developed in the anterior pituitary, which is derived from oral ectoderm.

    Answer C is incorrect. Neither the anterior nor the posterior pituitary is derived from neural crest cells. The patient's adenoma developed in the anterior pituitary, which is derived from oral ectoderm.

Answer D is incorrect. Neuroectoderm gives rise to the posterior pituitary, but the patient's adenoma is a prolactin-secreting tumor that develops in the anterior pituitary. The anterior pituitary is derived from oral ectoder.

40. **The correct answer is C.** Although a rare occurrence, fluoroquinolones have been reported to cause tendinitis, particularly Achilles' tendinitis. Occasionally the tendon will rupture, producing the clinical picture described in the stem. Those at increased risk for fluoroquinolone-induced tendinitis include those <50 years old and those with a history of renal disease, hemodialysis, renal transplant, or glucocorticoid use.

Answer A is incorrect. Amoxicillin is not associated with tendinitis. Adverse effects include hypersensitivity reactions, nausea, vomiting, and diarrhea.

Answer B is incorrect. Ceftriaxone is not associated with tendinitis. Adverse effects include hypersensitivity reactions, nausea, vomiting, diarrhea, elevated liver enzyme levels, pseudomembranous colitis, and nephrotoxicty.

Answer D is incorrect. Erythromycin is not associated with tendinitis. Adverse effects include gastrointestinal disturbances, jaundice, and ototoxicity.

Answer E is incorrect. Metronidazole is not associated with tendinitis. Adverse effects include nausea, vomiting, headache, dizziness, rash, urticaria, yellow discoloration of the skin, and optic nerve damage.

Answer F is incorrect. Penicillin G is not associated with tendinitis. Adverse effects include hypersensitivity reactions and diarrhea.

Answer G is incorrect. Vancomycin is not associated with tendinitis. Adverse effects include "red man" syndrome with rapid infusion, ototoxicity, nephrotoxicity, and phlebitis.

41. **The correct answer is E.** As seen in the image, the presence of many lymphocytes and few Reed–Sternberg cells with collagen bands that circumscribe the lymphoid tissue into discrete nodules is consistent with the nodular sclerosing subtype of Hodgkin's disease (HD). This is the subtype with the best prognosis, and it is also the most common. Nodular sclerosing Hodgkin's lymphoma is more common in women. This histologic picture also resembles the lymphocyte predominance subtype, which is much less common but has an excellent prognosis and is also found in women.

Answer A is incorrect. Acute myelogenous leukemia does not affect the lymph nodes, but rather, produces abnormalities in the blood and bone marrow. This disease usually affects patients of middle age (35–50 years) and is characterized by the presence of numerous myeloid precursor cells with the presence of Auer rods.

Answer B is incorrect. Burkitt's lymphoma is a non-Hodgkin's type lymphoma that is predominantly a B-lymphocyte lymphoma. It is associated with Epstein–Barr virus infections that can lead to activating mutations of *c-myc* caused by chromosomal translocation t(8;14). Histologically, Burkit's lymphoma is characterized by sheets of lymphocytes with interspersed macrophages; this is commonly referred to as a "starry sky" appearance.

Answer C is incorrect. Any type of HD involving many Reed–Sternberg cells and no or few lymphocytes describes the rare lymphocyte depletion subtype. This has the worst prognosis of any type of HD and is generally present in elderly men with disseminated disease.

Answer D is incorrect. The heterogenous mixture of many mononuclear cells, many Reed–Sternberg cells, and many lymphocytes is consistent with mixed cellularity HD. This subtype is more common in men and more likely to be diagnosed at a later stage. The overall prognosis is good.

42. **The correct answer is D.** Phosphoenolpyruvate carboxykinase functions as a regulatory enzyme in gluconeogenesis. It acts in the cytosol to convert oxaloacetate to phosphoenolpyruvate.

Answer A is incorrect. Pyruvate dehydrogenase converts pyruvate to acetyl-CoA.

Answer B is incorrect. Malate is converted to oxaloacetate by malate dehydrogenase.

Answer C is incorrect. Phosphoenolpyruvate carboxykinase produces phosphoenolpyruvate, not oxaloacetate.

Answer E is incorrect. Pyruvate is formed by the action of pyruvate kinase on phosphoenolpyruvate during glycolysis.

43. **The correct answer is E.** This patient has a metabolic alkalosis as her pH is >7.4 and partial pressure of carbon dioxide is >40 mm Hg. This is secondary to her dehydration (which is apparent by her symptoms of orthostatic hypotension). Her frequent emesis results in the loss of large quantities of protons from the body in the form of stomach acid. In addition, rapid loss of bicarbonate-free fluids such as stomach contents or urine can result in a net increase in plasma bicarbonate concentration; this effect is termed "contraction alkalosis." Finally, volume depletion leads to stimulation of the renin-angiotensin-aldosterone system, causing (1) an angiotensin-mediated increase in hydrogen secretion via the sodium-hydrogen antiporter in the proximal tubule, and (2) an aldosterone-triggered influx of sodium (and water) and an efflux of potassium and protons in the distal tubule. The loss of protons and build-up of bicarbonate in this patient causes metabolic alkalosis.

Answer A is incorrect. Consumption of antacids can contribute to metabolic alkalosis but is not the cause in this patient.

Answer B is incorrect. Dehydration causes an increase, not decrease, in hydrogen excretion in the distal tubule.

Answer C is incorrect. Total bicarbonate reabsorption in the setting of metabolic alkalosis and volume depletion is likely to be reduced. Acutely, volume depletion will result in a net decrease in the filtered load of bicarbonate, despite an increase in bicarbonate concentration. In addition, increased plasma levels of bicarbonate will impair the ability of the proximal tubule cells to secrete acid necessary for bicarbonate reabsorption. Although angiotensin II stimulation serves to partially counteract these effects, the proximal tubule is not the primary site of acid loss in this patient.

Answer D is incorrect. ADH does not have direct effects on acid-base status because the aquaporin channels it mobilizes to the cell membrane are permeable only to water.

44. **The correct answer is E.** The superficial arch is a continuation of the ulnar artery and forms anastomoses with branches of the radial artery, while the deep arch is a continuation of the radial artery that forms anastomoses with branches of the ulnar artery. Together, these palmar arches ensure good collateral flow to the hand even if the radial artery becomes occluded. The Allen test is a way to determine if there is adequate arterial supply to the hand if the radial artery is occluded. This test is performed prior to inserting a catheter into this artery for blood pressure monitoring purposes or during coronary procedures. The radial and ulnar arteries are occluded while the patient makes a fist. The hand is relaxed and will appear pale. The pressure on the ulnar artery is released and the hand is visualized for uniform pink color return and normalization of the pulse oximetry reading within 8–10 seconds.

Answer A is incorrect. The interosseous arteries branch from the radial and ulnar arteries proximal to the wrist, forming anastomoses between the two arteries more proximal in the arm.

Answer B is incorrect. The arcuate artery is a branch of the dorsal artery of the foot and gives off perforating branches to the plantar artery. This artery helps ensure collateral flow in the foot so that if either the posterior or anterior tibial artery becomes occluded, the foot will have adequate circulation.

Answer C is incorrect. The palmar digital arteries branch from the palmar arches to supply the fingers.

Answer D is incorrect. The dorsalis pedis is found in the foot.

45. **The correct answer is D.** The condition described in this vignette is polycystic ovarian disease (Stein–Leventhal syndrome), which is a syndrome of multiple ovarian cysts, amenorrhea, infertility, obesity, and hirsutism caused by excess LH and androgens. In some women, this is associated with insulin resistance and hyperinsulinemia, which increases androgen production and, secondarily, LH production. The insulin resistance also leads to hyperglycemia.

Answer A is incorrect. Abdominal striae are signs of adrenocortical excess or Cushing's syndrome. This syndrome includes central obesity, muscle wasting, virilization, hypertension, round facies, buffalo hump, and striae due to high levels of glucocorticoids, mineralocorticoids, and androgens secondary to adrenal hyperplasia. Ovaries are not affected. The name Cushing's disease applies when these effects are due to elevated levels of ACTH.

Answer B is incorrect. Exophthalmos, or bulging eyes, is a sign of Graves' hyperthyroidism. Hyperthyroidism can present with amenorrhea, fine hair growth, restlessness, heat intolerance, diarrhea, and tachycardia. However, high thyroid levels usually result in low TSH levels and do not affect the ovaries.

Answer C is incorrect. Amenorrhea and galactorrhea are signs of hyperprolactinemia. Prolactin is controlled by dopamine secretion from the hypothalamus and inhibits gonadotropin secretion. This would not explain the high level of LH, elevated androgen levels, or enlarged ovaries.

Answer E is incorrect. Weak pulses in the lower extremities is a sign of coarctation of the aorta, which is associated with Turner's syndrome. Turner's syndrome is the most common cause of primary amenorrhea, and patients present with short stature, webbed neck, and infantile genitalia. Ovaries are replaced with fibrous streaks.

46. **The correct answer is A.** The suspicion of child abuse arises when the injury and the story of the injury do not match. Spiral fractures generally do not occur with a simple fall down the stairs. The physician should look for other signs such as multiple bruises in varying states of healing, old fractures on x-ray, subdural hematoma, retinal detachment/hemorrhage, and cigarette burns. Child abuse must be reported in all states of the United States.

Answer B is incorrect. Normal play is an insufficient explanation for a serious injury such as a spiral fracture of the femur.

Answer C is incorrect. Children with osteogenesis imperfecta can certainly present with spiral fractures due to seemingly benign accidents; however, the time delay from the accident to presentation in the emergency department is more suspicious for child abuse.

Answer D is incorrect. Fracture can be a complication associated with osteosarcoma; however, osteosarcomas are generally seen in male adolescents. The common finding on x-ray is a lytic lesion with or without soft tissue calcification in the proximal tibia or distal femur.

Answer E is incorrect. Rickets can present with fractures of the long bones; however, they tend to be greenstick fractures. These children are also typically bowlegged or knock-kneed due to the softening of the bony structure associated with vitamin D deficiency.

47. **The correct answer is B.** Volvulus is a common result of malrotation of the midgut but may also be associated with other congenital anomalies, such as Meckel's diverticulum and Hirschsprung's disease. Malrotation occurs when the midgut undergoes only partial rotation during development instead of rotating the normal 270 degrees counterclockwise between weeks 10 and 12 of gestation. Volvulus can result when malrotation leads to intestinal twisting and vascular congestion or ischemia. The presentation of volvulus varies depending on the age of the child and the severity of the twisting, but it is generally associated with vomiting, bloody diarrhea, abdominal distention, and tenderness to palpation. In the x-ray film, note the twisting and overdistention of the colon with its coffee-bean shape and lack of septa

and haustra, all indicative of obstruction due to volvulus. This is a dangerous condition, since ischemia can lead to gangrene and midgut necrosis; necrosis of the entire midgut is incompatible with life. Definitive treatment is corrective surgery.

Answer A is incorrect. Hirschsprung's disease occurs when neural crest cells fail to migrate, leading to aganglionosis of the distal colon. Although Hirschsprung's disease may cause similar radiographic findings and symptoms of obstruction, it would not cause symptoms of ischemia and is not the result of malrotation.

Answer C is incorrect. Intussusception is a cause of intestinal obstruction, and occurs when one segment of the intestine suddenly becomes telescoped into the immediately distal segment of bowel.

Answer D is incorrect. Although a normal physiologic umbilical herniation occurs around week 6 of gestation, an omphalocele will develop if the midgut loop fails to return to the abdominal cavity. An omphalocele appears as a shiny gray sac protruding from the base of the umbilical cord and is evident in the newborn.

Answer E is incorrect. Meckel's diverticulum is a blind pouch near the terminal ileum that represents a remnant of the vitelline duct. It is often associated with volvulus but is not a result of malrotation. It is often asymptomatic but may become inflamed and ulcerated.

48. **The correct answer is A.** Acyclovir is a guanosine analog used in the treatment of active herpes virus infections. Acyclovir causes premature DNA chain termination and limits the length of a herpes outbreak, although it does not change the frequency with which they occur.

Answer B is incorrect. Didanosine (ddl) is an antiretroviral drug also classified as a nucleoside analog.

Answer C is incorrect. Foscarnet is a viral DNA polymerase inhibitor that binds to the pyrophosphate binding site of the enzyme. It is used to treat cytomegalovirus retinitis

Answer D is incorrect. Stavudine (d4T) is a nucleoside analog of thymidine that inhibits reverse transcriptase when biotransformed to its active form.

Answer E is incorrect. Zalcitabine (ddC) is a nucleoside analog that inhibits viral reverse transcriptase when converted to its active form.

Test Block 5

1. A 47-year-old man with a history of hyperparathyroidism presents to the physician with a thyroid mass. Laboratory studies show elevated serum calcitonin levels. The patient reports that multiple family members have had similar health problems. Which of the following is the most likely pathology of this patient's thyroid mass?

   (A) Atrophic follicles with lymphocyte infiltrate and germinal centers
   (B) Nests of hormone-secreting tumor cells in an amyloid-filled stroma
   (C) Papillary pattern with ground-glass nuclei and psammoma bodies
   (D) Sheets of undifferentiated, pleomorphic cells
   (E) Uniform follicles with sparse colloid and a large cell lining

2. A 65-year-old man with cancer gives his best friend durable power of attorney. However, the patient also has a living will with the condition that all measures should be undertaken to maintain his life. As his condition worsens, he goes into respiratory failure and is intubated. He is now on a ventilator in a coma. The friend believes the patient would have wished for life support to be withdrawn. The patient's son, however, believes the father's living will is closest to this father's wishes and wants extreme measures taken to maintain his life. What is the legal course of action?

   (A) Advise the friend to listen to the son's wishes
   (B) Appoint a new power of attorney
   (C) Keep the patient on life support
   (D) Poll all the family members present
   (E) Withdraw life support

3. Three days after eating in a fast-food hamburger restaurant, a 12-year-old boy develops abdominal pain and bloody diarrhea. He is admitted to the hospital. His stool smear shows many leukocytes; a Gram stain shows many gram-negative rods. The organism forms pink colonies on MacConkey agar. The responsible organism is thought to be associated with development of which of the following conditions?

   (A) Fever, migratory polyarthritis, and carditis
   (B) Fever, new murmur, small erythematous lesions on the palms, and splinter hemorrhages on the nail beds
   (C) Petechial rash and bilateral hemorrhage into the adrenal gland
   (D) Symmetric ascending muscle weakness beginning in the distal lower extremities
   (E) Thrombocytopenia, anemia, and uremia

4. A 65-year-old man suffers an acute myocardial infarction (MI). His right coronary artery is stented, and the patient is started on a cardioprotective regimen of drugs. Three weeks later, laboratory studies show:

   Alanine aminotransferase (ALT): 62 U/L
   Aspartate aminotransferase (AST): 42 U/L
   Bilirubin, total: 1.4 mg/dL
   Albumin: 3.6 g/dL

   Which of the following agents was most likely included in this patient's drug regimen?

   (A) Aspirin
   (B) Clopidogrel
   (C) Lisinopril
   (D) Metoprolol
   (E) Pravastatin

5. A 42-year-old African-American woman with a history of sarcoidosis presents to a neurologist with evidence of a Bell's palsy. The muscles involved in this condition are derived from which of the following embryologic structures?

   (A) First branchial (pharyngeal) arch
   (B) Second branchial (pharyngeal) arch
   (C) Third branchial (pharyngeal) pouch
   (D) Fourth branchial (pharyngeal) pouch
   (E) Thyroglossal duct

6. A 22-year-old woman presents to the emergency department with lethargy, anorexia, loss of pubic and axillary hair, and inability to

nurse her newborn twins. Her past medical history is significant for a recent spontaneous vaginal delivery of twins complicated by postpartum bleeding. Physical examination reveals hypotension, and laboratory studies show hyponatremia. A CT scan of the head is performed and shows no tumors or masses. Which of the following sets of laboratory values is most likely to be seen in this patient?

CHOICE	CORTISOL	PROLACTIN	THYROID-STIMULATING HORMONE
A	↑	↑	↑
B	No change	No change	No change
C	No change	↑	No change
D	No change	↓	No change
E	↓	↓	↓

(A) A
(B) B
(C) C
(D) D
(E) E

7. While working in a microbiology lab, a research come across an unlabeled cryotub0° freezer. She deduces that it contains a strain of *Escherichia coli* and decides to test whether this strain has an intact lactose (*lac*) operon. After growing the cells in media containing both glucose and lactose, she observe that the β-galactosidase, encoded by *lac* operon, is expressed. However, no protein products are produced when the *E. coli* is grown only with glucose. Based on this observation, where is the mutation most likely located?

(A) cAMP receptor protein
(B) Inducer-binding site
(C) Promoter
(D) Repressor
(E) RNA polymerase

8. A 14-month-old boy presents with recurrent viral and fungal infections, congenital heart defects, tetany, and anatomic malformations in the neck. The abnormal cells in his spleen would be found in which of the following areas?

(A) Periarterial lymphoid sheath
(B) Splenic artery
(C) Splenic capsule
(D) Splenic vein
(E) White pulp follicles

9. Prior to the advent of antibiotics, patients suffering from life-threatening bacterial infections often received injections of serum from horses that were immunized with the disease-causing bacteria. A severe adverse event with this treatment occurred 7–10 days later and included fevers, rash, arthritis, and glomerulonephritis. Today, the same adverse event is seen with certain drugs or with delivery of large amounts of foreign protein. Why does it take 7–10 days for symptoms to occur?

(A) It usually takes the immune system 7–10 days to mount a mature antibody response against foreign proteins
(B) Symptoms begin to occur much earlier, but they often go unnoticed for 1 week
(C) Symptoms occur when the life-threatening bacterial infection worsens; this happens about 1 week after an unsuccessful course of treatment
(D) The foreign protein or drug must be metabolized before the immune system recognizes it, which takes about 1 week
(E) This is a T-cell-mediated adverse effect, and it takes about 1 week to activate the T cells

10. A woman whose mother had cancer in both breasts develops breast cancer at age 26 years. Her identical twin sister would like to know how likely it is that she, too, will develop the disease, and she decides to undergo testing for mutations in the *BRCA* gene. What mechanism causes *BRCA1* and *BRCA2* genes to become tumorigenic?

(A) Chromosomal rearrangement
(B) Dominant negative effect
(C) Gain of function
(D) Loss of function
(E) Viral insertion

11. A 53-year-old man is brought to the emergency department via ambulance after he began to feel heart palpitations. He has no significant past medical history. The ECG taken by paramedics shows an elevated heart rate and no apparent ventricular pathology. Which of the following antiarrhythmic agents should this patient be given intravenously?

(A) Adenosine
(B) Amiodarone
(C) Bretylium
(D) Lidocaine
(E) Procainamide

12. A 3-year-old boy is brought to his pediatrician with difficulty breathing and wheezing. His mother states that he recently had a cold. The boy has a heart rate of 95/min, a blood pressure of 130/85 mm Hg, a respiratory rate of 20/min, and an oxygen saturation of 94%. The boy appears to be having difficulty breathing, and on lung examination, wheezing can be heard bilaterally throughout. Which of the following is contributing to this child's respiratory symptoms?

(A) Cyclooxygenase
(B) Leukotriene B_4
(C) Leukotriene C_4
(D) Prostaglandin I_2

13. A 26-year-old Mexican immigrant presents to the clinic with a 3-month history of right upper quadrant abdominal pain. The patient denies any history of fever, vomiting, or diarrhea in the last 6 months. An ultrasound of the right upper quadrant reveals a well-circumscribed circular lesion that is 3 cm in diameter. Laboratory studies show:

WBC count: 9000/mm³
Segmented neutrophils: 56%
Band forms: 4%
Eosinophils: 10%
Basophils: 0.6%
Lymphocytes: 26%
Monocytes: 3%

Which of the following is the most likely morphology of the offending agent?

(A) Aerobic gram-negative bacteria
(B) Nonmotile gram-negative bacteria
(C) Pear-shaped protozoan
(D) Tapeworm
(E) Trophozoite

14. A 25-year-old woman presents with hypersecretion from the organ shown in the image. Increased levels of which of the following neurotransmitters might cause this patient's condition?

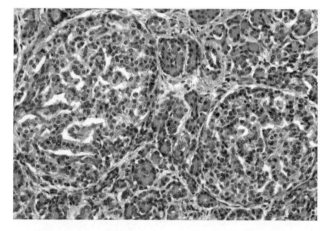

Reproduced, with permission from PEIR Digital Library (http://peir.net).

(A) Acetylcholine
(B) GABA
(C) Glycine
(D) Norepinephrine
(E) Serotonin

15. A 57-year-old man is brought to the emergency department in respiratory failure and dies shortly after his arrival. Paramedics report that the patient's examination was initially notable for meningeal signs and left-sided hemiplegia and hyperreflexia; he then vomited and became obtunded. The patient had reported suffering from a severe headache for the past 5 hours but had no history of neurologic disease and had not experienced any traumatic events recently. According to the wife's report, the patient's only medical problem was chronic renal insufficiency because "like his father, he has large kidneys." Which of the following is the most likely cause of death?

(A) Disruption of the middle meningeal artery
(B) Disruption of the sigmoid sinus
(C) Hypertensive cerebrovascular disease
(D) Rupture of a saccular aneurysm
(E) Thromboembolization of the right middle cerebral artery

16. A 3-year-old boy presents to his pediatrician with irritability, an ataxic gait, and regression of speech to single words. During the interview, the patient is constantly putting objects in his mouth. Laboratory values are significant for a hemoglobin level of 8.3 g/dL. Which of the following etiologies should be suspected in this patient?

(A) Acetaminophen toxicity
(B) Aspirin toxicity
(C) Button battery ingestion
(D) Lead poisoning
(E) Organophosphate absorption
(F) Tricyclic antidepressant overdose

17. A mother brings her 1-month-old infant to the pediatrician. She says the baby is crying more than usual and is vomiting and does not want to eat. Meningitis is suspected, and a lumbar puncture is done, which shows the following results:

Opening pressure: 240 mm H_2O (normal 100–200 mm H_2O)

WBC count: 1200/mm³
Protein: 200 mg/dL
Glucose: 30 mg/dL
Gram stain: gram-positive rods

Which of the following is most likely responsible for this infant's meningitis?

(A) *Escherichia coli*
(B) Herpes simplex virus
(C) *Listeria monocytogenes*
(D) *Neisseria meningitides*
(E) *Streptococcus agalactiae*

18. A 10-year-old boy with an x-linked immunodeficiency disease suffers from chronic recurrent gut inflammation, which modestly improves with cyclosporine therapy. The child has had previous laboratory evaluation that showed a negative reaction to the nitroblue-tetrazolium test. The patient's father wants to know how his son can have both an immunodeficiency disease as well as an autoimmune disease. Deficiencies in which of the following immunologic processes or molecules provides a logical link between this child's immunodeficiency and his autoimmune gut inflammation?

(A) Antibodies
(B) IgA
(C) IgM
(D) Lysosomes
(E) Neutrophils

19. A 60-year-old man is found to have advanced adenocarcinoma of the stomach. The tumor is centered at the pyloric zone just near the pyloric sphincter, on the lesser curvature. By mass effect, the neoplasm impinges on the omental (epiploic) foramen. Which of the following is most likely to be seen in this patient due to the mass effect of the tumor?

(A) Anemia
(B) Constipation
(C) Hoarseness
(D) Jaundice
(E) Seizures

20. Genetic analysis of multiple members in a family shows that they all have the same mutant gene. However, not all members display the characteristic phenotype; some members are more obviously affected than others. This is an example of which of the following?

(A) Anticipation
(B) Dominant negative mutation
(C) Mosaicism
(D) Pleiotropy
(E) Variable penetrance

21. A 16-year-old boy with sickle cell disease has complained of a weak right leg for the past 10 days. He is unable to put much weight on it. On physical examination, the area over the right tibia is found to be swollen and erythematous. The organism responsible for this patient's infection most likely has which of the following features that makes it particularly pathogenic?

(A) Capsule
(B) Flagella
(C) Lack of cell wall
(D) Mycolic acids
(E) Pili

22. A 44-year-old woman presents with extreme fatigue that has worsened over the past two month. She recently overcame her battle against alcoholism, and says her next goal is to improve her "horrible diet." Physical examination is unremarkable. Laboratory studies are significant for a hemoglobin level of 8 g/dL and a mean corpuscular volume of 110 mm³. A folic acid deficiency is suspected. Which of the following is the function of folic acid?

(A) Catalyzes γ-carboxylation of glutamic acid residues
(B) Hydroxylates prolyl- and lysyl- residues
(C) Increases intestinal calcium and phosphate absorption
(D) Makes up the constituents of the visual pigments
(E) Transfers one carbon intermediates between biochemical reactions

23. A 32-year-old woman with a history of schizophrenia presents to the physician with amenorrhea and a milky discharge from both nipples. A pregnancy test is negative. Laboratory results show an increased level of prolactin, decreased gonadotropin levels, and normal thyroid function tests. Which of the following medications is the most likely cause of this patient's symptoms and laboratory findings?

(A) Amantadine
(B) Bromocriptine
(C) Cabergoline
(D) Chlorpromazine
(E) Clozapine

24. A 20-year-old woman is referred to an endocrinologist for lack of menarche. On physical examination, breast tissue is found to be present, no cervix is palpable, the vagina ends in a blind pouch, and small atrophic testes are palpated in the inguinal canal. Laboratory studies reveal elevated levels of testosterone, estrogen, and luteinizing hormone (LH). The karyotype is 46,XY. Which of the following is responsible for this patient's condition?

(A) CGG triplet repeat expansion
(B) Deficiency of 5α-reductase
(C) Deletion of the X-linked dystrophin gene
(D) Excessive early gestational androgenic exposure
(E) Unresponsive testosterone receptors

25. A 40-year-old man will undergo a cholecystectomy during surgery to remove a small intestine adenocarcinoma. Before surgery, the surgeon explains to the patient the biliary system and the production, storage, and secretion of bile. He mentions that the gallbladder is involved only in storage, but not production, of bile. In which of the following locations is bile produced?

(A) Brush border of colon
(B) Brush border of terminal ileum
(C) Hepatocytes
(D) Kupffer cells
(E) Space of Disse

26. A 26-year-old woman is diagnosed with a congenital uterine malformation after several miscarriages. The gross specimen shown in the image is from a patient with the same uterine malformation who died of unrelated causes. Which of the following is the most likely etiology of this malformation?

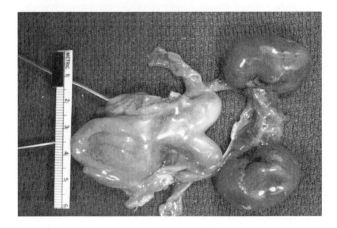

Reproduced, with permission from PEIR Digital Library (http://peir.net).

(A) Complete lack of fusion of the paramesonephric (müllerian) ducts
(B) Excessive resorption of mesonephric (wolffian) ducts
(C) Failure of the vaginal plates to canalize
(D) Incomplete fusion of mesonephric (wolffian) ducts
(E) Incomplete fusion of paramesonephric (müllerian) ducts

27. A previously healthy 5-year-old boy is brought to the pediatrician with a 3-day history of sore throat, conjunctivitis, rhinitis, and cough. His mother explains that more than 10 children in his class at school have similar symptoms, particularly conjunctivitis. No cultures are ordered, and the mother is assured that her son's illness will go away on its own. One week later, the mother reports that her son is healthy and back at school. Which of the following is the most likely cause of this child's illness?

(A) Adenovirus
(B) Coxsackie A virus
(C) Cytomegalovirus

(D) Herpes simplex virus type 1
(E) Rotavirus

28. A 40-year-old woman presents with progressive fatigue and bilateral joint inflammation characterized by pain, swelling, warmth, and morning stiffness. The patient says that the symptoms began in her hands over 1 year ago but have now begun to affect her knees. Which of the following agents would be most useful in her treatment?

(A) Ceftriaxone
(B) Cyclophosphamide
(C) Methotrexate
(D) Probenecid
(E) Tamoxifen

29. An 83-year-old man is brought to the family physician by his daughter because the patient has become "increasingly forgetful" over the past few months. The patient's only complaints are that his joints hurt a bit and he feels "run down lately." His past medical history is remarkable only for mild hypertension. A neurologic examination is notable for impaired short-term recall, but motor and sensory functioning are intact with no ataxia and a negative Romberg's sign. CT scan of the head shows mild cerebral atrophy. Which of the following is a treatable and reversible cause of this patient's dementia?

(A) Alzheimer's dementia
(B) Hypothyroidism
(C) Multi-infarct dementia
(D) Neurosyphilis
(E) Normal aging

30. A 7-year-old girl presents with a 5-month history of persistent weakness despite taking vitamins and supplements. Her mother denies that she has a significant medical history of any kind. Physical examination is completely benign, with normal blood pressure and no peripheral edema. Laboratory studies show hyponatremia, hypokalemia, metabolic alkalosis, and an increased plasma renin level. Renal biopsy reveals juxtaglomerular cell hyperplasia. Bartter's syndrome, a defective cotransporter in the thick ascending loop of Henle, is suspected. Which of the following diuretics acts at the same location as the defect in Bartter's syndrome?

(A) Acetazolamide
(B) Furosemide
(C) Hydrochlorothiazide
(D) Spironolactone
(E) Triamterene

31. A 6-year-old boy presents to the physician with poor exercise tolerance. Physical examination shows a wide pulse pressure and a continuous murmur. He is diagnosed with a congenital disorder of a structure that shunts fetal blood from the pulmonary artery to the aorta. Which of the following therapies for the mother would have reduced the risk of conceiving a child with this disorder?

(A) Amantadine
(B) Ganciclovir
(C) Pertussis vaccine
(D) Rubella vaccine
(E) Spectinomycin

32. A 53-year-old woman notices that her menstrual periods are becoming irregular, and sometimes she goes for 2 to 3 months without a period. She also complains of vaginal dryness and hot flashes. Blood tests reveal an estrogen level of 22 pg/mL, follicle-stimulating hormone (FSH) level of 100 mIU/L, and LH level of 50 mIU/mL (without surge). Which of the following is responsible for this patient's symptoms?

(A) Decreased estrogen levels
(B) Decreased feedback on the anterior pituitary
(C) Decreased hormone inhibition
(D) Increased progesterone levels
(E) Increased testosterone levels

33. A young couple presents to a fertility clinic because they have been unable to conceive despite trying for the past 18 months. On examination, the 27-year-old husband is found to have small testes and mild gynecomastia. He is 188 cm (6' 2") tall and weighs 64.4 kg (142 lb) (body mass index = 18.2 kg/m^2). Further cytogenetic testing reveals the presence of an additional X chromosome in his cells. Which of the following laboratory results is consistent with this man's condition?

(A) Decreased follicle-stimulating hormone level
(B) Decreased gonadotropin-releasing hormone level
(C) Decreased thyroid-stimulating hormone level
(D) Increased luteinizing hormone level
(E) Increased testosterone level

34. A 63-year-old woman develops tachyarrhythmia after recovering from an MI. Her physician prescribes a new medicationn. Five months later she presents to the clinic complaining of difficulty breathing and dry coughing, neither of which she has experienced previously. Physical examination reveals decreased breath sounds. After ruling out cardiac causes for her symptoms, her physician conducts a series of tests. X-ray of the chest shows decreased lung volume. Lung function tests show decreased vital capacity. Which agent most likely caused her current condition?

(A) Amiodarone
(B) Busulfan
(C) Flecainide
(D) Procainamide
(E) Propranolol
(F) Quinidine
(G) Verapamil

35. A large study is conducted in a Middle Eastern country to observe the renal function of subjects with the nephritic disease shown in the image. Which of the following is a common finding in this disease?

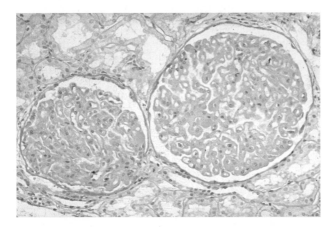

Reproduced, with permission from PEIR Digital Library (http://peir.net).

(A) Foot process effacement
(B) Linear immunofluorescence
(C) Mesangial deposits of IgA
(D) Split basement membrane
(E) Subendothelial humps

36. A 27-year-old woman is involuntarily committed to a psychiatric ward. Her physicians note persistently elevated blood pressure with a mean arterial pressure of 120 mm Hg over a week. The patient has been asymptomatic. Her physicians would like to begin a standard treatment regimen but the patient refuses. She understands the risks, benefits, and outcomes that would result either with or without treatment. What has priority in the care of this patient?

(A) Beneficence
(B) Duty to other patients
(C) Informed consent
(D) Nonmaleficence
(E) Patient autonomy

37. A 19-year-old woman with no significant past medical history presents to her primary care physician for a sports physical. Her examination is notable for a brachial artery pressure of 160/110 mm Hg and a weak femoral pulse. Prompted by the weak pulse, her physician measures her blood pressure in the lower extremity and finds it to be 80/40 mm Hg. An x-ray film of the chest shows rib notching. This woman is presenting with a congenital condition that places her at high risk for bacterial endocarditis and which of the following other conditions?

(A) Acute lymphocytic leukemia
(B) Boot-shaped heart
(C) Cerebral hemorrhage
(D) Cor pulmonale
(E) Eisenmenger's syndrome

38. A 25-year-old man is brought to the emergency department by his next-door neighbor after being found unconscious. The neighbor reports having last seen the man working in his yard about 4 hours earlier. No medical history is available. On physical examination, the patient has a blood pressure of 60/40 mm Hg, a pulse of 150/min, and respirations of 10/min. Despite the efforts of the emergency department staff, the man cannot be resuscitated. On autopsy, he is noted to have extremely flexible joints and skin. A number of bruises are noted on his thorax that were not present on admission. The cause of death is determined to be rupture of the abdominal aorta. This patient suffered from defective synthesis of which of the following structural proteins?

(A) Collagen
(B) Elastin
(C) Fibrillin
(D) Keratin
(E) Myosin

39. A 56-year-old man who is undergoing chemotherapy for colorectal carcinoma develops profound nausea and vomiting 4 hours after receiving treatments. The drug most likely to relieve the patient's symptoms functions by which of the following mechanisms?

(A) Acetylcholine antagonist
(B) Dopamine agonist
(C) Norepinephrine reuptake inhibitor
(D) Serotonin agonist
(E) Serotonin antagonist

40. A 15-month-old boy is brought to the pediatrician by his parents because they have noticed that he has difficulty walking. On physical examination, the child exhibits a broad-based waddling gait. Laboratory studies show a serum calcium level of 6.0 mg/dL, a serum phosphate level of 2.0 mg/dL, and a serum alkaline phosphatase activity of 85 U/L. Which of the following processes is most likely deficient in this child?

(A) Degradation of serum alkaline phosphatase
(B) Demineralization of osteoid matrix
(C) Hydroxylation of proline and lysine in collagen synthesis
(D) Intestinal absorption of calcium and phosphate
(E) Renal absorption of calcium and phosphate

41. A 24-year-old tall, thin man complains of sudden unilateral pleuritic chest pain and shortness of breath after playing a game of basketball. Being suspicious of a spontaneous pneumothorax, an x-ray film is made, which confirms the suspicion. A chest tube is placed. Which of the following is a likely physical finding before chest tube placement?

(A) Bilateral chest expansion
(B) Bronchial breath sounds
(C) Hyperresonance on percussion
(D) Increased tactile fremitus
(E) Tracheal deviation away from the affected lung

42. A 20-year-old mother is unsure of the paternity of her newborn son. To determine the father of her child, a genetic test based on DNA restriction fragment length polymorphism was performed. Blood was drawn from the four men suspected to be the father (F1, F2, F3, F4) as well as from the mother (M) and the infant (C). DNA extracted from the samples was amplified using polymerase chain reaction and then treated with the restriction enzyme EcoRI. The resulting fragments were separated with gel electrophoresis and a Southern blot analysis was performed. According to the Southern blot shown in the image, who is most likely the father of the child?

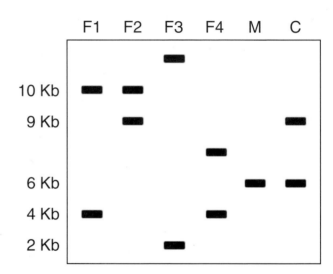

Reproduced, with permission from USMLERx.com.

(A) F1
(B) F2
(C) F3
(D) F4

43. Taxonomists categorize the RNA viruses according to the shape of their nucleocapsid and the characteristics of their RNA. Which of the following pairs of RNA viruses have RNA that is described as double-stranded segmented?

(A) Bunyavirus and Orthomyxovirus
(B) Paramyxovirus and Morbillivirus

(C) Picornavirus and Calicivirus
(D) Rotavirus and Coltivirus
(E) Togavirus and Flavivirus

44. A 28-year-old woman comes to the physician's office complaining of anxiety and a recent 4.5-kg (9.9 lb) weight loss. Her physical examination is significant for an inability to fully cover her eyes with her eyelids and swelling on the anterior surface of both legs. The skin of her anterior legs appears dry and waxy and has several diffuse, slightly pigmented papules. Laboratory studies show low levels of serum thyroid-stimulating hormone (TSH) and high levels of serum total thyroxine (T_4) and serum free T_4. Which of the following drug therapies should be used to treat this patient?

(A) Levothyroxine
(B) Mercaptopurine
(C) Procainamide
(D) Propofol
(E) Propylthiouracil

45. The symptoms of thiamine deficiency were first described over 4,000 years ago. In adults, these symptoms commonly include polyneuropathy of the distal extremities, resulting in paresthesias and motor dysfunction. In addition to neuropathy, how else can isolated thiamine deficiency present in adults?

(A) Chronic infection
(B) Convulsions, hyperirritability, and jaundice
(C) Excessive diarrhea, dermatitis, and dementia
(D) Kidney failure
(E) Peripheral edema and congestive heart failure

46. A 42-year-old man comes to the physician complaining of heartburn for the past 3 months. His pain is sharp, and is worse after meals and when lying down. He also mentions having black, tarry stools for the past month. Laboratory tests show a hemoglobin level of 11.2 g/dL, a hematocrit of 35%, mean corpuscular volume of 98 fL, a WBC count of 7000/mm³, and platelet count of 260,000/mm³. Endoscopy reveals a small flat lesion on the fundus; it has smooth

borders and is filled with exudate. Which of the following is a risk factor for his condition?

(A) Celecoxib usage
(B) Diabetes
(C) *Helicobacter pylori* infection
(D) Hypertension
(E) Stress

47. A patient with long-standing renal failure secondary to focal segmental glomerulosclerosis undergoes parathyroid biopsy that shows marked hyperplasia. On physical examination, tapping over the cheek elicits facial muscle spasm. Which of the following sets of laboratory values is most likely to be seen in this patient?

CHOICE	PARATHYROID HORMONE	SERUM CA²⁺	SERUM PHOSPHATE	ALKALINE PHOSPHATASE
A	↑	↑	↑	↑
B	↑	↑	↓	↑
C	↑	↓	↑	↑
D	↑	↓	↑	↓
E	↑	↓	↓	↑

(A) A
(B) B
(C) C
(D) D
(E) E

48. A 40-year-old nonsmoking woman comes to the physician complaining of a persistent cough and loss of weight and appetite over the past 3 months. On radiography, a well-demarcated subpleural mass is found on the right lung. Which of the following types of carcinoma does this patient most likely have?

(A) Adenocarcinoma of the lung
(B) Carcinoid of the lung
(C) Metastases to lung from a distant primary tumor
(D) Small-cell carcinoma of the lung
(E) Squamous cell carcinoma of the lung

1. **The correct answer is B.** This patient has multiple endocrine neoplasia (MEN) type II (formerly known as type IIA), a condition characterized by tumors of the parathyroid gland, medullary carcinoma of the thyroid, and tumors of the adrenal medulla. All MEN syndromes follow an autosomal dominant mode of inheritance with incomplete penetrance, thought to be inherited through activating mutations in the proto-oncogene Ret. MEN type I involves parathyroid hyperplasia, pancreatic islet cell tumors, and pituitary adenomas, whereas MEN type III (formerly known as type IIB) involves medullary thyroid carcinomas, mucosal neuromas, and pheochromocytomas. Medullary carcinoma of the thyroid is a calcitonin-secreting tumor of parafollicular thyroid cells. Microscopically, the tumor consists of nests of tumor cells in an amyloid-filled stroma.

Answer A is incorrect. Atrophic follicles with prominent germinal center formation and lymphocyte infiltrate is characteristic of Hashimoto's thyroiditis.

Answer C is incorrect. A papillary branching pattern of epithelial cells with ground-glass nuclei and psammoma bodies (laminated concentric calcified spherules) is seen in papillary carcinoma of the thyroid, the most common form of thyroid cancer and the one with the best prognosis.

Answer D is incorrect. Sheets of undifferentiated pleomorphic cells are seen in anaplastic, or undifferentiated, thyroid cancer. This form of thyroid cancer is more common in older patients and has a very poor prognosis.

Answer E is incorrect. Follicular carcinoma of the thyroid can resemble normal thyroid tissue. It is composed of relatively uniform follicles lined with cells that are typically larger than those seen in a normal thyroid. Colloid is sparse.

2. **The correct answer is E.** The appointed durable power of attorney is truly durable and supersedes even a living will. The patient, in good state of mind, believed that the friend would make decisions with which he agreed. It is always appropriate to facilitate a discussion between people involved in the decision, but it is unethical to sway the friend by making the choice for him or telling him to listen to the patient's son or the living will.

Answer A is incorrect. The friend should be advised to decide what he believed the patient would have wanted.

Answer B is incorrect. A patient's chosen power of attorney can only be changed by the patient. If a patient is noncommunicative, the power of attorney cannot be changed.

Answer C is incorrect. The durable power of attorney is the ultimate decision maker and their decision to withdraw life support will be upheld despite the existence of a living will.

Answer D is incorrect. The durable power of attorney was appointed as such to make decisions in accordance with the patient's wishes and should act accordingly. Input from family members is important and may be appropriate but is not legally necessary or in accordance with the patient's wishes.

3. **The correct answer is E.** *E. coli* O157:H7 is an enterohemorrhagic bacterium that can cause bloody diarrhea, abdominal pain, and (in some cases) mild fevers. It is often ingested in undercooked hamburger. Hemolytic-uremic syndrome is associated with infection with this organism. It is characterized by a low platelet count (thrombocytopenia), anemia, and renal failure, often manifested by uremia.

Answer A is incorrect. Rheumatic fever is characterized by fever, migratory polyarthritis, and carditis. It may follow group A streptococcal pharyngitis.

Answer B is incorrect. Fever, a new murmur, Janeway lesions, and nail-bed hemorrhages are all signs of bacterial endocarditis. Acute endocarditis is caused by *Staphylococcus aureus*;

subacute infection can be caused by viridans streptococci.

Answer C is incorrect. Waterhouse–Friderichsen syndrome is characterized by high fever, shock, purpura, and adrenal insufficiency classically associated with meningococcemia, although virtually any bacterial cause of septic shock can trigger the same findings.

Answer D is incorrect. Guillain–Barré syndrome is characterized by rapidly progressing ascending paralysis. It is thought to follow a variety of infectious diseases, such as cytomegalovirus, Epstein–Barr virus, HIV, and gastroenteritis caused by *Campylobacter jejuni*.

4. **The correct answer is E.** The 5-hydroxy-3-methylglutaryl-coenzyme A reductase inhibitors can cause an elevation of the transaminases, AST and ALT. Levels of these enzymes should be monitored following commencement of any statin. If the levels of AST and ALT increase, the drug should be discontinued.

Answer A is incorrect. Aspirin is associated with renal toxicity and gastrointestinal bleeds.

Answer B is incorrect. Clopidogrel is used to reduce the incidence of stent restenosis. It is associated with an increased risk of bleeding.

Answer C is incorrect. Lisinopril is an angiotensin-converting enzyme inhibitor and is associated with angioedema, cough, and hyperkalemia.

Answer D is incorrect. Metoprolol is a beta blocker that is important in the treatment of myocardial infarction but is not associated with elevation of hepatic enzymes. Its adverse effects include impotence, depression, bradycardia, and sedation.

5. **The correct answer is B.** A Bell's palsy is a lesion of cranial nerve VII (facial nerve) and affects the muscles of facial expression. These muscles are derived from the second branchial pharyngeal) arch. Patients with sarcoidosis, tumors, diabetes, AIDS, and Lyme disease are at increased risk for Bell's palsy, although most cases are idiopathic. Important signs of Bell's

palsy are ptosis and facial droop. The second arch also gives rise to the posterior belly of the digastric, the stylohyoid, and the stapedius muscles.

Answer A is incorrect. The first branchial arch gives rise to the muscles of mastication, the mylohyoid, the anterior belly of the digastric, the tensor veli palatini, and the tensor tympani. These muscles are innervated by cranial nerve V and are not affected by Bell's palsy.

Answer C is incorrect. The third branchial pouch gives rise to the inferior parathyroid glands and the thymus. It is implicated in DiGeorge's syndrome but has no relation to Bell's palsy.

Answer D is incorrect. The fourth branchial pouch gives rise to the superior parathyroid glands. It is implicated in DiGeorge's syndrome but is not related to Bell's palsy.

Answer E is incorrect. The thyroglossal duct connects the thyroid diverticulum to the foregut in the embryo but is obliterated during development. Its only remnant in the adult is the foramen cecum.

6. **The correct answer is E.** The patient is most likely suffering from Sheehan's syndrome, a state of postpartum panhypopituitarism that can develop after severe uterine hemorrhage during or after childbirth. A lack of blood supply to the enlarged pituitary leads to ischemic necrosis and destruction of hormone-producing tissue of the pituitary gland. Thus, patients with Sheehan's syndrome frequently have decreased levels of all hormones made in the anterior lobe of the pituitary gland, including a decreased prolactin level, which makes them incapable of breastfeeding after delivery.

Answer A is incorrect. Elevated cortisol, prolactin, and TSH would result in significantly different symptoms from those described in the patient above. Such a patient might have a hypothalamic hypersecretory lesion that would not be accompanied by the symptoms of lethargy, low blood pressure, and hyponatremia.

Answer B is incorrect. Changes in cortisol, prolactin, and TSH levels would be expected in this patient.

Answer C is incorrect. An isolated increase in prolactin levels suggests a prolactinoma, which was not seen on CT scan, or treatment with a drug that decreases dopamine levels, such as chlorpromazine. An isolated increase in prolactin would not be expected to cause hypotension and hyponatremia.

Answer D is incorrect. An isolated decrease in prolactin levels would also not be expected to cause hypotension and hyponatremia.

7. **The correct answer is A.** The lactose *(lac)* operon is an example of an inducible operon. Glucose is the preferred energy source for the *E. coli* bacterium and in the presence of glucose, *lac* operon transcription is inhibited by a repressor protein that binds to the operator region of the *lac* operon and blocks RNA polymerase. In the absence of glucose and the presence of *lac*, *lac* binds the repressor molecule and changes its shape so that it can no longer bind to the operator, allowing transcription to occur. Furthermore, as glucose levels decrease, cAMP levels rise and bind to the cAMP receptor protein (CRP). The CRP-cAMP complex binds to the operon and promotes the binding of RNA polymerase to the promoter. When the cells are exposed to both glucose and *lac*, *lac* does bind the repressor and release its repression. However, because the presence of glucose decreases levels of cAMP, the CRP-cAMP complex formation decreases consequently and RNA polymerase does not efficiently bind the promoter. Thus, under normal conditions, if the bacterium is grown in the presence of both *lac* and glucose, the *lac* operon should be mostly inactive. In this vignette, glucose fails to suppress transcription of the *lac* operon. Therefore, the mutation is most likely located in the CRP.

Answer B is incorrect. *Lac* is the inducer of the lactose operon. *Lac* binds tightly to the repressor so that the repressor can no longer bind to the operator and block the RNA polymerase from transcribing the products of the *lac* operon. If the inducer-binding site were mutated, the *lac* operon would not be expressed in the presence of *lac*.

Answer C is incorrect. A mutation in the promoter of the *lac* operon is not consistent with the above observation. If the promoter were mutated, the ability of RNA polymerase to bind to it would be altered regardless of the presence of glucose or *lac*.

Answer D is incorrect. In the absence of *lac*, the *lac* operon repressor binds to the operator and halts transcription. In this case, a mutation in the repressor protein would either increase or decrease repressor binding to the operator, which would alter the amount of products produced. No such changes were observed, which makes it unlikely that the mutation is located in the repressor.

Answer E is incorrect. If RNA polymerase were mutated in these bacterial cells, all gene expression would be affected.

8. **The correct answer is A.** The patient described has many of the classic hallmarks of DiGeorge's syndrome, or thymic aplasia. Due to a 22q11 deletion that causes maldevelopment of the third and fourth pharyngeal pouches, this disease is marked by T lymphocyte deficiency secondary to thymic aplasia. Failure of parathyroid development creates a setting of hypocalcemia that leads to tetany. The periarterial lymphoid sheath is a sheet of lymphoid tissue that surrounds the central arteries in the spleen. This sheath and the splenic red pulp contain T lymphocyte and would have different appearances in the setting of T lymphocyte deficiency. This location of T lymphocytes allows pathogens in the blood to come in close contact with lymphoid cells for antigen recognition.

Answer B is incorrect. The splenic artery is the only artery supplying oxygen-rich blood to the spleen. This blood is important for carrying antigens to the lymphoid cells within the spleen. The splenic artery is not affected by DiGeorge's syndrome.

Answer C is incorrect. The splenic capsule is a layer of connective tissue that covers and holds the splenic tissue together. It is covered by a thin layer of mesothelium that is a covering of the visceral peritoneum over the spleen. It is not affected by DiGeorge's syndrome.

Answer D is incorrect. The splenic vein is the only vein that drains the spleen and it empties into the hepatic portal vessels. The splenic vein is not affected by DiGeorge's syndrome.

Answer E is incorrect. The splenic white pulp contains follicles of B lymphocytes. B lymphocytes are deficient in Bruton's agammaglobulinemia and selective immunoglobulin deficiencies, not in DiGeorge's syndrome.

9. **The correct answer is A.** This adverse effect, known as serum sickness, is mediated by immune complex formation and deposition (in the skin, they cause a rash; in the kidney, they cause glomerulonephritis). The patient mounts a humoral immune response against the foreign protein or drug, thus forming antibodies that bind with high avidity to the foreign protein. The induction of an affinity-matured antibody response usually takes 7–10 days and requires T-cell help.

Answer B is incorrect. This is not usually true. It takes about 1 week to mount a mature antibody response.

Answer C is incorrect. Symptoms are likely to occur after the body has had a chance to mount a humoral-mediated response. While symptoms may worsen if an infection worsens, this does not explain why there would be fevers, rash, arthritis, and glomerulonephritis 7 to 10 days after administration of a certain drug.

Answer D is incorrect. Since it takes time for the antibody-mediated response to be mounted, symptoms do not typically occur until this time.

Answer E is incorrect. While T-cell help is needed to make the pathogenic antibodies and thus immune complexes, this is a type III hypersensitivity reaction, which is mediated by antibodies, not T cells.

10. **The correct answer is D.** *BRCA1* and *BRCA2* are tumor suppressor genes whose protein products act as inhibitors of tumor growth. Frameshift or nonsense mutations commonly occur in *BRCA1* and *BRCA2* and produce truncated protein products. Both alleles of these tumor suppressor genes must be inactivated to cause loss of function of these genes.

Answer A is incorrect. The chromosomal alterations in human solid tumors are heterogeneous and complex and allow for selection of the loss of tumor suppressor genes on the involved chromosome. However, in leukemias and lymphomas, the chromosomal alterations are often simple translocations, in which the breakpoints of chromosomal arms occur at the site of cellular oncogenes. For example, the Philadelphia chromosome in chronic lymphocytic leukemia is produced from a reciprocal translocation involving the *ABL* oncogene (a tyrosine kinase on chromosome 9) being placed in proximity to the *BCR* (breakpoint cluster region) on chromosome 22. The expression of the *BCR-ABL* gene product leads to tumorigenic growth.

Answer B is incorrect. Dominant negative effects occur when the loss of one allele leads to disease because the body cannot produce enough of the necessary protein product from just one functioning allele. An example of this is osteogenesis imperfecta, caused by mutations in the *COL1A1* gene.

Answer C is incorrect. Oncogenes acquire gain-of-function mutations that lead to increased activity of the gene product, which causes uninhibited cellular proliferation. This mutational event typically occurs in a single allele of the oncogene and acts in a dominant fashion. An example of this is the *c-myc* gene.

Answer E is incorrect. The first oncogene (*src*) was discovered as a cellular homolog of a viral gene capable of causing cancer. However, the *BRCA1* and *BRCA2* genes are tumor suppressor genes, and have not been shown to be inactivated by viral insertion.

11. **The correct answer is A.** Intravenous adenosine is the drug of choice in a case of acute su-

praventricular tachycardia. Because adenosine slows the conduction velocity and increases refractoriness at the atrioventricular node, it can convert an acute supraventriclular tachycardia into a normal rhythm.

Answer B is incorrect. Amiodarone, a class III antiarrhythmic, slows repolarization or phase 3 of the action potential. Because it does not cause atrioventricular nodal block, it is not indicated for patients in acute supraventricular tachycardia.

Answer C is incorrect. Bretylium, a class III antiarrhythmic, slows repolarization or phase 3 of the action potential and is not indicated for cases of acute supraventricular tachycardia because it does not achieve atrioventricular nodal block.

Answer D is incorrect. Lidocaine, a class IB drug, is indicated for ventricular arrhythmias because it has a greater effect on inactivated sodium channels. Because the action potential in atrial cells is short, lidocaine is not effective in treating atrial arrhythmias.

Answer E is incorrect. As a class IA antiarrhythmic, procainamide decreases sodium conduction and thus increases the duration of the action potential, makes the action potential less negative, and increases the QT interval. However, it is not indicated in cases of SVT because it does not achieve atrioventricular nodal block.

12. **The correct answer is C.** This child has the symptoms of asthma. Leukotriene (LT) C_4, LTD_4, and LTE_4 are bronchoconstrictors and are believed to contribute to symptoms of asthma. 5-Lipoxygenase is the enzyme that converts arachidonic acid to 5-hydroperoxy-eicosatetraenoic acid, which is then used to produce leukotrienes.

Answer A is incorrect. Cyclooxygenase (COX) is the enzyme that catalyzes the formation of prostaglandins, thromboxanes, and prostacyclins. Nonsteroidal anti-inflammatory drugs, COX-2 inhibitors, and acetaminophen exert their effects by inhibiting the cyclooxygenase

pathway. Products of the COX pathway cause inflammation, but are not directly responsible for bronchoconstriction.

Answer B is incorrect. Leukotriene B_4 is a neutrophil chemotactic agent. It is produced via the 5-lipoxygenase pathway; however, it does not cause bronchospasm.

Answer D is incorrect. Prostaglandin I_2 (PGI_2) inhibits platelet aggregation and vasoconstriction. PGI_2 is a product of the cyclooxygenase pathway.

13. **The correct answer is D.** This patient has *Echinococcus granulosus*, presenting with a classic hydatid cyst lesion of the liver. Hydatid cysts contain larvae of the tapeworm *E. granulosus*, whose eggs are carried from the intestinal tract to the liver via the portal circulation. *Echinococcus* is a dog tapeworm that incidentally infects humans and causes walled-off granulomatous lesions that result in anaphylactoid reactions when they erupt. Treatment is surgical excision. Note that the patient's lab values show eosinophilia, a common finding when infected by a parasite.

Answer A is incorrect. Aerobic gram-negative bacteria such as Pseudomonas species do not cause mass lesions. Also of note, an infection by a gram-negative bacterium would not cause the eosinophilia seen in the patient's lab data.

Answer B is incorrect. Nonmotile gram-negative bacteria such as Shigella species do not cause mass lesions. Also of note, an infection by a gram-negative bacterium would not cause the eosinophilia seen in the patient's lab data.

Answer C is incorrect. Although pear-shaped protozoans such as *Entamoeba histolytica* can cause hepatic abscesses, a patient with *E. histolytic* infection would present more acutely with a 1- to 2-week history of fever and abdominal pain. Less than one third of patients infected with a liver abscess have concurrent diarrhea.

Answer E is incorrect. Trophozoites such as *Trichomonas* species present with dysuria and genital discharge.

14. The correct answer is A. The organ shown in the image is the pancreas. The pancreas is divided into lobules that contain acini, or clusters of exocrine cells. Within the lobules are islets of Langerhans, which contain the endocrine tissue of the pancreas. Pancreatic secretions are stimulated by the parasympathetic nervous system (PNS). The major neurotransmitter of the PNS is acetylcholine. Thus, increased levels of acetylcholine would lead to increased activity of the PNS and increased pancreatic secretions.

Answer B is incorrect. GABA is a major inhibitory neurotransmitter commonly found in the brain. It does not cause hypersecretion of the pancreas.

Answer C is incorrect. Glycine is an inhibitory neurotransmitter released by spinal interneurons. It does not cause hypersecretion of the pancreas.

Answer D is incorrect. Norepinephrine is the primary neurotransmitter for postganglionic sympathetic neurons. It does not cause hypersecretion of the pancreas.

Answer E is incorrect. Serotonin is a neurotransmitter in nuclei in the brainstem. It does not cause hypersecretion of the pancreas.

15. The correct answer is D. This patient has suffered a rupture of a saccular or berry aneurysm. Although the etiology of these aneurysms is mostly unknown, an increased occurrence is found in patients with certain heritable conditions, such as polycystic kidney disease, connective tissue disorders, and coarctation of the aorta. Rupture of these aneurysms is associated with clinically significant subarachnoid hemorrhage that most often occurs in the fifth decade and involves the onset of severe headache followed by rapid deterioration in mentation. Because the patient has renal insufficiency, "large kidneys," and a positive family history, polycystic kidney disease, which is associated with intracranial aneurysms, is the most probable etiology. The patient's severe headache and the nausea/vomiting with signs of nuchal rigidity and deteriorating level of consciousness are consistent with this diagnosis.

Answer A is incorrect. Disruption of the middle meningeal artery would result in an epidural hematoma, which is almost always the result of a traumatic event. It is frequently associated with skull fractures.

Answer B is incorrect. Disruption of the sigmoid sinus would result in a subarachnoid hemorrhage and would almost certainly be the result of a traumatic event, as is the case with epidural hematoma. The extremely rapid progression of symptoms is also uncharacteristic of venous bleeding that would result from injury to bridging veins.

Answer C is incorrect. Hypertensive cerebrovascular disease can result in massive hemorrhages, lacunar infarcts, and slit hemorrhages as well as hypertensive encephalopathy. However, in the absence of a history of hypertension, atherosclerotic disease, or diabetes, this is a less likely cause, especially given the patient's likely history of polycystic kidney disease.

Answer E is incorrect. Thromboembolization of the middle cerebral artery would result in a stroke syndrome with associated hemiplegia (affecting the arm and face more often than the leg), hemianesthesia, and possibly drowsiness or stupor. However, it would not result in a rapidly progressive decrease in mentation and death.

16. The correct answer is D. A diagnosis of lead poisoning should be considered in young patients living in an environment with high lead levels (such as old houses with lead paint) and with a history of pica (eating non-nutritive substances) These patients present with the findings described in this case, including irritability, anorexia, ataxia, and regression of speech. These findings are due to acute encephalopathy secondary to lead poisoning as well as a microcytic anemia from inhibition of the heme synthetic pathway by lead. Treatment should includED ethylenediamine tetra-acetic acid (EDTA) or, for more severe cases, dimercaprol.

Answer A is incorrect. Acetaminophen toxicity can be a "time bomb" because patients may initially be asymptomatic. In the first 24 hours, nausea, vomiting, and malaise are common. At 24–48 hours, the patient's symptoms subside with possible right upper quadrant pain. At day 3–4, there is onset of jaundice and hepatic failure. N-acetylcysteine (Mucomyst) should be given within 8 hours of ingestion but is useful as late as 36 hours after ingestion.

Answer B is incorrect. Aspirin (salicylic acid) toxicity is associated with tinnitus, abdominal pain, vomiting, and tachypnea at low doses. At higher doses, respiratory alkalosis, metabolic acidosis, hypotension, coma, and death can occur. Urine can be alkalinized with sodium bicarbonate infusion to promote excretion of salicylate. Salicylate toxicity can be confused with diabetic ketoacidosis.

Answer C is incorrect. Button battery ingestion is a concern only if the battery becomes lodged in the esophagus, because leakage of alkali can lead to perforation. If the battery is past the esophagus, the child can be sent home and the parents can be instructed to screen for the battery in the patient's stool.

Answer E is incorrect. Organophosphate toxicity found in insecticides and carbamates can be absorbed through the skin. Symptoms include excess cholinergic activity (due to block of anticholinesterase by the organophosphate) leading to miosis, salivation, lacrimation, diarrhea, urination, and sweating. Treatment includes atropine and pralidoxime.

Answer F is incorrect. Tricyclic antidepressant overdose can result in anticholinergic symptoms such as hallucinations, dry mouth, flushing, urinary retention, and mydriasis ("mad as a hatter, dry as a bone, red as a beet"). However, the most severe complication of tricyclic antidepressant overdose is tachyarrhythmias, which can result in death.

17. **The correct answer is C.** The cerebrospinal fluid findings (CSF) described in the question point toward a bacterial cause of the infant's meningitis. In infants between the ages of 0 and 3 months, the most common organisms causing meningitis are *Listeria monocytogenes*, *E. coli*, and group B streptococcus. *Listeria monocytogenes* is the only gram-positive rod in the group.

Answer A is incorrect. *E. coli* can cause bacterial meningitis in infants, but a Gram stain of CSF would show gram-negative rods.

Answer B is incorrect. Herpes simplex virus (HSV) has also been shown to cause meningitis in infants. In viral meningitis, the CSF findings would show far fewer leukocytes (11–500/mm³), protein levels between 50 and 200 mg/dL, and normal glucose levels; a Gram stain would not show any organisms.

Answer D is incorrect. *Neisseria meningitides* also causes bacterial meningitis but is commonly seen in older children.

Answer E is incorrect. *Streptococcus agalactiae* can cause bacterial meningitis in infants, but a Gram stain of CSF would show gram-positive cocci.

18. **The correct answer is E.** Chronic granulomatous disease (CGD) is a disorder in which neutrophils are unable to completely eradicate certain phagocytosed bacteria and fungi. As a result, the chronic immune response to these lingering pathogens leads to the development of self-tissue damage. This answer provides a logical link between a correct description of CGD (a disorder of neutrophil production of nicotinamide adenine dinucleotide phosphatase oxidase, which results in neutrophils that are unable to completely eradicate certain phagocytosed bacteria and fungi) and the development of autoimmune disease. This answer points to theories questioning why 50% of patients with CGD suffer a chronic gut inflammation that is similar to Crohn's disease.

Answer A is incorrect. Common variable immunodeficiency, the most common symptomatic primary antibody deficiency syndrome, is a disorder characterized by differing degrees of deficiency of antibody production, leading to recurrent sinopulmonary and gastrointestinal infections.

Answer B is incorrect. This choice is not the correct immunologic deficiency of CGD. The disorder characterized by a deficiency of IgA antibodies is called IgA deficiency, the most common primary immunodeficiency disease in the Western hemisphere.

Answer C is incorrect. Wiskott–Aldrich syndrome is an X-linked disorder that results in the body being unable to mount an IgM response to capsular polysaccharides or bacteria. It is associated with low levels of IgM, high levels of IgA, and normal levels of IgE.

Answer D is incorrect. Chédiak–Higashi syndrome is an autosomal recessive disease affecting a lysosomal trafficking regulator gene; it leads to defective microtubular function and lysosomal emptying of phagocytic cells. This disease is characterized by a partial oculocutaneous albinism, abnormally large granules found in many different cell types, and recurrent pyogenic staphylococcal and/or streptococcal infections.

19. **The correct answer is D.** This question tests the concept of mass effect of tumors, as well as anatomy. These two topics are inseparable and are necessary to understanding the etiology of some symptoms seen in the context of neoplasms. The adenocarcinoma impinges on the omental foramen, which is formed partly by the hepatoduodenal ligament. This ligament contains the common bile duct along with the hepatic artery proper and the hepatic portal vein. Obstruction of the common bile duct would lead to cholestasis and subsequently conjugated hyperbilirubinemia.

Answer A is incorrect. Anemia may be a sign of gastrointestinal bleeding (seen with stomach or colonic cancers) or that bone marrow is dysfunctional and/or being replaced with malignant cells. Although anemia may be seen in this patient due to bleeding into the stomach, anemia is not a direct result of mass effect of the tumor.

Answer B is incorrect. Constipation may be a symptom of obstruction of the left colon.

Answer C is incorrect. Persistent hoarseness could be a manifestation of impingement of the recurrent laryngeal nerve. This symptom may be seen with thyroid or lung cancer.

Answer E is incorrect. Seizures may be a symptom of a tumor mass in the brain.

20. **The correct answer is E.** Variable penetrance indicates that not all individuals with a mutant genotype exhibit the mutant phenotype. Treacher Collins syndrome (an autosomal dominant disease that presents with numerous craniofacial deformities) is an example of a disease with variable penetrance.

Answer A is incorrect. Anticipation is the term used when a disease worsens or the age of onset of the disease is earlier in successive generations. Huntington's disease and fragile X syndrome (both of which involve trinucleotide repeats) show anticipation.

Answer B is incorrect. Dominant negative mutation is a mutation in which the mutant product interferes with the function of the normal gene product, leading to pathology.

Answer C is incorrect. Mosaicism occurs when cells in the body have a different genetic make-up. Patients with Turner's syndrome can have a mosaic genotype, with some cells having 45,XO and some having 46,XX.

Answer D is incorrect. Pleiotropy is a term used when one gene has more than one effect on a person's phenotype.

21. **The correct answer is A.** Since sickle cell disease leads to autosplenectomy, a condition in which fibrosis results from repeated infarcts of the spleen due to adherence of sickled RBCs. The spleen is unable to perform its normal functions, such as sequestering capsulated organisms. Since the spleen is the major defender against these organisms, patients without splenic function are susceptible to infection by encapsulated organisms such as *Salmonella typhi*. The symptoms suggest that the boy has osteomyelitis of the tibia, and the most important determinant of virulence in sickle cell patients with osteomyelitis is the

presence of a capsule. *S. aureus* is the most common cause of osteomyelitis in all groups, but *Salmonella* osteomyelitis has a particular association with sickle cell disease, and it is this association that is often tested on the Step 1 USMLE.

Answer B is incorrect. The flagellum of *Salmonella* is indeed a virulence factor that acts as an antigen that can be varied (antigenic variation or switching). However, it is not the presence of the flagellum that makes *Salmonella* more pathogenic in sickle cell patients.

Answer C is incorrect. *Mycoplasma* species are bacteria that lack a cell wall and that most often cause pneumonia (*M. pneumoniae*) or nongonococcal urethritis (also *Ureaplasma urealyticum*).

Answer D is incorrect. Mycolic acids are found in the outer cell membrane of mycobacteria. Mycobacteria can cause osteomyelitis, but autosplenectomy does not particularly put sickle cell patients at a higher risk.

Answer E is incorrect. Pili are structures on some bacteria that aid in adhesion to host cells.

22. **The correct answer is E.** Folic acid plays a key role as a coenzyme for one carbon transfer as seen in methylation reactions and is essential for the biosynthesis of purines and the pyrimidine thymidine. Deficiency of the vitamin is characterized by growth failure in children and macrocytic megaloblastic anemia. The anemia is a result of diminished DNA synthesis in erythropoietic stem cells. Large cells are seen with mean cell volumes of 100–150 mm³ and reduced levels of hemoglobin. Folic acid is a water-soluble vitamin stored in small amounts by the body; thus a continuous supply is need from foods such as green, leafy vegetables, lima beans, and whole grain cereals. Nutrient deficiency can commonly lead to folate deficiency. The deficiency is usually seen in pregnant women and alcoholics.

Answer A is incorrect. Vitamin K serves as a coenzyme in the γ-carboxylation of glutamic acid residues in blood clotting proteins. A vitamin K deficiency is rarely seen because adequate amounts are generally produced by intestinal bacteria or easily obtained from the diet. Decreased bacterial production in the gut (as with antibiotics, for example) can lead to hypoprothrombinemia and, subsequently, hemorrhage. Newborns have sterile intestines and cannot initially synthesize vitamin K. Because human milk fails to provide the adequate daily requirement of vitamin K, it is recommended that all newborns receive a single dose of vitamin K as prophylaxis against hemorrhagic diseases.

Answer B is incorrect. Ascorbic acid (vitamin C) acts as a coenzyme in hydroxylation of prolyl- and lysyl- residues of collagen, allowing collagen fibers to crosslink and providing greater tensile strength to the assembled fiber. A deficiency of ascorbic acid results in scurvy, a disease characterized by sore, spongy gums, loose teeth, fragile blood vessels, swollen joints, anemia, and poor wound healing.

Answer C is incorrect. 1,25-Dihydroxycholecalciferol, the active molecule of vitamin D, produces its effect at the DNA level to produce proteins in intestinal cells that allow for greater calcium and phosphate absorption. Vitamin D deficiency causes a net demineralization of bone, resulting in rickets in children and osteomalacia in adults. Rickets is characterized by continuous formation of collagen matrix of bone but incomplete mineralization, resulting in soft, pliable bones. In osteomalacia, demineralization of preexisting bones increases their susceptibility to fracture.

Answer D is incorrect. Vitamin A (retinol) is a component of the visual pigments of rod and cone cells. This fat-soluble vitamin plays an essential role in vision, growth, maintenance of epithelial cells, and reproduction. Night blindness is one of the earliest signs of vitamin A deficiency as a result of a loss in the number of visual cells. Further deficiency can lead to dryness of conjunctiva and cornea, leading to corneal ulceration and ultimately blindness.

23. **The correct answer is D.** Chlorpromazine is an antipsychotic used in the treatment of

schizophrenia and psychosis. Chlorpromazine blocks dopamine D_2 receptors and thus blocks the effects of excess dopamine associated with schizophrenia. Because dopamine inhibits the secretion of prolactin, a dopamine antagonist such as chlorpromazine can cause hyperprolactinemia by decreasing the inhibitory effects of dopamine.

Answer A is incorrect. Amantadine is used for influenza A prophylaxis, and because it causes release of dopamine from intact nerve terminals, it is also used in the treatment of Parkinson's disease.

Answer B is incorrect. Bromocriptine is a dopamine agonist that decreases, rather than increases, prolactin levels and is actually used for the treatment of hyperprolactinemia.

Answer C is incorrect. Cabergoline, like bromocriptine, is a dopamine agonist that decreases prolactin levels.

Answer E is incorrect. One of the atypical antipsychotics, clozapine blocks 5-HT_2 and dopamine receptors. It tends to have fewer extrapyramidal adverse effects than drugs such as chlorpromazine, including hyperprolactinemia. However, one of the more worrisome adverse effects of clozapine is agranulocytosis.

24. **The correct answer is E.** This patient has testicular feminization syndrome (androgen insensitivity), which is due to unresponsiveness on the part of the testosterone receptor protein to androgenic stimulation.

Answer A is incorrect. Fragile X syndrome, which is associated with congenital mental retardation, large ears, and macro-orchidism, is due to a CGG triplet repeat disorder.

Answer B is incorrect. A deficiency of 5α-reductase presents with ambiguous genitalia until puberty, when there is masculinization of the genitalia. Testosterone and estrogen levels are normal.

Answer C is incorrect. Duchenne's muscular dystrophy, a disorder of skeletal muscle, is due to the deletion of the dystrophin gene.

Answer D is incorrect. Excessive exposure to androgenic steroids during early gestation leads to female pseudohermaphroditism (XX), a condition in which ovaries are present but the external genitalia are virilized.

25. **The correct answer is C.** Bile is produced in liver hepatocytes, where primary bile acids are synthesized. They are then conjugated with taurine or glycine to form bile salts. In the gallbladder, bile is concentrated as solutes and water is reabsorbed.

Answer A is incorrect. Bacteria exist in the colon, where they help to deconjugate and dehydroxylate bile acids. Production of bile, however, takes place in the liver.

Answer B is incorrect. The brush border of the terminal ileum is the site of uptake for conjugated and unconjugated bile acids. Bacteria in the terminal ileum also function to deconjugate and dehydroxylate bile acids. Bile, however, is produced in the liver.

Answer D is incorrect. Kupffer cells line the sinusoids of the liver. These cells are tissue macrophages that ingest foreign particles, recycle old and damaged RBCs, and mediate inflammatory responses in the liver.

Answer E is incorrect. The space of Disse in the liver is located between hepatocytes and sinusoids. Rather than producing bile, it is responsible for lymphatic drainage.

26. **The correct answer is E.** The image shows a bicornuate uterus in which the uterus has two horns entering a common vagina. The embryologic cause of this is incomplete fusion of the paramesonephric (müllerian) ducts. Normally, in the absence of müllerian-inhibiting substance, the paramesonephric (müllerian) ducts develop into the uterine tubes and fuse caudally to form a single uterus, cervix, and superior third of the vagina. A bicornuate uterus is associated with infertility and urinary tract abnormalities.

Answer A is incorrect. Complete lack of fusion of the paramesonephric (müllerian) ducts leads to a double uterus with a double vagina.

However, in this patient and in the autopsy specimen, there is a common vagina due to partial fusion of the paramesonephric (müllerian) ducts.

Answer B is incorrect. In the male, the mesonephric (wolffian) duct develops into the seminal vesicles, epididymis, ejaculatory duct, and ductus deferens. In the female, the mesonephric (wolffian) duct is not stimulated to develop and it forms only vestigial structures (the appendix vesiculosa and the duct of Gartner), but the mesonephric (wolffian) duct is not resorbed.

Answer C is incorrect. If the vaginal plates fail to canalize, atresia of the vagina results. This leads to blockage of the vaginal lumen. The vaginal plates play no role in the development of the uterus, normal or bicornuate.

Answer D is incorrect. The mesonephric (wolffian) ducts play no role in the development of female reproductive organs and thus are unrelated to a bicornuate uterus. Normally, in the presence of müllerian-inhibiting substance and testosterone in the male, these ducts develop into the **S**eminal vesicles: **E**pididymis, **E**jaculatory duct, and **D**uctus deferens (remember the mnemonic **SEED**).

27. **The correct answer is A.** Adenovirus is a major cause of epidemic keratoconjunctivitis (pink eye). It is the fourth most common cause of childhood respiratory tract infections, after respiratory syncytial virus, parainfluenza, and rhinovirus. It is a naked, icosahedral, double-stranded linear DNA that results in a self-limited illness that requires no treatment.

Answer B is incorrect. Coxsackie A virus causes cold symptoms and rashes. It is also the causative agent of herpangina and hand, foot, and mouth disease.

Answer C is incorrect. Cytomegalovirus can reactivate and cause a variety of illnesses in the immunocompromised but is usually asymptomatic in healthy individuals.

Answer D is incorrect. HSV type 1 causes gingivostomatitis, herpetic keratitis of the eye, and encephalitis.

Answer E is incorrect. Rotavirus is the most common cause of diarrhea in infants less than 3 years old.

28. **The correct answer is C.** This patient is presenting with signs suggestive of rheumatoid arthritis. Methotrexate, a folic acid analog antimetabolite that inhibits dihydrofolate reductase, is often used as treatment due to reduction of adenosine-mediated inflammatory changes. Methotrexate is used in a number of neoplastic conditions, including breast carcinoma, head and neck carcinoma, lung carcinoma, choriocarcinoma, acute lymphoblastic leukemia, and non-Hodgkin's lymphoma. Other non-oncologic uses of methotrexate include ectopic pregnancy, psoriasis, and inflammatory bowel disease.

Answer A is incorrect. Ceftriaxone is a third-generation cephalosporin antibiotic that inhibits bacterial transpeptidase and cell wall synthesis. It is most commonly used to treat serious gram-negative infections, including meningitis and gonorrhea. Although gonorrhea can present with unilateral arthritis of the knee, this patient's clinical presentation is more consistent with rheumatoid arthritis. Ceftriaxone would therefore not be an effective treatment for this patient. Notably, tetracyclines **can** be used to inhibit the activity of metalloproteinases involved in joint destruction by the rheumatoid synovium, and are therefore effective agents in patients with early rheumatoid arthritis.

Answer B is incorrect. Cyclophosphamide is an alkylating agent that is useful in the treatment of non-Hodgkin's lymphoma and breast and ovarian carcinomas. It is also used as an immunosuppressant in systemic lupus erythematosus, multiple sclerosis, and autoimmune hemolytic anemia. It is not generally used as a treatment for rheumatoid arthritis.

Answer D is incorrect. Probenecid is an organic acid that is used most commonly for the treatment of chronic tophaceous gout or increasingly frequent gouty attacks. The drug acts at the anionic transport sites in the renal tubule to inhibit the reabsorption of uric acid, promoting its secretion. Gout normally presents with intermittent acute inflammatory arthritis, most often at only one site. In more chronic disease, more joints become involved and the intervals between attacks become shorter. Advanced gout results in chronic arthropathy, characterized by persistent asymmetric and asynchronous joint inflammation accompanied by uric acid deposits known as tophi, and can occasionally resemble rheumatoid arthritis. Nevertheless, the progressive and steady nature of this patient's disease strongly suggests a diagnosis of rheumatoid arthritis rather than gout. Probenecid would therefore be an ineffective pharmacologic therapy.

Answer E is incorrect. Tamoxifen is an estrogen receptor mixed agonist-antagonist that is most useful against estrogen-sensitive breast cancers.

29. **The correct answer is B.** This patient's fatigue and joint pain may be indications of hypothyroidism. Untreated hypothyroidism in the elderly, although uncommon, is a treatable cause of dementia. The work-up for a patient with dementia includes a complete blood cell count, liver function tests, thyroid function tests, renal function tests, electrolytes, glucose, vitamin B_{12}, folate, rapid plasma reagin, HIV testing, and urinalysis along with ECG, CT/MRI, and/or electroencephalography if clinically indicated. It is also important to talk with family members and friends because patients may not relate an accurate or complete history.

Answer A is incorrect. Alzheimer's disease is not reversible. Its course can be temporarily slowed by cholinergic therapies such as donepezil, galantamine, and rivastigmine, but dementia and finally death are inevitable.

Answer C is incorrect. Multi-infarct dementia is irreversible. By the time a patient has had enough mini-strokes to manifest neurologic deficits, the brain tissue is permanently damaged. Progression of the dementia can be slowed or even halted by statins and antiplatelet agents, but a full recovery is not possible.

Answer D is incorrect. Neurosyphilis is a late-stage complication of *Treponema pallidum* in-

fection. Typical manifestations include a decline in memory, changes in personality, and tabes dorsalis (degeneration of the posterior columns of the spinal cord), leading to a sensory ataxia. It is screened for with the rapid plasma reagin assay and treated with intravenous penicillin G.

Answer E is incorrect. Normal aging is not a cause of dementia. The mild memory changes associated with aging are irreversible but do not qualify for a diagnosis of dementia.

30. **The correct answer is B.** Bartter's syndrome has three variants, each with a different defective channel. The three channels that can be involved are the Na^+-K^+-$2Cl^-$ (NKCC) channel, the K^+ channel, and the Cl^- channel. In all three variants, the defective channels are found in the thick ascending limb. Furosemide is a loop diuretic that acts on the NKCC channel in the thick ascending limb. Patients with Bartter's syndrome have both hypokalemia and metabolic alkalosis.

Answer A is incorrect. Acetazolamide acts at the proximal convoluted tubule, inhibiting carbonic anhydrase. It causes a reduction in total body bicarbonate.

Answer C is incorrect. Hydrochlorothiazide is a thiazide diuretic that acts early in the distal tubule.

Answer D is incorrect. Spironolactone is a potassium-sparing diuretic that acts as a competitive aldosterone receptor antagonist in the cortical collecting tubule.

Answer E is incorrect. Triamterene is a potassium-sparing diuretic that blocks sodium channels in the cortical collecting tubule.

31. **The correct answer is D.** The child has a patent ductus arteriosus (PDA), identified in this question by its role in fetal circulation. This causes exercise intolerance, a wide pulse pressure, and a continuous "machine-like" murmur. Indomethacin may be used to close it in the neonate, but older children will require surgery or catheter placement. An important

risk factor for a PDA is congenital rubella. Rubella is a mild, self-limited illness in adults but is one of the ToRCHeS organisms that can cross the placenta and cause congenital disease. There is no specific treatment for rubella, but a vaccine exists that can prevent maternal infection and thus significantly reduce the risk of a congenital PDA induced by rubella. Note that the Centers for Disease Control and Prevention warn that rubella vaccine should not be given to a pregnant woman because of a possible risk to the fetus; administering the rubella vaccine to a woman before she becomes pregnant, however, would lower the risk of congenital PDA in any future offspring. The other ToRCHeS infections are toxoplasma, CMV, HSV/HIV, and syphilis. Most of these may present as mild or asymptomatic infections in the mother, but can cause a variety of congenital defects when transmitted to the fetus.

Answer A is incorrect. Amantadine is effective in the treatment and prevention of influenza A. It is commonly used in nursing home settings as prophylaxis during flu outbreaks. Influenza does not cross the placenta and is thus not a risk factor for a patent ductus arteriosus.

Answer B is incorrect. Ganciclovir is active against all herpes viruses, although its toxicity is much greater than that of acyclovir. Its use is therefore reserved for cytomegalovirus (CMV) infections in the immunocompromised, as CMV is not susceptible to acyclovir. CMV is one of the ToRCHeS organisms, but it typically causes mental retardation, microcephaly, and deafness; CMV does not commonly cause a patent ductus arteriosus.

Answer C is incorrect. While a vaccine does exist to prevent infection by *Bordetella pertussis*, this is not one of the organisms known to cause congenital disease and is not a risk factor for a patent ductus arteriosus. Infection causes whooping cough in the adult.

Answer E is incorrect. Spectinomycin effectively kills strains of *Neisseria gonorrhoeae* that are resistant to penicillin and tetracycline. Gonorrhea is an important cause of pelvic inflammatory disease, infertility, and ectopic pregnancies but does not cross the placenta and is not associated with a patent ductus arteriosus.

32. **The correct answer is A.** Menopause is the cessation of estrogen production due to a decreased number of available ovarian follicles. The average age of menopause onset is 51 years, with a normal range of 45–55 years. Remember, menopause causes **HAVOC**: **H**ot flashes, **A**trophy of the **V**agina, **O**steoporosis, and **C**oronary artery disease. Estrogen is necessary for the maintenance and development of the vagina and bone deposition, so a decrease leads to vaginal atrophy and osteoporosis. There is no direct link between estrogen and heart disease, but the incidence of coronary artery disease following menopause is two to three times higher than in premenopausal women, suggesting some protective effect of endogenous estrogen. Hot flashes are thought to be related to changes in the ability of the hypothalamus to recognize body temperature. As estrogen replacement therapy alleviates these symptoms, there may be a role for estrogen in body temperature regulation. Therefore, a decreased estrogen level will cause decreased maintenance of body organs and structures. The given value of estrogen in this case is low (<100 pg/ml), and the FSH and LH levels are high compared to reference values.

Answer B is incorrect. Decreased negative feedback on the pituitary would lead to increased levels of FSH and LH and therefore increased levels of estrogen. However, the patient described above shows symptoms of decreased estrogen.

Answer C is incorrect. Decreased estrogen inhibition would lead to increased levels of estrogen, resulting in weight gain, fluid retention, breast swelling, hypertension, fatigue, and endometriosis. However, the patient described above shows symptoms of decreased estrogen.

Answer D is incorrect. High levels of progesterone may result in fatigue, depression, and vaginal dryness. However, this woman's symptoms are more characteristic of menopause, which is due to low levels of estrogen.

Answer E is incorrect. Increased testosterone levels in a woman are classically seen in congenital adrenal hyperplasia and lead to masculine features such as hirsutism. This is not the case in this patient.

33. **The correct answer is D.** The man has Klinefelter's syndrome, a common cause of male infertility. His karyotype is 47,XXY, thus accounting for the additional X chromosome found on cytogenetic analysis. In Klinefelter's syndrome, the testicles are nonfunctional, and therefore testosterone levels are decreased, resulting in a secondary increase in gonadotropin levels (FSH and LH) due to lack of negative feedback.

Answer A is incorrect. Because of testicular dysfunction, FSH secondarily becomes increased, not decreased, in Klinefelter's syndrome.

Answer B is incorrect. Gonadotropin-releasing hormone will be increased secondary to the diminished testosterone level.

Answer C is incorrect. TSH, a measure of thyroid function, has no clinical application in diagnosing Klinefelter's syndrome.

Answer E is incorrect. Klinefelter's syndrome causes testicular atrophy. This results in decreased, not increased, testosterone.

34. **The correct answer is A.** Amiodarone is a class III antiarrhythmic that acts as a potassium channel blocker. One of its potential adverse effects is pulmonary fibrosis. This woman's symptoms of shortness of breath and dry cough, as well as her pulmonary function test results, are consistent with pulmonary fibrosis.

Answer B is incorrect. Although busulfan also has the potential adverse effect of pulmonary fibrosis, it is a chemotherapeutic drug that was not indicated in this woman's case.

Answer C is incorrect. Flecainide is a class IC antiarrhythmic that is used only as a last resort in refractory tachyarrhythmia because it is potentially proarrhythmic.

Answer D is incorrect. Procainamide is a class IA antiarrhythmic that can induce a systemic lupus erythematous-like syndrome.

Answer E is incorrect. Propranolol is a class II antiarrhythmic that acts as a β-blocker. Its adverse effects include impotence, exacerbation of asthma, and bradycardia.

Answer F is incorrect. Quinidine is a class IA antiarrhythmic that acts as a sodium channel blocker. Its major adverse effects include cinchonism and torsades des pointes.

Answer G is incorrect. Verapamil is a class IV antiarrhythmic that acts as a calcium channel blocker. Its adverse effects include constipation, flushing, and edema.

35. **The correct answer is E.** Membranoproliferative glomerulonephritis (MPGN) is an uncommon autoimmune renal disorder that mainly affects young individuals (ages 8–30 years). The diagnosis is based on histologic findings as shown in the image, including mesangial proliferation, thickening of the peripheral capillary walls by subendothelial "hump-like" immune deposits, and mesangial interposition into the capillary wall, giving rise to a tramtrack appearance on light microscopy (type I). MPGN is caused by a variety of factors. Primary MPGN is idiopathic and can be treated with aspirin and/or dipyridamole. Secondary MPGN can be caused by hepatitis C and B, cryoglobulinemia, lupus, rheumatoid arthritis, and malignancy. Due to significant complement activation, decreased completement levels is a characteristic finding with all types of MPGN. Diagnosis is confirmed by kidney biopsy.

Answer A is incorrect. Minimal change disease (lipoid nephrosis) is the most common cause of childhood nephrotic syndrome. It is characterized by lipid-laden renal cortices and demonstrates normal-appearing glomeruli by light microscopy. However, on examination by electron microscopy, fusing of epithelial foot processes (podocytes) can be seen. This disease responds well to steroid therapy.

Answer B is incorrect. Goodpasture's syndrome (anti-glomerular basement membrane disease)is caused by antibodies directed against antigens in glomerular and alveolar basement membranes. It demonstrates linear immunofluorescence by fluorescent antibody staining. It is manifest clinically by nephritic syndrome, pneumonitis with hemoptysis, and hematuria.

Answer C is incorrect. IgA nephropathy (Berger's disease) is a common cause of nephritic syndrome with a deposition of IgA in the mesangium. It is most often characterized by a mild postinfectious hematuria in children.

Answer D is incorrect. Alport's syndrome is hereditary nephritis associated with nerve deafness and ocular disorders such as lens dislocation and cataracts. It is caused by a mutation in the gene for the α-5 chain of type IV collagen. It demonstrates a split basement membrane on electron microscopy.

36. **The correct answer is E.** Patient autonomy in a legally competent patient is paramount. Understanding the risks and benefits of a treatment, as well as outcomes, with and without the treatment are defining characteristics of competence. A physician is obligated to respect patient autonomy over the principals of nonmaleficence and beneficence. Patients who are involuntarily admitted are done so for treatment of psychiatric conditions only. Even then, unless they pose a risk to themselves or others, competent patients can refuse psychiatric treatment.

Answer A is incorrect. Beneficence implies that an intervention is in a patient's best interest. All interventions have this characteristic in modern medicine but cannot be instituted without patient consent.

Answer B is incorrect. The duty to other patients involves patients who are a potential harm to other patients. Psychiatric patients have an increased potential to be physically dangerous to other patients as well as the normal potential to be a carrier of infectious disease. This patient's condition is not a threat to other patients.

Answer C is incorrect. Informed consent implies patient acknowledgement of the risks, benefits, and alternatives of a procedure or treatment. However, it is the patient's autonomy (of informed consent) that must be respected and that should take priority.

Answer D is incorrect. Nonmaleficence implies that risks of a treatment are less than benefits. Such a treatment can be offered by physicians but cannot be instituted without patient consent.

37. **The correct answer is C.** A blood pressure in the upper extremity significantly greater than in the lower extremity, a weak to nonexistent femoral pulse, and rib notching on chest x-ray are all consistent with postductal coarctation of the aorta. This condition is associated with a high risk of bacterial endocarditis and cerebral hemorrhage. Postductal coarctation is caused by an abnormal constriction of the aorta distal to the ductus arteriosus during fetal development.

Answer A is incorrect. Acute lymphocytic leukemia is associated with Down's syndrome, which is also associated with an increased risk of an atrial septal defect. However, this is not associated with coarctation of the aorta.

Answer B is incorrect. A boot-shaped heart refers to the cardiac silhouette produced in cases of isolated right ventricular hypertrophy, classically seen in tetralogy of Fallot. While aortic coarctation may theoretically lead to right ventricular hypertrophy, it will do so only after the left ventricle has hypertrophied and thus will not produce the boot-shaped silhouette.

Answer D is incorrect. Cor pulmonale is defined as heart failure secondary to lung disease. If lung disease produces pulmonary hypertension, it will lead to right-sided failure. Since aortic coarctation is not lung disease, it cannot be associated with cor pulmonale.

Answer E is incorrect. Eisenmenger's syndrome is the secondary development of cyanosis in conditions that produce a left-to-right shunt, such as ventricular septal defects. The increased blood flow in the pulmonary circulation leads to pulmonary hypertension, which raises the pressure on the right side of the heart, eventually reversing the shunt. Because blood is now shunted right to left, avoiding the pulmonary circulation, cyanosis develops. Aortic coarctation does not produce a left-to-right shunt and thus does not lead to Eisenmenger's syndrome.

38. **The correct answer is A.** Aortic aneurysms (both abdominal and thoracic) are sequelae of Ehlers–Danlos syndrome, a group of disorders characterized by joint hypermobility, skin hyperelasticity, easy bruising, and tissue weakness. The disorders can be traced to a genetic defect in collagen, which results in the observed joint laxity and poor tissue integrity.

Answer B is incorrect. Elastin is another structural protein found in the body. While collagen provides structural rigidity to the tissues, elastin allows them to distend and recoil. A defect in elastin synthesis might be observed as an increase in tissue rigidity as opposed to an increase in elasticity, as observed in this patient.

Answer C is incorrect. Fibrillin is a glycoprotein that forms a sheath around elastin to facilitate its normal function. Mutations in fibrillin lead to Marfan's syndrome. Although hyperflexible joints can be seen in patients with Marfan's syndrome the skin findings here are not consistent with this syndrome. Cardinal signs include ectopia lentis, arachnodactyly, and scoliosis. Aortic dissection is a possible complication of Marfan's syndrome.

Answer D is incorrect. Keratin is a structural protein found in hair, nails, and skin. However, it is not a component of arterial walls and is not implicated in Ehlers–Danlos syndrome.

Answer E is incorrect. Myosin is a component of skeletal, cardiac, and smooth muscle. It interacts with actin to produce muscle contraction but is not implicated in Ehlers–Danlos syndrome.

39. **The correct answer is E.** The first-line therapy for treating severe nausea and vomiting due to chemotherapy is ondansetron. It is the strongest available antiemetic, surpassing more common agents, such as metoclopramide, in its ability to decrease symptoms. The mechanism of action of ondansetron is blockade of serotonin 5-HT$_3$ receptors. Adverse effects of ondansetron are headache and constipation.

Answer A is incorrect. Anticholinergic drugs include atropine, benztropine, scopolamine, and ipratropium. These drugs decrease parasympathetic activity by blocking muscarinic receptors. Scopolamine is commonly used to treat motion sickness but would not be the first-line therapy for chemotherapy-induced nausea and vomiting.

Answer B is incorrect. Dopamine agonists include bromocriptine, L-dopa, pramipexole, and amantadine. These drugs are mainly used for the treatment of Parkinson's disease and are not indicated for nausea and vomiting.

Answer C is incorrect. Tricyclic antidepressants such as imipramine and amitriptyline act by inhibiting presynaptic reuptake of norepinephrine, thus augmenting their effect on postsynaptic receptors. These drugs are primarily used to treat depression. Their adverse effects include sedation, α-blocking effects, and anticholinergic properties.

Answer D is incorrect. Serotonin agonists include selective serotonin reuptake inhibitors such as paroxe tine and sertraline, which are antidepressants.

40. **The correct answer is D.** The vignette describes a patient with rickets, the clinical syndrome that results from vitamin D deficiency. Hallmarks of this condition include a broad-based waddling gait, bending of long weight-bearing bones on radiographs, and hypocalcemia with low to normal serum phosphate and elevated alkaline serum phosphatase activity. Vitamin D functions in its active form, 1,25-dihydroxycholecalciferol, to increase intestinal absorption of calcium and phosphate. A deficiency in this nutrient will result in a deficiency in intestinal calcium and phosphate absorption.

Answer A is incorrect. A deficit in serum alkaline phosphatase degradation would result in increased alkaline serum phosphatase activity with hypercalcemia and hyperphosphatemia as a consequence. This is not consistent with the clinical manifestations of vitamin D deficiency described in this vignette.

Answer B is incorrect. A deficit in the demineralization of bone would result in brittle bones with an increased frequency of fractures, which is inconsistent with the syndrome described in the vignette.

Answer C is incorrect. A deficiency in the hydroxylation of proline and lysine in collagen synthesis is typically a result of ascorbic acid, or vitamin C, deficiency. This usually results in the clinical syndrome known as scurvy, which is not consistent with this clinical scenario.

Answer E is incorrect. Although this patient does have vitamin D deficiency, vitamin D is not important in renal absorption of calcium and phosphate. A deficiency in this process is typically the result of renal failure.

41. **The correct answer is C.** Since air is filling up the space previously occupied by the lung, there will be hyperresonance on percussion on the side of the lesion.

Answer A is incorrect. Primary pneumothorax presents with unilateral chest expansion, indicating that one side is not being filled with air during inspiration.

Answer B is incorrect. Lobar pneumonia may have bronchial breath sounds over the lesion, while pneumothorax will have decreased breath sounds over the lesion.

Answer D is incorrect. Lobar pneumonia would present with increased tactile fremitus, while pneumothorax will have absent tactile fremitus.

Answer E is incorrect. Tension pneumothorax will have tracheal deviation away from the side with the lesion. Spontaneous pneumothorax will often deviate toward side of the lesion.

42. **The correct answer is B.** F2 is most likely the father of this child. The child could have received the 9-kb fragment from the mother (M) and the 6-kb fragment from F2.

Answer A is incorrect. F1 is unlikely to be the father of this child. The child could have received the 6-kb fragment from his mother (M), but he could not have received the 9-kb fragment from either the mother or F1.

Answer C is incorrect. F3 is unlikely to be the father of this child. The child could have received the 6-kb fragment from his mother (M), but he could not have received the 9-kb fragment from either the mother or F3.

Answer D is incorrect. F4 is unlikely to be the father of this child. The child could have received the 6-kb fragment from his mother (M), but he could not have received the 9-kb fragment from either the mother or F4.

43. **The correct answer is D.** Rotavirus and Coltivirus are two types of reoviruses. They have icosahedral nucleocapsids and are nonenveloped, double-stranded RNA viruses.

Answer A is incorrect. Bunyavirus and Orthomyxovirus have helical nucleocapsids and are enveloped, single-stranded, segmented RNA viruses.

Answer B is incorrect. Paramyxovirus and Morbillivirus are both from the Paramyxoviridae family. They have helical nucleocapsids and possess single-stranded, nonsegmented RNA.

Answer C is incorrect. Picornavirus and Calicivirus are single-stranded, nonsegmented RNA viruses. They have icosahedral nucleocapsids and are nonenveloped.

Answer E is incorrect. Togavirus and Flavivirus have icosahedral nucleocapsids and are enveloped with single-stranded, nonsegmented RNA.

44. **The correct answer is E.** This patient has Graves' disease, an autoimmune disorder resulting from the presence of elevated levels of thyroid-stimulating immunoglobulin (TSI), an IgG immunoglobulin that binds to and stimulates the TSH receptor of the thyroid gland. This causes an increase in the production and release of thyroid hormone. The presence of TSI is relatively specific for Graves' disease. While the exact trigger for this autoimmune response is unknown, Graves' disease is associated with the HLA-B8 subtype. The three classic findings associated with Graves' disease are hyperthyroidism, ophthalmopathy (ex-

ophthalmos), and dermopathy/pretibial myxedema (i.e., nonpitting edema on the anterior surface of both legs, with overlying skin that is dry and waxy and may have several diffuse, slightly pigmented papules). Propylthiouracil is used to treat hyperthyroidism. It works by blocking many of the steps of endogenous thyroid hormone synthesis and decreasing peripheral conversion of T_4 to tri-iodothyronine. Methimazole is another possible treatment for Graves' disease, and it acts via a similar pathway as propylthiouracil.

Answer A is incorrect. Levothyroxine, a synthetic thyroxine analog, is not indicated for Graves' disease. Please note that this drug is indicated for certain cases of hypothyroidism.

Answer B is incorrect. Mercaptopurine, an adenine analog that functions as an immunosuppressant/antineoplastic drug, is not indicated for Graves' disease.

Answer C is incorrect. Procainamide, a class IA antiarrhythmic drug commonly used for ventricular arrhythmias, is not indicated for Graves' disease.

Answer D is incorrect. Propofol, a hypnotic agent used for anesthesia and sedation, is not indicated for Graves' disease.

45. **The correct answer is E.** Adult beriberi is classified as dry or wet. Dry beriberi includes the described polyneuritis while wet beriberi includes the polyneuritis plus cardiomegaly, cardiomyopathy, peripheral edema, and ultimately high-output cardiac failure. Infant beriberi manifests as tachycardia, vomiting, seizures, and death. Beriberi was first described in Chinese medical texts used where the diet of thiamine-deficient rice was the culprit.

Answer A is incorrect. Chronic infection is not a direct manifestation of vitamin B_1 deficiency.

Answer B is incorrect. Convulsions and hyperirritability are symptoms of vitamin B_6 deficiency. The additional symptom of jaundice suggests alcohol abuse and withdrawal, but the three are not seen in isolated thiamine deficiency.

Answer C is incorrect. While dry skin and disordered thought can also be seen in adult beriberi, diarrhea, dermatitis, and dementia are the triad associated with vitamin B_3 deficiency, called pellagra. It is worth noting that Wernicke–Korsakoff syndrome is associated with thiamine deficiency in malnourished alcoholics.

Answer D is incorrect. Kidney failure is not associated with vitamin B_1 deficiency.

46. **The correct answer is C.** This patient has peptic ulcer disease (PUD), which presents as a burning epigastric pain worsened by eating. Bleeding from the ulcer may lead to black, tarry stools and abnormal findings on a complete blood cell count indicating anemia. The gold standard for diagnosis is endoscopy. Benign lesions are flat and have smooth borders, unlike malignant lesions, which may protrude into the lumen and have irregular borders. *H. pylori* infection is a major cause of PUD; >70% of patients with PUD have concurrent *H. pylori* infection.

Answer A is incorrect. Although the use of nonsteroidal anti-inflammatory drugs is a risk factor associated with PUD, celecoxib spares cyclooxygenase isoform 1 found in gastric mucosa. Thus celecoxib use is not a risk factor for PUD.

Answer B is incorrect. Diabetes is not a risk factor for PUD.

Answer D is incorrect. Hypertension is not associated with PUD.

Answer E is incorrect. In the past, PUD was attributed to stress. It was not until the discovery of the relationship between *H. pylori* infection and PUD that the theory of stress inducing PUD was dispelled.

47. **The correct answer is C.** The patient is suffering from hyperparathyroidism secondary to renal disease, also known as renal osteodystrophy. As the glomerular filtration rate (GFR) decreases, excretion of phosphate also decreases, leading to hyperphosphatemia. This in turn causes an increase in parathyroid hormone

(PTH) secretion, leading to secondary hyperphosphatemia and a decrease in blood calcium levels (and seen as a positive Chvostek's sign, in which tapping on the cheek causes facial muscle spasm). Additionally, conversion of vitamin D to its active form is impaired in patients with renal disease. As a result, calcium absorption from the gut is decreased, which then further increases levels of PTH. The patient's lab findings, therefore, reflect an increased PTH, a decreased serum calcium level, and an increased phosphate level. The increase in PTH activates osteoclasts, leading to bone resorption and increased levels of alkaline phosphatase.

Answer A is incorrect. Patients with renal disease have decreased serum calcium levels secondary to impaired activation of vitamin D to $1,25(OH)_2D_3$. Lack of biologically active vitamin D results in decreased absorption of calcium from the gastrointestinal tract. Thus, these lab values would not be consistent with this patient.

Answer B is incorrect. This set of lab values is characteristic of a patient with primary hyperparathyroidism. The major difference between the lab results for a patient with primary versus secondary hyperparathyroidism is the relationship between PTH and serum calcium. Patients with primary hyperparathyroidism will have a resultant increase in serum calcium levels, while those with secondary hyperparathyroidism have a decreased serum calcium level, which then leads to the increase in PTH.

Answer D is incorrect. Increased levels of PTH in patients with secondary hyperparathyroidism leads to osteoclast activation, increased bone resorption, and an increase in alkaline phosphatase.

Answer E is incorrect. Patients with renal disease have increased, not decreased, levels of phosphate.

48. **The correct answer is A.** The two most important points in this question are that the patient is a nonsmoker and that the lesion is located peripherally (subpleural mass). Lung cancers are typically divided into two types: small-cell lung cancers and non-small-cell lung cancer consisting of adenocarcinoma, squamous cell carcinomas, and other histologic types. These two types are treated with different chemotherapy regimens. The most common lung cancer subtype in nonsmokers and women in general (independent of smoking status) is adenocarcinoma. Adenocarcinomas are peripherally located and are more amenable to (possibly curative) surgical removal than other more centrally located primary lung tumors.

Answer B is incorrect. Carcinoid tumors are found in major bronchi and may cause carcinoid syndrome (flushing due to excessive histamine release).

Answer C is incorrect. Although metastases from other organs are by far the most common malignancy found in the lung, they would likely present as multiple foci rather than a single peripheral nodule.

Answer D is incorrect. Small-cell carcinoma of the lung is an undifferentiated tumor usually in a central location. It is clearly linked to smoking and tends to be widespread at diagnosis, with frequent brain metastases. Small-cell lung cancer is often not amenable to surgical removal and is treated primarily with chemotherapy and radiation.

Answer E is incorrect. Squamous cell carcinoma of the lung often presents as a centrally located hilar mass. This lung cancer subtype is more common in men, and it is clearly linked to smoking.

Test Block 6

1. A 45-year-old man presents to his physician with occasional burning mid-epigastric pain that is ameliorated when he eats food. The patient has been experiencing this symptom intermittently for the past 5 months. A drug that inhibits which of the following receptors would be helpful in treating this patient's symptoms?

(A) α_1
(B) β_1
(C) β_2
(D) Histamine$_1$
(E) Histamine$_2$

2. A 24-year-old man presents to the emergency department with nausea, vomiting, low-grade fever, and crampy abdominal pain that has gotten progressively worse over the past 12 hours. He is otherwise healthy except for a 6-month history of a previously nonpainful, reducible bulge in his right groin that worsened with lifting. The physician diagnoses a strangulated indirect hernia with resulting bowel obstruction and necrosis. Which of the following is the underlying cause of this type of hernia?

(A) Congenital defect in diaphragmatic membrane
(B) Enlarged external inguinal ring
(C) Enlarged femoral ring
(D) Patent processus vaginalis
(E) Weak abdominal wall musculature

3. A 42-year-old man comes to the physician because of a 2-day history of a low-grade fever. He also says that he has been feeling weak and tired recently. He says that he went to the dentist last week, but did not complete the course of prophylactic medication prescribed by his doctor prior to the dentist appointment. His physical examination is unremarkable except for a grade III/VI blowing systolic murmur heard best at the apex. His laboratory findings are significant for a mild anemia. Which of the following is most likely responsible for this man's condition?

(A) *Clostridium difficile*
(B) *Staphylococcus aureus*
(C) *Staphylococcus epidermidis*
(D) *Streptococcus mutans*
(E) *Streptococcus pneumoniae*

4. A 70-year-old African-American man with a 50-pack-year history of smoking comes in complaining of shortness of breath. While sitting, the patient is leaning forward and breathing with his lips pursed. Auscultation of his lungs reveals decreased breath sounds. Which of the following statements describes the type of gas exchange occurring in his condition?

(A) It is illustrated by CO and O_2 under healthy, resting conditions
(B) It is illustrated by N_2O and CO_2 concentrations in the blood during strenuous exercise and at rest
(C) It is only increased by an increase in blood flow
(D) It is present when there is a decreased surface area for gas exchange
(E) It is when oxygen equilibrates early along the length of the pulmonary capillary
(F) It is when the gas partial pressure of alveolar air and pulmonary capillary blood equalizes

5. A 60-year-old man with recurrent bacterial sepsis is hospitalized in order to receive intravenous antibiotics. He is started on his fourth course of broad-spectrum antibiotics within the past month. Three days into the admission, his nurse notes that his venous access is oozing blood. Laboratory tests reveal a prolonged prothrombin time, a prolonged partial thromboplastin time, and a normal platelet count. Which of the following coagulation cofactors would most likely be deficient first in this patient?

(A) Factor II
(B) Factor V
(C) Factor VII
(D) Factor VIII
(E) Factor XI
(F) Factor XII

6. A 27-year-old man dies of acute respiratory distress syndrome 1 day after presenting to the hospital with shortness of breath and a fever of 38° C (100.4° F). On the second hospital day, he developed extreme pulmonary edema and hypotension before he died. His family says that he had recently gone hiking and caving in an area known to be heavily populated with rodents. Which of the following is the most likely cause of death?

(A) Dengue virus
(B) Ebola virus
(C) Hantavirus
(D) Marburg virus
(E) Rhabdovirus

7. A 32-year-old woman presents to her primary care physician with a 3-week history of fever, weakness, and petechiae on her abdomen. Laboratory studies show:

WBC count: 125,000/mm³
Hemoglobin: 7.8 g/dL
Hematocrit: 23.4%
Platelet count: 17,000/mm³

A peripheral blood smear is shown in the image. Which of the following is the most likely diagnosis?

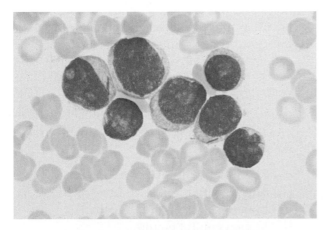

Image courtesy of Armed Forces Institute of Pathology.

(A) Acute lymphocytic leukemia
(B) Acute myelogenous leukemia
(C) Chronic myelogenous leukemia

(D) Multiple myeloma
(E) *Streptococcus pyogenes* (Group A) infection

8. Intravenous administration of drug X to an anesthetized animal produces an increase in its blood pressure. After administration of drug Y, re-administration of drug X produces a decrease in the animal's blood pressure. Which of the following pairs of drugs could produce this sequence of events?

(A) Drug X = acetylcholine;
    Drug Y = neostigmine
(B) Drug X = epinephrine;
    Drug Y = phentolamine
(C) Drug X = isoproterenol;
    Drug Y = atropine
(D) Drug X = norepinephrine;
    Drug Y = propranolol
(E) Drug X = phenylephrine;
    Drug Y = hexamethonium

9. An 82-year-old man comes to the physician because of a 3-week history of progressively worsening nonlocalizing, nonradicular low back pain that is not relieved by sitting or sleeping. He describes urinary hesitancy and a long history of benign prostatic hyperplasia that has recently worsened. He has been afebrile throughout this time. Physical examination is notable for perianal hyperesthesia with slightly decreased rectal tone, a uniformly enlarged prostate, and diminished ankle jerk reflexes bilaterally. No pain is elicited with straight leg raises in the supine position. X-ray films of the thoracic and lumbosacral spine show moderate osteoarthritis. Laboratory studies are unremarkable. Which of the following is the most likely cause of the patient's symptoms?

(A) Conus medullaris tumor
(B) Guillain-Barré syndrome
(C) L4–L5 disc herniation
(D) Spinal epidural abscess
(E) Vertebral osteomyelitis

10. A newborn girl presents to the neonatologist with an inability to swallow, coughing, choking, and vomiting when fed. Work-up reveals a tracheoesophageal fistula. Which of the following may have been present during the mother's pregnancy with this child?

   (A) Abnormal vaginal bleeding
   (B) Hematosalpinx
   (C) Oligohydramnios
   (D) Polyhydramnios
   (E) Preeclampsia

11. A 6-year-old boy with recurrent otitis media is being treated with oral antibiotics by his pediatrician. His father notices he has been bruising easily on his legs and bleeding heavily when he brushes his teeth. Examination reveals splinter hemorrhages in the fingertips. A micronutrient deficiency is suspected. Which of the following describes the correct function of the micronutrient the boy is missing?

   (A) It is required to carboxylate glutamic acid residues in inactive clotting molecules
   (B) It is required to counter exchange with sodium in a common membrane pump
   (C) It is required to hydroxylate proline residues in procollagen synthesis
   (D) It is required to maintain prothrombic antibiotic-sensitive intestinal flora
   (E) It is required to reduce anti-thrombic antibiotic breakdown intermediates

12. A 67-year-old man presents to the emergency department with diaphoresis and crushing chest pain that radiates down his left arm. An ECG shows ST-segment elevations and inverted T waves in leads V_1 through V_3. His troponin I level is high. He is taken to the cardiac catheterization unit, where he is diagnosed with an obstructive myocardial infarction. Which of the following best describes the area of myocardium supplied by the blocked artery?

   (A) Anterior wall and interventricular septum
   (B) Atrioventricular node and posterior septum
   (C) Left atrium and left ventricle
   (D) Right atrium and posterior wall
   (E) Right ventricle and apex

13. A 32-year-old man with a history of atrial fibrillation, gastroesophageal reflux disease, type 1 diabetes mellitus, and mitral valve stenosis was recently started on a new medication. He presents to the physician with easy bruising and palpable petechiae on his arms. He has been taking warfarin for 4 years without any complications. An ECG reading reveals a new arrhythmia. A coagulation panel shows the following results:

   Prothrombin time: 45 seconds
   Partial thromboplastin time: 38 seconds
   Platelet count: 300,000/mm³
   Bleeding time: 7 minutes
   D-dimer: 0.4 µg/mL (normal <0.5 µg/mL)

   Which of the following medications is most likely responsible for these symptoms?

   (A) Cimetidine
   (B) Insulin lispro
   (C) Metoprolol
   (D) NPH insulin
   (E) Omeprazole

14. A 40-year-old woman presents to the physician with a 5-year history of morning stiffness, intermittent low-grade fever, and fatigue. The morning stiffness is most pronounced in the distal joints of her arms and legs, and the pain improves throughout the day. The physician notes that there is swelling and redness of the proximal interphalangeal joints in both hands but not the distal interphalangeal joints. The patient reports that her maternal aunt and cousin both suffer from similar symptoms. Which of the following therapies, correctly paired with a possible adverse effect of treatment, is most likely to directly benefit this patient?

   (A) Abciximab; thrombocytopenia
   (B) Aldesleukin; fever
   (C) Etanercept; myelosuppression
   (D) Etanercept; tuberculosis
   (E) Infliximab; myelosuppression

15. A 25-year-old woman presents to her physician because she has been feeling fatigued. She states the fatigue has been getting progressively worse for the past 3 months and is not relieved

by sleep, although she has been averaging 12–16 hours of sleep per day over the past few months. She also complains of difficulty concentrating at work, weight loss without dieting, and reduced interest in socializing with her friends. The patient is diagnosed with a major depressive episode and given a prescription for an antidepressant. Which of the following antidepressants most strongly inhibits norepinephrine uptake?

(A) Escitalopram
(B) Fluoxetine
(C) Nortriptyline
(D) Reserpine
(E) Sertraline
(F) Trazodone

16. A 13-year-old boy is brought to the physician because of swelling and pain of his right leg. He says he first noticed these symptoms about 3 months ago, but the pain has gotten much worse over the past few weeks. An x-ray film of the leg shows a large lytic lesion with an onion-skin appearance located midway along the femur. Malignancy is suspected, and a karyotype of the biopsied bone tumor cells is ordered. Which of the following chromosomal translocations would most likely be found in the karyotype of this patient?

(A) t(8;14)
(B) t(9;22)
(C) t(11;14)
(D) t(11;22)
(E) t(14;18)
(F) t(15;17)

17. A 19-year-old woman comes to the emergency department after losing a large amount of blood in a motor vehicle collision. The patient requires large amounts of intravenous fluids, blood replacement, and medications to maintain her blood pressure. On the third day of her hospitalization, she becomes severely acidotic with a tense, tender abdomen. Bowel ischemia is suspected. Which of the following is the most likely site of infarcted bowel?

(A) Cecum
(B) Hepatic flexure, large bowel

(C) Ileum
(D) Jejunum
(E) Splenic flexure, large bowel
(F) Stomach

18. The table below shows a mutation that can be caused by a hemoglobinopathy. This is an example of which type of mutation?

mRNA transcript of normal gene	UCU UCA CGU
mRNA transcript of mutation	UCU UAA

(A) Frameshift mutation
(B) Insertion mutation
(C) Missense mutation
(D) Nonsense mutation
(E) Silent mutation

19. A 35-year-old woman from Arizona comes to the physician with an x-ray film of her chest taken during a routine health insurance examination. The x-ray film shows bilateral hilar adenopathy. The patient is completely asymptomatic. Sarcoidosis is suspected. She was told that her serum levels of angiotensin-converting enzyme (ACE) were elevated. The sensitivity and specificity of using ACE levels to test for the disease in question are 80% and 50%, respectively. Assuming that sarcoidosis is highly prevalent among residents in the southwestern United States, how would the patient's place of residence affect the positive predictive value (PPV) and negative predictive value (NPV) of the test?

(A) In areas of higher prevalence, both the PPV and the NPV are higher
(B) In areas of higher prevalence, both the PPV and the NPV are lower
(C) In areas of higher prevalence, the PPV is higher and the NPV is lower
(D) In areas of higher prevalence, the PPV is lower and the NPV remains the same
(E) Regardless of the prevalence, the PPV and NPV are unchanged

20. A tall, lanky 13-year-old boy presents to the ophthalmologist with a sudden change in vision. Examination shows lens subluxation. The patient has always been tall and thin for his age, and a family history reveals that his uncle died from a ruptured aortic aneurysm. On physical examination, the patient is found to have long and slender fingers, ligament laxity, an abnormal ratio of arm length to height, and a diastolic murmur over the aortic area. Which of the following is most likely deficient in this patient?

(A) Dystrophin
(B) Elastase
(C) Fibrillin
(D) LDL cholesterol receptor
(E) Type I collagen

21. A pathologist examines a section of bronchial tissue obtained during a transbronchial biopsy performed on an individual who smokes. She notes that the bronchial lining consists of several layers of well-differentiated, organized squamous epithelia contained above the basement membrane. Which of the following terms best describes the pathologist's finding?

(A) Anaplasia
(B) Dysplasia
(C) Hyperplasia
(D) Metaplasia
(E) Neoplasia

22. A 51-year-old man with a history of Cushing's syndrome undergoes surgery for resection of an adrenal adenoma. During the operation, the patient becomes hypotensive. Despite aggressive fluid resuscitation, the patient remains hypotensive and requires therapy with intravenous pressors to maintain his blood pressure. Which of the following medications should have been administered intraoperatively to avoid this complication?

(A) Octreotide
(B) Phenylephrine
(C) Phenoxybenzamine
(D) Prednisone
(E) Vasopressin

23. Following antibiotic treatment for a respiratory infection, a 35-year-old woman experiences vaginal itching along with a vaginal discharge that has a cheese-like consistency. Her doctor explains that the "good bacteria" of the vagina have been killed, in addition to the bacteria that were causing her respiratory infection. Suppressing the normal flora made conditions favorable for the overgrowth of more virulent organisms already present in the vagina. Species from which of the following genera constitute the largest portion of the normal flora of the vagina?

(A) *Bacteroides*
(B) *Candida*
(C) *Lactobacillus*
(D) *Staphylococcus*
(E) *Trichomonas*

24. β-Thalassemia major results from a homozygous genotype that leads to complete absence of both of the β-globin chains. An intrauterine screening test has been used on 100,000 patients, 87 of whom tested positive for β-thalassemia major, with the remaining 99,913 testing negative. Of those 87 cases, seven were shown to be false positives. Ultimately, 100 of those originally screened were found to have the disease. Which of the following is the correct sensitivity of the intrauterine screening test?

(A) 8%
(B) 80%
(C) 87%
(D) 92%
(E) 99.99%

25. A 30-year-old man presents to the emergency department complaining of shortness of breath, dizziness, nausea, and vomiting. He also says that his heart feels "like it is jumping out of my chest." Two days ago, while he was out for his daily run, he passed a burning house and stopped to help the residents evacuate. He made multiple trips into the house, inhaling a lot of smoke each time. He declined medical assistance because aside from a mild cough, he felt fine at the time. Yesterday, however, he felt fatigued and stayed in bed for most of the day. His pulse is 90/min, blood pressure is

100/60 mm Hg, and respiratory rate is 22/min. He is slumped in a chair in the examination room, taking deep gasps of air. The rest of the examination is unremarkable with the exception of bright red vessels in both of his eyes. Also, there is a smell of bitter almonds on his breath. What is the mechanism of action of the toxic agent that resulted in this patient's symptoms?

(A) Direct tissue injury
(B) Increased epinephrine release
(C) Inhibition of cellular respiration
(D) Inhibition of cholinesterase
(E) Interference with DNA synthesis

26. The human leukocyte antigen (HLA)-DR4 and HLA-DR3 molecules are known to confer greater-than-average susceptibility to type 1 diabetes. In fact, epidemiologic studies suggest that a carrier of both HLA-DR4 and HLA-DR3 is 50 times more susceptible to type 1 diabetes than a noncarrier. For the pedigree shown in the image, what is the probability that the proband harbors both of these high-risk alleles (HLA-DR3 and HLA-DR4)? (Note that the two DR alleles possessed by the proband's grandparents are shown above their pedigree symbols.)

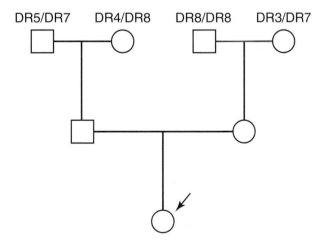

DR5/DR7   DR4/DR8   DR8/DR8   DR3/DR7

Reproduced, with permission, from USMLERx.com.

(A) 1/16
(B) 1/8
(C) 1/4

(D) 1/2
(E) 1

27. A 26-year-old woman and her husband have been trying to conceive a child for the past 14 months and have been unsuccessful. They visit the woman's obstetrician/gynecologist to learn more about their options for increasing their fertility. The physician decides to prescribe a medication for the woman that induces ovulation. Which of the following is a common adverse effect of this medication?

(A) Disturbances in color vision
(B) Nasal congestion
(C) Nausea and vomiting
(D) Vasomotor flushes
(E) Weight gain

28. An intoxicated man is found unresponsive in the woods and is brought to the emergency department. On examination, he is found to have animal bite marks on his lower left extremity. He is unable to explain how they appeared. Which of the following is the most likely recommended course of action?

(A) Administer human immune globulin immediately, and follow-up with injections of killed virus vaccine only if the patient develops symptoms
(B) Administer human immune globulin immediately, and give a series of five injections of killed virus vaccine
(C) Administer human immune globulin in a series of five doses
(D) Administer killed virus vaccine immediately, and follow-up with injections of human virus vaccine only if the patient develops symptoms
(E) Administer killed virus vaccine immediately, and give a series of five injections of human immune globulin
(F) Do nothing

29. An 82-year-old woman presents to the emergency department with a 3-week history of fever, weight loss, and malaise in the setting of hip and shoulder girdle pain that is most severe in the morning. She also reports a 1-week history of headaches and left-sided jaw pain that occurs at every meal. The patient's temperature is 38.2° C (100.8° F), her pulse is 104/min, and her blood pressure is 140/80 mm Hg. Laboratory studies show a hemoglobin level of 11.8 g/dL, a WBC count of 11,900/mm³, and an erythrocyte sedimentation rate of 121 mm/h. Physical examination is unremarkable except for moderate synovitis of the ankles and wrist. Which of the following procedures is most likely to be diagnostic in this patient?

(A) Arthrocentesis
(B) Mesenteric angiogram
(C) Temporal artery biopsy
(D) Testing for anti-double-stranded DNA and antinuclear antibody levels
(E) Testing for rheumatoid factor and anti-cytidine cyclic phosphate levels

30. A patient with a known allergy to sulfa drugs presents to the emergency department with severe shortness of breath and rapid, shallow breathing. A pulmonary examination reveals bilateral crackles halfway up from the bases, and x-ray film of the chest shows pulmonary vascular redistribution and bilateral interstitial markings. The attending physician chooses to treat the patient with a high dose of a diuretic agent. Subsequently, the patient develops muscle weakness and difficulty hearing his wife's voice. Which of the following diuretics is this patient most likely taking?

(A) Acetazolamide
(B) Ethacrynic acid
(C) Furosemide
(D) Hydrochlorothiazide
(E) Spironolactone

31. A 65-year-old previously healthy man comes to the physician with a high temperature, neck stiffness, nausea, and vomiting. He is lethargic and shows definite signs of mental status changes. Physical examination shows a positive Kernig's sign. The patient notes that he has just returned from a business trip in a town located on the Mississippi River. Which of the following would most likely be found on lumbar puncture?

Choice	Opening Pressure	Protein Level	Glucose Level	Cells
A	↓	↓	↑	↑ poymorphonuclear leukocytes and lymphocytes
B	Normal	Normal	Normal	↑ lymphocytes
C	↑	No charge	No charge	↑ RBCs
D	↑	↑	↓	↑ lymphocytes
E	↑	↑	↓	↑ polymorphonuclear leukocytes

(A) A
(B) B
(C) C
(D) D
(E) E

32. The hemoglobin tetramer is composed of two identical dimers, αβ1 and αβ2. The dimers, which are held together by polar bonds, are able to move with respect to each other to assume either a taut or a relaxed form of the hemoglobin tetramer. An experimenter is attempting to isolate hemoglobin in its taut form. Where in the body would one find the highest concentration of the taut form of hemoglobin?

(A) Alveolar capillaries
(B) Coronary arteries
(C) Femoral arteries
(D) Peripheral capillaries
(E) Pulmonary veins

33. A 60-year-old man comes to the physician because of persistent headaches and increased clumsiness; he cites repeated collisions into

door frames. He says that he has experienced decreased libido and impotence over the same period. Which of the following is most likely on physical examination of this patient?

(A) Bitemporal hemianopsia
(B) Dysphagia
(C) Hydrocephalus
(D) Right facial droop
(E) Right hand weakness

34. A 39-year-old man who is treated for schizophrenia begins to experience muscular rigidity, decreased perspiration, hyperthermia, and signs of autonomic instability. Which of the following drugs should be administered to the patient immediately?

(A) Dantrolene
(B) Diazepam
(C) Flumazenil
(D) Haloperidol
(E) Phenobarbital

35. The mother of a 3-year-old boy is referred to genetic counseling after her son is diagnosed with an enzyme deficiency. Recently, the mother noticed that her son has an abnormal facial appearance as well as pearly papular skin lesions over the scapulae and on the lateral upper arms and thighs, however, his corneas are clear bilaterally. She has also noticed that her son is hyperactive compared to other children of the same age. This patient carries a diagnosis of which of the following syndromes?

(A) Hunter's syndrome
(B) Hurler's syndrome
(C) Morquio's syndrome
(D) Sanfilippo's syndrome
(E) Sly syndrome

36. A 31-year-old man comes to the physician with a 5-day history of shortness of breath. The patient says that he also has had a nonproductive cough in the same time period. X-ray film of the chest reveals bilateral diffuse infiltrates, and laboratory results show a WBC count of 2500/mm3. An enzyme-linked immunosorbent assay is positive for HIV infec-

tion, and methenamine silver stain shows the causative organism. The patient is started on sulfamethoxazole-trimethoprim. Which of the following is the mechanism of action of the antibiotic used to treat this patient's infection?

(A) Blockade of cell wall synthesis through inhibition of transpeptidase
(B) Blockade of ergosterol synthesis through inhibition of 14-demethylase
(C) Blockade of the pathway that utilizes pteridine and PABA in nucleotide formation
(D) Inhibition of the 50S ribosomal subunit and subsequent protein chain elongation
(E) Inhibition of the 30S ribosomal subunit, which halts protein synthesis

37. A 30-year-old male drug user with a history of methylphenyltetrahydropyridine (MTPT) exposure presents to the clinic with a tremor at rest, cogwheel rigidity, and postural instability. Direct innervation from the site of the lesion to which nuclei has been damaged?

(A) Caudate and putamen (striatum)
(B) Globus pallidus externus
(C) Globus pallidus internus
(D) Lateral geniculate nucleus
(E) Subthalamic nucleus

38. A 59-year-old man with type 2 diabetes presents to the emergency department with nausea, vomiting, and abdominal pain. On examination his blood pressure is 130/93 mm Hg, respiratory rate is 32/min, arterial oxygen saturation is 99%, and pH is 7.28; he is disoriented to time and place. Laboratory tests show:

Na^+: 138 mEq/L
K^+: 4.2 mEq/L
Cl^-: 103 mEq/L
HCO_3^-: 8 mEq/L
Blood urea nitrogen: 25 mg/dL
Creatinine: 2.0 mg/dL

Which of the following medications has this patient most likely been taking?

(A) Acarbose
(B) Metformin
(C) Miglitol
(D) Tolbutamide
(E) Troglitazone

39. An outbreak of infection in Ghana has nearly wiped out an entire village. A group of scientists travels to Ghana to determine the cause of this disease. As a result of their work, they discover that a new toxin-producing bacterium caused the outbreak. The toxin appears to inhibit the Na^+-K^+-ATPase pump. Which of the following compounds has a mechanism of action similar to that of the newly isolated toxin?

(A) Albuterol
(B) Botulinum toxin
(C) Cocaine
(D) Ouabain
(E) Procainamide

40. Mr. Smith is a 66-year-old man who was diagnosed with diabetes mellitus 15 years ago. Over the past 3 years his serum creatinine levels have increased from 1.3 to 2.2 mg/dL. In an effort to slow diabetes-induced damage to his kidneys, he was started on an ACE inhibitor 2 years ago, without much change in his nephropathy. His most recent laboratory tests show:

K^+: 5.5 mEq/L
Na^+: 140 mEq/L
HCO_3^-: 18 mEq/L

Cl^-: 110 mEq/L
Arterial blood pH: 7.33
Partial carbon dioxide pressure: 40 mm Hg
Urine pH: 5.2

Which of the following conditions does this patient most likely have?

(A) Anion-gap metabolic acidosis
(B) Hyperreninemic hyperaldosteronism
(C) Type I renal tubular acidosis
(D) Type II renal tubular acidosis
(E) Type IV renal tubular acidosis

41. A pregnant woman comes to the physician for a check-up before the beginning of her third trimester. It is learned that she has been exposed to an infectious disease. Fortunately, the infections disease caused no morbidity to the fetus, and the resulting pregnancy is uncomplicated. The woman later gives birth to a healthy child. To which of the following pathogens was the woman most likely exposed?

(A) Cytomegalovirus
(B) Epstein-Barr virus
(C) Herpes simplex virus
(D) HIV
(E) Rubella
(F) Syphilis
(G) Toxoplasmosis

42. Carcinoma in situ (CIS) refers to neoplastic cells that have not yet invaded the basement membrane. In many cases, CIS can be surgically removed, providing curative treatment. An invasive carcinoma occurs when a CIS invades through the basement membrane. The aberrant expression of what factor could allow the neoplastic cells to invade through the basement membrane?

(A) Collagenase
(B) α-Fetoprotein
(C) γ-Glutamyl transpeptidase
(D) Keratin
(E) Mucin

43. A 41-year-old man comes to the physician complaining of crampy, bloating abdominal discomfort. He also reports changes in his

bowel habits and recently noticed dark stool. His father, sister, and uncle all died of colorectal cancer. At the physician's office, a fecal occult blood test is positive. A colonoscopy is performed and reveals 15–20 polyps in the distal colon. Which of the following is the most likely cause of these findings?

(A) A defect in base excision repair
(B) A defect in mismatch repair
(C) A translocation between chromosomes 15 and 17
(D) Exposure to benzo(a)pyrene
(E) The bcr-abl hybrid gene

44. A 75-year-old man comes to the physician because he recently began experiencing seizures. A CT scan shows an irregular ring-enhancing lesion with central necrosis. A biopsy taken from a mass in one of his cerebral hemispheres is shown in the image. Which of the following is the most likely diagnosis?

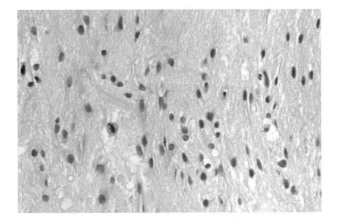

Reproduced, with permission, from PEIR Digital Library (http://peir.net).

(A) Glioblastoma multiforme
(B) Medulloblastoma
(C) Meningioma
(D) Neurilemmoma
(E) Oligodendroglioma

45. A 19-year-old college student developed sore throat, palatal petechiae, splenomegaly, fever, and generalized lymphadenopathy after she began dating her first serious boyfriend. The symptoms were self-limiting and lasted approximately 2–3 weeks. Upon presentation at the campus health clinic, a blood sample tests positive for heterophil antibodies and she is diagnosed with symptomatic primary Epstein-Barr virus (EBV) infection. Which of the following innate immune cell types plays a direct and important role in controlling the early stages of the systemic response to EBV infection?

(A) Eosinophils
(B) Mast cells
(C) Megakaryocytes
(D) Microglia
(E) Natural killer cells
(F) Plasma cells
(G) Regulatory T lymphocytes

46. A 4-month-old girl who was born full-term presents to her pediatrician with an upper respiratory infection. Her mother notes that this is the fifth time her daughter has had an upper respiratory infection since birth. Her past medical history is significant for seizures shortly after birth. In addition to pulmonary findings, the physical examination is notable for oropharyngeal candidiasis that the patient's mother says has been occurring regularly. This child is presenting with a syndrome that is due to aberrant development of which of the following embryonic structures?

(A) First and second aortic arches
(B) First and second branchial arches
(C) Fourth and sixth pharyngeal arches
(D) Second and third branchial clefts
(E) Third and fourth branchial pouches

47. A major problem in hospitals is the risk of needle sticks and the accidental transmission of hepatitis C, hepatitis B, and HIV to health care personnel. Although different circumstances can make the likelihood of infection higher or lower, it is well known that the chance of infection transmission from a needle is not the same for each of these diseases. From greatest chance of infection to least, which of the following is the order of infection among these three diseases?

(A) Hepatitis B, hepatitis C, HIV
(B) Hepatitis C, hepatitis B, HIV
(C) Hepatitis B, HIV, hepatitis C
(D) Hepatitis C, HIV, hepatitis B
(E) HIV, hepatitis B, hepatitis C

48. Four inhaled anesthetics (drugs A-D) have the properties indicated in the chart. Which of the following statements best describes the properties of these drugs?

	MINIMUM ALVEOLAR CONCENTRATION	BLOOD SOLUBILITY
Drug A	7.3	0.5
Drug B	3.1	1.0
Drug C	2.0	0.1
Drug D	4.4	0.15

(A) Drug A is more potent than drug D
(B) Drug B is less soluble in blood than drug C
(C) Drug C will have both the highest potency and the most rapid induction
(D) Drug D will induce anesthesia more rapidly than drug C
(E) Patients treated with drug B will recover more quickly from anesthesia than drug A

1. **The correct answer is E.** This patient's symptoms are consistent with those of a duodenal ulcer. A duodenal ulcer can be caused by hypersecretion of stomach acid, *Helicobacter pylori* infection, or use of nonsteroidal anti-inflammatory drugs. The initial treatment of a duodenal ulcer involves a trial of a histamine$_2$ blocker such as cimetidine. Activation of histamine$_2$ receptors leads to increased gastric acid production. Thus, by inhibiting the histamine$_2$ receptor, gastric acid secretion is decreased, allowing the ulcer to heal. Other treatments for ulcers involve inhibiting the H^+-K^+-ATPase pumps on parietal cells (using proton pump inhibitors such as omeprazole) or neutralizing stomach acid (using antacids). If a biopsy of the ulcer is positive for *H. pylori*, then the patient should be treated with a triple regimen of bismuth, metronidazole, and either amoxicillin or tetracycline.

Answer A is incorrect. Activation of α_1 receptors results in vasoconstriction and increased blood pressure. α_1 Receptors are typically found in blood vessel walls and are not involved in the production of gastric acid. Thus, inhibition of these receptors would result in vasodilation and decreased blood pressure.

Answer B is incorrect. Activation of β_1 receptors leads to inotropy (increased contractility) and chronotropy (increased heart rate). β_1 Receptors are typically located in the heart. Inhibition of the receptors would thus lead to decreased contractility and decreased heart rate.

Answer C is incorrect. Activation of β_2 receptors located in blood vessel walls and respiratory epithelium leads to vasodilation and bronchodilation, respectively. Thus, inhibition of the receptors would lead to vasoconstriction and bronchoconstriction.

Answer D is incorrect. Activation of histamine$_1$ receptors results in pruritus, bronchoconstriction, and increased nasal and bronchial mucus production. Thus, inhibition of the receptors results in inhibition of histamine release, decreased itchiness and mucous production.

2. **The correct answer is D.** Indirect inguinal hernias are the most common type of hernia and are the result of a congenital defect of the processus vaginalis. If the processus vaginalis remains patent, this provides a potential space through the internal inguinal ring for abdominal contents to herniate. In autopsy specimens, up to 20% of men have some degree of patency of their processus vaginalis, so other factors contribute to the development of an indirect hernia. One factor is increased abdominal pressure (from lifting heavy objects, chronic cough, or constipation) that can force intestine into this space. Potential complications of any hernia include strangulation and infarction of bowel, as has occurred in this case.

Answer A is incorrect. A congenital defect in the development of the pleuroperitoneal membranes of the diaphragm would lead to a hiatal hernia, which is characterized by the esophageal-gastric junction pulling upward through the diaphragm into the thorax. A classic sign for this is the hourglass sign on abdominal radiographs.

Answer B is incorrect. An enlarged external inguinal ring can be seen in hernias but is not the cause of a hernia. The external ring is a superficial structure that is separated from the intestines by the thick abdominal wall. Abdominal contents must first penetrate the abdominal wall or enter the internal ring before reaching the external ring.

Answer C is incorrect. An enlarged femoral ring may predispose people to the development of a femoral hernia, which is characterized by abdominal contents entering the femoral sheath at the femoral canal.

Answer E is incorrect. A weakness in the abdominal wall musculature can lead to a direct inguinal hernia, where abdominal contents protrude directly through the abdominal wall. Direct hernias are often seen in Hesselbach's triangle, which is the area bound by the inguinal ligament, the inferior epigastric vessels, and the lateral border of the rectus abdominis muscle. Both direct and indirect hernias can exit through the external ring and enter the scrotum. The distinction between these two types of hernias lies in whether the abdominal contents enter the internal ring (indirect) or not (direct).

3. **The correct answer is D.** *Streptococcus mutans* is a viridans group streptococcus. Members of this group of bacteria are known to cause subacute bacterial endocarditis. After the bacteria gain entry into the bloodstream, they seed the surface of a previously damaged heart valve. The bacteria slowly pile up and cause the slow development of low-grade fevers, fatigue, anemia, and a new heart murmur. This patient most likely had his mitral valve damaged by rheumatic fever, for which his doctor prescribed antibiotic prophylaxis before his dental procedure.

Answer A is incorrect. *Clostridium difficile* causes severe nonbloody diarrhea associated with pseudomembranes. It is associated with previous antibiotic treatment. It does not cause bacteremia and, consequently, is virtually unknown as a cause of endocarditis.

Answer B is incorrect. *Staphylococcus aureus* causes acute bacterial endocarditis, which manifests as acute onset of high fever, other flu-like symptoms, new-onset murmur, and petechiae. *S. aureus* is a common cause of right-sided endocarditis, which is associated with intravenous drug abuse.

Answer C is incorrect. *Staphylococcus epidermidis*, a common skin flora, most commonly causes endocarditis on prosthetic heart valves or right-sided valves in intravenous drug users..

Answer E is incorrect. *Streptococcus pneumoniae* is a rare cause of bacterial endocarditis in the post-antibiotic era.

4. **The correct answer is D.** Emphysema is an obstructive lung disease in which alveoli are destroyed. This decreases surface area for gas exchange, and illustrates diffusion-limited exchange.

Answer A is incorrect. Diffusion-limited exchange is illustrated by CO and O_2 during strenuous exercise.

Answer B is incorrect. N_2O and CO_2 under strenuous conditions are not illustrative of diffusion-limited exchange.

Answer C is incorrect. Diffusion-limited exchange is not related to blood flow, it is related to the borders of gas exchange (type I pneumocytes, basement membrane, and capillary endothelial cells).

Answer E is incorrect. Oxygen does not equilibrate by the time blood reaches the end of the capillary.

Answer F is incorrect. Gas partial pressure difference is maintained between alveolar air and pulmonary capillary blood.

5. **The correct answer is C.** Vitamin K is synthesized by the intestinal flora; therefore long-term treatment with broad-spectrum antibiotics can induce a vitamin K deficiency by clearing intestinal flora. Vitamin K is a necessary cofactor for hepatic production of clotting factors II, VII, IX, and X and proteins C and S. Factor VII has the shortest half-life of all clotting factors (4–6 hours), which is why the prothrombin time is prolonged first in vitamin K deficiency.

Answer A is incorrect. Factor II requires vitamin K as a cofactor, and early factor II deficiency would result in prolongation of prothrombin time and partial thromboplastin time. However, the half-life of factor II is 42–72 hours, and thus it would not be deficient before factor VII is deficient.

Answer B is incorrect. Vitamin K is not required for factor V synthesis and would not be deficient in this patient.

Answer D is incorrect. Factor VIII is not a vitamin K dependent clotting factor.

Answer E is incorrect. Factor XI is not a vitamin K dependent clotting factor.

Answer F is incorrect. Factor XII is not a vitamin K dependent clotting factor.

6. **The correct answer is C.** Hantavirus pulmonary syndrome is a rare viral cause of acute respiratory distress syndrome. Hantavirus is a Bunyavirus that has been found in rodents throughout the United States. It is thought to be transmitted via rodent droppings and saliva.

Answer A is incorrect. Dengue virus is an *Aedes* mosquito-transmitted virus that causes a hemorrhagic fever. It is found in tropical regions of Asia and has spread to South and Central America. Patients present with rash and bleeding from mucous membranes.

Answer B is incorrect. Ebola virus and Marburg virus are members of the *Filovirus* genus, which cause hemorrhagic fever. Both are found only in central and southern Africa. They have an animal reservoir that has not been found. Treatment is supportive, and symptoms include massive hemorrhage from the mucous membranes accompanied by high fevers.

Answer D is incorrect. Ebola virus and Marburg virus are members of the *Filovirus* genus, which cause hemorrhagic fever. Both are found only in central and southern Africa. They have an animal reservoir that has not been found. Treatment is supportive, and symptoms include massive hemorrhage from the mucous membranes accompanied by high fevers.

Answer E is incorrect. Rhabdovirus is the causative agent of rabies. It is possible to become infected with rabies from a rodent; however, the incubation period is much longer (weeks to a year), and the later stages of the disease are classically acute encephalitis.

7. **The correct answer is B.** Acute myelogenous leukemia (AML) typically presents with rapid-onset symptoms of bone marrow suppression, including anemia (weakness), thrombocytopenia (petechiae), and poor immunity (suscepti-bility to infection) in the context of leukocytosis. The peripheral blood smear demonstrates myeloblasts with Auer rods, which are present in many cases of AML, particularly acute promyelocytic leukemia (type M3).

Answer A is incorrect. Acute lymphocytic leukemia (ALL) presents with clinical symptoms that are often indistinguishable from AML. Thus, the only way to tell these two apart with the information in the question is the image, which shows myeloblasts with Auer rods. If it were ALL, the image would show lymphoblasts. Another clue to differentiating ALL from AML is the patient's age: Of course both AML and ALL can be seen in all age groups, however AML is more common in adults 15–40 years old, whereas ALL is usually seen in patients younger than 15 years. ALL is also more common in individuals with Down's syndrome (mnemonic: We **ALL** fall **DOWN**).

Answer C is incorrect. Chronic myelogenous leukemia (CML) follows a more insidious course than AML, with symptoms of bone marrow suppression developing slowly. Additionally, it presents with fewer myeloblasts and increased neutrophils, myelocytes, and metamyelocytes.

Answer D is incorrect. Multiple myeloma can present with leukocytosis, but the peripheral blood smear would not show myeloblasts with Auer rods. Renal failure and lytic lesions in the bones are also common. Additionally, it follows a more chronic progressive course.

Answer E is incorrect. *Streptococcus pyogenes* (Group A) infection can present with scarlet fever, which could produce symptoms similar to these. However, the presence of myeloblasts with Auer rods is diagnostic of AML. In addition, the WBC is not likely to be as high as in the leukemias.

8. **The correct answer is B.** Epinephrine is an agonist at α_1, α_2, β_1, and β_2 receptors; phentolamine is an antagonist at α_1 and α_2 receptors. Therefore, after the administration of phentolamine, epinephrine administration stimulates only β receptors, which results in decreased blood pressure. This is called epinephrine

reversal because epinephrine originally increased blood pressure and then produced the opposite effect after phentolamine administration.

Answer A is incorrect. Acetylcholine stimulates the non-innervated muscarinic (M_3) receptors that are located on endothelial cells of the vasculature. Stimulation of these receptors releases endothelial-derived relaxing factor (nitric oxide), which produces a relaxation of the neighboring smooth muscle cells, leading to a decrease in blood pressure. Neostigmine, an acetylcholinesterase inhibitor, would simply prolong the action of acetylcholine at its receptors and would thus indirectly cause a decrease in blood pressure.

Answer C is incorrect. This choice should be eliminated because isoproterenol, a nonspecific β agonist, decreases blood pressure by stimulation of $β_2$ receptors in the vasculature. Epinephrine, norepinephrine, and phenylephrine all increase blood pressure, so the remaining answers must be eliminated by examining the effects of drug Y on drug X.

Answer D is incorrect. Norepinephrine is an agonist at $α_1$, $α_2$, and $β_1$ receptors; propranolol is a nonselective β antagonist. After administration of propranolol, norepinephrine can stimulate only α receptors, which will still cause vasoconstriction (primarily via $α_1$ stimulation in the vasculature) and therefore increase blood pressure.

Answer E is incorrect. Phenylephrine is an $α_1$ agonist, and hexamethonium is a nicotinic ganglionic blocker. Hexamethonium administration will eliminate the baroreceptor response after the second phenylephrine administration by blocking the peripheral ganglia. However, phenylephrine will still reach the $α_1$ receptors on the vasculature to produce an increase in blood pressure.

9. **The correct answer is A.** This patient is suffering from a cord compression syndrome due to a conus medullaris tumor. These tumors are relatively uncommon and can be very difficult to diagnose because they are difficult to differentiate from tumors of the cauda equina. Pa-

tients can manifest symptoms of one or both syndromes. Night and rest pain is an immediate red flag for metastatic disease, multiple myeloma, or spinal infections. The x-ray films and normal laboratory values help to make metastatic disease or myeloma less likely. The examination is consistent with conus medullaris syndrome because of the relatively rapid, bilateral onset of moderate back pain with a minimal radicular component and preserved ankle reflexes. These patients tend to have perianal numbness and urinary retention with an atonic rectal sphincter, as opposed to the saddle anesthesia more typically found in cauda equina syndrome. This patient's presentation warrants empiric steroids and emergent MRI.

Answer B is incorrect. Guillain-Barré syndrome is a symmetrical ascending weakness that commonly follows diarrheal or flu-like illness in young adults. It is not associated with focal neurological pain and is much less common in elderly patients.

Answer C is incorrect. The physical examination largely excludes the possibility of disc herniation as a cause of the patient's symptoms because of absent positive straight leg raises and pain that is neither aggravated by activity nor relieved by resting. Furthermore, the perianal region is innervated by sacral nerve roots that would not be impinged by a disc herniation at the L4–L5 level.

Answer D is incorrect. The triad for spinal epidural abscess includes back pain, fever, and progressive weakness. This patient does not have the second two symptoms, making abscess a less likely possibility.

Answer E is incorrect. Vertebral osteomyelitis would most likely present in a patient that was suffering constitutional signs and symptoms, as opposed to the relatively focal findings presented in this case. Characteristically, a patient with osteomyelitis would have night sweats and fever. The patient would have symptoms that would point to the source of the hematogenous dissemination of the infectious agent to the spine (e.g., urinary tract infection).

10. **The correct answer is D.** A tracheoesophageal fistula (TEF) will cause polyhydramnios during pregnancy in approximately 80% of cases, as the fetus is unable to swallow amniotic fluid. The defect occurs when the lateral walls of the foregut fail to fuse after separating from the trachea. Treatment is immediate surgical repair.

Answer A is incorrect. Abnormal vaginal bleeding is a nonspecific sign but is not associated with TEF.

Answer B is incorrect. Hematosalpinx refers to bleeding into the fallopian tubes most commonly caused by an ectopic pregnancy. It is not associated with TEF in the fetus.

Answer C is incorrect. Oligohydramnios occurs when fetal urine is not produced or cannot be excreted, as in bilateral renal agenesis. There is no evidence of urinary obstruction or renal defects in this case.

Answer E is incorrect. Preeclampsia is a syndrome of hypertension, albuminuria, and edema. Its etiology is not well understood, but it is not specifically associated with TEF.

11. **The correct answer is A.** Vitamin K dependent gamma-glutamyl carboxylase converts glutamic acid residues to gamma-carboxyglutamic acid residues. Gamma-glutamyl carboxylase residues are formed in clotting factors II, VII, IX, and X, as well as protein C and S. They function to bind the calcium which is required to activate the factors. Vitamin K deficiency is rare because it is synthesized by gut flora. This patient's deficiency is probably secondary to oral antibiotic use that destroyed those organisms. Deficiency is also seen in neonates who have sterile guts and a relatively new liver. Easy bruisability, melena, hematuria, and splinter hemorrhages can be seen with vitamin K deficiency.

Answer B is incorrect. This is the function of potassium, abbreviated as K, which has nothing to do with vitamin K.

Answer C is incorrect. The hydroxylation of proline and lysine residues requires the coenzyme ascorbic acid, or vitamin C. Deficiency results in a defective connective tissue syndrome called scurvy. Vitamin C has not been shown to cure the common cold or prevent coronary heart disease. Vitamin C is a water-soluble vitamin and oral antibiotic use does not lead to its deficiency.

Answer D is incorrect. The antibiotics have resulted in a decrease in gut flora and subsequent synthesis of vitamin K. The intestinal flora themselves have no effect on blood clotting.

Answer E is incorrect. The antibiotics have resulted in a decrease in gut flora and subsequent synthesis of Vitamin K. Metabolism of antibiotics does not generate significant anti-thrombic intermediates.

12. **The correct answer is A.** The left anterior descending artery branches from the left main coronary artery as it approaches the atrioventricular junction. It descends towards the apex on the anterior wall of the heart between the right and left ventricles and supplies the anterior wall of both ventricles and most of the interventricular septum.

Answer B is incorrect. The right main coronary artery courses around to the posterior wall of the heart and supplies the atrioventricular node and posterior interventricular septum.

Answer C is incorrect. The circumflex artery branches from the left main coronary and courses superiorly-posteriorly between the left atrium and ventricle to supply both of these areas.

Answer D is incorrect. The right main coronary artery branches from the aorta near the superior vena cava and hugs the right atrium as it courses toward the posterior side of the heart. It is the main supply to the right atrium and posterior wall of the heart.

Answer E is incorrect. The right marginal artery is a branch of the right main coronary on the inferior-anterior surface of the heart and supplies the right ventricle and apex.

13. **The correct answer is A.** Cimetidine is an H_2 blocker associated with P-450 inhibition, antiandrogenic effects, decreased renal excretion of creatinine, and arrhythmias. As a result of P-450 inhibition, cimetidine decreases hepatic metabolism of many drugs oxidized by the P-450 system, including warfarin, increasing their systemic toxicities. This results in a prolonged prothrombin time.

Answer B is incorrect. Insulin lispro can cause hypoglycemia.

Answer C is incorrect. Metoprolol can be associated with decreased perception of hypoglycemia in diabetics. However, it does not affect warfarin levels.

Answer D is incorrect. NPH insulin can cause hypoglycemia or idiopathic allergic and anaphylactoid reactions.

Answer E is incorrect. Omeprazole is a proton pump inhibitor that is relatively free of adverse effects.

14. **The correct answer is D.** The patient is suffering from rheumatoid arthritis, an autoimmune disorder that targets the synovial lining of distal joints, leading to cartilage destruction, microscopic pannus formation, and eventual bony deformation. Both an antibody- and a T-lymphocyte-mediated immune response have been implicated in the pathogenesis of this disease. In particular, proinflammatory cytokines such as tumor necrosis factor (TNF)-α are believed to play an important role in the maintenance of the immune response within the joint. Etanercept is a recombinant TNF-α receptor:Fc fusion protein that binds TNF-α in vivo, thereby neutralizing its activity. Some patients respond quite well to this treatment, with both drops in subjective pain scores and objective improvements within the joints. Unfortunately, TNF-α plays a major role in the host defense response against certain pathogens, and the occurrence/reactivation of tuberculosis in some patients treated with anti-TNF therapy attests to this.

Answer A is incorrect. Abciximab is a monoclonal antibody that binds to the glycoprotein receptor IIb/IIIa on activated platelets, thus inhibiting interaction between platelets and fibrinogen. While thrombocytopenia is often a side effect of this treatment, abciximab is not an antirheumatic.

Answer B is incorrect. Aldesleukin is recombinant interleukin (IL)-2 and is used clinically as adjuvant therapy for renal cell carcinoma and metastatic melanoma. While fever is often a side effect of this treatment, it is unlikely that IL-2 therapy would benefit a patient suffering from rheumatoid arthritis (RA); thus, this is not the correct answer choice.

Answer C is incorrect. Myelosuppression is not a common side effect of etanercept treatment.

Answer E is incorrect. Infliximab is a monoclonal antibody to tumor necrosis factor-α and has shown efficacy in the treatment of RA. Like etanercept, it acts to neutralize the effect of this proinflammatory cytokine. However, myelosuppression is not a common side effect of infliximab treatment.

15. **The correct answer is C.** Nortriptyline is a tricyclic antidepressant that inhibits the reuptake of both norepinephrine and serotonin in the synaptic cleft of central nervous system (CNS) neurons. Serious adverse effects include arrhythmia, prolonged QT interval, seizures, and agranulocytosis. Anticholinergic adverse effects are common (dry mouth, urinary retention).

Answer A is incorrect. Escitalopram is a selective serotonin reuptake inhibitor and hence does not significantly affect the reuptake of norepinephrine.

Answer B is incorrect. Fluoxetine is a selective serotonin reuptake inhibitor and hence does not significantly affect the reuptake of norepinephrine.

Answer D is incorrect. Reserpine depletes catecholamines and serotonin. It can cause severe depression. It was originally developed for the treatment of hypertension.

Answer E is incorrect. Sertraline is a selective serotonin reuptake inhibitor and hence does not significantly affect the reuptake of norepinephrine.

Answer F is incorrect. Trazodone works by inhibiting serotonin reuptake and acting as a partial serotonin agonist. It is useful for the treatment of depression with insomnia. Male patients should be warned of the potential for priapism.

16. **The correct answer is D.** This is a case of Ewing's sarcoma, which can present with symptoms similar to an infection. However, the x-ray describes the classic location and appearance of the sarcoma. Ewing's sarcoma is a small blue cell tumor of childhood that arises in the medullary cavity in the diaphysis of long bones. It is most often found in boys younger than 15 years of age. The periosteal reaction results in reactive bone deposition in an onion-skin manner. The tumor cells carry the t(11;22) translocation, and this would be seen on karyotype.

Answer A is incorrect. t(8;14) is most commonly associated with Burkitt's lymphoma.

Answer B is incorrect. t(9;22), the Philadelphia chromosome, is most commonly associated with CML.

Answer C is incorrect. t(11;14) is associated with mantle cell lymphoma.

Answer E is incorrect. t(14;18) is most commonly associated with *bcl-2* activation in follicular lymphomas.

Answer F is incorrect. t(15;17) is associated with the M3 type of AML. This type is treatable by all-trans retinoic acid.

17. **The correct answer is E.** The splenic flexure of the large bowel is vulnerable to ischemia from hypoperfusion because it lies at the junction of two vascular areas, the superior and inferior mesenteric arteries. This watershed phenomenon also occurs in the brain.

Answer A is incorrect. The cecum is supplied by the superior mesenteric artery (SMA); it is not a watershed area.

Answer B is incorrect. The hepatic flexure of the large bowel is supplied by the SMA; unlike

the splenic flexure, it is not in a border zone between two vascular territories.

Answer C is incorrect. The ileum is supplied by the SMA; it is not in a watershed area.

Answer D is incorrect. The jejunum is supplies by the SMA; it is not a watershed area.

Answer F is incorrect. The stomach is richly supplied by the celiac trunk, it is not a watershed area.

18. **The correct answer is D.** A nonsense mutation occurs when a single base substitution in DNA (in this case, thymine to cytosine) results in a chain termination codon.

Answer A is incorrect. A frameshift mutation involves a deletion or insertion that is not an exact multiple of three base pairs and therefore changes the reading frame of the gene downstream of the mutation.

Answer B is incorrect. Insertion mutation is a chromosomal abnormality in which a DNA segment from one chromosome is inserted into a nonhomologous chromosome.

Answer C is incorrect. Missense mutation is a mutation that changes a codon specific for one amino acid to specify another amino acid.

Answer E is incorrect. A silent mutation produces a mutant gene that has no detectable phenotypic effect. The mutation is usually a point mutation often in the third position of the codon.

19. **The correct answer is C.** Sarcoidosis is a systemic granulomatous disease of unknown origin that particularly involves the lungs. The pathologic hallmark is the presence of noncaseating granulomas. Bilateral hilar adenopathy can be the presenting sign in asymptomatic patients with sarcoidosis. Sarcoidosis is associated with increased levels of ACE, but testing serum ACE levels does not provide a definitive diagnosis of sarcoidosis because of the relatively low specificity and sensitivity of the test. Nevertheless, for any given test, the PPV (i.e., the probability that a positive test result is truly positive for the disease one is looking for) in-

creases and the NPV (i.e., the probability that a negative test result is a truly negative for the disease one is looking for) decreases as the prevalence of the disease increases. In the United States, sarcoidosis used to be strongly associated with residence in the southeastern United States; however, recent studies have suggested that the disease may be common in other areas as well.

Answer A is incorrect. For any given test, as the prevalence of the disease increases, the PPV increases and the NPV decreases.

Answer B is incorrect. For any given test, as the prevalence of the disease increases, the PPV increases and the NPV decreases.

Answer D is incorrect. For any given test, as the prevalence of the disease increases, the PPV increases and the NPV decreases.

Answer E is incorrect. For any given test, as the prevalence of the disease increases, the PPV increases and the NPV decreases.

20. **The correct answer is C.** This patient most likely has Marfan's syndrome. Marfan's syndrome is due to a defect in the fibrillin gene, manifested by a deficiency of fibrillin (a glycoprotein constituent of microfibrils).

Answer A is incorrect. Dystrophin deficiency is seen in Becker's and Duchenne's muscular dystrophy, both of which are progressive degenerative muscular conditions. They are manifested by increasing weakness and paralysis.

Answer B is incorrect. Elastase is a neutrophil-elaborated protease that plays an important role in alveolar destruction in the lung disease emphysema. Elastase is inhibited by α_1-antitrypsin, so individuals with α_1-antitrypsin deficiency develop premature emphysema.

Answer D is incorrect. A deficient LDL cholesterol receptor manifests as familial hypercholesterolemia, which leads to accelerated atherosclerosis.

Answer E is incorrect. Mutations in one of two genes that code for proteins that combine to form type I collagen cause the skeletal disease osteogenesis imperfecta.

21. **The correct answer is D.** The pathologist has found an example of metaplasia, which is characterized by one adult cell type being replaced by another cell type. This change is reversible. Normal bronchi are lined with pseudostratified, columnar, ciliated epithelium. Squamous epithelia in the bronchi are not normal and are often a sign of environmental exposure and/or irritation (i.e., smoking).

Answer A is incorrect. Anaplasia, an irreversible change, describes abnormal cells lacking differentiation. Anaplasia is not the answer, since the squamous cells appear organized and differentiated, although they are in an abnormal location.

Answer B is incorrect. Dysplasia is abnormal growth with loss of cellular orientation, shape, and size in comparison to normal tissue maturation. Dysplasia is not the answer, since the squamous cells appear organized and differentiated, although they are in an abnormal location.

Answer C is incorrect. Hyperplasia is an increase in number of the normal cell type.

Answer E is incorrect. Neoplasia describes a clonal proliferation of cells that is uncontrolled and excessive, and in this case the growth is confined above the basement membrane. There is no sign of metastasis, nor is there a sign of uncontrolled proliferation, as there are only a few layers of squamous cells. Like anaplasia, neoplasia is not reversible.

22. **The correct answer is D.** Patients with Cushing's syndrome secondary to a hyperfunctioning adrenal adenoma suffer from symptoms secondary to excessive levels of cortisol in the blood. This results in negative feedback of the cortisol onto the anterior pituitary, leading to adrenal suppression. Such patients require exogenous cortisol to maintain hemodynamic stability in response to stresses such as surgery. Prednisone administered intraoperatively would be the most appropriate agent to prevent hemodynamic instability due to hypocortisolemia.

Answer A is incorrect. Octreotide is a somatostatin analog that can be used to inhibit secretion of growth hormone and prolactin from the anterior pituitary. It can also inhibit the secretion of gastrin, secretin, cholecystokinin, vasoactive intestinal polypeptide, insulin, glucagon, and pancreatic exocrine enzymes. Octreotide does not have any effect on adrenal cortisol secretion, nor does it have any intrinsic effect on the maintenance of hemodynamic stability.

Answer B is incorrect. Phenylephrine is an α-specific adrenergic agonist that primarily stimulates peripheral vasoconstriction, resulting in an increase in blood pressure. Like epinephrine, this agent is effective as a pressor in treating hypotension, but it is not the most appropriate selection because it does not address the primary problem of adrenal suppression.

Answer C is incorrect. Phenoxybenzamine is an α-specific adrenergic antagonist that acts primarily to cause peripheral vasodilation. Like metoprolol, this agent acts to reduce blood pressure and hence would not be appropriate in the treatment of hypotension, regardless of the cause. Phenoxybenzamine is classically indicated for the treatment of hypertension secondary to phcochromocytoma.

Answer E is incorrect. Vasopressin acts both to increase water absorption in the renal collecting duct via increased expression of aquaporin channels, and to stimulate peripheral vasoconstriction, although this latter effect is observed only at supraphysiologic concentrations. Although this agent can be used to provide blood pressure support in the treatment of septic shock, it does not address the core problem of adrenal suppression and would not be the most effective agent in this case.

23. **The correct answer is C.** Lactobacilli make up a majority of the normal flora of the vagina. The composition of the normal flora varies from premenarchal, childbearing, and menopausal stages, but a key feature of the normal vaginal environment is a low pH (3.5-4.2), which inhibits growth of other, possibly pathogenic, organisms. This pH is likely maintained by the lactobacilli, and when numbers of these bacteria are reduced during the course of anti-

biotic treatment (with, for example, tetracycline), the vaginal pH may increase, making conditions favorable for the yeast *Candida albicans* to grow. Symptoms of a yeast infection are as described, and diagnosis is made by 10% potassium hydroxide preparation on which pseudohyphae are seen.

Answer A is incorrect. *Bacteroides* is an anaerobe and a major colonizer of the colon.

Answer B is incorrect. *Candida* is the yeast that is most likely to cause the symptoms described in the stem. Although many women are colonized with *Candida* (specifically *C. albicans*), most do not experience symptoms unless conditions in the vagina change to allow overgrowth of the organism.

Answer D is incorrect. Staphylococci are not a majority of the flora in the vagina but may be found around the external vaginal opening, as staphylococci are normal skin flora.

Answer E is incorrect. *Trichomonas* is a pathogenic protozoan and is never considered normal flora. It is responsible for causing symptoms of frothy, foul-smelling discharge, along with itching and burning on urination. Motile parasites are seen on wet mount.

24. **The correct answer is B.** The screening test results were positive in 80 of the 100 patients with β-thalassemia. Sensitivity = 80 / 100 = 80%.

Answer A is incorrect. Calculation error.

Answer C is incorrect. Eighty-seven percent is the answer one would arrive at if the seven false-positives were not recognized.

Answer D is incorrect. Positive predictive value = 80 / 87 = 92%.

Answer E is incorrect. Specificity = 99,893 / 99,900 = 99.99%.

25. **The correct answer is C.** Cyanide is a very toxic compound that can be formed in the high temperature combustion of many materials such as polyurethane, acrylonitrile, nylon, wool, and cotton, thus making cyanide poisoning common in the setting of smoke inhalation. The most common cause of cyanide poi-

soning in industrialized countries is household fires. Cyanide modifies the iron within cytochrome oxidase (cytochrome aa$_3$) in the mitochondria, thereby abnormally interrupting the electron transport chain and halting cellular respiration. Tissues with the highest oxygen demands, such as the heart, brain, and liver, are most significantly affected because cyanide prevents oxygen from binding to cytochrome oxidase and serving as the final electron acceptor in the chain. On physical examination the retinal arteries and veins are bright red due to absent tissue oxygen extraction. Additionally, in some patients there is a smell of bitter almonds on their breath. These findings are not present with carbon monoxide inhalation, the other common toxin associated with smoke inhalation. Treatment includes induction of methemoglobinemia with a nitrite, then administration of a sulfate.

Answer A is incorrect. Substances such as ammonia or chlorine cause direct injury to exposed tissues. Symptoms include shortness of breath, severe throat pain, vomiting, and coughing up blood. The ocular symptoms in this patient are not characteristic of this type of poisoning.

Answer B is incorrect. While the patient's increased heart rate and tachypnea could be explained by an increase in sympathetic nervous system activity achieved by epinephrine release, this is not the mechanism of action of cyanide.

Answer D is incorrect. Sarin gas irreversibly inhibits acetylcholinesterase, resulting in an overload of acetylcholine at synapses. As a result, the body experiences a parasympathetic overload and flaccid paralysis. Symptoms of sarin poisoning depend on the degree of exposure and the form of the toxin; they resemble some of the symptoms this patient is experiencing. However, the circumstances of his injury point to an adverse effect of smoke inhalation as opposed to poisoning with a biological warfare agent.

Answer E is incorrect. Alkylating or blister agents are so called because they penetrate the skin and mucous membranes and cause large blisters to form all over the exposed person's

body. The mechanism of action is interference with DNA synthesis. However, this patient lacks the characteristic dermal symptoms.

26. **The correct answer is A.** While HLA-DR3- and/or HLA-DR4-positive individuals are at increased risk for developing type 1 diabetes, the causal nature of this association is still being researched. The DR locus is one of the class II major histocompatibility complex alleles, and therefore presents peptides to CD4$^+$ T lymphocytes. It should also be noted that carriers of the DR2 allele are less susceptible to type 1 diabetes. The answer to this question can be resolved based on genetic principles: (1) The proband's paternal grandmother and maternal grandmother carry a single copy of DR4 and DR3, respectively. The chance that the proband's father inherited the DR4 allele is 1/2. Similarly, the chance that the proband's mother inherited the DR3 allele is 1/2. (2) Since the proband's parents each have a 1/2 chance of contributing an allele to their offspring, the chance that the proband inherited DR4 from the father is 1/2 and the chance that the proband inherited DR3 from the mother is 1/2. (3) Thus, the probability of the proband inheriting the paternal grandmother's DR4 is $1/2 \times 1/2 = 1/4$, while the probability of the proband inheriting the maternal grandfather's DR3 is $1/2 \times 1/2 = 1/4$. (4) The probability that the proband inherited both of these alleles is thus, $1/4 \times 1/4 = 1/16$.

Answer B is incorrect. The probability is not 1/8, because the question is asking the chance that the proband inherits both alleles. If the question were asking the probability that the proband inherits either one of the DR3 or DR4 alleles from the grandparents, then the answer would be 1/8.

Answer C is incorrect. The probability is not 1/4.

Answer D is incorrect. The probability is not 1/2.

Answer E is incorrect. The probability is not 1.

27. **The correct answer is D.** Clomiphene acts by binding estrogen receptor sites in the hypothalamus and blocking the negative feedback of circulating estrogens. This results in increased folli-

cle-stimulating hormone and luteinizing hormone levels, which stimulate ovulation. It successfully treats women with anovulatory cycles but is not effective in women whose infertility is secondary to a pituitary abnormality. Hot flashes are a common adverse effect caused by hypoestrogenism at the hypothalamic level due to blockade of estrogen receptors. Other adverse effects of clomiphene include ovarian enlargement.

Answer A is incorrect. Disturbances in color vision are an adverse effect of sildenafil, a muscle relaxant used to treat erectile dysfunction.

Answer B is incorrect. Nasal congestion, orthostasis, nausea and headache may occur with cabergoline in the treatment of infertility due to hyperprolactinoma. Cabergoline is an ergoline derivative with potent inhibitory effects on prolactin secretion.

Answer C is incorrect. Nausea and vomiting are common adverse effects of estrogen therapy, not anti-estrogen therapy. Estrogen therapy can be used for postmenopausal hormone therapy and hypogonadism.

Answer E is incorrect. Weight gain and fluid retention are adverse effects of gonadotropins, which can be used to increase ovarian follicular maturation.

28. **The correct answer is B.** This man may have been bitten by a rabid animal. The best prophylaxis for rabies infection is immediate administration of human rabies immune globulin to provide passive immunity, followed with a series of five injections of killed rabies virus vaccinations to develop active immunity. The idea is to provide immunity while the patient is still in the incubation period.

Answer A is incorrect. If the patient develops symptoms, the disease will have progressed to an incurable stage.

Answer C is incorrect. The administration of human rabies immune globulin is not the best course of action, because it does not provide long-term active immunity.

Answer D is incorrect. If the patient develops symptoms, the disease will have progressed to an incurable stage.

Answer E is incorrect. Providing the killed rabies virus vaccine first and following with a series of human rabies immune globulin does not give immediate passive immunity and is not the standard of care.

Answer F is incorrect. Although rabies is not curable after symptoms develop, it is possible to provide immunity to a patient who has been exposed before the virus replicates enough to cause disease. Therefore, doing nothing is not the appropriate response.

29. **The correct answer is C.** This patient has symptoms consistent with polymyalgia rheumatica (PMR) and giant cell arteritis (temporal arteritis). She requires immediate steroids for treatment and subsequent temporal artery biopsy to confirm the diagnosis. PMR occurs in 50% of patients with temporal arteritis and involves symmetrical aching of the proximal muscles and girdle stiffness. The elevated erythrocyte sedimentation rate indicates a generalized inflammatory process, and additional evidence is provided by the new-onset jaw claudication and constitutional symptoms that usually present in patients with temporal arteritis.

Answer A is incorrect. Analysis of joint fluid would be neither diagnostic nor possible in this patient because she is only currently suffering from synovitis of her wrists and ankles.

Answer B is incorrect. Mesenteric angiography is the primary imaging modality used to determine the presence of aneurysms and vessel narrowing in patients with polyarteritis nodosa (PAN). PAN is a necrotizing vasculitis that typically presents with constitutional signs as well as with myalgias, arthralgias, and fatigue. This patient's girdle stiffness and jaw claudication are not consistent with this diagnosis.

Answer D is incorrect. Testing for anti-double-stranded DNA and antinuclear antibody levels would be appropriate to diagnose lupus, which is uncommon in patients this age and does not involve jaw claudication.

Answer E is incorrect. Testing for rheumatoid factor and anti-cytidine cyclic phosphate levels would be appropriate to diagnose RA, which may produce symmetrical and proximal joint symptoms. However, RA does not cause jaw claudication and does not usually present for the first time in someone this elderly.

30. **The correct answer is B.** This patient has a typical presentation of acute pulmonary edema. Common causes include myocardial ischemia, acute aortic insufficiency, acute mitral regurgitation, renovascular hypertension, or acute decompensation of chronic congestive heart failure. Loop diuretics such as furosemide are the normal treatments of choice for this condition. Ethacrynic acid is a diuretic similar in action to furosemide but without sulfa adverse effects such as rash or acute interstitial nephritis, and is therefore used in persons with a sulfa allergy. Other adverse effects, including ototoxicity, metabolic alkalosis, hypokalemia, hyperglycemia, and hyperuricemia are shared with furosemide. The patient is suffering from ototoxicity and hypokalemia, leading to the hearing and muscle disturbances, respectively.

Answer A is incorrect. Acetazolamide causes hyperchloremic metabolic acidosis and neuropathy.

Answer C is incorrect. Furosemide has an adverse event profile very similar to that of ethacrynic acid, but also causes sulfa allergy, and thus would be contraindicated in this patient.

Answer D is incorrect. Hydrochlorothiazide causes hypokalemic alkalosis, hyponatremia, hyperglycemia, hyperlipidemia, hyperuricemia, and hypercalcemia as well as sulfa allergy.

Answer E is incorrect. Spironolactone causes hyperkalemia and anti-androgen effects.

31. **The correct answer is B.** These are the expected findings for viral meningitis. St. Louis encephalitis virus, a flavivirus, is the most common cause of epidemic encephalitis in the United States and can cause meningitis. Treatment is supportive since there are no antiviral medications for this virus. It can occur throughout the United States but is more prevalent in the Mississippi-Ohio river valley. The clinical description is classic for meningitis, including a positive Kernig's sign, which is elicited by flexing the patient's leg at both the hip and knee; straightening the knee from this position elicits pain.

Answer A is incorrect. These findings are an unlikely combination in the context of meningitis.

Answer C is incorrect. These findings are consistent with a subarachnoid hemorrhage, in which case the patient would likely complain of "the worst headache of my life."

Answer D is incorrect. These findings suggest a fungal meningitis, such as due to *Cryptococcus* or *Coccidioides*. The patient's recent trip to the Mississippi River and previous healthy history should put St. Louis encephalitis virus higher on the differential diagnosis.

Answer E is incorrect. These findings suggest a bacterial meningitis, such as *Neisseria meningitidis*, *Streptococcus pneumoniae*, or *Listeria*. The patient's recent trip to the Mississippi River should put St. Louis encephalitis virus higher on the differential diagnosis.

32. **The correct answer is D.** The four polypeptide chains that make up hemoglobin are arranged in different relative positions, depending on whether the molecule is deoxyhemoglobin or oxyhemoglobin. The taut (T) form of hemoglobin is the deoxy form. The movement of the polypeptide chains is restricted hemoglobin is in its low-oxygen-affinity state. The T form predominates in environments with low oxygen tension, such as peripheral tissue, when it is favorable for oxygen to be released from hemoglobin for use by these tissues. In the relaxed

(R) form, the polypeptide chains have greater ability to move and also have a higher oxygen affinity. This R form predominates in environments with high oxygen tension, such as the pulmonary capillary bed, when it is favorable for oxygen to bind hemoglobin for later circulation throughout the body. A good way to remember this fact is that you get very **T**ense when you can't breathe, but you **R**elax when you can.

Answer A is incorrect. The alveolar capillary bed is characterized by high oxygen tension. Thus the high-affinity, R form of hemoglobin predominates. Oxygen binds readily to the R form, permitting the formation of oxyhemoglobin that be circulated throughout the body.

Answer B is incorrect. The coronary arteries originate from the root of the aorta. They are filled with oxygen-rich blood from the lungs that passed through the left atrium and ventricle and into the aorta. Because gas exchange occurs at the level of the capillary beds, the predominant form of hemoglobin will be the same as the form that exited the pulmonary capillary beds. This is the R form of hemoglobin, since the pulmonary capillary beds are characterized by high oxygen tension.

Answer C is incorrect. The femoral artery is a continuation of the external iliac artery. Femoral arteries are filled with oxygen-rich blood from the lungs that passed through the left heart and into the aorta, which bifurcates in the abdomen into the common iliac arteries. The common iliac arteries split to form the internal and external iliac arteries. Because gas exchange occurs at the level of the capillary beds, the predominant form of hemoglobin will be the same as the form that exited the pulmonary capillary beds. This is the R form of hemoglobin, since the pulmonary capillary beds are characterized by high oxygen tension. Hemoglobin has different oxygen affinities in its T versus its R form. In the R form, hemoglobin is in its oxygenated form with high oxygen affinity, whereas in its T form hemoglobin is in its deoxy form with a low oxygen affinity.

Answer E is incorrect. The pulmonary veins carry oxygen-rich blood from the lungs to the left atrium of the heart. They are filled with oxygen-rich blood that has just passed through the pulmonary capillary beds. Because gas exchange occurs at the level of the capillary, the predominant form of hemoglobin will be the same as the form that exited the pulmonary capillary beds. This is the R form of hemoglobin, since the pulmonary capillary beds are characterized by high oxygen tension.

33. **The correct answer is A.** The vignette describes a presentation of prolactinoma, the most common tumor of the pituitary gland. Signs and symptoms are a consequence of excessive prolactin secretion and local mass effects, specifically compression of suprasellar structures in the brain. Among these structures is the optic chiasm, which is situated just superior to the pituitary gland. Compression of the optic chiasm by pituitary tumors characteristically causes a bitemporal hemianopsia (or tunnel vision). This loss of the temporal visual fields is often asymmetric. This lesion often causes patients to miss objects that present in their temporal fields, such as door frames. Additional causes of bitemporal hemianopsia include meningioma, craniopharyngioma, and hypothalamic glioma. In this case, a prolactinoma is also causing the sexual adverse effects by inducing a hypogonadotropic hypogonadism. In this condition patients can also present with infertility and galactorrhea.

Answer B is incorrect. Dysphagia can occur with compression or ischemia of the medulla involving cranial nerves IX and X or the motor cortex within the frontal lobe. A tumor of the pituitary generally would not result in this finding.

Answer C is incorrect. Hydrocephalus usually occurs due to obstruction of cerebrospinal fluid (CSF) outflow from the cerebral ventricular system or due to impaired CSF absorption by the arachnoid granulations. Rarely, large pituitary adenomas can cause CSF outflow obstruction and hydrocephalus if left untreated. In this case, although hydrocephalus is plausible, it is not the most likely presenting symptom of the choices given.

Answer D is incorrect. Right facial droop can occur due to compression or ischemia of the motor cortex within the frontal lobe, as well as compression or damage to cranial nerve VII (Bell's palsy). However, a tumor of the pituitary generally would not result in this finding.

Answer E is incorrect. Right-handed weakness can occur as the result of tumor compression or infiltration into the motor cortex, or precentral gyrus, of the left frontal lobe. However, this finding is more likely in a transient ischemic attack or stroke of the same region. A tumor of the pituitary gland generally cannot cause this finding via local compression of surrounding structures.

34. **The correct answer is A.** This patient is likely suffering from neuroleptic malignant syndrome (NMS), a severe and potentially life-threatening extrapyramidal side effect of antipsychotic agents. Classic symptoms of this syndrome include hyperpyrexia, autonomic instability, and severe rigidity. Treatment requires rapid discontinuation of all neuroleptics, supportive care, and the administration of dantrolene, a skeletal muscle relaxant.

Answer B is incorrect. Diazepam is not indicated for the treatment of NMS.

Answer C is incorrect. Flumazenil, a competitive antagonist at the γ-aminobutyric acid receptor, is used to treat an overdose of benzodiazepines but is not indicated for the treatment of NMS.

Answer D is incorrect. Haloperidol, a neuroleptic agent, would worsen the symptoms of NMS and therefore should not be given.

Answer E is incorrect. Phenobarbital, a barbiturate, would not be helpful in a patient who is experiencing NMS.

35. **The correct answer is A.** Hunter's syndrome is an X-linked disorder that is caused by a deficiency of iduronate sulfatase. Although Hunt-

er's syndrome and Hurler's syndrome are similar, Hunter's syndrome is notable for the absence of corneal clouding, which is present in Hurler's syndrome.

Answer B is incorrect. Hurler's syndrome is a severe disorder with a broad spectrum of clinical findings. It is generally diagnosed within the first year of life and is characterized by a variety of musculoskeletal abnormalities, corneal clouding, hepatosplenomegaly, and severe mental retardation.

Answer C is incorrect. Morquio's syndrome is typically diagnosed around the age of 1 year and is characterized primarily by short stature and joint laxity. Other musculoskeletal abnormalities are also associated with this autosomally transmitted disorder. Some patients demonstrate hepatosplenomegaly, mild corneal clouding, and valvular heart disease.

Answer D is incorrect. There are multiple enzyme deficiencies associated with Sanfilippo's syndrome, but this class of disorders is primarily distinguished by the CNS symptoms in these patients. Some of the physical abnormalities seen in the other mucopolysaccharidoses are also observed in Sanfilippo's patients, but the hallmarks of this disease are developmental delay and behavioral problems such as aggressive tendencies and hyperactivity that manifest in early childhood. Sleep disorders are also common in these patients, and the physical findings typically develop after the behavioral and sleep pattern abnormalities.

Answer E is incorrect. Patients with Sly syndrome have a defect in the beta-glucuronidase enzyme and are generally diagnosed as toddlers. The disorder is autosomal recessive, and the presentation can resemble that of Hurler's syndrome. Mental retardation is not a significant component of Sly syndrome, although various musculoskeletal abnormalities are common.

36. **The correct answer is C.** The patient described is infected with *Pneumocystis jiroveci* pneumonia, which is commonly associated with AIDS and immunosuppression. It is diagnosed with

methenamine silver stain of lung biopsy tissue. *P. jiroveci* pneumonia is treated primarily with sulfamethoxazole-trimethoprim, but it can be treated with pentamidine or dapsone. Both sulfamethoxazole and trimethoprim inhibit the folate synthesis pathway. In the folate synthesis pathway, pteridine and para-aminobenzoic acid (PABA) are incorporated into folic acid, which is important in the formation of nucleic acids and certain amino acids.

Answer A is incorrect. Cell wall synthesis is blocked by many antibiotics, including penicillins, cephalosporins, and vancomycin. *P. jiroveci* is a fungus and does not have a cell wall.

Answer B is incorrect. Many antifungal agents inhibit ergosterol synthesis, including fluconazole and terbinafine. Although *P. jiroveci* is a fungus, antifungals that block ergosterol synthesis are not effective in the treatment of this infection.

Answer D is incorrect. Inhibition of the larger ribosomal subunit (50S) is the mechanism of action of chloramphenicol, erythromycin, clindamycin, and linezolid. None of these is used to treat *P. jiroveci* pneumonia.

Answer E is incorrect. Inhibition of the small ribosomal subunit (30S) is the mechanism of action for many antibiotics, including aminoglycosides and tetracyclines. None of these antibiotics is used for *P. jiroveci* pneumonia.

37. **The correct answer is A.** This patient has the classic signs of Parkinson's disease (PD). Acute PD in young patients has been associated with drug users who have had exposure to MPTP, a contaminant in some illicit street drugs that causes damage to the substantia nigra and induces early-onset PD. The site of the lesion is the substantia nigra, which sends direct projections to the striatum. The striatum is composed of the caudate and putamen, which are involved in both direct and indirect motor pathways of the basal ganglia. The direct pathway, promoted by dopamine release from the substantia nigra, facilitates movement, and the indirect pathway, inhibited by dopamine release

from the substantia nigra, inhibits movement. When the substantia nigra is damaged in PD, dopamine is no longer released in adequate amounts, so the direct pathway is inhibited and the indirect pathway is unchecked, leading to the paucity of movement characteristic of PD.

Answer B is incorrect. The globus pallidus externus is innervated by the striatum in the indirect pathway of the basal ganglia. It is not directly innervated by the substantia nigra.

Answer C is incorrect. The globus pallidus internus is a downstream nucleus in both direct and indirect pathways of the basal ganglia. It is not directly innervated by the substantia nigra.

Answer D is incorrect. The lateral geniculate nucleus is a thalamic nuclei involved in visual processing. It is not part of the basal ganglia motor pathway and is not innervated by the substantia nigra.

Answer E is incorrect. The subthalamic nucleus is innervated by the globus pallidus externus in the indirect pathway of the basal ganglia. It is not directly innervated by the substantia nigra.

38. **The correct answer is B.** This patient presents with a classic picture of anion gap metabolic acidosis caused by lactic acidosis. The anion gap is calculated by $([Na^+] - [Cl^-] - [HCO_3^-])$ or in this case, $138 - 103 - 8$, or 27. Normal anion gap is between 10 and 12. Metformin is an oral hypoglycemic medication classified as a biguanide. As it reduces glucose levels, there is a risk for lactic acidosis that is increased in patients with renal or cardiovascular disease. Its exact mechanism of action remains unknown, although it has been shown to increase insulin binding to its receptor.

Answer A is incorrect. Acarbose is an α-glucosidase inhibitor leading to delayed hydrolysis of sugars and absorption of glucose. Toxicity is generally limited to gastrointestinal disturbances.

Answer C is incorrect. Miglitol is an α-glucosidase inhibitor leading to delayed hydrolysis of sugars and absorption of glucose. Toxicity is generally limited to gastrointestinal disturbances.

Answer D is incorrect. Tolbutamide is a sulfonylurea that stimulates endogenous insulin release and is associated with disulfiram-like effects. Second-generation sulfonylureas such as glyburide and glipizide are more commonly associated with hypoglycemia.

Answer E is incorrect. Troglitazone increases peripheral sensitivity to insulin, and adverse effects include hepatotoxicity and weight gain.

39. **The correct answer is D.** Ouabain, like digoxin, is a Na^+-K^+-ATPase inhibitor similar to the newly isolated toxin. The Na^+-K^+-ATPase pump creates a necessary membrane gradient by pumping sodium out of the cell and bringing potassium into the cell. Na^+-K^+-ATPase pumps are located throughout the body and inhibition of these pumps has serious physiological consequences. For example, decreased activity of the Na^+-K^+-ATPase pump in vascular smooth muscle will lead to an increase in intracellular sodium concentration, which will in turn block Na^+-Ca^{2+} exchange. The ensuing accumulation of calcium inside the cell will then increase vascular resistance and raise systemic blood pressure. In the kidney, inhibition of the Na^+-K^+-ATPase pump will lead to an impairment in tubular sodium resorption.

Answer A is incorrect. Albuterol is a β_2 agonist. β_2 Receptors are located primarily in blood vessel walls and in the respiratory tract. Drugs that agonize β_2 receptors are used in the treatment of asthma.

Answer B is incorrect. Botulinum toxin blocks the release of acetylcholine from presynaptic vesicles and interrupts neuromuscular function. The toxin is produced by *Clostridium botulinum*, a gram-positive anaerobic bacterium. In addition, it exerts a blocking action on the parasympathetic nervous system and may inhibit other neurotransmitters or affect transmission of afferent neuronal impulses.

Answer C is incorrect. Cocaine is a catecholamine reuptake inhibitor. Since reuptake is the major mechanism by which neurotransmitters are removed from their active receptor sites, this inhibition results in potentiation of the response to sympathetic stimulation of innervated organs and to infused catecholamines.

Answer E is incorrect. Procainamide is a class Ia sodium channel blocker. It is used primarily as an antiarrhythmic drug. Procainamide decreases myocardial excitability and conduction velocity and may depress myocardial contractility by increasing the electrical stimulation threshold of the ventricle and His–Purkinje system as well as through direct cardiac effects.

40. **The correct answer is E.** Renal tubular acidosis (RTA) is a disorder of renal acidification characterized by non-anion-gap, hyperchloremic metabolic acidosis. There are several types of RTA. Type IV RTA is characterized by impaired ability to secrete sufficient acid into the urine due to hypoaldosteronism. The most common causes of this hyporeninemic hypoaldosteronism are diabetic nephropathy and chronic tubulointerstitial nephropathies. Hypoaldosteronism leads to decreased sodium reuptake in the distal convoluted tubule and collecting duct and therefore decreased excretion of potassium (and to some extent hydrogen ions) into the urine. The resulting hyperkalemia generates a shift in hydrogen ions to the extracellular fluid to maintain potassium balance, thus producing a metabolic acidosis. The alkalotic environment in the renal tubule cells, however, inhibits ammonia and hydrogen production and secretion, reducing the kidney's ability to excrete the generated acid. Specifically, low ammonia levels decrease the buffering capacity of the urine for hydrogen ions, and therefore the pH of the urine remains low although few hydrogen ions are secreted. Clinically, hypoaldosteronism therefore presents with elevated serum potassium levels, and urinary pH is below 5.5. Angiotensin-converting enzyme inhibitors, trimethoprim, and heparin can similarly reduce aldosterone production, producing an RTA IV picture.

Answer A is incorrect. This patient presents with a non-anion-gap metabolic acidosis. His anion gap (calculated as [serum Na^+] – [serum Cl^-] – [serum HCO_3^-]) is 12.

Answer B is incorrect. Hyperaldosteronism can promote alkalosis based roughly on the reversal of the arguments described in the correct answer.

Answer C is incorrect. In type I renal tubular acidosis, there is an inability to acidify urine due to inadequate transport of hydrogen ions (failure of the ATPase pump) or back diffusion of ions (increased tight junction permeability). Potassium levels are usually normal or reduced, and urine pH is greater than 5.5.

Answer D is incorrect. In type II renal tubular acidosis (RIA), impaired bicarbonate reabsorption in the proximal tubule is typically observed in childhood with other features of Fanconi's syndrome. Rickets and osteomalacia are commonly associated disorders.

41. **The correct answer is B.** Epstein–Barr virus, the virus that causes infectious mononucleosis, is a rare cause of congenital defects. The other answer choices make up the ToRCHeS diseases, a collection of serious infections of pregnancy that are associated with morbidity and mortality of the fetus and newborn. **ToRCHeS** stands for **To**xoplasmosis, **R**ubella, **C**ytomegalovirus, **H**erpes/HIV, and **S**yphilis.

Answer A is incorrect. Congenital cytomegalovirus can result in hepatosplenomegaly, jaundice, and brain calcifications.

Answer C is incorrect. Herpes simplex virus can result in a variety of congenital defects, spontaneous abortion, and neonatal encephalitis.

Answer D is incorrect. Congenital HIV results in neonatal AIDS.

Answer E is incorrect. Congenital rubella infection can result in deafness, patent ductus arteriosus, pulmonary artery stenosis, cataracts, and microcephaly.

Answer F is incorrect. Congenital syphilis can result in cranial nerve VIII deafness, mulberry molars, saber shins, saddle nose, and Hutchinson's teeth.

Answer G is incorrect. Congenital toxoplasmosis infection can result in mental retardation and chorioretinitis.

42. **The correct answer is A.** Collagen is a major component of the basement membrane. Neoplastic cells bound to the basement membrane can potentially escape if they can break through it into the underlying tissue. Aberrant expression of collagenase and hydrolase can confer that ability, leading to an invasive neoplasm. Metastasis occurs when these cells escape the confines of the basement membrane, find their way to the lymph or bloodstream, and subsequently adhere to tissues in another part of the body.

Answer B is incorrect. α-Fetoprotein is a normal serum protein produced by fetal yolk sac and liver. In the context of oncology, α-fetoprotein levels can be used to follow the progression of hepatocellular carcinoma.

Answer C is incorrect. γ-Glutamyl transpeptidase (GGT) participates in the transfer of amino acids across the cellular membrane and in the metabolism of glutathione. High concentrations are found in the liver, bile ducts, and kidney. A test for serum GGT is used to detect diseases of the liver, bile ducts, and kidney and to differentiate liver or bile duct (hepatobiliary) disorders from bone disease.

Answer D is incorrect. Keratin is a marker of epithelial differentiation and is not a factor in metastasis.

Answer E is incorrect. Mucin is a nitrogenous substance found in mucous secretions that serves as a lubricant that protects body surfaces. It is often produced by colonic-type adenocarcinomas.

43. **The correct answer is B.** This patient has hereditary nonpolyposis colorectal cancer (HNPCC), which can be caused by an inherited mutation

in one of the five DNA mismatch repair genes. The mismatch repair mechanism replaces segments of DNA that include mismatched bases. Without this proofreading function, errors can accumulate in crucial areas, such as inactivating mutations in cancer suppressor genes or activating mutations in proto-oncogenes. HNPCC is associated predominantly with an increased risk for cancers of the colorectum and endometrium, but cancers may also occur in the stomach, ovary, pancreas, ureter and renal pelvis, biliary tract, small bowel, and brain.

Answer A is incorrect. A defect in base excision repair results in xeroderma pigmentosum, a disease characterized by extreme sensitivity to sunlight, skin damage, and a predisposition to malignancies such as melanoma.

Answer C is incorrect. t(15;17) is characteristic of acute promyelocytic leukemia. This translocation causes the polymorphonuclear leukocytes and RAR α genes to fuse, arresting the development of myeloid lineage cells at the promyelocyte stage.

Answer D is incorrect. Benzo(a)pyrene is a carcinogen found in cigarette smoke. This carcinogen binds to DNA and forms bulky adducts with guanine residues. Bulky lesions are repaired by nucleotide excision.

Answer E is incorrect. The *bcr-abl* hybrid gene is the result of a translocation between chromosomes 9 and 22, t(9,22). CML is associated with t(9,22), or the Philadelphia chromosome..

44. **The correct answer is A.** Glioblastoma multiforme (GBM) is the most common primary intracranial neoplasm and is typically seen in older patients. Although this neoplasm arises from glial cells, it is impossible to differentiate the specific line. The characteristic features shown in the image include a central area of necrosis surrounded by a hypercellular zone called palisading necrosis. There is also a high degree of anaplasia and pleomorphism. The tumor as a whole shows vascular proliferation and areas of necrosis. Patients with GBM have a very poor prognosis regardless of management.

Answer B is incorrect. Medulloblastomas are tumors that preferentially affect children in the first decade of life and do not typically affect adults. The cells have a characteristic blue appearance and crowd together to form perivascular rosettes or pseudorosettes. They arise from the cerebellum, not the cerebral hemispheres, and commonly block the fourth ventricle, resulting in an obstructive hydrocephalus.

Answer C is incorrect. Meningiomas are the second most common primary intracranial tumors in adults and are typically benign and slow-growing. They commonly affect people in the fourth and fifth decades of life but can affect younger adults as well and are seen more frequently in women than men. They can arise from any portion of the meninges and classically exhibit calcified whorls called psammoma bodies on histologic examination.

Answer D is incorrect. Neurilemmomas are benign tumors arising from Schwann cells associated with cranial nerve VIII (appropriately, they are also called acoustic schwannomas). They are the third most common primary intracranial tumor in adults and, if bilateral, are associated with neurofibromatosis type 2. The two typical patterns seen histologically are either a compact palisading nuclei (Antoni A) or a loose arrangement of cells (Antoni B).

Answer E is incorrect. Oligodendrogliomas are generally benign, slow-growing tumors that arise from oligodendrocytes, which are found in the cerebral hemispheres. They are the fourth most common primary intracranial tumors and typically have the appearance of a fried egg with interspersed chicken wire.

45. **The correct answer is E.** Natural killer (NK) cells are a component of the innate immune system. These cells have a battery of germline-encoded activating and inhibitory receptors that can detect and distinguish virally infected cells from uninfected cells. For example, virally infected cells often express less major histocompatibility complex class I on their surface, and this absence is detected by the NK

cell. Detection of a virally infected cell signals the NK cell to release cytotoxic granules onto the infected cell; thus they play a direct and important role in controlling the early stages of systemic response to viral infection. NK cells express CD16 and CD56 among other markers. It should be noted that individuals with defective NK cell function are particularly susceptible to herpes virus infection. This suggests that NK cells play an important, nonredundant physiologic function in the control of this family of viral infections. EBV binds to CD21 on B lymphocytes, which become infected. In addition to the NK cell-mediated response, CD8+ T lymphocytes mediate the main cellular immune response to this infection.

Answer A is incorrect. Eosinophils are important effector cells in host defense against parasites.

Answer B is incorrect. Mast cells control the early inflammatory response by release of potent vasoactive granules.

Answer C is incorrect. Megakaryocytes are resident bone marrow cells that give rise to platelets.

Answer D is incorrect. Microglia are tissue macrophages located within the CNS and do not play as direct a role in the control of systemic viral infections as NK cells do.

Answer F is incorrect. Plasma cells are antibody-producing B lymphocytes and an important component of the adaptive immune system.

Answer G is incorrect. Regulatory T lymphocytes are components of the adaptive immune response that suppress effector T-lymphocyte functions in both an antigen-specific and antigen-nonspecific manner.

46. **The correct answer is E.** The child is presenting with DiGeorge's syndrome, which is due to abnormal development of the third and fourth branchial (pharyngeal) pouches. This leads to hypoplasia of the thymus and parathyroid glands. Without a properly functioning thymus, T lymphocyte maturation fails, resulting in impaired cell-mediated immunity. Thus, patients with DiGeorge's syndrome often present

with recurrent viral and fungal infections, as in this patient. Without adequate production of parathyroid hormone, these patients are often hypocalcemic, leading to tetany and seizures. DiGeorge's syndrome can be summarized by the mnemonic **CATCH-22: C**ardiac defects, **A**bnormal facies, **T**hymic hypoplasia, **C**left palate, and **H**ypocalcemia due to a microdeletion on chromosome **22**.

Answer A is incorrect. The first aortic arch gives rise to part of the maxillary artery, while the second aortic arch gives rise to the stapedial artery and the hyoid artery. They are not involved in DiGeorge's syndrome.

Answer B is incorrect. The first and second branchial arches play no role in DiGeorge's syndrome. For first-arch derivatives, think "**M**": **M**andible, **M**alleus, spheno**M**andibular ligament; muscles of **M**astication (te**M**poralis, **M**asseter, **M**edial and lateral pterygoids). The first arch is associated with cranial nerve V. For second-arch derivatives, think "**S**": **S**tapes, **S**tyloid process, **S**tylohyoid ligament, muscles of facial expression, **S**tapedius, **S**tylohyoid. Cranial nerve VII is associated with the second arch.

Answer C is incorrect. The fourth and sixth pharyngeal arches do not play a role in DiGeorge's syndrome. The fourth arch is responsible for muscles of the soft palate (but not the tensor veli palatini, a first arch derivative), the muscles of the pharynx (except the stylopharyngeus), the cricothyroid, and the aortic arch. Fourth-arch muscles are innervated by the superior laryngeal branch of cranial nerve X. The sixth arch produces the muscles of the larynx (except for the cricothyroid) as well as the pulmonary arteries. These muscles are innervated by the recurrent laryngeal branch of cranial nerve X.

Answer D is incorrect. The second through fourth branchial clefts form temporary sinuses but are obliterated before maturation. Thus, they have no derivatives in the adult.

47. **The correct answer is A.** The Centers for Disease Control and Prevention reports that if

stuck by an infected needle, there is up to a 30% chance of contracting hepatitis B, while there is only a 10% chance of contracting hepatitis C. The Occupational Safety and Health Adminstration reports that the chance of actually becoming infected with HIV if you are accidentally stuck with a needle used on an HIV patient is between 0.3% and 0.45%.

Answer B is incorrect. One has a 10% chance of being infected with hepatitis C if accidentally stuck, versus up to a 30% chance of infection if stuck with a needle contaminated with hepatitis B.

Answer C is incorrect. One has only a 0.3%–0.45% chance of being infected with HIV if accidentally stuck, versus a 10% chance of infection if stuck with a hepatitis C–infected needle.

Answer D is incorrect. One has a 10% chance of being infected with hepatitis C if accidentally stuck, versus up to a 30% chance of infection if stuck with a hepatitis B–infected needle.

Answer E is incorrect. One has up to a 30% chance of being infected with hepatitis B if accidentally stuck, versus a 0.3%–0.45% chance of being infected with HIV if accidentally stuck.

48. **The correct answer is C.** The potency of inhaled anesthetics is quantified as the minimum alveolar concentration (MAC). This is the concentration of inhaled gas that is needed to eliminate movement among 50% of patients who are challenged by surgical incision. For potent anesthetics, the MAC will be numerically small, meaning that it is inversely proportional to the anesthetic's potency. Drug C, which has the smallest MAC value, is thus the most potent. The blood solubility of an anesthetic is the physical property that determines both speed of induction and time to recovery. Drugs with low blood solubility, such as nitrous oxide, will rapidly induce anesthesia, and patients will recover quickly. In contrast, an anesthetic gas with high blood solubility, such as halothane, will have a longer time to induction and a slower time to recovery. Therefore, drug C, which has the lowest blood solubility, will have the most rapid induction.

Answer A is incorrect. The MAC for a drug is inversely related to its potency. Drug A has a larger MAC than drug D and will be less potent than drug D.

Answer B is incorrect. Drug B, with a solubility of 1.0 (100% soluble in blood), will dissolve completely in the bloodstream, whereas drug C, with its solubility value of 0.1, will be only 10% dissolved in blood. Drug B is more soluble than Drug C.

Answer D is incorrect. An anesthetic with greater blood solubility will have a more rapid induction time. Drug D, which is more soluble in blood than drug C, will therefore induce anesthesia less rapidly than drug C.

Answer E is incorrect. Recovery time from anesthesia is based on the blood solubility of a gas. Gases with high blood solubility result in slower recovery when compared with drugs that have lower blood solubility. Drug B has the highest blood solubility of all those that are listed and thus will have the slowest recovery time of all.

Test Block 7

1. A 23-year-old G1P0 woman who is 39 weeks' pregnant has dysuria with increased urinary frequency, and becomes febrile. She takes some medication prescribed for a previous urinary tract infection (UTI), and continues to use it through delivery. At term she gives birth to a mildly jaundiced boy who is otherwise healthy. Five days later, however, she brings the infant to the emergency department stating that the baby has become fussy, refuses feeding, and wails at a high pitch. He soon becomes extremely lethargic and stops producing urine. Which of the following medications did the mother most likely take to treat her UTI?

(A) Amoxicillin
(B) Ampicillin
(C) Nitrofurantoin
(D) Ofloxacin
(E) Trimethoprim-sulfamethoxazole

2. A physician is performing blood work on another physician. Through the blood work, the physician discovers that the patient is HIV-positive. The physician is practicing medicine in a state that does not require routine reporting of HIV-positive results. What is the appropriate course of action regarding reporting of his HIV status?

(A) No reporting is necessary
(B) Report his status to his sexual partner
(C) Report his status to other patients
(D) Report his status to the appropriate medical association
(E) Report his status to the appropriate medical licensing board

3. A 9-year-old boy with no vaccine history presents with an erythematous maculopapular rash that erupted about 5 days after the onset of cough, conjunctivitis, coryza, high fever, and white spots on the buccal mucosa. The patient's immune system is activated to combat the infecting virus. Which of the following types of cells are the most capable of providing the two signals necessary for T-lymphocyte activation?

(A) Activated B lymphocytes, other T lymphocytes, and natural killer cells
(B) Activated CD8+ T lymphocytes, B lymphocytes, and dendritic cells
(C) Activated macrophages, epithelial cells, and B lymphocytes
(D) Activated macrophages, Langerhans cells, and B lymphocytes
(E) Activated macrophages, Langerhans cells, and natural killer cells

4. An Ashkenazi Jewish couple expecting their first child presents to the physician with concerns about their baby's health. The woman says that she had a sister who died at age 2 years. She says that her sister was healthy at birth but weakened over the first few months of her life and died of pneumonia. When questioned further, she says she remembers her sister having a "large head" as an infant. The man adds that he had an uncle who also died as a toddler. He had been told that the baby was blind and developed seizures toward the end of his life. Genetic testing reveals both parents are heterozygous carriers of an autosomal recessive disease. Which of the following represents the likelihood that this couple's child will be affected by this condition?

(A) 3%
(B) 25%
(C) 50%
(D) 100%
(E) Same as the population prevalence

5. A 29-year-old woman who is 36 weeks pregnant presents to the emergency department experiencing contractions that are 5 minutes apart. She is somewhat distraught because her first pregnancy 2 years ago ended in a miscarriage. Nevertheless, she delivers an apparently healthy baby boy. During the initial survey, the physician notes that the baby has good color and is crying loudly but seems unable to move either of his legs very well. Radiography reveals healing fractures bilaterally in the femoral shaft

and new fractures in the right tibia. Which of the following conditions exhibits a defect in the same molecule as this child?

(A) Alport's syndrome
(B) Goodpasture's syndrome
(C) Marfan's syndrome
(D) Osteomalacia

6. A 42-year-old woman comes to the physician with red papular lesions along her arm, some of which have ulcerated. She reports that the lesions appeared 1 week ago, a day after she worked in her garden. Initially there were only a couple of lesions on her right forearm. Since then more lesions have appeared along her arm approaching her axilla. The physician cultures material from one of the lesions, which grows the organism shown in the image. This patient is most likely infected with which of the following fungi?

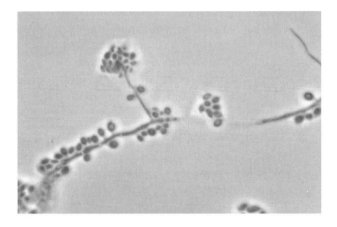

Image courtesy of Centers for Disease Control and Prevention's Public Health Image Library; content provider Dr. Libero Ajello.

(A) *Blastomyces species*
(B) *Coccidioides species*
(C) *Malassezia furfur*
(D) *Pneumocystis jiroveci*
(E) *Sporothrix schenckii*

7. A 63-year-old man presents to his primary care physician complaining of weakness, weight loss,

and left upper quadrant pain. Physical examination demonstrates diffuse lymphadenopathy and splenomegaly. Peripheral blood analysis demonstrates a WBC count of 40,000/mm³, with increased neutrophils, eosinophils, and basophils on peripheral smear. Polymerase chain reaction analysis of his blood demonstrates a t(9;22) chromosomal translocation. Which of the following would most likely be used to treat his condition?

(A) Imatinib mesylate
(B) Infliximab
(C) Paclitaxel
(D) Propylthiouracil
(E) Tamoxifen

8. A 56-year-old woman with a history of advanced cervical cancer that was treated with radiotherapy and chemotherapy is admitted to the hospital for worsening symptoms of abdominal pain and vomiting over a 3-day period. The patient's blood pressure is 108/75 mm Hg supine and 95/60 mm Hg standing. Laboratory studies show:

Serum pH: 7.64
Blood urea nitrogen: 31 mg/dL
Creatinine: 1.2 mg/dL
Na⁺: 141 mEq/L
K⁺: 3.3 mEq/L
Cl⁻: 90 mEq/L
Total CO_2: 35 mEq/L
Urine pH: 5.1
Urine Na⁺: 10 mEq/L

Which of the following is the most likely cause of the acidic urine?

(A) The paraneoplastic effects of the cancer
(B) The patient has a history of chemotherapy
(C) The patient is hypokalemic
(D) The patient is in prerenal failure due to hypotension
(E) The patient's hypotension has led to a lactic acidosis

9. A 54-year-old woman with a history of breast cancer recently underwent surgical lumpectomy with radical axillary node dissection. A neck exploration was performed for an enlarged cervical node on the right side of the neck secondary to concern about metastatic disease. Several weeks into her subsequent radiation treatment, she presents with a swollen right arm and fingers, right facial edema that is most pronounced around the orbit, and shortness of breath. X-ray of the chest reveals some accumulation of fluid in the right pleural cavity. Which of the following is the most likely cause of these findings?

(A) Deep venous thrombosis of the cephalic vein
(B) Disruption of the right lymphatic duct
(C) Disruption of the thoracic duct
(D) Metastatic disease to the humerus
(E) Normal adverse effect of radiation

10. A 35-year-old woman and her husband come to the physician because she has been acting strangely. The husband explains that approximately 3 weeks ago his wife stopped showing up for work, spent most of their life savings during this time, and seemed very irritable when he questioned her about this behavior. He also reports that she is no longer sleeping through the night and that she is now claiming to be the most intelligent woman in the world. Which of the following is the most likely diagnosis?

(A) Amphetamine intoxication
(B) Bipolar disorder
(C) Hyperthyroidism
(D) Schizoaffective disorder
(E) Schizophrenia

11. A 60-year-old man who is being treated for multiple myeloma develops osteonecrosis of his maxilla. His presentation is significant for a molar tooth extraction site that has displayed poor healing 4 months after surgery. Localized swelling, exposed bone, erythema, and a purulent discharge are noted on intraoral examination. Which of the following drug classes is most likely associated with this lesion?

(A) Angiotensin converting enzyme inhibitors
(B) Bisphosphonates
(C) Cephalosporins
(D) Osmotic diuretics
(E) Vinca alkaloids

12. A 12-year-old girl presents to her pediatrician with recent onset of bruising. Complete blood cell count reveals pancytopenia. Bone marrow biopsy shows hypercellularity with fatty infiltration. The patient's mother says her daughter received a course of antibiotics 3 weeks ago. Which of the following is most likely to cause the findings seen in this patient?

(A) Chloramphenicol
(B) Ciprofloxacin
(C) Clindamycin
(D) Erythromycin
(E) Gentamicin
(F) Tetracycline

13. A couple has four children. One of the children suffers from severe erythema and scaling on the sun-exposed areas of his body. The other three children and both parents are unaffected. The affected child later develops melanomas and squamous cell carcinoma. The affected child most likely has a genetic defect in which of the following pathways?

(A) DNA excision repair
(B) Double-stranded DNA break sensing
(C) Glycolytic
(D) Heme synthesis
(E) Purine salvage pathway

14. An infant is born with a defect in his abdominal wall. Studies confirm that the discharge from this defect is urine. Which of the following is the postnatal derivative of the structure with the defect?

(A) Fossa ovalis
(B) Ligamentum teres hepatis
(C) Medial umbilical ligament
(D) Median umbilical ligament
(E) Nucleus pulposus

15. A physician is setting up to perform a therapeutic thoracentesis on a patient with stage IV

ovarian cancer. She drapes the patient and inserts the needle in the midaxillary line on the right side, immediately superior to the tenth rib. Which of the following structures is the physician trying to avoid by inserting the needle here instead of higher in the intercostal space?

(A) Ninth intercostal nerve, artery, and vein
(B) Phrenic nerve
(C) Right pericardiophrenic artery and vein
(D) Right recurrent laryngeal nerve
(E) Tenth intercostal nerve, artery, and vein

16. A 55-year-old man with no past medical history is found to have a singular thyroid nodule during a routine visit to his physician. A section from the resected mass is shown in the image and is consistent with a neoplasm. The patient is informed that this type of thyroid cancer has a better prognosis than other forms of thyroid cancer and that resection of the mass is frequently curative. In which of the following tumors can the histologic finding shown in the image also be found?

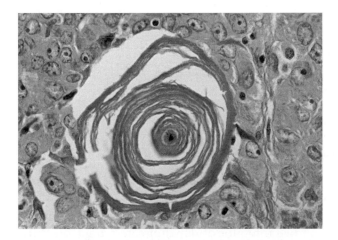

Image courtesy of Armed Forces Institute of Pathology.

(A) Adenocarcinoma of the lung
(B) Dysgerminoma
(C) Follicular carcinoma of the thyroid
(D) Medullary carcinoma of the thyroid
(E) Mesothelioma

17. A woman is concerned about her risks for developing cervical cancer. Which of the following factors poses the largest risk for developing cervical cancer?

(A) Alcoholism
(B) Early sexual activity
(C) Low-fiber diet
(D) Nulliparity
(E) Prolonged estrogen use

18. A 12-year-old boy with moderate mental retardation comes to the physician because of painful swollen joints. During the examination, the physician notices that the boy makes several uncontrolled spastic muscle movements. Past medical history includes a diagnosis of muscular hypotonia at 5 months of age. At 3 years of age, the patient was referred to a pediatric dentist for severe repetitive biting of his lip and tongue. Which of the following is the most likely cause of these findings?

(A) A deficiency of adenosine deaminase
(B) A deficiency of β-glucocerebroside
(C) A mutation of an enzyme in the de novo biosynthetic pathway
(D) Absence of hypoxanthine guanine phosphoribosyltransferase
(E) An excision repair enzyme deficiency

19. A 40-year-old woman visits her physician with complaints of dry mouth, chronic cough, difficulty swallowing, and dry eyes, especially in the morning. The patient's physical examination and review of systems are unremarkable except for low-grade fevers and recent onset of joint pain. Which of the following additional conditions is this patient most likely to develop?

(A) Dental caries
(B) Hyperglycemia
(C) Jaundice
(D) Septic joints
(E) Vision loss

20. A 59-year-old man presents to his physician with complaints of proximal muscle weakness evolving over the past 2 months, accompanied by a 5-kg (11 lb) weight loss and fatigue. He is no longer able to navigate the stairs in his home. His medical history is significant for hypertension and a 50-pack-year history of smoking. Electromyography shows impulse abnormalities following repeated stimulation. CT of the thorax shows a 2-cm nodule in the left lung. Which of the following is the most likely mechanism for this patient's muscle weakness?

(A) Ectopic ACTH production by tumor cells
(B) Ectopic ADH production by tumor cells
(C) Production of IgG autoantibodies against the acetylcholine receptor at the neuromuscular synapse
(D) Production of IgG autoantibodies against the voltage-dependent calcium channels at the neuromuscular synapse
(E) Tumor infiltration into skeletal muscle

21. When conducting a clinical trial on a new asthma drug, a nonblinded physician participating in the study has noticed benefits in patients who are taking the drug rather than the placebo. Knowing that the experimental drug is actually beneficial, he begins to unconsciously assign newly enrolled patients with more severe asthma to the experimental group rather than the placebo group. Which of the following types of bias is this?

(A) Late-look bias
(B) Length bias
(C) Recall bias
(D) Sampling bias
(E) Selection bias

22. A 68-year-old white man with a history of diabetes mellitus, hypertension, increased cholesterol, sedentary lifestyle, and 40-year smoking history comes into the office complaining of severe substernal chest pressure that resolved when he sat down and relaxed. The patient states that he has "always" had episodes like this but they have not caused this much distress. Angina caused by silent myocardial ischemia is suspected. An ECG is performed and the patient is recommended to have an exercise stress test. Which of the following is a physiologic response to exercise?

(A) Decreased arterial pH with strenuous exercise
(B) Decreased oxygen consumption
(C) Increased hypoxic vasoconstriction
(D) No change in venous partial carbon dioxide pressure
(E) Pulmonary blood flow remains unchanged

23. The sexually indifferent embryo contains several structures that will develop into male or female reproductive organs depending on hormonal influence. From which of the following embryonic structures is the clitoris derived?

(A) Genital tubercle
(B) Labioscrotal swellings
(C) Mesonephric (wolffian) duct
(D) Paramesonephric (müllerian) duct
(E) Urogenital folds

24. A town with 1,000 citizens has a 10% prevalence of disease X. A screening test for disease X was just developed, with a sensitivity of 80% and a specificity of 70%. How many people without disease X will be falsely diagnosed positive by this screening test?

(A) 20
(B) 80
(C) 100
(D) 270
(E) 630

25. A 54-year-old woman has had longstanding rheumatoid arthritis. Her rheumatologist recently started her on methotrexate, a competitive inhibitor of dihydrofolate reductase. What effect does methotrexate have on dihydrofolate reductase (DHFR)?

(A) Methotrexate acts on DHFR by decreasing its Michaelis-Menten constant
(B) Methotrexate acts on DHFR by increasing its Michaelis-Menten constant
(C) Methotrexate does not affect DHFR's Michaelis-Menten constant

(D) The maximum reaction rate is decreased

(E) The maximum reaction rate is increased

26. While watching an episode of her favorite television show, an 82-year-old woman with hypertension and hyperlipidemia suffers an episode of lightheadedness that is associated with double vision and the inability to speak. On her way to use the phone to dial 911 she knocks over a lamp and falls to the ground twice. Which of the following vessels is most likely affected in this patient?

(A) Anterior cerebral artery

(B) Anterior choroidal artery

(C) Lacunar artery

(D) Middle cerebral artery

(E) Vertebral artery

27. A 45-year-old man comes to the physician because of a fever of 39.6° C (103.2° F) that developed suddenly the previous night. On physical examination, the physician notes a new-onset murmur along with white spots on the retina. The appearance of his hands is shown in the image. Which agent, if used alone, is most likely to be used to treat this patient prior to the results of blood culture?

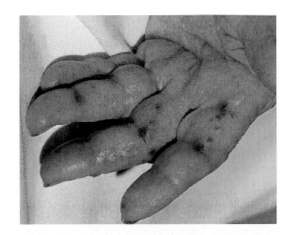

Reproduced, with permission, from Wolff K, Johnson RA, Suurmond D. *Fitzpatrick's Color Atlas & Synopsis of Clinical Dermatology*, 5th ed. New York: McGraw-Hill, 2005: Figure 22.38.

(A) Ceftriaxone

(B) Ciprofloxacin

(C) Erythromycin

(D) Gentamicin

(E) Vancomycin

28. When a peripheral nerve fiber is transected, degenerative changes occur in the injured neuron. Which of the following mechanisms is most likely involved?

(A) Degeneration of dendrites proximal to the lesion

(B) Degeneration of neuronal cell body

(C) Degeneration of neuronal target cells

(D) Degeneration of the axon distal to the lesion

(E) Degeneration of the axon proximal to the lesion

29. A 47-year-old man with chronic asthma who has been treated with high-dose steroids for many years develops a productive cough, weight loss, and night sweats. Imaging studies reveal the presence of abscesses in the lungs and brain. Cultures show gram-positive filaments that are weakly acid-fast. Which of the following organisms is responsible for this patient's condition?

(A) *Actinomyces israelii*

(B) *Bacillus anthracis*

(C) *Mycobacterium tuberculosis*

(D) *Nocardia asteroids*

(E) *Streptococcus pneumoniae*

30. A 76-year-old woman presents to the emergency department with blurry vision and a headache that started 5 hours ago. She has a past medical history of chronic essential hypertension and asthma. She is afebrile with a pulse of 75/min and a blood pressure of 210/120 mm Hg. Which of the following medications should be prescribed immediately?

(A) Captopril

(B) Hydrochlorothiazide

(C) Labetalol

(D) Losartan

(E) Sodium nitroprusside

31. DNA is extracted from cells and cut by restriction enzymes. The resulting fragments of DNA are run on an electrophoresis gel. Bands of DNA are transferred from a gel to a nitrocellulose sheet, which is then treated with a labeled DNA probe. Which of the following laboratory techniques does this describe?

(A) Enzyme-linked immunosorbent assay
(B) Gel electrophoresis
(C) Northern blot
(D) Polymerase chain reaction
(E) Sequencing
(F) Southern blot
(G) Western blot

32. A 15-year-old boy is brought to his pediatrician because he feels short of breath and has to stop and walk after brief runs. He underwent cardiac surgery when he was an infant for a congenital heart defect. An inspiratory chest x-ray shows an intact right hemidiaphragm that is much higher than the left one. This boy's exertional dyspnea is probably caused by which of the following conditions?

(A) Damaged left phrenic nerve
(B) Damaged right phrenic nerve
(C) Eisenmenger's syndrome
(D) Left diaphragmatic hernia
(E) Right diaphragmatic hernia

33. Nutrients such as fats and proteins are both produced by the body and consumed in the diet. On the other hand, many other nutritional components cannot be synthesized by the body and must be obtained in food. Which of the following substances can a healthy adult synthesize?

(A) The fatty acid linoleic acid
(B) The glucogenic amino acid histidine
(C) The ketogenic amino acid leucine
(D) The micronutrient folic acid
(E) The micronutrient vitamin K

34. A 52-year-old man presents to the emergency department because of nocturia, dysuria, and crippling back pain. X-ray of the spine is shown in the image. Laboratory studies are notable for a hemoglobin level of 10.2 mg/dL, calcium of 13.1 mg/dL, and increased total protein. Which of the following is the most likely explanation of the increased total protein observed in this man?

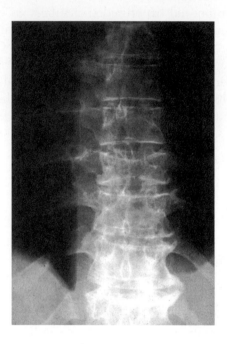

Reproduced, with permission, from the PEIR Digital Library (http://peir.net).

(A) Inability to clear chylomicron particles from the blood
(B) Increased production of albumin
(C) Increased production of clotting factors and acute-phase reactants
(D) Increased production of IgG molecules
(E) Increased production of IgM molecules

35. A 33-year-old man who is HIV-positive presents to the physician with a 3-week history of sore throat and dysphagia. On physical examination his oral mucosa is erythematous and friable, with white patches that bleed when removed. Laboratory tests reveal a CD4+ cell count of 100/mm³ (normal: 440–1600/mm³) and a CD8+ cell count of 300/mm³ (normal: 180–850/mm³). Which of the following is most likely responsible for this patient's condition?

(A) *Candida albicans*
(B) Cytomegalovirus

(C) Herpes simplex virus type 1

(D) JC virus

(E) *Pneumocystis jiroveci*

36. A 3-month-old girl is brought to her pediatrician because she has a high fever and cough. The patient is started on an antibiotic regimen. Over the next 24 hours her condition deteriorates and she is brought to the emergency department. Further history reveals that the child's birth was complicated by a delayed umbilical separation. This patient most likely has which of the following immune deficiencies?

(A) Chronic granulomatous disease

(B) Leukocyte adhesion deficiency syndrome

(C) Selective IgA deficiency

(D) Severe combined immunodeficiency

(E) Wiskott–Aldrich syndrome

37. A 20-year-old college student who is 4 weeks pregnant goes to her local Planned Parenthood to obtain information on her options for her pregnancy. She is interested in having an abortion, but is fearful of an operation and asks about medical abortion. She is told that mifepristone is a drug that can be used early in pregnancy to terminate gestation, with an efficacy around 85%. When administered with a particular drug, the efficacy rises to almost 100%. Which of the following is the coadministered drug?

(A) Clomiphene

(B) Diethylstilbestrol

(C) Ethinyl estradiol

(D) Progesterone

(E) Prostaglandin E_1

38. In a discussion with his therapist, a student at a local university reveals an affection for a fellow student that seems obsessive. He also notes he has an intent to purchase a gun but does not clearly state why. With whom must the physician be sure contact is made?

(A) Another physician who knows the fellow student

(B) Another physician who knows the patient

(C) Law enforcement authorities and the fellow student

(D) Law enforcement authorities only

(E) No one; do not break confidentiality

(F) The fellow student only

39. A 16-year-old girl presents to the clinical concerned that she is "becoming too hairy." Physical examination reveals a 167 cm (5'6"), 85.5 kg (188 lb) teenager with coarse facial hair on her upper lip, chin, shoulders, and back. She says that she's always "been heavy," but reports gaining 20 pounds in the past 3 months as well. She says that she developed this unusual hairiness over the past 6 months, and is very concerned about her outward physical appearance. Physical examination reveals hyperpigmented, velvety patches of skin on the nape of her neck and around her axillae. When questioned, she admits that while she has never been sexually active, she has always had irregular, spotty menstrual periods, often missing them completely. What laboratory finding is most likely to be present in this patient?

(A) Hypercalcemia

(B) Hyperglycemia

(C) Hyperkalemia

(D) Hyperuricemia

40. In order to ascertain the specific genetic defect in patients with cystic fibrosis, scientists obtained buccal smears from several patients and isolated DNA from these cells. The DNA was amplified by polymerase chain reaction and then sequenced. The region of the sequencing gel where the normal gene differs from the mutated gene is shown in the image. Which of the following types of DNA mutations caused this disease?

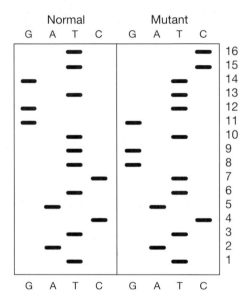

Reproduced, with permission, from USMLERx.com.

(A) Deletion mutation
(B) Frameshift mutation
(C) Insertion mutation
(D) Missense mutation
(E) Nonsense mutation
(F) Point mutation
(G) Silent mutation

41. A new experimental cancer drug for treating acute lymphocytic leukemia has just been discovered. The drug is designed to prevent microtubule spindle formation. This new drug's mechanism of action is most similar to that of which of the following?

(A) Busulfan
(B) Cisplatin
(C) Cytarabine

(D) Paclitaxel
(E) Vincristine

42. An 82-year-old man is brought to the emergency department by ambulance with complaints of severe dyspnea and altered mental status. He is obtunded and tachypneic with moist mucous membranes, and his blood pressure is 70/40 mm Hg. Bilateral rales are auscultated, and a new soft decrescendo systolic murmur is heard at the apex of the heart, as is an S_4 gallop. Of the following, which medication would be most effective in this patient?

(A) Amrinone
(B) Dopamine
(C) Epinephrine
(D) Isoproterenol
(E) Phenylephrine

43. A 65-year-old man with a history of hypertension and hyperlipidemia comes to the physician because of constant, dull groin pain. The patient has noticed a slight decrease in his urine output but denies fever or hematuria. The right kidney is palpable in the right flank region. A CT scan of the pelvis is performed and confirms the diagnosis. Which of the following is the most likely cause of this patient's findings?

(A) Abdominal aortic aneurysm
(B) Right bladder calculus
(C) Right common iliac artery aneurysm
(D) Right ureteral calculus
(E) Urinary tract infection

44. A 5-year-old boy is expected to be discharged from the pediatric intensive care unit after sustaining an intraventricular hemorrhage following a motor vehicle accident. Maintenance fluids have been discontinued, and intravenous (IV) access has been kept open by flushing with heparin. The intern asks the third-year medical student to draw blood off the patient's IV line for coagulation studies. The third-year student, however, neglects to discard the first 5 cc of blood before collecting blood for the sample. He then sends this sample to the hematology laboratory for a coagulation panel but neglects to tell the intern about the error.

Which of the following laboratory results would be expected in this situation?

(A) Decreased activated partial thromboplastin time
(B) Decreased international normalized ratio
(C) Decreased prothrombin time
(D) Increased activated partial thromboplastin time
(E) Increased international normalized ratio
(F) Increased prothrombin time

45. A 43-year-old woman in a psychiatry ward is admitted from a medical floor after attempting suicide by medication overdose. She states that she recently broke up with her boyfriend, who disapproved of her cocaine and marijuana use. This is the fifth time they have broken up. She also states that she and her ex-boyfriend fought constantly; however, she adds that the only times she did not feel "empty" were when they were fighting. She also states that she has made "hundreds" of suicide attempts and has been hospitalized numerous times. Which of the following personality disorders best describes this patient?

(A) Avoidant
(B) Borderline
(C) Dependent
(D) Narcissistic
(E) Schizoid
(F) Schizotypal

46. A term infant is born after an uncomplicated pregnancy to a 35-year-old woman. On cutting the umbilical cord, the pysician notes an abnormality that leads him to consult a pediatric cardiologist. Which of the following abnormalities did this physician most likely observe?

(A) Single allantoic duct
(B) Single umbilical artery
(C) Single umbilical vein
(D) Two umbilical arteries
(E) Two umbilical veins

47. A construction worker accidentally drives a nail into his thigh with a nail gun. The nail is removed, but the area remains painful and edematous. A diagnosis of cellulitis is made. After a few days, the skin over the affected area becomes spongy and, on palpation, exhibits crepitus. A blood-tinged exudate is also observed. To which of the following organisms was this man most likely exposed?

(A) *Actinomyces israelii*
(B) *Bacillus anthracis*
(C) *Clostridium perfringens*
(D) *Clostridium tetani*
(E) *Sporothrix schenckii*

48. A 64-year-old woman presents to the physician because of vaginal bleeding. Ultrasonography reveals a small mass in the left adnexa, along with a thickened endometrial stripe. A biopsy of her left ovary reveals the presence of Call-Exner bodies. Which of the following is the most likely diagnosis?

(A) Endometrioid tumor
(B) Granulosa cell tumor
(C) Krukenberg's tumor
(D) Serous cystadenocarcinoma
(E) Teratoma

1. **The correct answer is E.** Trimethoprim-sulfamethoxazole is one of the most common treatments for simple UTIs, most of which in the general population are caused by *Escherichia coli.* Sulfamethoxazole binds to, and will displace, unconjugated bilirubin from albumin. In a newborn, this can lead to kernicterus (bilirubin encephalopathy), a disorder of newborns caused by deposition of bilirubin in the brain. The basal ganglia are particularly affected. Common early symptoms include lethargy, poor feeding, and absent Moro reflex. If the infants survive, they can develop seizures, mental retardation, deafness, choreoathetoid movements, and decreased upward eye movements.

   Answer A is incorrect. Amoxicillin is not associated with kernicterus.

   Answer B is incorrect. Ampicillin is not associated with kernicterus.

   Answer C is incorrect. Nitrofurantoin, commonly used to treat UTIs, is not associated with kernicterus.

   Answer D is incorrect. Ofloxacin is not associated with kernicterus.

2. **The correct answer is A.** All states have a requirement to report cases of AIDS, but not all states have a requirement to report HIV-positive results.

   Answer B is incorrect. Reporting to a sexual partner is a requirement of all HIV patients, but a physician is only required to do so if he or she believes that the patient will not.

   Answer C is incorrect. A physician who practices infection control is not at risk for infecting his other patients.

   Answer D is incorrect. Medical associations do not require HIV-positive result reporting.

   Answer E is incorrect. Medical licensing boards do not require HIV-positive result reporting.

3. **The correct answer is D.** T-lymphocyte activation requires two signals: (1) T-lymphocyte receptor recognition of major histocompatibility complex/peptide, and (2) CD28-B7 interaction. Only professional antigen-presenting cells (APCs) are capable of delivering both of these signals. The three types of professional APCs are the dendritic cells, macrophages, and B lymphocytes. Langerhans cells are a type of dendritic cells present within the skin.

   Answer A is incorrect. T lymphocytes and natural killer cells are not professional APCs.

   Answer B is incorrect. T lymphocytes are not professional APCs.

   Answer C is incorrect. Epithelial cells are not professional APCs.

   Answer E is incorrect. Natural killer cells are not professional APCs.

4. **The correct answer is B.** Twenty-five percent of heterozygous parents' offspring will be affected with autosomal recessive diseases such as Tay–Sachs disease, which is the condition described in this couple's family histories.

   Answer A is incorrect. Three percent is the approximate recurrence risk for the offspring of an individual with a multifactorial genetic disorder (e.g., cleft lip). This also applies to siblings of an affected child; each subsequent birth in a family with one affected child has a 3% risk of also being affected.

   Answer C is incorrect. Fifty percent of heterozygous parents' offspring will be affected in autosomal dominant inheritance.

   Answer D is incorrect. In the case of mitochondrial inheritance, 100% of an affected mother's children receive the disease, and none of an affected father's children receive it (children inherit their mother's mitochondrial DNA).

   Answer E is incorrect. When a disease is due to somatic mutations, the chance of a child being affected will depend on the population prevalence of the somatic mutation that causes the disease to occur. There is no transmission from one generation to the next, and therefore it is not considered an inherited condition.

5. **The correct answer is A.** This child has osteogenesis imperfecta, an inherited defect in type I collagen. There is a spectrum of severity observed with osteogenesis imperfecta, ranging from prepubertal fractures with mild deformity and normal stature to frequent childhood fractures and even severe in utero fractures that result in perinatal death. Alport's syndrome is another disease by which mutations in (type IV) collagen cause problems in the kidney, inner eye, and ear. Patients with Alport's syndrome often have a history of nephritis and sensineural hearing loss.

    Answer B is incorrect. Autoantibodies against the structures typically hidden in the recesses of collagen IV cause Goodpasture's syndrome.

    Answer C is incorrect. Marfan's syndrome involves an inherited defect in fibrillin, a glycoprotein that forms a sheath around elastin to ensure its proper function. The condition is characterized by ocular defect, arachnodactyly, and a predisposition to aortic dissection due to a weakened aortic wall.

    Answer D is incorrect. Osteomalacia refers to softening of the bones and is often caused by vitamin D deficiency. Collagen defect is not implicated in this condition.

6. **The correct answer is E.** *Sporothrix schenckii* is the cause of sporotrichosis. When *S. schenckii* is introduced into the skin, usually by a thorn prick, it causes a local pustule or ulcer with nodules along draining lymphatics (ascending lymphangitis). *S. schenckii* is a dimorphic fungus that has cigar-shaped budding yeast visible in pus. Itraconazole or potassium iodide is used for the treatment of *S. schenckii* infection.

    Answer A is incorrect. Blastomycosis can present with flu-like symptoms, fevers, chills, productive cough, myalgia, arthralgia, and pleuritic chest pain. Some patients will fail to recover from an acute infection and progress to develop chronic pulmonary infection or widespread disseminated infection. Fluconazole or ketoconazole is used for the treatment of local blastomycosis, and amphotericin B is used for the treatment of systemic infections.

    Answer B is incorrect. Coccidioidomycosis is the second most common fungal infection encountered in the United States. About 60% of these infections cause no symptoms, and in the remaining 40% of cases the symptoms can range from mild to severe. Severe forms of the infection can present with blood-tinged sputum, loss of appetite, weight loss, a painful red rash on the legs, and change in mental status.

    Answer C is incorrect. *Malassezia furfur* infection is the cause of tinea versicolor. Symptoms of this infection include hypopigmented skin lesions that occur in hot and humid conditions. *M. furfur* is treated with topical miconazole or selenium sulfide.

    Answer D is incorrect. *Pneumocystis jiroveci* (formerly carinii), like most fungal infections, does not present with any symptoms in the immunocompetent host. In children or patients afflicted with AIDS, cancer, or inherited immune deficiencies, *P. jiroveci* can present with pneumonia. Symptoms begin suddenly in this form of pneumonia. The patient develops a fever and begins to cough and breathe abnormally fast. Often the patient's lips, fingernails, and skin turn blue or gray because the patient has difficulty drawing in air. The diffuse interstitial pneumonia gives a ground-glass appearance on x-ray of the chest. *P. jiroveci* infection is treated with trimethoprim-sulfamethoxazole.

7. **The correct answer is A.** Weakness, weight loss, and left upper quadrant pain in a middle-aged person with an increased number of cells of myeloid lineage and a t(9;22) chromosomal translocation (Philadelphia chromosome) suggests chronic myeloid leukemia (CML). CML is a stem cell disorder that results in the overproduction of myeloid cells. Although not specified in the question, bone marrow and pe-

ripheral myeloid cells would be left-shifted toward a higher proportion of mature forms, with <5% blasts. Imatinib mesylate inhibits the abnormal bcr-abl tyrosine kinase found in >90% of cases of CML. It does not cure patients, but can result in quiescent disease and restoration of normal blood cell counts. As a first-line single agent for chronic-phase disease, imatinib mesylate prevents the progression of CML to the accelerated- or blast-phase (acute leukemia transformation) in most patients for several years. It is the first successful targeted molecular therapy for cancer and is the model for a new era of drug design.

Answer B is incorrect. Infliximab is a monoclonal antibody to tumor necrosis factor- that is used in the treatment of refractory Crohn's disease.

Answer C is incorrect. Paclitaxel is an antimitotic agent that binds to tubulin and stabilized polymerized microtubules so that they cannot break down. It is used in ovarian and breast cancers.

Answer D is incorrect. Propylthiouracil is used in the treatment of hyperthyroidism and acts by blocking thyroid hormone synthesis and conversion of thyroxine to triiodothyronine.

Answer E is incorrect. Tamoxifen is a selective estrogen receptor modulator used in the treatment of breast cancer.

8. **The correct answer is C.** Acidic urine in the presence of metabolic alkalosis, known as paradoxical aciduria, is primarily a result of hypokalemia in the presence of volume contraction. The loss of hydrochloric acid due to vomiting leads to a transient increase in pH. The kidney responds by excretion of sodium and/or potassium bicarbonate. As the vomiting persists, the alkalemic and dehydrated patient tries to conserve sodium by activation of the renin-angiotensin-aldosterone system. Therefore, while bicarbonate excretion persists due to the alkalosis, it is primarily excreted with potassium rather than sodium due to the dehydration. Compensating by conserving sodium and excreting bicarbonate at the expense of po-

tassium soon fails because in the presence of severe hypokalemia, the kidney begins to exchange hydrogen ions in the distal convoluted tubule in order to conserve potassium. Therefore, acidic urine in the setting of volume contraction and alkalosis is primarily due to the loss of potassium.

Answer A is incorrect. Cervical cancer is not associated with any common paraneoplastic effects.

Answer B is incorrect. A history of chemotherapy would have no effect on the present state of this patient's urine.

Answer D is incorrect. The patient is hypotensive, and her blood urea nitrogen/creatinine (BUN:Cr) ratio shows prerenal failure (defined as BUN:plasma creatinine >20:1). Renal failure leads to an inability to excrete hydrogen ions (as seen in renal tubular acidosis). Therefore, although she is suffering from prerenal disease due to a drop in her blood pressure, it does not account for the loss of hydrogen ions in her urine.

Answer E is incorrect. Lactic acidosis normally occurs in the setting of shock. There is reduced tissue oxygenation and, as the oxygen requirements of cells are not met, they begin to metabolize anaerobically, leading to a buildup of lactic acid and a subsequent metabolic acidosis. However, this patient is not in shock because her systolic blood pressures are >90 mm Hg and sufficiently perfusing her peripheral tissues. Therefore, she does not need to excrete hydrogen ions to counteract a metabolic acidosis.

9. **The correct answer is B.** Most of the lymph in the body is drained via the thoracic duct. It passes through the diaphragm with the aorta and azygous vein posteriorly at the level of T12. The right chest, back, arm, neck, and head, however, are drained via the right lymphatic duct, which empties into the angle between the internal jugular and subclavian veins. With symptoms of swelling in the right upper quadrant of the body, one must consider disruption of this structure, especially with a history of surgery in the axilla and neck.

Answer A is incorrect. Symptoms of deep venous thrombosis (DVT) include swelling, redness, and tenderness of the areas distal to the thrombosis. DVT can develop in the axillary or subclavian veins as a complication of venous catheters in these sites and may present as in this patient. A DVT in the cephalic vein, however, does not explain the facial edema.

Answer C is incorrect. The thoracic duct drains all the lymph in the body except that from the right upper quadrant, which includes the right arm and right side of the face.

Answer D is incorrect. Metastatic disease to bone is common in advanced breast cancer, and most metastatic disease occurs in the central skeleton (vertebrae, pelvis, ribs, upper legs, and arms). Bone metastases may cause pain and pathologic fractures but does not best explain the symptoms of swelling and edema in the face and arm.

Answer E is incorrect. Radiation has many adverse effects, including systemic effects, such as a decreased WBC count, as well as local effects, such as skin irritation. Local radiation to the right breast does not explain this patient's edema of the arm and face. These symptoms should prompt a more thorough work-up.

10. **The correct answer is B.** The manic phase of bipolar disorder is characterized by an elevated, expansive, or irritable mood for more than 1 week; marked impairment in functioning socially, at work, or at home; and three or more of the following symptoms: inflated self-esteem/grandiosity, decreased need for sleep, increased rate of speech/talkativeness, flight of ideas/racing thoughts, distractibility, increased activity/psychomotor agitation, and an increase in pleasurable activities without regard for consequences.

Answer A is incorrect. Amphetamine intoxication can present with manic-type symptoms, but the duration of this patient's symptoms rules out drug intoxication. Routine drug screening would also confirm such findings.

Answer C is incorrect. Hyperthyroidism can present with agitation and decreased sleep, but patients with this disorder are unlikely to exhibit other symptoms of mania, including grandiosity and flight of ideas.

Answer D is incorrect. Schizoaffective disorder is schizophrenia with a prominent component of mood disorder, either depression or mania.

Answer E is incorrect. Schizophrenia typically does not have a clinical picture similar to that of bipolar disorder. Schizophrenia classically presents as a persisting chronic illness, often with residual psychotic symptoms, but it lacks the periodicity seen in bipolar disorder and usually has no evidence of manic symptoms.

11. **The correct answer is B.** Osteonecrosis of the jaw, (avascular necrosis of the jaw) has been associated with dental extraction, local infection, and pathologic fracture of the jaw. Osteonecrosis of the jaw has also been described in patients receiving chronic bisphosphonate therapy. Bisphosphonates such as aledronate and risedronate are used to treat metastatic bone diseases such as multiple myeloma. Multiple myeloma causes bone destruction due to increased osteoclast activity; this can cause pain, spinal cord compression, and fractures. Bisphosphonates decrease pain and fractures by inhibiting bone resorption through reducing the number and activity of osteoclasts. Gastrointestinal toxicity has been the primary concern for patients taking oral bisphosphonates. Treatment with an oral bisphosphonate lowers serum calcium concentrations, but clinically important hypocalcemia has been reported only in patients with hypoparathyroidism.

Answer A is incorrect. Angiotensin converting enzyme (ACE) inhibitors, such as enalapril, inhibit angiotensin-converting enzyme and are utilized in the treatment of hypertension. ACE inhibitor toxicity can include cough, angioedema, proteinuria, taste changes, rash, and hyperkalemia. Osteonecrosis is not associated with use of ACE inhibitors.

Answer C is incorrect. Cephalosporins are β-lactam antibiotics used to treat infections caused by gram-positive and gram-negative bacteria. Use of cephalosporins does not cause osteonecrosis.

Answer D is incorrect. Osmotic diuretics such as mannitol are used to treat shock and drug overdose. Osmotic diuretics are not associated with causing osteonecrosis.

Answer E is incorrect. The vinca alkaloids, such as vincristine and vinblastine, are microtubule inhibitors used in the treatment of testicular carcinoma and Hodgkin's and non-Hodgkin's lymphomas. Vinca alkaloids are not associated with osteonecrosis.

12. **The correct answer is A.** The answer is chloramphenicol, which is no longer widely used due to its toxicities, including gray baby syndrome and aplastic anemia. Aplastic anemia secondary to chloramphenicol is a rare, dose-dependent adverse event that can occur after only a short course of therapy and can be fatal. The challenge with using this medication is that it is difficult to predict which patient will have this serious complication.

Answer B is incorrect. Ciprofloxacin is associated with gastrointestinal upset, superinfections, skin rashes, headache, and dizziness. The most notable complications include tendonitis and tendon rupture in adults, and cartilage malformation in children and in utero.

Answer C is incorrect. Clindamycin is classically associated with intestinal colonization with *Clostridium difficile* (leading to pseudomembranous colitis).

Answer D is incorrect. Erythromycin is associated with gastrointestinal discomfort, cholestatic hepatitis, eosinophilia, and skin rashes. Azithromycin, a related macrolide, is better tolerated and has fewer adverse events.

Answer E is incorrect. Gentamicin is associated with nephrotoxicity and ototoxicity with prolonged use.

Answer F is incorrect. Tetracycline is associated with gastrointestinal distress, tooth discoloration, and inhibition of bone growth in children. Photosensitivity can also result, leading to sun-exposed tetracycline skin rash.

13. **The correct answer is A.** The condition described is xeroderma pigmentosum (XP), a genetic defect in the DNA excision repair pathway. In XP, there is a defective excision repair that results in the inability to repair thymidine dimers, which form in DNA exposed to ultraviolet light, XP is associated with dry skin, and individuals that have XP are much more likely to develop both melanoma and nonmelanoma skin cancers. Clinically, XP manifests as a sunburnlike reaction, and individuals with XP often die by age 30 years. XP is autosomal recessively inherited, which is demonstrated by the frequency of occurrence of XP in the vignette family.

Answer B is incorrect. A defect in double-stranded DNA break repair leads to ataxia-telangiectasia, which renders the individual's cells susceptible to x-ray damage. The primary features of ataxia-telangiectasia include progressive gait and truncal ataxia with onset between the ages of 1 and 4 years. The most common malignancies among these patients are leukemia and lymphoma.

Answer C is incorrect. The various glycolytic enzyme deficiencies are associated with hemolytic anemia and are not associated with an increased risk of cancer.

Answer D is incorrect. A defect in heme synthesis results in a type of porphyria and is not associated with an increased risk of cancer.

Answer E is incorrect. Purine salvage deficiencies such as adenosine deaminase deficiency (leading to severe combined immunodeficiency) and Lesch–Nyhan syndrome (excess uric acid production) do not lead to an increased risk of cancer.

14. **The correct answer is D.** This vignette describes an urachal cyst or sinus, which is a remnant of the allantois and continues to drain urine from the bladder. The allantoic duct eventually becomes the median umbilical ligament. Remember, "alla**N**tois" has an "**N**," as does "media**N**."

Answer A is incorrect. The fossa ovalis is the remnant of the foramen ovale, which allowed shunting of blood from the right to left atrium but did not communicate with the bladder.

Answer B is incorrect. The ligamentum teres hepatis is the remnant of the umbilical vein, which carried blood from the mother to the baby but did not communicate with the bladder.

Answer C is incorrect. The medial umbilical ligaments are the remnants of the fetal umbilical arteries, which carried blood from the baby to the mother but did not communicate with the bladder.

Answer E is incorrect. The nucleus pulposus is the remnant of the notochord, which induced differentiation during development but did not directly communicate with the bladder.

15. **The correct answer is A.** Ovarian cancer is difficult to detect, and unfortunately the presenting symptom may be large pleural effusions from metastatic disease. The intercostal vessels and nerve run in the intercostal groove on the inferior surface of each rib. When thoracentesis is performed, the needle is always inserted immediately superior to a rib to avoid these structures.

Answer B is incorrect. The phrenic nerve is found deep in the thorax, running along the mediastinum and pericardium; it is too deep to be injured by thoracentesis.

Answer C is incorrect. The pericardiophrenic vessels travel with the phrenic nerve along the mediastinum and pericardium. These vessels are too deep to be injured by this procedure.

Answer D is incorrect. The recurrent laryngeal nerve is a branch of the vagus nerve and is found in the neck. This nerve can be injured during a thyroidectomy or other neck surgeries but is not in danger of being damaged during a chest procedure.

Answer E is incorrect. The needle here is inserted above the tenth rib, in the ninth intercostal space. The tenth intercostal vessels and nerve run below the tenth rib, in the tenth intercostal space.

16. **The correct answer is E.** The patient has papillary thyroid carcinoma, which accounts for approximately 80% of thyroid carcinomas and can usually be cured by resection of the primary tumor. The diagnosis can usually be made with a fine needle biopsy. The histologic finding depicted in the slide is a psammoma body, which is found in approximately 50% of papillary adenocarcinomas of the thyroid. Psammoma bodies are laminated, concentric calcified spherules that are also found in serous papillary cystadenocarcinoma of the ovary, meningiomas, and mesotheliomas.

Answer A is incorrect. Psammoma bodies are not found in adenocarcinomas of the lung. Well differentiated adenocarcinomas of the lung are characterized microscopically by mucin-producing glands lined by cuboidal or columnar cells, while poorly differentiated adenocarcinomas have a papillary or solid structure that usually does not produce mucin.

Answer B is incorrect. Dysgerminoma tumors of the ovary do not contain psammoma bodies; however, as previously mentioned, serous papillary cystadenocarcinoma of the ovary does. Dysgerminoma tumors of the ovary often have cells with clear cytoplasm in large sheets. The cells contain regular nuclei with a background of fibrous stroma.

Answer C is incorrect. Follicular carcinomas of the thyroid are less common but more malignant than papillary carcinomas of the thyroid. Unlike papillary carcinoma, in which hematogenous metastasis is rare, follicular carcinomas commonly metastasize via the blood to lungs or bones. Histologically, follicular carcinomas tend to form acini or follicles lined with cells that are larger than those found in normal thyroid. Psammoma bodies are not found in follicular carcinoma.

Answer D is incorrect. Medullary carcinoma of the thyroid arises from the C cells of the thyroid, which produce calcitonin. It is a rare cancer of the thyroid and can be associated with multiple endocrine neoplasia types IIA and IIB. Histologic examination of medullary carcinomas reveals sheets of tumor cells in an amyloid stroma. Psammoma bodies are not found in medullary carcinoma.

17. **The correct answer is B.** Risk factors for developing cervical cancer include early sexual activity, multiple sex partners, smoking, and low socioeconomic status. Furthermore, cervical cancer is almost always associated with human papillomavirus infection. Cervical cancers are most often squamous cell and arise from disordered epithelial growth, classified as cervical intraepithelial neoplasia 1, 2, or 3, depending on the extent of epithelial involvement from the basal layer. Papanicolaou smears have reduced the mortality of these cancers.

Answer A is incorrect. Alcoholism has little relation to cervical cancer but is strongly associated with chronic pancreatitis and pancreatic adenocarcinoma. Smoking is also a risk factor for these conditions.

Answer C is incorrect. A low-fiber diet has little relation to cervical cancer, but it is a risk factor for developing colorectal cancer. Other risk factors for developing colorectal cancer include villous adenomas, familial adenomatous polyposis, hereditary nonpolyposis colorectal cancer, inflammatory bowel disease, and a positive personal or family history.

Answer D is incorrect. Nulliparity is a risk factor for breast cancer. Other risk factors for breast cancer include gender, early first menarche (<12 years), delayed first pregnancy (>30 years), late menopause (>50 years), and a positive family history.

Answer E is incorrect. Prolonged estrogen use is a risk factor for endometrial carcinoma. Other risk factors for endometrial carcinoma include obesity, diabetes, and hypertension.

18. **The correct answer is D.** Lesch–Nyhan syndrome is an X-linked recessive disorder caused by a deficiency in the production of hypoxanthine guanine phosphoribosyltransferase that leads to the overproduction of purine and the accumulation of uric acid. This rare biochemical disorder is characterized clinically by hyperuricemia, excessive production of uric acid, and certain characteristic neurologic features, including self-mutilation, choreoathetosis, spasticity, and mental retardation.

Answer A is incorrect. A deficiency of adenosine deaminase would result in severe combined immunodeficiency disease (SCID), which prevents development of both the humoral and cell-mediated immune systems. Therefore individuals with SCID are faced with recurrent devastating bacterial, viral, and fungal infections.

Answer B is incorrect. A deficiency of b-glucocerebroside would result in Gaucher's disease. There are several types of Gaucher's disease based on the type of mutation, but most forms are marked by lipid-laden macrophages (termed Gaucher cells) that invade the bone marrow and cortex, leading to bone infarction, vertebral collapse, and anemia and thrombocytopenia.

Answer C is incorrect. This boy's findings can best be explained by Lesch–Nyhan syndrome, which is caused by a deficiency in the production of hypoxanthine guanine phosphoribosyltransferase, not a mutation of an enzyme in the de novo biosynthetic pathway, which would result in deficiencies in nucleotides needed for DNA synthesis. Symptoms may resemble conditions in which dietary deficiencies impede de novo nucleotide synthesis, such as megaloblastic anemia due to folic acid and/or vitamin B_{12} deficiency.

Answer E is incorrect. An excision repair enzyme deficiency would result in XP, which is marked by dry and hyperpigmented skin that is extremely sensitive to exposure to ultraviolet radiation. Therefore, individuals with this disease are at increased risk for severe sunburns and skin cancer.

19. **The correct answer is A.** The patient's complaints of dry mouth, difficulty swallowing, dry eyes in the eyes, and associated joint pain are consistent with the clinical presentation of Sjögren's syndrome. Sjögren's syndrome is characterized by dry eyes (keratoconjunctivitis sicca) and dry mouth (xerostomia) resulting from autoimmune destruction of lacrimal and salivary glands. It can occur as an isolated disorder or as an association with another autoimmune disease (secondary form). Among associ-

ated disorders, rheumatoid arthritis is the most common, explaining the recent onset of joint pain in this patient. Since patients with Sjögren's syndrome have decreased salivary secretions, the defense against pathogenic bacteria that cause dental caries is compromised.

Answer B is incorrect. Hyperglycemia is most commonly associated with insulin resistance and/or absence of insulin production associated with diabetes mellitus. It is not a common phenomenon in Sjögren's syndrome.

Answer C is incorrect. Jaundice is usually associated with pathologic processes involving liver or hemolytic anemias. These pathologies are relatively uncommon in Sjögren's syndrome.

Answer D is incorrect. Septic joints are usually a consequence of an infectious process and generally have no association with Sjögren's syndrome.

Answer E is incorrect. Although development of vision loss could be a potential consequence of Sjögren's syndrome due to the lack of lacrimal gland secretions, it is not the most likely condition that these patients will develop.

20. **The correct answer is D.** This patient has Lambert–Eaton syndrome, a paraneoplastic syndrome commonly associated with small cell lung cancer. In Lambert–Eaton syndrome, patients produce IgG autoantibodies against voltage-dependent calcium channels at the neuromuscular synapse, inhibiting acetylcholine release and leading to muscle weakness, particularly in the lower extremities.

Answer A is incorrect. Ectopic ACTH production can occur in small cell lung cancer, but this patient does not have typical symptoms of ACTH overproduction, such as hyperpigmentation, glucose intolerance, and hypokalemia.

Answer B is incorrect. Ectopic ADH production can occur in some cases of lung cancer. Patients present with symptoms of the syndrome of inappropriate secretion of ADH, such as hyponatremia, fatigue, and excessive water retention.

Answer C is incorrect. Myasthenia gravis is caused by production of IgG autoantibodies that target the acetylcholine receptor. Cases typically occur in women and are associated with thymoma, not lung cancer.

Answer E is incorrect. Although infiltration of skeletal muscle can occur in some tumors, the abnormal electromyogram and CT scan suggest a paraneoplastic syndrome involving muscle that is secondary to lung cancer.

21. **The correct answer is E.** Selection bias occurs when patients in a study are not randomly assigned to a treatment group. This can occur because either the patients or the investigators select the group that an individual patient will enter.

Answer A is incorrect. Late-look bias concerns information gathered at an inappropriate time of the study. It results in selection of patients of less severe disease because those with more severe disease died before detection.

Answer B is incorrect. Length bias (and lead-time bias) occurs when a disease's characteristics are ignored. For instance, a disease with more aggressive symptoms may progress to death more quickly and be falsely underrepresented by a cross-sectional look for prevalence. In evaluating 1,000 patients with thyroid biopsies on follow-up visits each month, it would appear that fewer patients with anaplastic carcinoma have survived each month. Looking in cross-section 1 year after biopsy without considering patients who have died, the prevalence of anaplastic carcinoma would be falsely decreased.

Answer C is incorrect. Recall bias occurs when a patient's report of symptoms or past events is selective, either intentionally or not. It may be secondary to perceptions of the patient about their own treatment, disease, or symptom causes.

Answer D is incorrect. Sampling bias occurs when a sample group is not representative of the population from which it is taken.

22. **The correct answer is A.** With mild exercise, arterial pH does not change because the body is able to maintain aerobic metabolism. During strenuous exercise arterial pH is decreased secondary to anaerobic metabolism and generation of lactic acid.

Answer B is incorrect. During exercise, the increased oxygen need by the muscles is attained by increased oxygen consumption by the lungs through more rapid and deeper ventilation.

Answer C is incorrect. As a result of increased pulmonary blood flow, more pulmonary capillaries are perfused and more gas exchange occurs. The ventilation/perfusion ratio is more even throughout the lung during exercise.

Answer D is incorrect. Venous partial carbon dioxide pressure increases during exercise because the muscles give off excess carbon dioxide that is carried to the lungs by venous blood.

Answer E is incorrect. Pulmonary blood flow increases during exercise because cardiac output increases to ensure adequate O_2 delivery to muscles and carbon dioxide delivery to the lungs to be exhaled.

23. **The correct answer is A.** Up until the seventh week of development, the external genitalia, including the genital tubercle, labioscrotal swellings, and urogenital folds, is the same in both sexes and can develop into male or female structures, depending on hormonal influences. In the male, the genital tubercle develops into the glans penis; the labioscrotal swellings fuse to form the scrotum, and the urogenital folds become the penile urethra in the ventral shaft of the penis. In females, the absence of androgens ceases the growth of the genital tubercle and the presence of estrogens leads to the development of the clitoris; the labioscrotal swellings develop into the labia majora, and the urogenital folds become the labia minora.

Answer B is incorrect. The labioscrotal swellings normally develop into the labia majora in the female and the scrotum in the male.

Answer C is incorrect. The production of testosterone by the Sertoli cells of the testes causes the mesonephric (wolffian) ducts to develop into the seminal vesicles, epididymis, ejaculatory duct, and ductus deferens. The absence of testosterone in females leads to the regression of the mesonephric ducts.

Answer D is incorrect. The testes produce antimüllerian hormone, which leads to the regression of the paramesonephric (müllerian) ducts in a male. In a female, there is no antimüllerian hormone and the paramesonephric ducts develop into the fallopian tubes, the uterus, and the upper two thirds of the vagina.

Answer E is incorrect. The urogenital folds fuse in the male to form the penile urethra and the ventral shaft of the penis; in the female, the unfused portions of the urogenital folds become the labia minora.

24. **The correct answer is D.** The question is asking for the number of false-positives. Specificity = true-negatives/(true-negatives + false-positives). False-positive signifies the number of people without disease X who will be falsely diagnosed by the screening test. In this case, 900 people do not have the disease, represented by true-negatives + false-positives. Using a specificity of 70%, the number of true-negatives is 630, while the number of false-positives is 270. Thus, 270 people without disease X will be falsely diagnosed with this screening test (i.e., they will be false-positives).

Answer A is incorrect. The figure 20 is the number of people with the disease who will have an incorrect negative screening test result (i.e., false-negatives).

Answer B is incorrect. The figure 80 is the number of people who will have a correct positive screening test result (i.e., true-positives).

Answer C is incorrect. The figure 100 is the number of people in the town with disease X (i.e., the prevalence of disease X).

Answer E is incorrect. The figure 630 is the number of people who will have a correct negative screening test result (i.e., true-negatives).

25. **The correct answer is B.** The Michaelis–Menten constant (K_m) of an enzyme such as

DHFR reflects the enzyme's affinity for a particular substrate [S], such as methotrexate, in an inverse fashion. The K_m of an enzyme is the concentration of substrate required to achieve a reaction velocity equal to half of the maximum reaction rate (V_{max}). A competitive inhibitor binds reversibly to the same site that the substrate would normally occupy and thus competes with the substrate for that site. Therefore, in the presence of a competitive inhibitor, the concentration of methotrexate required to achieve half of V_{max} will be increased.

Answer A is incorrect. The Michaelis-Menten constant of an enzyme is increased by a competitive inhibitor.

Answer C is incorrect. The Michaelis-Menten constant of an enzyme is increased by a competitive inhibitor.

Answer D is incorrect. The maximum reaction rate of an enzyme is unchanged by a competitive inhibitor.

Answer E is incorrect. The V_{max} is the maximum rate or velocity in which substrate molecules are converted to product per unit time. At high substrate concentrations, the reaction rate levels off, reflecting the saturation of all available binding sites with substrate. At a sufficiently high substrate concentration, the reaction velocity reaches the V_{max} observed in the absence of inhibitor. Thus, the V_{max} of an enzyme is unchanged by a competitive inhibitor, as an increase in substrate outcompetes this type of inhibitor.

26. **The correct answer is E.** This patient is most likely suffering a cerebrovascular event due to decreased perfusion of the vertebrobasilar system. Clinical manifestations include diplopia, dysarthria, vertigo, and ataxia resulting from brain stem and cerebellar ischemia. Patients with vertebrobasilar insufficiency often present with ipsilateral cranial nerve deficits and contralateral motor weakness. Hypertension and hyperlipidemia are major risk factors for the development of both transient ischemic attack and stroke.

Answer A is incorrect. Ischemia in the distribution of the anterior cerebral artery often presents with contralateral motor weakness that is greater in the leg than in the arm and mild sensory deficits, not diplopia and dysarthria.

Answer B is incorrect. Ischemia in the anterior choroidal artery often leads to contralateral homonymous hemianopsia, hemiparesis, and hemisensory loss.

Answer C is incorrect. Lacunar ischemia is often due to long-standing hypertension. The most common clinical manifestation of ischemia in these small penetrating arteries is dementia, but acute ischemia can result in pure motor deficits (face, arm, and leg paralysis) or sensory deficits (sensory loss in face, arm, and leg). The basal ganglia and pons are the regions most likely to be affected in lacunar ischemia.

Answer D is incorrect. Ischemia in the distribution of the middle cerebral artery often presents with contralateral motor and sensory deficits that are greater in the face and arms than in the leg. Diplopia and dysarthria are not characteristic of ischemia in the distribution of the middle cerebral artery.

27. **The correct answer is E.** *Staphylococcus aureus* causes acute bacterial endocarditis, which presents with an acute onset of high fever, other flu-like symptoms, new-onset murmur, petechiae, Roth's spots (white spots on the retina formed by microemboli), Janeway lesions (painless macules on the palms or soles), Osler's nodes (small, painful nodules on the pads of the fingers or toes), and nail bed (subungual) hemorrhages. The bacteria can attack healthy valves and result in vegetations that are much larger than those of subacute bacterial endocarditis. Vancomycin is typically used to treat *S. aureus* endocarditis, and provides coverage in the case of methicillin-resistant *S. aureus*.

Answer A is incorrect. Ceftriaxone is not used to treat *S. aureus* endocarditis.

Answer B is incorrect. Ciprofloxacin is not used to treat *S. aureus* endocarditis.

Answer C is incorrect. Erythromycin is not used to treat *S. aureus* endocarditis.

Answer D is incorrect. Gentamicin may be used in combination with vancomycin to treat *S. aureus* endocarditis, but not alone.

28. **The correct answer is D.** After transection of a nerve fiber, degeneration of nerve terminals begins almost immediately. Wallerian degeneration (also called orthograde degeneration) refers specifically to the process whereby peripheral nerve fibers (generally the axon) distal to the site of transection are lost as they are cut off from the soma, the source of metabolic nourishment. After the nerve fibers die, calcium is liberated, which activates enzymes that destroy the axon. Wallerian degeneration becomes apparent about 1 week after the injury to the axon and continues over the next 1–2 months.

Answer A is incorrect. While it is possible that changes to the dendrites of a neuron with a transected axon may occur, the most likely mechanism remains degeneration of the distal axon.

Answer B is incorrect. Following a transection the cell body is spared from degeneration, but it may be altered due to loss of neurotrophic factors from the axon to the soma.

Answer C is incorrect. The most likely consequence of peripheral nerve transection is degeneration of the axon distal to the lesion. Target cells are cells that receive postsynaptic stimuli (i.e., neurotransmitters) from the damaged axons. The target cells (i.e., neurons, endocrine cells, muscle cells) may be spared, although in some cases transneuronal or transynaptic changes may occur. Transneuronal degeneration is referred to as anterograde if the targets of the damaged cell are affected. Although anterograde degeneration is a possibility, the most likely mechanism remains degeneration of the distal axon as that will definitely occur.

Answer E is incorrect. In Wallerian degeneration the proximal fibers are spared since they maintain communication with the soma.

29. **The correct answer is D.** *Nocardia asteroides* is a filamentous gram-positive organism that is weakly acid-fast. Infection with this organism is typically seen in immunocompromised individuals, such as someone who has chronically taken steroids. *Nocardia* inhaled by an immunocompromised person produces lung abscesses and cavitations. The bacteria may erode blood vessels and disseminate humorally, leading to abscesses in the brain and elsewhere. *Nocardia* infection is commonly misdiagnosed as tuberculosis because of its acid-fast nature and its similar disease process.

Answer A is incorrect. *Actinomyces israelii* is also a filamentous organism but is not weakly acid-fast. It is part of the normal flora of the mouth and gastrointestinal tract. It is classically associated with "sulfur granules" seen on microscopy. It can cause abscesses and invasive infections, most commonly in the head/neck, oropharynx, and abdomen. It easily traverses tissue planes, so it is known for causing draining sinus tracts.

Answer B is incorrect. *Bacillus anthracis* can cause inhalation anthrax. It is a gram-positive rod that is not acid-fast.

Answer C is incorrect. *Mycobacterium tuberculosis* causes tuberculosis, the symptoms of which are similar to the disease caused by *Nocardia asteroides*. Unlike *N. asteroides*, *M. tuberculosis* is an acid-fast bacillus (it is not filamentous).

Answer E is incorrect. *Streptococcus pneumoniae* causes pneumonia. It is a gram-positive coccus.

30. **The correct answer is E.** This patient has the signs and symptoms of hypertensive emergency; she has symptoms of end-organ involvement (blurry vision and headache) as well as a significantly elevated blood pressure. Sodium nitroprusside, a first-line medication for hypertensive emergencies, acts by direct vasodilation of both arteries and veins. Adverse affects of nitroprusside therapy include reflex tachycardia as well as cyanide toxicity, especially in patients with liver disease.

Answer A is incorrect. Captopril, an angiotensin-converting enzyme inhibitor, is an extremely effective medication in controlling chronic hypertension. However, it is not useful in acute hypertensive emergencies because its mechanism of action is too slow.

Answer B is incorrect. As a diuretic, hydrochlorothiazide is an effective medication for the treatment of chronic essential hypertension. However, due to its mechanism of action, it does not cause a rapid enough reduction in blood pressure and thus is not useful in an emergent situation.

Answer C is incorrect. Labetalol, a nonselective β-blocker, is also a first-line agent for hypertensive emergencies as it decreases blood pressure by direct cardiac effects. In addition, β-blockers avoid the reflex tachycardia often associated with vasodilating drugs. However, the patient's past history of asthma makes labetalol a suboptimal choice, as adrenergic blockade in the airways could precipitate bronchospasm.

Answer D is incorrect. As an angiotensin receptor blocker, losartan is a useful drug with which to control chronic hypertension; however, it has no role in the acute management of hypertensive emergency because of its slow onset of effect.

31. **The correct answer is F.** This question describes a Southern blot. In a Southern blot procedure, DNA is separated with electrophoresis, denatured, transferred to a filter, and hybridized with a labeled DNA probe. Regions on the filter that base-pair with the labeled DNA probes can be identified when the filter is exposed to film that is sensitive to the radiolabeled probe.

Answer A is incorrect. Enzyme-linked immunosorbent assay (ELISA) is an immunologic technique used in laboratories to determine whether a particular antibody is present in a patient's blood. Labeled antibodies are used to detect whether serum contains antibodies against a specific antigen precoated on an ELISA plate. This is not the technique described above.

Answer B is incorrect. Gel electrophoresis uses an electric field to separate molecules based on their sizes. This is not the technique described above.

Answer C is incorrect. Northern blots are similar to Southern blots except that in Northern blotting, mRNA is separated by electrophoresis instead of DNA. This is not the technique described above.

Answer D is incorrect. Polymerase chain reaction is a laboratory technique used to produce many copies of a segment of DNA. In the procedure, DNA is mixed with two specific primers, deoxynucleotides and a heat-stable polymerase. The solution is heated to denature the DNA and is then cooled to allow synthesis. Twenty cycles of heating and cooling amplify the DNA over a million times. This is not the procedure described above.

Answer E is incorrect. Sequencing is a laboratory technique that utilizes dideoxynucleotides to randomly terminate growing strands of DNA. Gel electrophoresis is used to separate the varying lengths of DNA. The DNA sequence can then be read based on the position of the bands on the gel. This is not the technique described above.

Answer G is incorrect. In a Western blot procedure, protein is separated by electrophoresis and labeled antibodies are used as a probe. This technique can be used to detect the existence of an antibody to a particular protein.

32. **The correct answer is B.** An x-ray film of the chest indicates that the boy has a paralyzed right hemidiaphragm. It is possible for the phrenic nerve to become damaged during heart surgery, since it runs along the pericardium. It is not unusual for a patient to remain asymptomatic until starting to run long distances.

Answer A is incorrect. When a patient holds his or her breath during a chest x-ray, a contracted diaphragm will move downward, and a paralyzed diaphragm will paradoxically move upward because of the negative pressure generated on the left side of the thorax pulling the mediastinal structures towards the left.

Answer C is incorrect. Eisenmenger's syndrome is the cyanosis and symptoms that occur when a prior left-to-right shunt reverses and becomes a right-to-left shunt. Cyanosis does not occur in a left-to-right shunt because oxygenated arterial blood simply reenters the pulmonary circulation. After years of arterial blood overloading the right side of the heart, however, pulmonary pressures can increase above systemic pressures and the shunt reverses. When this occurs, deoxygenated blood enters systemic circulation and cyanosis results. Although the question states that this patient had a cardiac defect repaired in infancy, there is no evidence of cyanosis, which is the hallmark of Eisenmenger's syndrome.

Answer D is incorrect. An x-ray film of a left diaphragmatic hernia would also reveal abdominal viscera in the thoracic cavity, which is not reported in this scenario.

Answer E is incorrect. An x-ray film of a right diaphragmatic hernia would also reveal abdominal viscera in the thoracic cavity, which is not reported in this scenario.

33. **The correct answer is B.** The eight essential amino acids (those that the body cannot synthesize and must be supplied by diet) are leucine, lysine, isoleucine, phenylalanine, tryptophan, methionine, threonine, and valine. Arginine and histidine can be synthesized, but can become essential during times of intense anabolic states such as infancy, growth spurts, and recovery from infection.

Answer A is incorrect. The essential fatty acids are linoleic and linolenic acid. They are ubiquitous in natural diets.

Answer C is incorrect. Both ketogenic amino acids are essential and begin with the letter "**L**" (Leucine and Lysine). They must be supplied by dietary intake.

Answer D is incorrect. Folic acid is produced by symbiotic bacteria from the precursor p-aminobenzoic acid. This production is inhibited by sulfa antibiotics. Folic acid cannot be produced through cellular metabolism. Folic acid is also obtained from leafy vegetables and cereal. Supplementation is recommended for pregnant women to prevent congenital neural tube defects.

Answer E is incorrect. Vitamin K is synthesized by the microflora in the gut. It is also found in green leafy vegetables. Patients on warfarin therapy should be advised to maintain a stable intake of these vegetables from day to day, in order to achieve a therapeutic International Normalized Ratio that does not fluctuate.

34. **The correct answer is D.** This question describes the most common symptoms of multiple myeloma. The increased total protein could be further studied by ordering a serum protein electrophoresis, which would show increased gamma-globulin fraction. Multiple myeloma is a neoplastic proliferation of plasma cells, which produce immunoglobulins. The most common molecule that is produced by the plasma cells is IgG.

Answer A is incorrect. The inability to clear chylomicron molecules from the blood is the primary pathologic process in type I family dyslipidemias. However, these typically present at a young age with increased lipids, not increased total protein.

Answer B is incorrect. The production of albumin typically is normal in multiple myeloma.

Answer C is incorrect. There can be increased clotting factors and acute-phase reactants in a variety of conditions, but this is not the main cause of increased total protein in multiple myeloma.

Answer E is incorrect. IgM molecules are produced in Waldenström's macroglobulinemia, a condition related to multiple myeloma. Waldenström's typically presents with hyperviscosity syndrome, adenopathy, and hepatosplenomegaly. Hypercalcemia, lytic lesions, and renal insufficiency are much less common in this condition.

35. **The correct answer is A.** *Candida* stomatitis (often called thrush) and esophagitis classically

present with sore throat and dysphagia with friable white plaques and erythematous buccal mucosa present on physical exam. *Candida albicans* is an opportunistic fungal pathogen that is most commonly found in the oropharynx of immunosuppressed patients. It can also be present as diaper rash in infants or as a diffuse mucocutaneous fungal infection in severely immunosuppressed individuals. Nystatin "swish and swallow" is often used to treat oral candidiasis; however, amphotericin B or fluconazole is used for serious systemic infection.

Answer B is incorrect. Cytomegalovirus esophagitis has a presentation similar to that of herpes simplex virus (HSV) esophagitis, with punched-out mucosal lesions and "owl's-eye" inclusion bodies on light microscopy.

Answer C is incorrect. HSV stomatitis and esophagitis present with vesicular lesions and punched-out mucosal erosions characterized by intranuclear inclusion bodies on light microscopy.

Answer D is incorrect. Latent JC virus can be reactivated when a patient is immunosuppressed, developing into progressive multifocal leukoencephalopathy. Multifocal lesions in the white matter are seen on MRI.

Answer E is incorrect. *Pneumocystis jiroveci* infection classically causes a mixed alveolar and interstitial pneumonia in patients with CD4$^+$ cell counts <400/mm^3. It is associated with hypoxia, elevated LDH, and systemic symptoms such as fever and chills.

36. **The correct answer is B.** Leukocyte adhesion deficiency (LAD) syndrome is caused by a defect in the LFA-1 adhesion protein on the surface of neutrophils. The disease usually presents with marked leukocytosis and localized bacterial infections that are difficult to detect until they have progressed to an extensive life-threatening level. Since neutrophils are unable to adhere to the endothelium and transmigrate into tissues, infections in patients with LAD syndrome act similarly to those observed in neutropenic patients. There are two types of LAD: I and II. LAD I is far more common than

LAD II, and is associated with delayed umbilical separation beyond the normal range of 3 to 45 days. Fever is usually the initial presentation, and local infection in LAD I may include cellulitis and necrosis. Patients affected with LAD II have a characteristic facial appearance, short stature, limb malformations, and severe developmental delay. LAD II is not associated with delayed umbilical separation.

Answer A is incorrect. Chronic granulomatous disease presents with an increased susceptibility to infections by microbes that produce their own catalase (e.g., *Staphylococcus* and *Candida*). It results from defective neutrophil phagocytosis due to a lack of NADPH oxidase (or similar enzyme) activity. A negative nitroblue tetrazolium dye reduction test confirms the diagnosis of chronic granulomatous disease.

Answer C is incorrect. Selective immunoglobulin deficiency is a deficit in a specific class of immunoglobulins. IgA deficiency is the most common of these diseases. Since IgA is the most prominent immunoglobulin found in mucous membranes, patients suffering from a deficiency of it often present with sinus and lung infections.

Answer D is incorrect. Severe combined immunodeficiency is a defect in early stem cell differentiation that can have many causes. The typical presentation of this disease includes recurrent bacterial, viral, protozoal, and fungal infections.

Answer E is incorrect. Wiskott–Aldrich syndrome is an X-linked defect associated with elevated IgA levels, elevated IgE levels, normal IgG levels, and low IgM levels. It involves a defect in the ability to mount an IgM response to bacteria. Recurrent pyogenic infections, eczema, and thrombocytopenia are the typical triad of symptoms in this disease.

37. **The correct answer is E.** Mifepristone is a progesterone antagonist with partial agonist activity. Progesterone is necessary to maintain a pregnancy, so mifepristone's interference with this hormone causes abortion of the fetus. Prostaglandin E$_1$ is synergistic with mifepristone by

acting directly on the myometrium to induce contractions.

Answer A is incorrect. Clomiphene is used to treat infertility. It is a partial estrogen receptor agonist. It interferes with the negative feedback of physiologic estrogen on the hypothalamus and pituitary, thus increasing the secretion of gonadotropin-releasing hormone and the gonadotropins. This leads to increased stimulation of ovulation.

Answer B is incorrect. Diethylstilbestrol (DES) is a synthetic compound with estrogen-like activity that is used to treat primary hypogonadism. Clear cell adenocarcinoma of the vagina has been linked to DES use in patients' mothers during pregnancy.

Answer C is incorrect. Ethinyl estradiol is a synthetic estrogen analog that is used in combination oral contraceptives. The estrogen component of the combination pill suppresses ovulation using a constant low dose of estrogen for 21 days. High doses of ethinyl estradiol plus a progesterone analog such as norgestrel can be used for contraception up to 72 hours postcoitus.

Answer D is incorrect. Mifepristone is a progesterone antagonist. The addition of exogenous progesterone would decrease its efficacy, not increase it.

38. **The correct answer is C.** Confidentiality must be maintained in most circumstances, but harm to other persons or patients themselves warrants breach of confidentiality. The information presented in this question is based on *Tarasoff vs. Regents of the University of California* (1976). This landmark case involved a situation as described in this question. A student's therapist notified the police verbally and in writing. The police questioned the student and found him to be harmless. Two months later, the victim (Tarasoff) was murdered. In a rehearing in the Supreme Court, they ruled that "confidentiality ends with public peril" and that third parties must be informed.

Answer A is incorrect. Notifying another physician is never necessary.

Answer B is incorrect. Notifying another physician is never necessary, regardless of their relationship with the potential perpetrator.

Answer D is incorrect. The physician must notify the potential victim.

Answer E is incorrect. This choice is perhaps the most seductive but is also the most frankly inappropriate. A physician has a legal obligation to protect the public from "peril" according to the Supreme Court of the United States, regardless of the breach of confidentiality required to do so.

Answer F is incorrect. The physician must also notify law enforcement officials.

39. **The correct answer is B.** This patient has the clinical stigmata of polycystic ovarian syndrome (PCOS). PCOS results from hormone derangements (luteinizing hormone hypersecretion is the hallmark of PCOS) that manifest as obesity, hirsuitism, oligo- or amenorrhea, and acanthosis nigricans the velvety hyperpigmentation described. PCOS is often associated with insulin resistance, hyperglycemia, and hyperlipidemia. Diagnosis is made by ultrasound of the ovaries, which will reveal 10 or more follicles per ovary. Oral contraceptive pills are often used as treatment to reduce the levels of circulating androgens that result in the hirsuitism, and to help regulate ovulation.

Answer A is incorrect. Although acanthosis nigricans is sometimes seen in occult visceral malignancies, which are associated with hypercalcemia, this patient does not exhibit any of the clinical signs or symptoms of hypercalcemia ("stones, bones, groans, and moans"). Hyperglycemia is far more likely in this case.

Answer C is incorrect. Although insulin resistance and hyperglycemia can result in diabetic ketoacidosis, which in turn can lead to hyperkalemia, this patient is in no acute distress, and would be unlikely to exhibit high potassium levels.

Answer D is incorrect. Hyperuricemia is not associated with PCOS.

40. The correct answer is A. This is a deletion mutation. Bases 7–9 of the normal gene are missing from the mutant gene. Because three nucleotides are missing, there is no change in the reading frame.

Answer B is incorrect. A frameshift mutation is an insertion or deletion of nucleotides that results in a misreading of all codons downstream. Deletions or insertions in multiples of three do not cause a shift in the reading frame.

Answer C is incorrect. An insertion mutation is an addition of one or more nucleotides to the DNA.

Answer D is incorrect. A missense mutation occurs when a point mutation causes one amino acid in a protein to be replaced by a different amino acid.

Answer E is incorrect. A nonsense mutation occurs when a point mutation results in an early stop codon. This type of mutation causes a truncated protein.

Answer F is incorrect. A point mutation is the change of a single base in the DNA sequence.

Answer G is incorrect. A silent mutation occurs when a point mutation does not change the amino acid sequence of the protein. The point mutation is often in the third position of the codon.

41. The correct answer is E. This experimental drug is exerting its effects by preventing microtubule polymerization. Vincristine is a vinca alkaloid that also acts to prevent microtubule polymerization by binding to β-tubulin. Other drugs that prevent microtubule polymerization are vinblastine, colchicines, and griseofulvin.

Answer A is incorrect. Busulfan is used in the treatment of chronic myelogenous leukemia. It acts by alkylating DNA, thereby interfering with cell cycle function.

Answer B is incorrect. Cisplatin is an alkylating agent used to treat testicular, bladder, ovarian, and lung cancers.

Answer C is incorrect. Cytarabine is used in the treatment of acute myeloid leukemia and acts as a pyrimidine analog, inhibiting the action of DNA polymerase.

Answer D is incorrect. Although paclitaxel does affect microtubules, its effect is to inhibit depolymerization, rather than polymerization. It binds to β-tubulin at a site distinct from where vinca alkaloids bind and causes stabilization, thus freezing cells in mitosis. Another drug in the taxane class is docetaxel.

42. The correct answer is B. This patient is experiencing cardiogenic shock secondary to acute mitral regurgitation, presumably due to mitral valve leaflet rupture. At higher doses, dopamine exerts α-adrenergic effects in addition to its β_1 effects; it will thus cause positive inotropy with vasoconstriction, which would be supportive in this hypotensive patient with pump failure.

Answer A is incorrect. Amrinone, a phosphodiesterase inhibitor, causes an increase in cardiac inotropy but also causes vasodilation. Thus, its use would be inappropriate in this hypotensive patient.

Answer C is incorrect. Epinephrine is a potent α and β agonist and thus acts as a cardiac inotrope and chronotrope. It is also a vasoconstrictor that will increase blood flow to skeletal muscle and visceral organs from a combination of different receptors. However, the use of epinephrine can also induce cardiac arrhythmias, and this is not a first-line agent for the treatment of cardiogenic shock.

Answer D is incorrect. Isoproterenol is a potent β_1 agonist that increases the heart's chronotropy and inotropy. However, it is also a β_2 agonist and thus has vasodilatory effects that would be contraindicated in this hypotensive patient.

Answer E is incorrect. Because phenylephrine is a pure α agonist, it will cause vasoconstriction without any effect on the heart. Because this patient has pump failure, this drug would not be as effective as dopamine.

43. **The correct answer is C.** The cause of this patient's findings is an aneurysm of the right common iliac artery. The common iliac arteries lie posterior and medial to the ureters. Common iliac artery aneurysms are uncommon but can present with unilateral hydronephrosis if the ureters are compressed by the growing aneurysm. The patient's age and sex, his long history of hypertension and hyperlipidemia, and his constant dull pain suggest an aneurysm as the etiology.

Answer A is incorrect. The abdominal aorta is medial but not in close proximity to the ureters. An abdominal aortic aneurysm could not compress either of the ureters.

Answer B is incorrect. The clinical presentation does not suggest a ureteral or bladder calculus. Typical symptoms would include sharp, intermittent, excruciating pain in the lower back, abdomen, or testicular region. Fever, nausea, vomiting, and hematuria are usually present as well.

Answer D is incorrect. The clinical presentation does not suggest a ureteral or bladder calculus. Typical symptoms would include sharp, intermittent, excruciating pain in the lower back, abdomen, or testicular region. Fever, nausea, vomiting, and hematuria also are usually present.

Answer E is incorrect. UTIs can lead to the development of calculi, but due to the lack of fever and hematuria, it is highly unlikely that this is the etiology responsible for this presentation.

44. **The correct answer is D.** Heparin contamination is the most common cause of spuriously elevated activated partial thromboplastin time (aPPPT) values. IV lines, not running fluids, are flushed with heparin to prevent coagulation and obstruction of the line (i.e., keeping the line open). When drawing blood from a heparinized line, the first 5 cc should be discarded before collecting blood for laboratory testing.

Answer A is incorrect. Heparin would prolong, not shorten, the aPTT.

Answer B is incorrect. The International Normalized Ratio (INR) is a standardized measure derived from the prothrombin time (PT), adjusted for the particular assay type and the machine used to measure the PT. INR is increased if PT is increased.

Answer C is incorrect. PT would not decrease with heparin and warfarin treatment. If already prolonged, vitamin K treatment would lower the PT.

Answer E is incorrect. The INR is a standardized measure derived from the prothrombin PT, adjusted for the particular assay type and the machine used to measure the PT. INR is decreased if PT is decreased.

Answer F is incorrect. Heparin would increase the PT.

45. **The correct answer is B.** Cluster B personality disorders include antisocial, borderline, histrionic, and narcissistic, and are characterized as dramatic or wild behavior. Patients with these types of personality disorders are characterized by persistent violation of social norms, impulsivity, emotionality, grandiosity, and "acting out." There is a genetic association with mood disorders. Patients with borderline personality disorder are impulsive, unpredictable, and labile and have fluctuations in intense moods.

Answer A is incorrect. Patients with avoidant personality disorder are sensitive to rejection, socially inhibited, and timid with overwhelming feelings of inadequacy.

Answer C is incorrect. Patients with dependent personality disorder are submissive and clinging, have low self-confidence, and have an excessive need of nurturance.

Answer D is incorrect. Patients with narcissistic personality disorder are grandiose and have a sense of entitlement. They frequently demand the "best" of everything, including physicians and health care.

Answer E is incorrect. Patients with schizoid personality disorder exhibit voluntary social withdrawal and have limited emotional expressions.

Answer F is incorrect. Patients with schizotypal personality disorder demonstrate interpersonal awkwardness, odd thought patterns, and an odd appearance.

46. **The correct answer is B.** A single umbilical artery is a nonspecific finding but suggests an underlying cardiovascular abnormality. Normally, two umbilical arteries are present to carry deoxygenated blood out of the fetal circulation back to the mother.

    Answer A is incorrect. Having a single allantoic duct is normal.

    Answer C is incorrect. Having a single umbilical vein is normal. This vessel carries oxygenated blood from the maternal circulation to the fetus.

    Answer D is incorrect. Having two umbilical arteries is normal.

    Answer E is incorrect. Having two umbilical veins is abnormal but is extremely rare and is not known to be associated with any condition requiring consultation by a cardiologist.

47. **The correct answer is C.** *Clostridium perfringens* can infect necrotic tissues and produce toxins. Hemolysis results because the organism destroys erythrocytes. Crepitation is present as a result of degenerative enzymes producing gas in the tissues; this process has given the disease the name of "gas gangrene."

    Answer A is incorrect. The infection caused by *Actinomyces israelii* typically presents as a chronic, slowly progressing mass that eventually evolves into a draining sinus tract. It also produces sulfur granules.

    Answer B is incorrect. *Bacillus anthracis* can cause cutaneous anthrax, which is characterized by a painless ulcer with a black scab, called an eschar.

Answer D is incorrect. *Clostridium tetani* causes tetanus, which presents with severe muscle spasms. It is not associated with cellulitis. It is also called "lock jaw."

Answer E is incorrect. *Sporothrix schenckii* is a fungus typically seen after a prick with a thorn, which accounts for the nickname: "rose gardener's disease."

48. **The correct answer is B.** The classic histologic finding in a granulosa cell tumor of the ovary is the presence of Call-Exner bodies, which are follicles filled with eosinophilic secretions. The clinical presentation also supports this diagnosis. About two-thirds occur in postmenopausal women. Granulosa cell tumors are estrogen-secreting tumors, but occasionally produce androgens, masculinizing the patient. Secretory tumors in young women can produce precocious puberty. In adults, they may be associated with endometrial hyperplasia, cystic breast disease, and endometrial carcinoma. Up to 15% of patients with secretory tumors develop an endometrial carcinoma. This increase in estrogen stimulates the endometrium to undergo hyperplasia with subsequent sloughing off, resulting in the vaginal bleeding with which this patient presents.

    Answer A is incorrect. An endometrioid tumor, as the name suggests, histologically resembles endometrium. Call-Exner bodies would not be present, nor would vaginal bleeding.

    Answer C is incorrect. Krukenberg's tumors are tumors that are metastatic to the ovaries from the gastrointestinal system, most commonly the stomach. The classic histologic finding is a mucin-secreting signet-ring cell, not a Call-Exner body.

    Answer D is incorrect. Call-Exner bodies would not be found in a serous cystadenocarcinoma. Instead, one would expect to see a tumor lined with epithelium resembling that of the fallopian tube. These types of tumors are very common and account for 50% of ovarian carcinomas. They do not, however, classically present with vaginal bleeding.

Answer E is incorrect. A teratoma contains tissue derived from at least two different embryonic layers. For example, thyroid tissue, neural tissue, muscle tissue, bone, and even teeth may be present. The immature teratomas are more aggressive and are always malignant, while the mature teratomas are more well differentiated and benign. One would not expect to see Call-Exner bodies or vaginal bleeding with a teratoma.

Common Laboratory Values

* = Included in the Biochemical Profile (SMA-12)

Blood, Plasma, Serum	Reference Range	SI Reference Intervals
* Alanine aminotransferase (ALT, GPT at 30°C)	8–20 U/L	8–20 U/L
Amylase, serum	25–125 U/L	25–125 U/L
* Aspartate aminotransferase (AST, GOT at 30°C)	8–20 U/L	8–20 U/L
Bilirubin, serum (adult)		
Total // Direct	0.1–1.0 mg/dL // 0.0–0.3 mg/dL	2–17 μmol/L // 0–5 μmol/L
* Calcium, serum (Total)	8.4–10.2 mg/dL	2.1–2.8 mmol/L
* Cholesterol, serum	140–250 mg/dL	3.6–6.5 mmol/L
* Creatinine, serum (Total)	0.6–1.2 mg/dL	53–106 μmol/L
Electrolytes, serum		
Sodium	135–147 mEq/L	135–147 mmol/L
Chloride	95–105 mEq/L	95–105 mmol/L
* Potassium	3.5–5.0 mEq/L	3.5–5.0 mmol/L
Bicarbonate	22–28 mEq/L	22–28 mmol/L
Gases, arterial blood (room air)		
P_{O_2}	75–105 mmHg	10.0–14.0 kPa
P_{CO_2}	33–44 mmHg	4.4–5.9 kPa
pH	7.35–7.45	[H+] 36–44 nmol/L
* Glucose, serum	Fasting: 70–110 mg/dL	3.8–6.1 mmol/L
	2-h postprandial: < 120 mg/dL	< 6.6 mmol/L
Growth hormone - arginine stimulation	Fasting: < 5 ng/mL	< 5 μg/L
	provocative stimuli: > 7 ng/mL	> 7 μg/L
Osmolality, serum	275–295 mOsm/kg	275–295 mOsm/kg
* Phosphatase (alkaline), serum (p-NPP at 30°C)	20–70 U/L	20–70 U/L
* Phosphorus (inorganic), serum	3.0–4.5 mg/dL	1.0–1.5 mmol/L
* Proteins, serum		
Total (recumbent)	6.0–7.8 g/dL	60–78 g/L
Albumin	3.5–5.5 g/dL	35–55 g/L
Globulins	2.3–3.5 g/dL	23–35 g/L
* Urea nitrogen, serum (BUN)	7–18 mg/dL	1.2–3.0 mmol urea/L
* Uric acid, serum	3.0–8.2 mg/dL	0.18–0.48 mmol/L
Cerebrospinal Fluid		
Glucose	40–70 mg/dL	2.2–3.9 mmol/L
Hematologic		
Erythrocyte count	Male: 4.3–5.9 million/mm³	$4.3–5.9 \times 10^{12}$/L
	Female: 3.5–5.5 million/mm³	$3.5–5.5 \times 10^{12}$/L
Hematocrit	Male: 41–53%	0.41–0.53
	Female: 36–46%	0.36–0.46
Hemoglobin, blood	Male: 13.5–17.5 g/dL	2.09–2.71 mmol/L
	Female: 12.0–16.0 g/dL	1.86–2.48 mmol/L
Hemoglobin, plasma	1–4 mg/dL	0.16–0.62 μmol/L
Leukocyte count and differential		
Leukocyte count	4500–11,000/mm³	$4.5–11.0 \times 10^9$/L
Segmented neutrophils	54–62%	0.54–0.62
Band forms	3–5%	0.03–0.05
Eosinophils	1–3%	0.01–0.03
Basophils	0–0.75%	0–0.0075
Lymphocytes	25–33%	0.25–0.33
Monocytes	3–7%	0.03–0.07
Mean corpuscular hemoglobin	25.4–34.6 pg/cell	0.39–0.54 fmol/cell
Platelet count	150,000–400,000/mm³	$150–400 \times 10^9$/L
Prothrombin time	11–15 seconds	11–15 seconds
Reticulocyte count	0.5–1.5% of red cells	0.005–0.015
Sedimentation rate, erythrocyte	Male: 0–15 mm/h	0–15 mm/h
(Westergren)	Female: 0–20 mm/h	0–20 mm/h
Proteins, total	< 150 mg/24 h	< 0.15 g/24 h

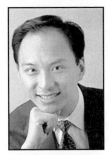

Tao Le, MD, MHS

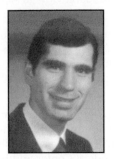

Seth K. Bechis, MS

Tao Le, MD, MHS

Tao has been a well-recognized figure in medical education for the past 15 years. As senior editor, he led the expansion of *First Aid* into a global educational series. In addition, he is the founder and editor-in-chief of the *USMLERx* online test bank series as well as a co-founder of the *Underground Clinical Vignettes* series. As a medical student, he was editor-in-chief of the University of California, San Francisco *Synapse,* a university newspaper with a weekly circulation of 9000. Tao earned his medical degree from the University of California, San Francisco in 1996 and completed his residency training in internal medicine at Yale University and fellowship training at Johns Hopkins University in allergy and immunology. In addition, he earned a Master of Health Science degree at the Johns Hopkins Bloomberg School of Public Health. At Yale, he was a regular guest lecturer on the USMLE review courses and an adviser to the Yale School of Medicine curriculum committee. Tao subsequently went on to co-found Medsn and served as its chief medical officer. He is currently pursuing research in asthma education at the University of Louisville.

Seth K. Bechis, MS

Seth grew up in Concord, Mass., and attended Harvard University, earning a Bachelor of Arts degree in chemistry and chemical biology. He took two years during medical school to complete a Master of Science degree in biomedical science, studying cancer biology, and is now in his third year of medical school at the University of California, San Francisco. Seth wants to become a practicing clinician-scientist in cardiology or potentially a surgical subspecialty. He also has interests in medical education and biotechnology development and hopes to combine these in his future practice. When not in school, Seth spends his time outdoors skiing, hiking, golfing, and traveling to faraway places.

ABOUT THE EDITORS

Karen A. Adler, MD

Karen grew up in the small town of Bel Air, Md., until she was 18 years old, when she moved to Providence, R.I., to attend Brown University. It was at Brown that Karen was first exposed to the world of academic publishing when she spent many months assisting a professor in preparing a textbook on complex cognition for publication. Karen majored in neuroscience and then pursued graduate work in clinical psychology in San Diego, focusing on the neurobiology of stress and disease. She earned her medical degree at Weill Medical College of Cornell University and is beginning a residency in psychiatry at Massachusetts General Hospital.

Jacob S. Appelbaum

Jacob grew up in Seattle, Wash., working in laboratories at the University of Washington and the Fred Hutchinson Cancer Research Center before moving to Amherst College, where he majored in biology and chemistry. Following graduation he moved to Washington, D.C., where he was a predoctoral fellow at the National Cancer Institute. In 2004 he began the MD/PhD program at Yale School of Medicine in the department of cell biology. He has no idea what he will specialize in.

Carina H.G. Baird, MD	Carina is from Riverside, Calif. She attended the University of California, Los Angeles for her undergraduate education, where she majored in psychobiology and minored in music history. As a student she worked as an emergency medical technician for UCLA Emergency Medical Services. She graduated from the University of California, San Francisco School of Medicine, where she was a member of the Alpha Omega Alpha honor society. She is pursuing her residency training in pediatrics at UCSF as well, and will be an intern in the critical care track. Carina will likely specialize in neonatology.
Xuemei Cai	Xuemei grew up in Tucson, Ariz. She received the Flinn Scholarship in 2001, which led to her decision to stay instate at the University of Arizona, where she earned a Bachelor of Science degree in biochemistry and molecular biophysics as well as a Bachelor of Arts degree in East Asian studies. She is currently in her fourth year at Harvard Medical School and is considering a career in a surgical subspecialty or interventional radiology.
Phillip J. Gray, Jr.	Phil graduated summa cum laude from the University of Arizona and is pursuing his medical degree at Johns Hopkins University School of Medicine. He recently completed a Howard Hughes Medical Research Training Fellowship with the department of radiation oncology at the Beth Israel Deaconess Medical Center and Harvard Medical School. Phil plans to pursue a career in academics in the field of radiation oncology.
Christopher R. Kinsella, Jr.	"Topher" was born and raised in St. Louis, Mo., and found his way to Drexel University College of Medicine after spending two years in the Caribbean at St. George's University School of Medicine. He has gone inner-tubing in Laos, climbed the world's largest religious structure in Cambodia, ran into drug smugglers on the lip of a volcano in St. Vincent, and placed his first sutures in the mountains of Vietnam. How he came to work for the *First Aid* team is anyone's guess. He hopes to become a plastic surgeon and thanks his family and friends for everything. The rest he owes to chance.
Gabriel J. Martinez-Diaz	Gabriel was born and raised in Mayagüez, Puerto Rico. He attended the College of Engineering at the University of Wisconsin-Madison, where he earned his Bachelor of Science degree with honors in research in biomedical engineering. Upon graduation, and after a short teaching experience through the PEOPLE program at the University of Wisconsin, Gabriel moved to Bethesda, Md., to work at the National Institutes of Health in the Academy Fellowship Program. During 2007–08 he completed a Doris Duke Clinical Research Fellowship at the University of California, San Francisco School of Medicine. He is entering his clinical rotations in the summer of 2008, hoping to find a specialty field where he can work toward improving the quality of health care received by medically underserved communities.

ABOUT THE AUTHORS

Rebecca Ahrens
Rebecca grew up in St. Louis, Mo. She attended Duke University and Cambridge University for her undergraduate work. She is currently working on her Doctor of Philosophy degree in the Physiology, Biophysics and Systems Biology program at Weill Medical College of Cornell University. Her work focuses on exploring mechanisms of cardiac arrhythmogenesis through computational and electrophysiological techniques. In her free time Rebecca likes to cook, dance, read, spend time with friends, and watch Duke basketball.

Sara Alcorn
Sara grew up in the Central Valley of California. She earned her undergraduate degree at Cornell University, where she studied sociology and wetland ecology. After spending four very cold years in upstate New York, she decided to endure five more in Boston, working toward a dual MD/MPH degree at Harvard. Her future goals include providing health care to vulnerable communities while finding time to write prose and poetry, preferably in a warm location.

Vijay Babu, MD
Vijay is a native of State College, Pa., and a life-long Penn State fan. He earned a Bachelor of Science degree in premedicine with honors in biochemistry and molecular biology at Penn State. He went on to complete his medical education at the Penn State College of Medicine. Currently he is an internal medicine intern at The Reading Hospital in Reading, Pa., and will begin a residency in anesthesiology at the Albert Einstein College of Medicine/Montefiore Medical Center in July 2009. After completing residency, Vijay plans to pursue a career in academic medicine.

Paula Borges, MS
Paula attended Florida Atlantic University to earn a Bachelor of Science degree in biotechnology and her Master of Science degree in biochemistry. She is currently pursuing her medical degree at Stanford University, where she is involved with pain research. She hopes possibly to pursue a career in a surgical subspecialty.

Rachel Bortnick, MPhil
Rachel is a fifth-year MD/PhD candidate at Harvard Medical School. She graduated from the University of Chicago with Bachelor of Arts degrees in biology and philosophy and from the University of Cambridge with a Master of Philosophy degree in neuroscience. Her current research focuses on neurodevelopment, and in the future she hopes to combine her interests in neuroscience, medicine, writing, and global health.

Steven Chen
Steven, originally from Saratoga, Calif., graduated from Johns Hopkins University in 2005 with a Bachelor of Science degree in cellular and molecular biology. He is currently a third-year medical student at Hopkins and will be taking a year off to pursue a Master of Public Health degree before graduating in 2010. He plans to ultimately go into academic medicine; however he has yet to decide on a specialty. Steven enjoys traveling, tennis, playing piano and guitar, and trying new restaurants and bars.

John Childress III
John is originally from Washington, D.C., and attended the University of Maryland for his undergraduate education, majoring in physiology and neurobiology. After graduation he completed a year-long Postbaccalaureate Intramural Research Training Award program at the National Institutes of Health. John is currently pursuing a career in academic medicine at the University of Maryland Medical School.

Raghu Chivukula
Raghu grew up in New York, attended high school in Kansas, and subsequently graduated with an undergraduate degree in neuroscience from Johns Hopkins University. He is currently a fourth-year student in the Medical Scientist Training Program at Hopkins, where he also enjoys auto racing, fitness, and "Law and Order" marathons. Raghu plans residency training in general surgery after graduation.

Justin Brent Cohen
Justin was raised in Westchester, N.Y., and attended Princeton University, where he earned a degree in molecular biology. His thesis work there involved developing a transgenic mouse line to allow easier access to specific stem cell populations. He is currently attending Yale School of Medicine and will spend next year as a Howard Hughes Fellow investigating epithelial engraftment of bone marrow stem cells. Justin plans to pursue a surgical residency.

Ana Costa, MD
Ana grew up in Sao Paulo, Brazil, and moved to New York City after completing high school. She attended Hunter College, where she earned undergraduate degrees in history and biology. She recently graduated from Weil Medical College of Cornell University and is beginning a residency in anesthesiology at Cornell. Ana has done extensive research in neuroscience at Hunter College and Rockefeller University. She plans to subspecialize in pain medicine or regional anesthesiology. Ana enjoys cycling, ballet, and playing board games. She has also traveled extensively and plans to volunteer her medical expertise in developing countries.

Andres E. Cruz-Inigo
Andres was born and raised in Mayaguez, Puerto Rico. He graduated magna cum laude from Boston University with a Bachelor of Arts degree in biology. Currently he is a medical student at Weill Medical College of Cornell University and works on clinical translational research in immunology at The Rockefeller University. After completing his medical training, Andres plans to pursue a career in academic medicine. During his free time, you will find him traveling the world to remote locations in order to treat those in need of medical care and to fulfill his passions for surfing, snowboarding, scuba diving, and photography.

Martin H. Dominguez
Martin was raised in Indianapolis, Ind., and attended school there until he was 18 years old. He graduated from Yale College in 2005 with an intensive Bachelor of Science degree in molecular, cellular, and developmental biology. He is currently undertaking joint MD/PhD graduate studies at Yale School of Medicine. His graduate work has focused on the development of the cerebral cortex, and he wishes to pursue a career in medicine and science.

Allen Omid Eghrari
Allen is currently a fourth-year medical student at Johns Hopkins University School of Medicine. He earned undergraduate degrees in economics and psychology from the University of Illinois at Urbana-Champaign. His interests include international health, community development, medical education, and technological innovation.

Sharifeh (Sheri) Farasat
Sheri is a fourth-year student at Johns Hopkins University School of Medicine. During the 2007–08 academic year she was a research fellow of the National Institutes of Health Clinical Research Training Program. She graduated from the University of California, Los Angeles with undergraduate degrees in neuroscience and political science.

James A. Feinstein, MD
James is a resident pediatrician at Seattle Children's Hospital and Regional Medical Center. He attended Dartmouth College for his undergraduate studies and the University of Pennsylvania for medical school. He plans a career in pediatric cardiology and will continue to be highly involved in medical student education.

Shennen Floy
Shennen was born and raised on a farm in Iowa and attended Creighton University in Omaha, Neb., majoring in biology and chemistry. She is currently pursuing her medical degree at Harvard Medical School and hopes to eventually practice in either a surgical subspecialty or gynecologic oncology. Her current research interests include international health systems and clinical research in trauma/orthopedic surgery.

Ariella Friedman
Ariella grew up in Woodmere, N.Y., and attended The University of Pennsylvania, earning Bachelor of Arts degrees in psychology and biology. She is a fourth-year student at Weill Medical College of Cornell University. In her spare time Ariella sings and composes music. She is a big fan of all things related to steak, poker, Johnny Depp, and weather/natural disaster movies.

Robert J. Gianotti, MD
Robert attended Cornell University as an undergraduate and earned a Bachelor of Science degree in biology. Following graduation he became a forest ranger with the United States Department of Agriculture Forest Service and worked as a research assistant in the Laboratory of Addictive Disease at Rockefeller University. He recently earned his medical degree from Weill Medical College of Cornell University and has begun a residency in internal medicine at New York University.

Philip Hall
Philip is from Cincinnati, Ohio. He graduated from Princeton University in 2005 with a Bachelor of Arts degree in classics. Currently Philip is in his third year at Yale School of Medicine.

Daniel M. Halperin
Daniel completed an undergraduate degree in biology at the Massachusetts Institute of Technology in 2004. He completed one year of research training as a medical student at Weill Medical School of Cornell University, funded by the Howard Hughes Medical Institute, in which he investigated signal transduction in a putative stem cell niche in multiple myeloma and glioblastoma. Daniel will be graduating in June 2009 with his wife, Jennifer, and will pursue training in internal medicine and likely hematology/oncology. In his spare time he enjoys playing and listening to jazz.

Colleen M. Harrison
Colleen grew up in the small mountain town of Nederland, Colo. She taught outdoor adventure courses in South Africa after high school. After two years away from academics, she began undergraduate work at the University of Colorado at Boulder, where she majored in international affairs. Colleen spent a year as a nurse's assistant at a nursing home before she began studies at Harvard Medical School. She received a National Health Service Corps scholarship, which involves a commitment to provide care to an underserved population after residency. Colleen plans to graduate from medical school in 2009 and train in family medicine.

Chloe Hill
Chloe is from Shaker Heights, Ohio. She studied neuroscience at Brown University, and is currently a third-year student at Weill Medical College of Cornell University. She is about to begin a Doris Duke Clinical Research Fellowship at the University of North Carolina in the field of gastroenterology. Chloe plans someday to have an integrative clinical practice while continuing to pursue clinical research.

Selena Liao
Selena grew up in Princeton Junction, N.J., and earned a Bachelor of Arts degree in history at Yale College, where she focused on the development of the Taiwanese identity and ethnic relations in Taiwan, as well as the history of the breath mint. She is currently a fourth-year medical student at Harvard Medical School and intends to apply for a residency in otolaryngology. Her interests in include eating strange foods, traveling to new places, and playing the bagpipes.

Ken Lin
Kenny grew up in Tainan, the oldest city in Taiwan and famous for its rich history and folk cuisine. He came to the United States during high school and studied biological sciences and Greco-Roman history at Stanford University as a undergraduate. Kenny is currently an MD/PhD student at Harvard Medical School and plans to graduate in 2010. He likes to travel to exotic places with his fiancée and enjoys nature and portrait photography. At present Kenny hasn't decided on a specialty, but he hopes to contribute to medicine through teaching and innovation.

Susan Mathai
Susan was born in Dallas, Texas, and attended Harvard College, where she concentrated in social studies, focusing on medical anthropology and Latin American studies. She graduated Phi Beta Kappa and magna cum laude. Susan is attending Yale School of Medicine, and plans to pursue a career in internal medicine. While at Yale, Susan served as one of the student directors of the HAVEN Free Clinic, Yale's student-run free clinic serving uninsured patients in the New Haven area. Susan speaks Spanish and Portuguese.

Heather McGee, MPhil

Heather grew up in Davis, Calif., and completed her undergraduate degree in molecular biology & biochemistry at the University of California, Berkeley. After an exciting semester abroad in London, she returned to the United Kingdom to work at the Welcome Trust Immunology Unit and earn a Masters of Philosophy degree from the University of Cambridge. She is now pursing her doctorate of philosophy in immunobiology as an MD/PhD student at Yale School of Medicine. In the future she hopes to incorporate immunology research into her career as a physician-scientist.

Leah McNally

Leah grew up in Fort Lauderdale, Fla., and earned a Bachelor of Science degree in evolutionary biology from Duke University. She is currently in her fourth year of medical school at Yale School of Medicine. She is still not sure what area of medicine she wants to go into, but plans to take a research year to study insulin signaling in type 2 diabetes mellitus.

Emily Pfeil

Emily grew up just north of Boston, Mass., and graduated from Tufts University with a Bachelor of Science degree in biology and a senior thesis in the field of developmental biology. She is currently a fourth-year student at Johns Hopkins University School of Medicine and is working on research in the field of endocrinology. Emily plans on a future in internal medicine and/or pediatrics.

Michelle Rios, MD

Michelle grew up in Bakersfield, Calif. She later attended the University of California, Los Angeles, earning a degree in psychobiology. She graduated medical school from the University of California, San Francisco. She recently began her internal medicine residency at UCLA Medical Center.

Maya Roberts

Maya is entering her fifth year in the MD/MPH program at Yale School of Medicine and the Harvard School of Public Health as a Reynolds Foundation Fellow for Social Entrepreneurship. For her thesis she is studying the physical health status of medical and surgical residents over the course of their postgraduate training. She is passionate about bridging the worlds of clinical medicine and public health through innovative efforts to improve efficiency and efficacy. In her free time she loves to cook, play squash, and train for triathlons.

Marianeli Rodriguez

Marianeli grew up in Havana, Cuba, and came to the United States for college. She received a Bachelor of Science degree from the University of Tulsa, where she was a biochemistry major. Currently Marianeli is doing research on the effects of retinoids in the development of the nervous system. Her goal is to pursue a career in neurology. In her spare time Marianeli enjoys traveling, reading, and dancing.

Sepideh Saber

Sepideh earned her Bachelor of Science degree in neurobiology from the University of California, Irvine. She is currently attending Stanford University School of Medicine and is involved with tissue engineering research at the Palo Alto Veterans Administration. Sepideh hopes to pursue a career in surgery.

Benjamin Smith

Ben grew up in Cambridge, Mass., and left home to attend Yale College, where he studied evolutionary patterns in plants. The draw of the Red Sox was too strong, however, and after spending two years in Wyoming working on a public health project, he returned to Boston for medical school. He now is a third-year student in the MD/MPH program at Harvard School of Medicine, and he plans to pursue a career in either primary care or psychiatry, with a focus on adolescent health.

Sara Stern-Nezer

Sara grew up moving between the west and east coasts of North America, and attended Columbia University for her undergraduate education. She is a currently a third-year student in the MD/MPH combined program between Stanford University School of Medicine and the University of California, Berkeley School of Public Health. For her master's thesis she evaluated the relationship between biomass fuel use and respiratory health, particularly its effect on women in developing countries. Sara plans to pursue a career in clinical and academic medicine, with a focus on the alleviation of gender-based health disparities and undergraduate medical education. She spent the summer of 2008 working on a cluster randomized trial of the nonpneumatic antishock garment, a device aimed at decreasing maternal mortality and morbidity caused by postpartum hemorrhage.

Tomeka L. Suber

Tomeka was born and raised in Wilmington, N.C., and earned her Bachelor of Science degree in chemistry from the University of North Carolina at Chapel Hill in 2002. She is now a sixth-year MD/PhD student in the Cellular and Molecular Medicine Graduate Program at Johns Hopkins University School of Medicine. She is currently studying the role of programmed cell death in autoimmunity and plans to pursue a career in rheumatology.

Carlos A. Torre

Carlos was born and raised in San Juan, Puerto Rico. When he was 18 years old he moved to Chestnut Hill, Mass., where he spent the next four years completing his Bachelor of Arts degree in philosophy at Boston College. He then returned to Puerto Rico to enroll as a medical student at the University of Puerto Rico. After completing his third year of medical school, Carlos interrupted his studies to participate in a research fellowship program at the University of California, San Francisco. He is presently studying the molecular mechanisms that mediate cancer progression and chemoresistance in the head and neck. Carlos plans to resume his medical studies next year and to become a physician-scientist in the field of otolaryngology.

Jonathan Tzu

Jonathan grew up in Houston, Texas, and attended Rice University, earning a Bachelor of Science degree in biochemistry and a Bachelor of Arts degree in kinesiology. He is currently a fourth-year medical student at Johns Hopkins University School of Medicine and hopes to pursue an academic career in ophthalmology.

Brant W. Ullery, MD

A native of Minnesota, Brant completed his undergraduate studies at Northwestern University, where he majored in neuropsychology. After graduating from Weill Medical College of Cornell University in May 2008, Brant started his general surgery residency at the Hospital of the University of Pennsylvania. His academic interests focus on cardiac surgery in the elderly, off-pump coronary artery bypass grafting, and robotic cardiac surgery.

Kelly Vranas, MD

Kelly grew up in Eugene, Ore., and attended Santa Clara University for her undergraduate studies. She recently graduated from Weill Medical College of Cornell University, and started her residency in internal medicine at the University of Pennsylvania this summer with her fiancé, who will be a resident in Penn's general surgery program. She is interested in both gastroenterology and critical care medicine. In her free time Kelly enjoys playing sports, going running, reading mystery novels, cooking, and playing the piano.

Frederick Wang

Frederick is a fourth-year medical student at Yale School of Medicine. He grew up in Plano, Texas, and graduated from the Massachusetts Institute of Technology with a double major in electrical engineering and biology. He will be a Howard Hughes Medical Institute Research Scholar at the National Institutes of Health for the 2008–09 year.

Marc Wein

Marc is currently a sixth-year student in the MD/PhD program at Harvard Medical School. After graduation he's thinking about either a residency in internal medicine, law school, or wizard academy. In his free time he enjoys cooking Indian food and rooting for the New York Mets.

Rasika Wickramasinghe, PhD

Rasika was born and raised in Colombo, Sri Lanka, and moved to the United States to begin his undergraduate work at Stanford University, where he earned his Bachelor of Science degree in biology. Thereafter he entered the MD/PhD program at Johns Hopkins University School of Medicine; he has currently completed his Doctor of Philosophy degree in neuroscience and is in the final year of earning his medical degree. He is planning to pursue a career in cardiology and will be entering residency training in internal medicine.

ABOUT THE ASSOCIATE AUTHORS

Jan Brown II
Jan is a third-year student at St. George's University School of Medicine. He aspires to practice emergency medicine. In his free time he enjoys baseball, fishing, and caring for bonsai trees.

Paul D. Di Capua
Paul will graduate in May 2009 from Yale School of Medicine with a medical degree and a Master of Business Administration degree. Born in Colombia, he grew up in South Florida and attended Harvard University, where he majored in neurobiology. After college he edited a neuroscience book in Lima, Peru, and then worked in art restoration in Rome before pursuing his career in medicine. He plans to attend residency and pursue a career in providing the highest quality health care for his patients.

Lars Grimm
Lars is a fifth-year medical student at the Yale University School of Medicine. He plans to graduate in 2009 with a dual MD/MHS degree. Over the past year he received funding to pursue his research interests in the fields of radiology and human physiology. Lars has been involved with *First Aid* publications for three years. When not in the hospital or lab he enjoys working out and spending time with his friends and family.

Nicole M. Hsu
Nicole is a fourth-year medical student at the Uniformed Services University of the Health Sciences, and is also an active-duty Second Lieutenant in the United States Air Force. Over the past three years she has enjoyed the opportunity to work as an author on several publications for *First Aid* and *USMLERx*. During her free time she enjoys visiting family, going to the movies, and catching up on sleep.

Benjamin Silverberg, MS
A freelance writer and photographer, Ben graduated with honors from the University of North Carolina at Chapel Hill with dual degrees in chemistry and dramatic arts. Next he earned his Masters of Science degree in biotechnology from Georgetown University, where he also volunteered as an emergency medical technician and worked as a science tutor. Prior to entering medical school Ben spent a year at a community college in Ecuador simultaneously teaching English and learning Spanish. He is currently a fourth-year medical student at the University of Connecticut and is looking forward to a career in emergency medicine.

Harras Zaid
Harras was born and raised in Fresno, Calif., where he spent much of his childhood in the countryside on the farm. He did his undergraduate work at the University of California, Davis, graduating summa cum laude in 2005 with a degree in genetics. He is now a third-year medical student at the University of California, San Francisco, completing a Howard Hughes Medical Institute fellowship in transplantation research. He hopes to pursue a career in academic surgery.

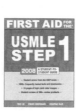
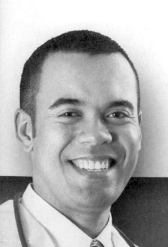